Excimer Laser Refractive Surgery

Practice and Principles

Jeffery J. Machat, MD
TLC The Laser Center
Windsor, Ontario, Canada

SLACK Incorporated, 6900 Grove Road, Thorofare, NJ 08086-9447

Publisher: John H. Bond
Acquisitions Editor: Amy E. Drummond
Associate Editor: Jennifer J. Cahill
Art Director: Linda Baker

Excimer laser refractive surgery: practice and principles/Jeffery J. Machat.

    p. cm.
Includes bibliographical references and index.
ISBN 1-55642-274-1.
1. Eye—Laser surgery. 2. Excimer lasers. I. Machat, Jeffery J.
[DNLM: 1. Myopia—surgery. 2. Astigmatism—surgery. 3. Keratectomy, Photorefractive, Excimer Laser—methods. WW 320 E96 1996]
RE86.E97 1996
617.7'55—dc20
DNLM/DLC
for Library of Congress   96-8007

Printed in the United States of America

Published by: SLACK Incorporated
               6900 Grove Road
               Thorofare, NJ 08086-9447 USA
               Telephone: 609-848-1000
               Fax: 609-853-5991

Contact SLACK Incorporated for more information about other books in this field or about the availability of our books from distributors outside the United States.

Dedication

This textbook must be dedicated to my wife, Marika, and my children, Justin and Hayley, because of the considerable time I spent thinking about them while writing.

Contents

Expanded Contents

SECTION II: LASIK

Acknowledgments

I must acknowledge the selfless efforts and offer my deepest appreciation to all my contributing authors without whom this textbook would not have achieved all that I had hoped for. I will also be forever indebted to Sandy Richards, who assisted me for untold hours in the creation of this textbook and for whom simple words of gratitude will never suffice. A final note of recognition must be given to Amy Drummond and Jennifer Cahill who endlessly listened and encouraged me, and then brought a magical order to my many months of chaos.

There are many people who directly and in many cases unknowingly contributed to this textbook as they provided me with the answers to many of my questions over the years. Stephen G. Slade opened my mind to LASIK and then emptied his as he taught me in 1 year what took him a decade to learn. Theo Seiler, who influenced me early and taught me what this technology was truly capable of achieving. Lucio Buratto, who invited me into his home to first learn what the future held for refractive surgery. Luis Ruiz mesmerized me with his surgical skill and showed me what was possible even today, making me a better refractive surgeon.

Marguerite McDonald, Richard Lindstrom, Jeffrey Robin, Stephen Trokel, Neal Sher, Bruce Grene, Lee Nordan, Ioannis Pallikaris, Roberto Zaldivar, John Marshall, David Gartry, Manus Kraff, Mickey Gordon, Dan Durrie, Chris Lohmann, David O'Brart, and George Waring were just a few of the people I listened to for hours with fascination and who I aspired to emulate.

When patients question me about the tremendous number of hours I have dedicated to refractive surgery, I tell them it is because I enjoy it. The only other feeling in my professional career that compares to it is when I delivered my first baby as an intern many years ago. I hope this textbook will serve as a source of inspiration and encouragement for others, as much as it will serve as a resource guide.

Contributing Authors

Jorge L. Alió, MD, PhD
Alicante, Spain

Maria Clara Arbelaez, MD
Cali, Colombia

Richard N. Baker, OD, FAAO
Houston, Texas

Andrew Bergin, BS
Minneapolis, Minnesota

Craig Beyer, DO
St. Petersburg, Florida

Lucio Buratto, MD
Milano, Italy

Thomas Burba, BA
Minneapolis, Minnesota

Enrique Suarez Cabrera, MD
Caracas, Venezuela

Richard A. Eiferman, MD, FACS
Louisville, Kentucky

Georgietta R. Gdovin, OD
Philadelphia, Pennsylvania

Ricardo Guimarães, MD, PhD
Belo Horizonte, Brazil

Mahmoud M. Ismail, MD
Alicante, Spain

Maurice John, MD
Jeffersonville, Indiana

Frederic B. Kremer, MD
Philadelphia, Pennsylvania

Michiel S. Kritzinger, MD
Johannesburg, South Africa

Shui T. Lai, PhD
Carlsbad, California

F. Linton Lavery, MCh, FRCSI, FRCS Ed DOMS
Dublin, Ireland

Richard Lindstrom, MD
Minneapolis, Minnesota

Eduardo Martines, MD
Sao Paulo, Brazil

Marguerite B. McDonald, MD, FACS
New Orleans, Louisiana

Ioannis Pallikaris, MD
Athens, Greece

Mihai Pop, MD
Hull, Quebec, Canada

Louis E. Probst V, MD
London, Ontario, Canada

Luis A. Ruiz, MD
Bogota, Colombia

Theo Seiler, MD, PhD
Dresden, Germany

Neal A. Sher, MD, FACS
Minneapolis, Minnesota

Stephen G. Slade, MD
Houston, Texas

Casimir A. Swinger, MD
New York, New York

Vance Thompson, MD
Sioux Falls, South Dakota

Stephen A. Updegraff, MD
Rapid City, South Dakota

D. Keith Williams, FRCSC, FACS, FRCOphth
London, England

Preface

Each textbook sets out to achieve certain goals and to enlighten the reader with concepts and ideas. This book is no different. This textbook is only unusual in that it reflects my personal experience in this rapidly evolving field of laser refractive surgery, a field in which I have become completely immersed both personally and professionally. After thousands of consultations, I have developed my own views as to what each candidate may be seeking. After several thousand laser refractive procedures with multiple excimer lasers, including over 2000 LASIK procedures, I have developed my own insight as to what this technology is capable of providing for these patients. This text is more than a guide to the principles for this rapidly evolving technology; it represents my personal philosophy.

The cover photo illustrates a human hair that has been etched with an excimer laser. When I first saw this photograph in my final year of residency, it changed my life immeasurably and prompted my quest for knowledge in this evolving field.

I started working with the Summit ExciMed in 1991, then the VisX 20/20 in early 1992. By mid-1992, I had already examined over 1000 cases of PRK and treated a few hundred cases on both the Summit and VisX. It was from my observation of the clinical differences between the laser systems that I theorized the Acoustic Shockwave model for central island formation and then developed the Pretreatment technique for improved ablation contour in July 1992. Pretreatment was incorporated into the software of both the Chiron Technolas 116 and VisX 20/20 Model B and STAR.

From my work with multiple laser systems I conceptualized the relationship of how the clinical profile is determined by the energy beam profile and treatment parameters of the various laser systems. Based upon a study of the clinical profiles, I created the bell curve model for describing patient healing types, developed guidelines for steroid titration as early as 1991, as we were free to alter our postoperative protocols in Canada, and put forth concepts of micro- and macrohomogeneity and beam testing.

I visited with Theo Seiler early in my career and learned more in hours from listening to his clinical observations than in months of reviewing articles. I spent time in Italy with Lucio Buratto, having my first introduction to keratomileusis and high myopia correction. Paolo Vinciguerra then taught me about scanning excimer lasers and demonstrated the refractive and therapeutic capabilities of the Aesculap-Meditec MEL 60.

I began working with the Chiron Technolas Keracor 116 in August 1993 and created the multi-multizone blending technique, using up to nine zones for improved surface contour. I developed the double pretreatment technique for forme fruste keratoconus and various retreatment techniques for topographical abnormalities, dense haze, and decentered ablations.

In August 1994, after having performed 3500 PRKs and on the advice of Stephen Slade, I traveled with him to Bogata, Colombia, and observed Luis Ruiz perform LASIK. We were joined by Charles Casebeer, who spoke to me of the challenges and limitations of PRK on the flight to South America. But what truly convinced me that

LASIK was the future was not the logical arguments Charles Casebeer proposed, not the 95 procedures I observed Luis Ruiz perform in that single first day, not even the theoretical benefits of combining lamellar surgery with the excimer laser, but simply the clinical appearance of the patients the following morning. The incredible comfort and the even more incredible vision of these quiet white eyes. On the long flight home I am sure I asked Stephen Slade more consecutive questions on lamellar surgery than he had ever been asked in his entire life. It did not take very long before I began incorporating this remarkable technique into my practice.

Over the following years, I added technologies as well as techniques to my armamentarium. In late 1994, I began utilizing the Sunrise holmium for laser thermokeratoplasty for primary hyperopia and consecutive hyperopia following PRK and LASIK. In late 1995, I began working with the Chiron Technolas PlanoScan program for myopic, toric, and hyperopic ablations utilizing flying spot technology. In 1996, I incorporated two more excimer lasers into my practice, a Nidek EC-5000 and a VisX STAR.

Just as I modified the ablation algorithms of PRK based upon my clinical observations, I began developing new intrastromal ablation algorithms and technique modifications to improve qualitative visual outcome after LASIK. LASIK is not ALK with a laser, just as it is not PRK simply in the deeper stroma; it is a procedure unto itself, based upon a unique set of principles and procedure nuances. LASIK clearly is in evolution and has become my overwhelming refractive procedure of choice, treating four out of every five of my patients.

Over these past several years, I have learned not only from my colleagues, but from my patients. I only wish that on occasion I had learned a little faster.

Foreword

More than 10 years ago, the excimer laser entered the ophthalmic world and initiated a revolution of refractive surgery. In the mid-1980s, only a few working groups worldwide investigated experimentally the potential of this laser and its interaction with ocular tissues. This period was followed by early preclinical and clinical applications in refractive (photorefractive keratectomy, or PRK) and curative corneal surgery (phototherapeutic keratectomy, or PTK) which led, finally, to scientific and administrative approvals of PTK and PRK in the years 1994 and 1995. During these studies we learned that PRK is not appropriate for corrections of high myopia and a new hybrid technique had to be developed, LASIK, merging the advantages of conventional keratomileusis and PRK. This evolution is still going on today, aiming toward the correction of astigmatism and hyperopia, as well as aspheric corrections of myopia to increase the optical performance of the operated eye. Experts expect the volume of refractive surgery to exceed that of cataract surgery within the next 10 years.

During the clinical evaluation and development of PRK techniques in Berlin, we had many visitors from all over the world. One of these visitors was a young Canadian ophthalmologist accompanied by his pregnant, lovely wife. He had many questions, and a fair amount of skepticism, but he also had many interesting ideas for further developments. After a few days, Dr. Jeffery Machat left Berlin, convinced that excimer laser surgery was the way to go and he started to do so immediately. He took advantage of the restrictions of refractive laser surgery in the United States and established a very successful refractive practice in Canada close to the border. Today, he is one of the most experienced laser surgeons in the world and now he is sharing his unique clinical experience with us in this book. I am sure that the reader will benefit from his insights.

Refractive surgery has historically created conflicts and still does. Also in this book, the reader will find proven scientific knowledge next to opinions and ideas. Although especially in refractive surgery, decisions are made by prospective studies, there must be also be space for such opinions and ideas of new approaches that will have to be judged by studies later. I hope that this book will stimulate many of us to commence such studies and to establish a broad fundamental of a new refractive surgery of which patients and physicians will benefit.

—*Theo Seiler, MD, PhD*

Introduction

Most of the concepts and instrumentation used in refractive surgery today were developed in Bogota, Colombia, the country of my birth. Jose Ignacio Barraquer, MD, widely acknowledged as the father of refractive surgery, brought an uncommon dedication to the pursuit of "plastic surgery of the eye" in his clinic in Bogota. The premise was simple: to remove or add sufficient material within the stroma to change the external curvature of the cornea without affecting Bowman's layer.

Shortly before 1949, Dr. Barraquer began work on the design of the instrumentation needed for refractive keratoplasty and made experimental resections on animal eyes. When he first began working on human eyes, the technique was still experimental and complex, and the instrumentation was in a primitive state of development. The microkeratome was not yet available, and the cryolathe for carving the frozen corneal tissue was actually a modified contact lens lathe, located in a laboratory some 3 km from the surgical suite. In freehand fashion with a Paufique knife or corneal dissector, he removed a corneal disc approximately 300 microns thick from the patient and transported the tissue by car to this laboratory for carving into a lenticule. He then brought this tissue back to the operating room and sutured it onto the patient's eye.

From these difficult beginnings, Barraquer proceeded to develop the computer-driven and automatic cryolathe, the motorized microkeratome, and the keratomileusis technique for the correction of myopia and hyperopia. He performed numerous successful keratomileusis procedures himself with promising results and formally taught his techniques to others. I had the good fortune to be one of his students at the Instituto Barraquer de Bogota, Colombia, and I continued the work necessary to make the keratome resections more predictable and irregular astigmatism less of a problem.

For a while I made resections with the BKS (Barraquer-Krumeich-Swinger) keratome and then carved the stromal side of these non-frozen discs of corneal tissue with the same keratome. For this technique, a thick resection of tissue was necessary because a thin section could not easily be carved. One day, the resection in one patient was too thin to be carved (approximately 130 microns). As luck would have it, this was a case that could not be canceled. After some thought, I decided that the only solution available was to change the plate of the microkeratome and resect a stromal disc from the bed. The result was excellent, and this surgery, which began with an undesirable result, turned out to be the birth of the keratomileusis in situ technique that today serves as the basis for the ALK and LASIK techniques.

The microkeratome that was available at that time had many shortcomings. Through the interaction with an engineer, we were able to develop the automated microkeratome which moves across the cornea at a constant speed and allows smooth-surface, predictable-thickness keratectomies to be made.

One of the principal benefits of mastering keratomileusis is that it allows the surgeon to correct refractive errors by working directly on the stromal bed while leaving the anterior surface intact. In this way, the wound healing problems associated with procedures that modify the corneal surface were avoided. In my experience, up to 33 D of myopia could be corrected.

With the automated microkeratome, the accuracy, predictability, and postoperative stability of keratomileusis in situ increased, but the accuracy of the second, refractive resection was still not of the level demonstrated by the excimer laser on corneal surface ablations. In addition, lost corneal caps were a concern.

The development of a corneal flap, instead of a free cap, as well as the combined use of the microkeratome for allowing access to the stromal bed and the excimer laser to ablate the exposed bed, addressed these problems. This modality, that came to be known as LASIK, allowed for the correction of high levels of myopia, eliminated the postoperative haze and refractive instability problems that can accompany laser corneal surface ablation patterns, and had greater predictability than the ALK technique.

In 1993, Stephen Slade and I performed some comparisons of results with ALK, PRK, keratomileusis with laser ablation of the underside of the cap, and LASIK in situ on the stromal bed. We found that LASIK definitely gave the best results. Since then, I perform only LASIK as a refractive procedure, and, to date, I have performed approximately 7000 LASIK cases.

One Venezuelan patient, on whom I had performed LASIK surgery 3 months before, had several postoperative follow-up visits in her hometown and then came back to my office. She was surprised because she was seeing very well but was confused by what her hometown doctor had told her. He said that her eyes showed no evidence that any surgery had been performed and that she had been cheated by paying a fee for non-existent surgery. I believe this anecdote illustrates the superb results that are possible with LASIK. At this time, I am trying to develop the laser algorithm for the correction of presbyopia, a condition that handicaps a very large percentage of the world's population. We have made much progress, but much can still be done.

—*Luis A. Ruiz, MD*

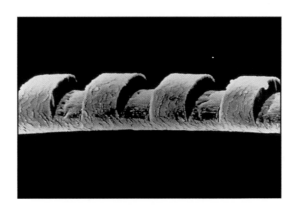

Section I
PRK

CHAPTER 1

PRK: Fundamental Concepts and Technology

EXCIMER LASER CONCEPTS

Refractive surgery, as with most forms of surgery, is as much an art as it is a science. It is often stated that there are as many techniques as there are surgeons. However, all surgical procedures are based upon certain fundamental principles which, when violated, result in less than satisfactory results or even complications. This basic belief is as true for laser refractive surgery as for any other form of surgery. The rapid evolution of the excimer laser has in many ways complicated the art of laser refractive surgery. The application of laser technology to refractive surgery has not only shortened the surgical learning curve, but has in a very real way obscured the surgical nature of the procedure itself. Clinical results are dependent not only upon the skill of the surgeon and the wound healing capabilities of the patient, but the proper application of this new technology. In fact, a level of sophistication has been added to the surgical process to enhance the surgical outcome, but it has also fostered a false sense of security. The utilization of the excimer laser for refractive procedures demands an understanding of the technology itself, in addition to the fundamental principles of proper surgical technique and perioperative care.

EXCIMER LASER SURGICAL PROCEDURES

There are two primary clinical applications of the excimer laser: refractive procedures and therapeutic procedures. Laser refractive procedures can either be surface ablation procedures, generally known as photorefractive keratectomy (PRK) (Figure 1-1), or intrastromal ablation procedures, referred to as laser in situ keratomileusis (LASIK). Photoastigmatic refractive keratectomy (PARK) has been used to designate the application of a toric ablation pattern (Figure 1-2). Therapeutic procedures, or phototherapeutic keratectomy (PTK) (Figure 1-3), may or may not alter refractive error, but are primarily designed to treat surface corneal pathology, such as corneal erosions, anterior corneal dystrophies, and superficial scars. The fundamental difference between PRK and PTK is that PTK delivers an equal amount of energy to all parts of the cornea within the area of ablation, whereas PRK myopia correction involves greater treatment or removal of tissue centrally.

FUNDAMENTAL ELEMENTS OF LASER REFRACTIVE SURGERY

The first two fundamental elements governing the limitations and capabilities of the excimer laser concern fluence and beam homogeneity. Fluence is defined as the amount of energy applied to the ablative zone, whereas homogeneity is defined as the pattern of energy distribution within the exposed area. Homogeneity can be subdefined into microhomogeneity and macrohomogeneity. The term microhomogeneity defines localized variability in energy beam density, that is, "hot" and "cold" areas within the beam. The hot areas represent the highest energy density areas or peaks; the cold

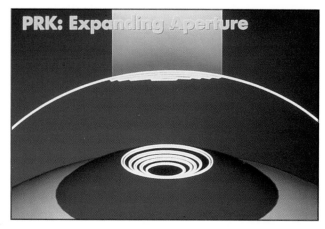

Figure 1-1.
Schematic diagram of myopic PRK removing more tissue centrally than peripherally.

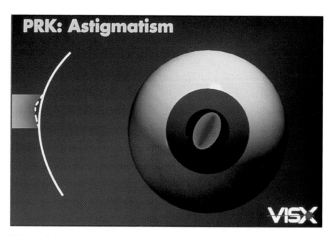

Figure 1-2.
Schematic representation of toric ablation.

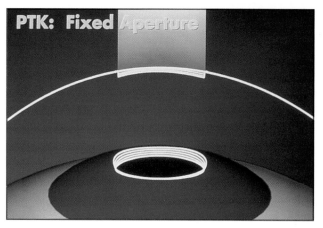

Figure 1-3.
Schematic of PTK removing equal amounts of tissue within area of ablation.

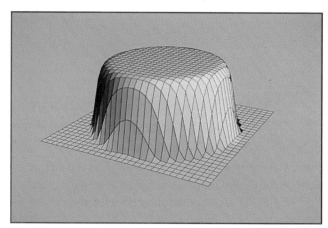

Figure 1-4.
Homogeneous (flat) energy beam profile of Coherent-Schwind Keratom laser system.

areas conversely represent the areas of lowest energy density or valleys. Microhomogeneity is best represented by the peak-to-valley ratio. The term macrohomogeneity, rather than defining localized energy patterns, tends to refer to the overall energy beam profile of a specific excimer laser system.

FLUENCE AND HOMOGENEITY

Each excimer laser system has a characteristic energy beam profile, which may be homogeneous, gaussian, or reverse gaussian. A homogeneous or flat beam profile indicates an overall equal distribution of energy density. A

> **Fluence relates to the *amount* of energy applied. Homogeneity relates to the *pattern* of energy applied.**

> **Homogeneity can be subdefined into:**
> - Microhomogeneity
> - Macrohomogeneity

gaussian energy beam profile, which is bell curved in nature, indicates that there is a greater energy density centrally within the beam, while reverse gaussian implies less energy density centrally. The importance of the energy beam profile is that it states the clinical profile, determining clinical factors such as refractive predictability and stability, as well as the incidence of certain complications, such as central island formation. The simplest way to envision the energy beam profile (Figure 1-4) is to imagine the shape of a single pulse being delivered to the surface of the cornea. In actuality it is a composite of many pulses. A homogeneous energy beam

PTK
Richard A. Eiferman, MD, FACS

The excimer laser is extremely useful in the treatment of recurring corneal erosions. The abnormal epithelium is debrided under topical anesthesia with a smooth curette or spatula. It is important to remove all affected areas even if they extend to the periphery (although 1 mm should be preserved at the limbus to retain stem cells). The laser is programmed to remove about 6 microns of Bowman's layer. All the debrided areas should be treated by scanning across the cornea or positioning the eye to treat the periphery. In general, the cornea heals uneventfully and rarely requires retreatment.

Reis-Buckler's dystrophy is best treated with a transepithelial approach. Since this dystrophy has marked thickening of Bowman's layer with curly filaments extending into the basal lamina, it is easier to simultaneously remove both tissues with the laser. Anterior basement membrane dystrophy and granular or lattice dystrophy can be handled by either mechanical or laser ablation.

Elevated corneal lesions, such as Salzmann's nodules or band keratopathy, should be debulked prior to PTK. The laser beam should be narrowed to smooth the residual lesion. The adjacent corneal epithelium serves as a natural modulator to protect the unaffected area and every effort should be made to preserve it.

Scars, corneal divots, and other irregular surfaces are far

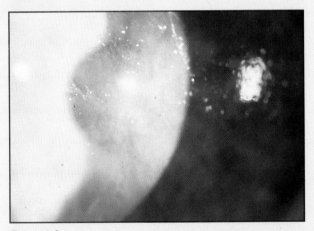

Figure A-1.
Preoperative corneal scar due to streptococcal ulcer.

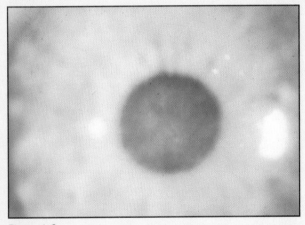

Figure A-2.
Postoperative excimer laser PTK. VA 20/20.

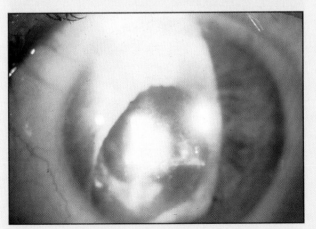

Figure A-3.
Preoperative corneal scar due to fish hook injury.

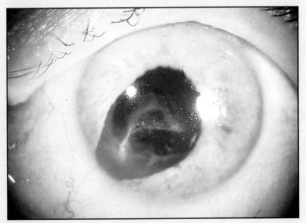

Figure A-4.
Postoperative excimer PRK. VA 20/50 with contact lens.

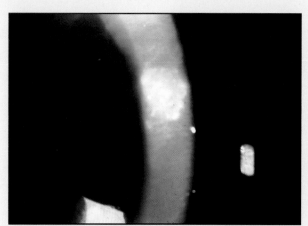

Figure A-5.
Intractable superficial corneal ulcer secondary to crystalline keratopathy.

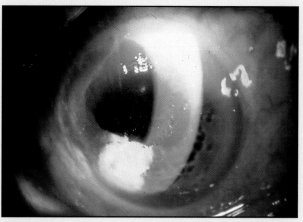

Figure A-6.
Postoperative PTK. VA 20/20.

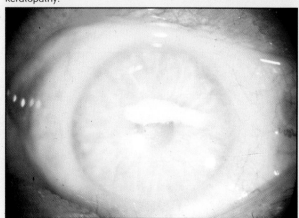

Figure A-7.
Preoperative band keratopathy.

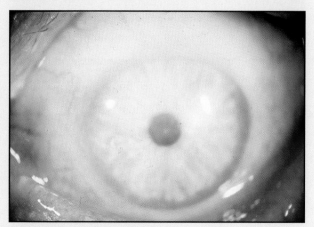

Figure A-8.
Postoperative PTK.

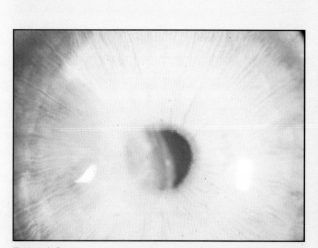

Figure A-9.
Preoperative corneal scar due to HSV.

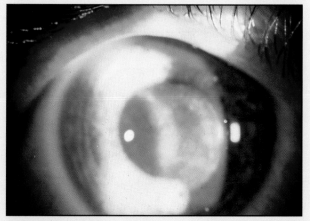

Figure A-10.
Poor postoperative result with increased scarring.

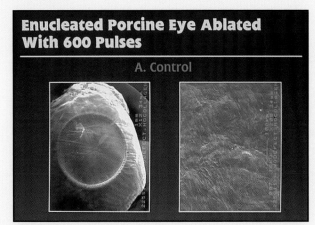

Figure A-11.
Rapidly polymerizing collagen modulator tested on porcine eye.

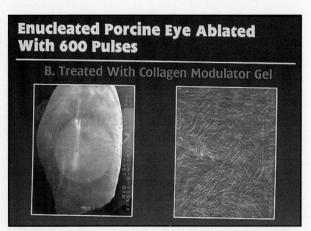

Figure A-12.
Postoperative PTK on porcine eye. Note the smooth surface.

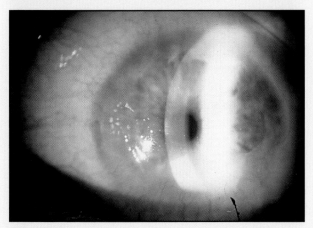

Figure A-13.
Superficial corneal scar. Preoperative VA 20/200.

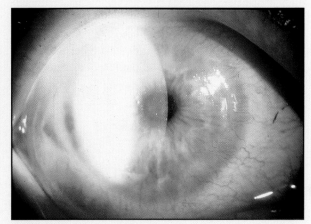

Figure A-14.
Postoperative PTK. VA 20/25.

more difficult to treat with the excimer laser. It should be noted that the excimer laser will reproduce an irregular surface deeper within the stroma without correcting the abnormality. Minor irregularities can be filled with artificial tears or viscoelastics, but these fluids are often unsatisfactory as they tend to form a meniscus and are affected by evaporation and effluent removers.

Various collagen gels are being developed to serve as modulators. In therapeutic procedures, the smoothing agent should protect the corneal tissue surrounding elevations removed by photoablation, thereby improving the corneal surface. Ideally, the modulator should be capable of absorbing 193-nm ultraviolet irradiation, flowing evenly across the corneal surface to fill in depressions with little to no meniscus, and resisting rippling effects due to vacuuming or gaseous flow which are sometimes used with excimer laser photoablation techniques. An addition-al benefit from a modulator might be its ability to maintain the hydration of the corneal surface. This is of particular importance since it is known that the pulse depth of excimer laser ablation depends on the level of tissue hydration.

It must be emphasized that scar tissue may not ablate evenly and may require repeated slit lamp biomicroscopy to determine the smoother corneal surface and not necessarily remove all interstitial opacities.

It is obvious that removal of stromal substance induces a hyperopic shift. While this may provide myopes with a double benefit, it can cause objectionable anisometropia.

An alternative approach is a superficial keratectomy using the ALK unit. Using the suction ring at its maximum diameter, a superficial cut induces minimal refractive power. This approach can be used to remove a large variety of anterior corneal pathology.

Each excimer laser system has a characteristic energy beam profile.

Energy beam profile can be:
- Gaussian
- Homogeneous
- Reverse gaussian

profile would look like a top hat with equal amounts of energy centrally and peripherally. Each part of the beam would therefore remove identical amounts of tissue from the corneal surface. A gaussian beam is hotter centrally, having more energy centrally than peripherally, thereby removing more tissue centrally than peripherally with each pulse.

Fluence, defined as energy applied to a given area, is expressed in units of millijoules per square centimeter and varies from approximately 100 to 250 mJ/cm^2 depending upon the specific excimer laser system discussed, for example:
- VisX: 160 mJ/cm^2
- Summit: 180 to 200 mJ/cm^2
- Technolas: 130 mJ/cm^2
- Nidek: 130 mJ/cm^2

Energy beam profile determines the clinical profile.

A simple way to understand the importance of fluence is that it is the primary determinant of the amount of tissue ablated with each pulse. Fluence determines the ablation rate, whereas the computer algorithm is merely programmed to apply a given number of pulses in a given manner for any given refractive error. The precise amount of energy delivered per pulse will help determine outcome predictability. With fluence below 50 mJ/cm^2 there is minimal ablative effect, and at 120 mJ/cm^2 the ablative effect appears to level off. As one increases fluence, the pulse-to-pulse variability decreases, improving overall beam quality. However, the

$$Fluence = \frac{Energy}{Area}$$

improvement in beam homogeneity from increased fluence is accompanied by increased thermal energy effect, increased optic degradation, and increased acoustic shockwave effect.

ENERGY OUTPUT

Excimer lasers should not be viewed merely as black boxes. The excimer must be understood, not only to achieve superior refractive results but to avoid complications. The laser head is at the heart of the black box and consists of the laser cavity and electrodes. The two primary determinants of energy output, or fluence, are the freshness of the laser gas and the voltage. The laser gas becomes consumed as pulses are produced. When the fluence is low, the voltage within the cavity can be increased. Once maximal voltage is obtained, a gas exchange must be performed, putting fresh gas within the cavity. Higher voltages also have the benefit of producing improved beam homogeneity; therefore, one can maintain high voltage within the laser cavity, and filter or attenuate beam energy later within the optical pathway to control fluence. To further complicate our developing insight into excimer lasers, the energy output from each laser varies and thus frequent recalibration is vital. The importance of recalibration to assess beam output, not only quantitatively but qualitatively, cannot be overstated.

Fundamental to understanding the excimer is that the energy output from this laser is inherently nonhomogeneous, and therefore requires sophisticated optical delivery systems to render these beams usable. An important fact to be elaborated on later in this chapter is that it is much more difficult to produce and maintain a homogeneous beam of large diameter, making wide area surface ablation more challenging.

Excimer lasers are divided into essentially two types based upon their delivery systems:
- Broad beam delivery systems
- Scanning beam delivery systems

There are two basic laser delivery systems: broad beam (wide field ablation) and scanning. Broad beam delivery systems, such as the Summit Excimed and OmniMed and the VisX 20/20 (Figure 1-5a) and STAR (Figure 1-5b) and the original Chiron Technolas Keracor 116 system (Figures 1-6a and 1-6b), utilize a computer-controlled variable iris diaphragm for myopic correction (Figures 1-7a and 1-7b), whereas the Coherent-Schwind Keratom broad beam system

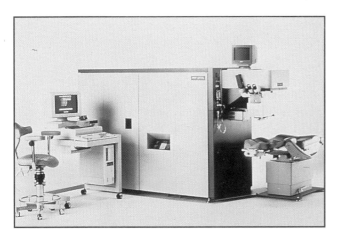

Figure 1-5a.
VisX 20/20 Model B excimer laser system.

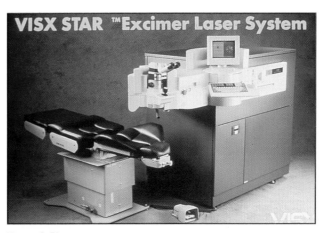

Figure 1-5b.
VisX STAR excimer laser system with substantially smaller footplate.

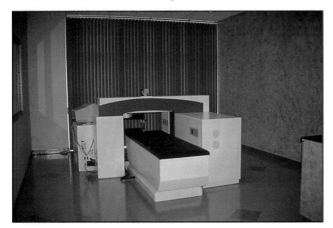

Figure 1-6a.
Chiron Technolas Keracor 116 excimer laser system.

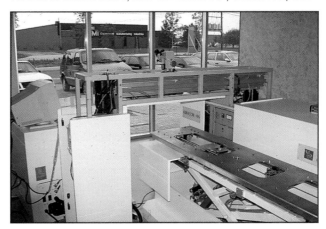

Figure 1-6b.
Chiron Technolas Keracor 116 partially assembled.

Broad beam delivery systems lasers:
- Summit ExciMed
- Summit OmniMed
- VisX 20/20
- VisX (Taunton) 20/15
- Chiron Technolas Keracor 116
- Coherent-Schwind Keratom

(Figure 1-8a) utilizes a series of round or elliptical apertures to produce the desired ablation pattern (Figure 1-8b). The beam is delivered at the maximal optical zone, but the diaphragm controls the area of the cornea exposed for each pulse. Scanning delivery systems such as the Aesculap-Meditec MEL 60 (Figure 1-9) and Nidek EC-5000 utilize a scanning slit to alter the corneal curvature, whereas the CIBA–Autonomous Technologies Corporation Tracker-

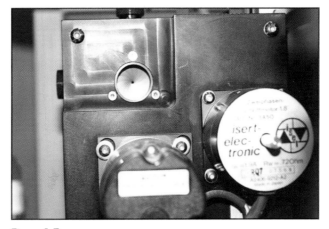

Figure 1-7a.
Chiron Technolas Keracor iris diaphragm in closed position, aperture size reduced to 0.8 mm.

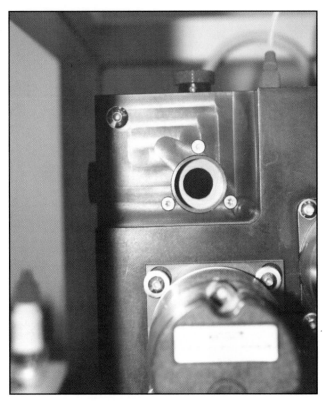

Figure 1-7b.
Chiron Technolas Keracor iris diaphragm in open position, aperture size expanded to 7.0 mm.

Scanning delivery system lasers:
- Aesculap-Meditec MEL 60
- Nidek EC-5000
- Chiron Technolas Keracor 116, 117
- LaserSight Compak-200 Mini-Excimer
- CIBA–Autonomous Technologies Corporation Tracker-PRK
- Novatec LightBlade solid-state (non-excimer)

PRK and LaserSight Compak-200 Mini-Excimer use a flying spot. The advantage of scanning systems is that they manipulate a small beam, typically 1 to 2 mm in diameter, which can be made highly homogeneous much more easily.

The energy output of an excimer laser system is actually rectangular initially and is manipulated through a series of lenses, prisms, and spatial integrators to improve beam quality (Figure 1-10). A tremendous amount of energy is lost through the optical pathway. It is important to recognize that these lasers are sensitive to optic misalignment and degradation, which can dramatically alter beam quality. Understanding that larger beams are more at risk for beam

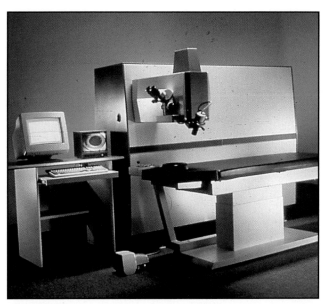

Figure 1-8a.
Coherent-Schwind Keratom excimer laser system.

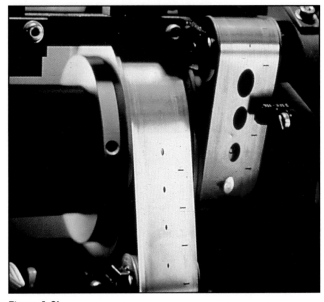

Figure 1-8b.
Series of oval and circular apertures on rotating belt utilized by Coherent-Schwind Keratom laser for toric and spherical ablations.

abnormalities is important for developing a realistic understanding of the excimer laser.

ESSENTIAL PHYSICS OF THE EXCIMER LASER

The excimer laser has been evolving for more than a decade, and continues to evolve. The fundamental element which allows for photoablation is that far ultraviolet light energy is capable of excising corneal tissue with submicron

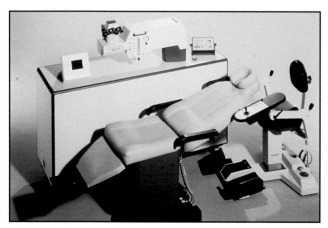

Figure 1-9.
Aesculap-Meditec MEL 60 excimer laser system utilizing scanning slit delivery system and hand-held mechanical mask.

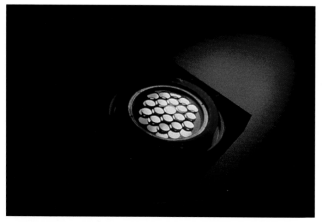

Figure 1-10.
Integrator of beam homogenization system of Coherent-Schwind Keratom excimer laser.

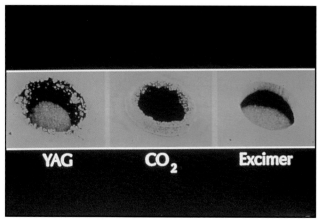

Figure 1-11.
Comparison of YAG, CO_2, and excimer laser effects on PMMA. The virtually non-thermal excimer laser ablation leaves a smooth contour compared to the thermal damage and disruption produced by the other lasers.

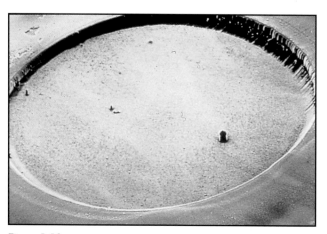

Figure 1-12.
This figure illustrates the incredible smoothness of excimer photoablation on PMMA plastic.

precision as well as submicron collateral damage. This alone has generated considerable interest in laser refractive surgery. It is the very minimal thermal energy effect produced by the 193-nm wavelength (Figure 1-11) that limits the degree of collateral damage to the surrounding tissue and provides the characteristic smooth ablative surfaces which are now familiar to all of us (Figures 1-12 and 1-13). The ablation rate is approximately 0.25 microns per pulse. Although the effects of thermal energy from an excimer laser emitting cool far ultraviolet light energy are very minimal, it is not zero and each pulse is associated with an area of collateral damage of less than 1 micron, usually in the range of 0.2 to 0.3 microns (Figures 1-14 and 1-15). Thus, the excimer laser removes 0.25 microns per pulse and damages an additional 0.25 microns of adjacent corneal tissue.

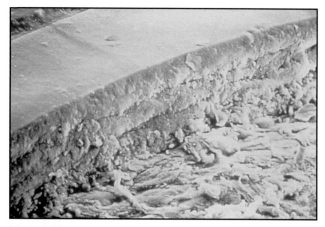

Figure 1-13.
Excimer photoablation may produce smooth tissue excision patterns with minimal disturbance to adjacent cells.

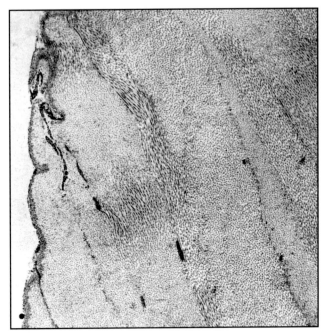

Figure 1-14.
Scanning electron micrograph of tissue treated with excimer photoablation, illustrating the most important element of PRK, removing tissue without damaging adjacent tissue. Courtesy of Dr. Stephen Trokel and Dr. John Marshall.

The excimer laser is therefore 50 to 1000 times more precise than any other ophthalmic laser in this regard. Considering that a human cell is 10 microns in diameter and a red blood cell 7 microns, this degree of precision is difficult to comprehend (Figures 1-16a and 1-16b). The repetition rate varies from 5 to 10 pulses per second, but the actual ablative process requires about 12 nanoseconds. The repetition rate could be increased, however, time for thermal energy and plume dissipation is necessary. Plume (Figure 1-17) consists of the tissue particles and debris liberated during the ablative process. Special high-speed photography has been used to capture the ablative process, which closely resembles a mushroom cloud from a nuclear explosion. The plume is

> Despite phenomenal submicron precision, PRK is still limited by variability of wound healing.

Excimer laser unique qualities:
- Submicron precision
- Submicron collateral damage
- Minimal thermal energy effect

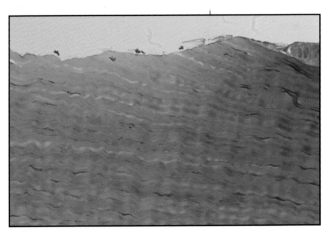

Figure 1-15.
Light microscopy examination of stromal tissue treated with the excimer laser. Minimal disruption of the lasered bed is observed with a well-contoured surface. Courtesy of Dr. Stephen Trokel.

ejected from the ablative surface at 1000 to 2000 m/second. Furthermore, the impact of each pulse and the recoil forces of plume ejection produce an acoustic shockwave that is both audible and visible with specialized videography and photography. The acoustic shockwave has a variety of clinical implications, from central island formation to endothelial cell loss. The average procedure removes tissue as slender as a human hair, approximately 50 microns, in less than 30 seconds. PRK (Figures 1-18a and 1-18b) typically removes between 15 to 150 microns of tissue, depending upon the degree of correction attempted. It is important to understand that it is not primarily the amount of tissue that is removed that may adversely affect wound healing, but the technique by which it is removed.

EVOLUTION OF PRK

In 1983, Trokel et al first described the removal of corneal tissue with an excimer laser for refractive surgery. Srinivasan et al coined the term *photoablative decomposition,* or *photoablation,* to describe the photochemical process by which far ultraviolet light energy produces tissue removal through the breakdown of molecular bonds. The process of photoablation is unlike any other ophthalmic laser interaction. Each pulse of ultraviolet light energy possesses 6.4 eV, more than double that of any other ophthalmic laser and more than adequate to cleave 3.5 eV carbon-carbon bonds (Figure 1-19). Whereas photocoagulation with an argon laser utilizes heat, and photodisruption with the YAG laser is dependent upon explosive shockwaves to produce its results, the effects of photoablation are related to direct breakdown of molecular bonds.

Evolution of PRK

Marguerite B. McDonald, MD, FACS

After Dr. Stephen Trokel's landmark paper published in the *American Journal of Ophthalmology* in 1983, the ophthalmic world realized the potential of the excimer laser. Dr. Trokel had correctly assumed that this wavelength, previously used to make computer chips in California's Silicon Valley, could be harnessed to remove corneal tissue with submicron precision and without thermal damage to surrounding tissue. However, Dr. Trokel was not a cornea specialist and did not have easy access to large numbers of rabbits and monkeys. Thus, he decided to collaborate with Dr. Charles Munnerlyn, a physicist based in California, and me, a corneal surgeon and research scientist at the LSU Department of Ophthalmology in New Orleans, where large numbers of experimental animals were housed. This three-way collaboration led to many laboratory experiments on cadaver, animal, and human eyes in an attempt to understand the depth per shot obtained with 160 mJ/cm^2 on corneal tissue. In addition, histological samples were studied to ensure that thermal damage to surrounding structures was not an impediment.

After cadaver eyes, live rabbits were treated with a very small, simple, non–computer-driven industrial laser from Questek. I changed the diaphragm position with a hand crank every few shots, creating ablations with only five steps. The rabbits responded with thick, hyperplastic scars within 2 to 3 weeks postoperatively, which sent the research team back to the drawing board. When the diaphragm of the laser closed automatically by means of a computer program, and 40 steps (instead of five) were utilized, the rabbit corneas healed beautifully, with a brief period of minimal haze. The histology further supported the improved clinical results.

Non-human primate studies were begun in 1984 by myself and my team at the Delta Primate Center. After numerous calibration studies, two large monkey trials were undertaken and the animals were followed for 1 year postoperatively. Elaborate preoperative examinations (consisting of slit lamp examination, slit lamp photography, cycloplegic retinoscopy, K-readings, corneal topography, ultrasonic pachymetry, and specular microscopy) were repeated at 1, 3, 6, and 12 months; timed histologic samples were also taken. These studies documented that excimer PRK could safely and permanently flatten the central cornea in a predictable fashion, without thermal

damage to surrounding tissues.

After the monkey studies in 1984 and 1985, one sighted human eye was ablated centrally early in 1987, 11 days prior to an exenteration for a conjunctival melanoma. The histological specimen showed a smoothly tapered (and then disappearing) Bowman's layer with new epithelium, not yet differentiated, adherent to the ablated stromal bed. Once again, no thermal damage was seen in the remaining corneal or adjacent ocular structures.

Several months later, in June 1987, the human blind eye study commenced; this study was the first indication that higher attempted corrections were less likely to be fully obtained. At this time, 4.25-, 4.50-, and 5.0-mm ablations were used, with smaller ablation zones reserved for higher attempted corrections.

One of the blind eye patients treated in June 1987 recovered her vision 7 weeks later. Though a chiasmal lesion and a previous retinal detachment had led to no light perception as documented in three well-known medical institutions, this patient apparently underwent the sudden reversal of hysterical blindness, originally described by Freud. She maintains her 4.5 D correction and 20/20 uncorrected visual acuity to this day.

The partially sighted trial followed, as did Phases IIa, IIb, and III, with an accompanying expansion of the number of investigative studies.

The original nitrogen-blow technique was used throughout the animal studies and Phases I, II, and the first half of III. The nitrogen was blown directly over the cornea through three small jets protruding from the inner aspect of a limbal suction ring which was attached to a handle. The handle was held by the surgeon to fixate the eye. Halfway through Phase III of the VisX multicenter clinical trial, anecdotal evidence from Canadian laser investigators indicated that if nitrogen blowing was stopped, patients would have less corneal haze and faster return and less loss of best corrected acuity. In addition, scanning electron micrographs taken by Stephen D. Klyce, PhD, of freshly ablated monkey corneas with and without nitrogen blowing indicated clearly that the no-blow technique led to much smoother post-ablation surfaces.

At the 1-year postoperative evaluation of the Phase III PRK patients in the VisX trial, the evidence was clearly in favor of the no-blow technique. There was much lower incidence of mild and moderate haze, and much less incidence of loss of two or more lines of best corrected vision (actually, this incidence dropped to zero). The only drawback was the sudden appearance of central islands on corneal topography, areas of under-ablated or completely unablated tissue in the center of the ablated zone. Though theories abound as to why these islands occur without nitrogen blowing, they are still poorly understood. They are not of immense clinical importance, however, as all islands disappeared by 1 year and no central island patient had a decrease in best corrected acuity at 1 year.

Toric ablations were the next to be attempted by VisX and other laser companies, with ever-improving success as more accurate and reproducible software and methods of identifying the cylinder axis are developed.

The treatment of hyperopia with the excimer laser is still in development. Currently, most of the major laser companies are struggling with the exact algorithms and hardware specifications required to provide a permanent correction. Most attempts to date have suffered from a large degree of dioptric regression. It is clear that 9-mm or larger diameter ablations will be required so that the ablation sites will not fill in with new collagen and epithelium.

Physicians are demanding smaller, less expensive lasers with lower maintenance costs. The only way to make a smaller, cheaper, more fuel-efficient, optics-sparing laser is to make a scanning and tracking small-beam laser. A smaller beam spares the optics and requires less gas. A small beam must also have a perfectly registered tracker so that irregular astigmatism is not induced. There are several efforts underway internationally; the Autonomous Technologies Corporation of Orlando, Florida, has made the most progress to date. I conducted extensive laboratory and monkey trials from 1993 through 1994. Blind and sighted eye studies have been conducted from 1994 through 1995 in Crete by Ioannis Pallikaris, MD, with well-documented safety and efficacy. US clinical trials should begin in early 1996 at my hospital in New Orleans.

Excimer lasers can produce ultraviolet light energy at various wavelengths depending upon the gas elements utilized. Ultraviolet light energy of 248 nm not only results in potentially mutagenic behavior as evidenced by unscheduled DNA synthesis, but requires a higher energy density to achieve similar ablative effects as 193 nm and produces greater collateral damage. Similarly, ultraviolet light energy of 308-nm wavelength is associated with an increased risk of cataract formation. Ultraviolet light energy of 193-nm wavelength was associated with smoother ablation effects at lower energy densities and did not exhibit mutagenic or cataractogenic behavior.

Excimer laser PRK utilizes controlled pulses of 193-nm ultraviolet light energy to ablate stromal tissue producing a refractive excision pattern. The term excimer is derived from "excited dimer", which consists of an inert gas and a halide, specifically argon and fluoride gaseous elements, which are excited to a higher energy state by thousands of volts of electricity. Dimer is actually a misnomer as it applies to two of the same element. The argon and fluoride elements are in very small concentrations in a helium mixture known as premix. The elements combine to form an unstable compound which rapidly dissociates, releasing the ultraviolet light energy.

The relationship between the refractive effect produced and the depth of ablation is depicted by an algorithm developed by Munnerlyn et al. The Munnerlyn formula was based

	TABLE 1-1		
	DEPTH OF ABLATION RELATIONSHIP WITH OPTICAL ZONE SIZE		
Optical Zone Size (mm)	Depth of Ablation (microns)		
	-3.00 D	-6.00 D	-9.00 D
3.00	9.00	18.00	27.00
3.50	12.25	24.50	36.75
4.00	16.00	32.00	48.00
4.50	20.25	40.50	60.75
5.00	25.00	50.00	75.00
5.50	30.25	60.50	90.75
6.00	36.00	72.00	108.00
6.50	42.25	84.50	126.75
7.00	49.00	98.00	147.00
8.00	64.00	128.00	192.00
9.00	81.00	162.00	243.00

upon effecting a theoretical lenticular curve within polymethylmethacrylate (PMMA) model, refined through in vivo animal models. The essentials of the Munnerlyn formula are found in the following boxed aside:

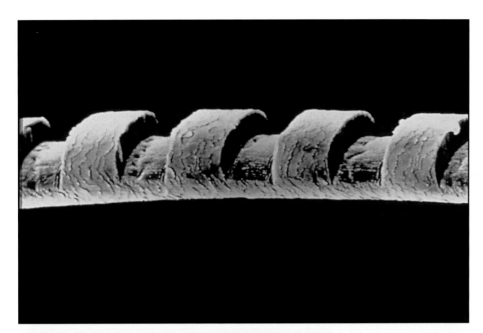

Figure 1-16a.
Human hair etched with the excimer laser demonstrating exceptional precision. Provided by VisX. Courtesy of IBM.

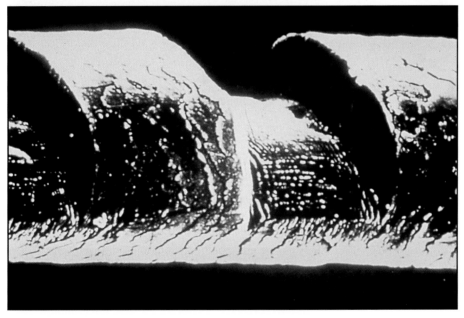

Figure 1-16b.
Magnification of human hair etched with the excimer laser. Provided by VisX. Courtesy of IBM.

$$\text{Depth of ablation} = \frac{(\text{optical zone})^2 \times \text{refractive change}}{3}$$

The essential principle to be drawn from the formula is that the depth of ablation increases exponentially with the square of the optical zone size. That is, a small increase in the optical zone results in a large increase in the amount of tissue ablated for any dioptric correction (Table 1-1). For example, the amount of tissue ablated for a -4.00 D correction increases from 12 to 48 microns, a four-fold increase, when the optical zone is doubled from 3 to 6 mm.

Munnerlyn and other investigators demonstrated in animal studies that deeper ablations were more likely to produce a loss of corneal transparency secondary to stromal scarring.

When PRK was first performed, small optical zones were utilized in order to minimize the depth of ablation. In clinical studies, Seiler, utilizing a 4.00-mm optical zone with the Summit ExciMed UV 200, and McDonald, utilizing a 4.25-

The depth of ablation increases exponentially with the square of the optical zone size.

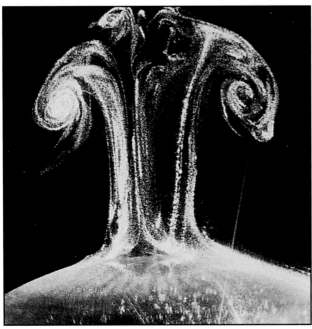

Figure 1-17.
High speed photography demonstrating plume generated by each excimer laser pulse. The plume contains photoablative debris which is ejected from the surface of the cornea at 1000 to 2000 m/second secondary to recoil forces.

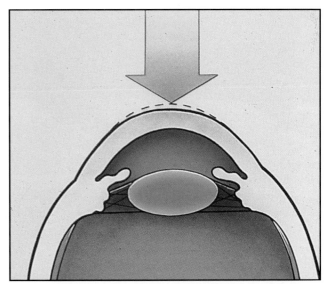

Figure 1-18a.
Schematic diagram illustrating excimer laser photoablation.

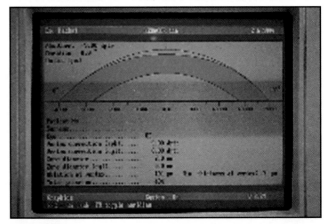

Figure 1-18b.
Graphic representation of PRK.

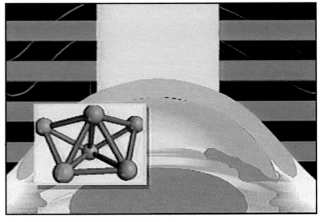

Figure 1-19.
Graphic illustration of surface PRK photoablation. Excimer laser utilizes 193-nm far ultraviolet wavelength which acts upon carbon-carbon molecular bonds to achieve photoablation.

mm optical zone with a VisX 20/20 excimer laser, both demonstrated that attempted corrections greater than -6.00 D resulted in an increased incidence of clinically significant haze, myopic regression, and loss of best corrected visual acuity. Of equal clinical significance, smaller optical zones produced clinically significant night glare. Night glare introduces

Large optical zones reduce:
- Regression
- Night glare

the concept of qualitative vision as being an essential target to achieve beyond merely quantitative vision. Investigators at the Phillips Eye Institute, using the Taunton 20/15 excimer laser, compared high myopia treatment results with optical zones less than 5.8 mm to results of those greater than 5.8 mm. It was discovered that patients treated with larger optical zones achieved more stable clinical results with a lower incidence of clinically significant haze. An evolution of technique toward larger optical zones continues despite the greater depth of ablation required. Larger optical zones have two primary benefits—reduced night glare and reduced regression of effect—leading to more stable high myopia results.

Piovella and Dossi developed a multizone technique

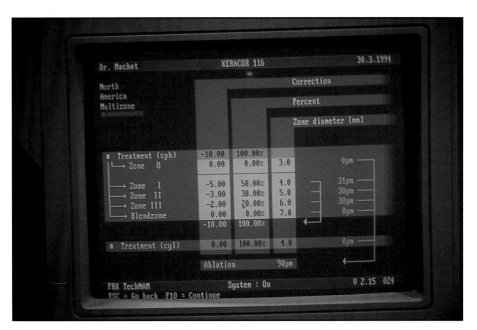

Figure 1-20a.
Multi-multizone computer screen of the Chiron Technolas Keracor 116 outlining the amount of pretreatment, dioptric distribution, micron distribution, and optical zones. The system allows the surgeon flexibility in customizing the program for his or her personal technique.

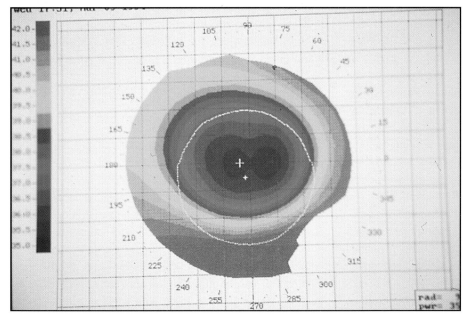

Figure 1-20b.
Corneal videokeratography of postoperative PRK patient treated for -12.50 D with multi-multizone technique demonstrating stable central corneal flattening at 1 year with 20/20 uncorrected vision. The fellow eye healed identically.

which limits the depth of ablation while providing a larger optical zone. In their multizone approach, the attempted correction for high myopia was divided into three steps with equal thirds of the total correction performed at 4-, 5-, and 6-mm optical zones. Since only part of the treatment is performed at the largest optical zone, the overall depth is significantly reduced. In an evolution of the multizone technique, I developed the multi-multizone technique, which utilized several optical zones increasing from 3 to 7 mm, in August 1993 with the Chiron Technolas Keracor 116 (Figures 1-20a through 1-20c). The primary benefit of the

Multi-multizone technique:
- Reduces depth of ablation while maximizing optical zone size to reduce night glare and regression
- Improves blending to provide a smoother surface to reduce haze formation and also regression
- Improves centration and reduces central island formation.

multizone approach is that it provides for an improved, more aspheric wound contour, reducing the depth of ablation

Figure 1-20c.
Treatment screen of Chiron Technolas Keracor 116. Each zone states the dioptric correction, number of seconds, and zone size. As each zone is treated, a blue bar advances across the screen allowing the surgeon or assistant the ability to monitor progress.

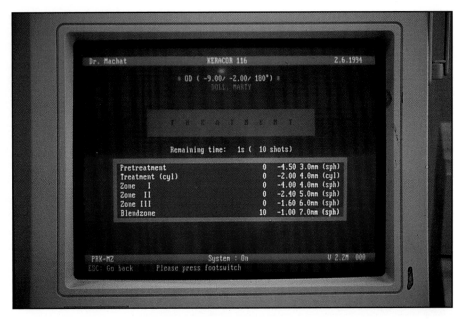

while maximizing the optical zone. The multi-multizone technique improves blending, promoting a smoother ablative surface and thereby reducing haze formation. Multizone itself also reduces central island formation as each zone starts centrally improving the treatment effect achieved centrally. The multipass/multizone technique presented by Mihai Pop, MD, at the American Society of Corneal and Refractive Surgeons in 1994 with the VisX 20/20 laser is equally efficacious and divides the treatment into steps of both increasing and identical optical zone sizes, thus providing the same smoothing benefits as the multi-multizone technique but with less reduction of ablation depth and slightly less wound edge blending (see Chapter 3).

In July 1992, using the VisX 20/20, I developed pretreatment, a technique to counteract central island formation, which also improves central qualitative vision. Pretreatment applies additional pulses to the central 2 to 3 mm of corneal tissue, in addition to the full refractive treatment. It compensates for the relative central undercorrection which occurs as a result of applying the Munnerlyn formula to hydrated stromal tissue rather than PMMA plastic or a theoretical lenticular curve. The concept of pretreatment (Figure 1-21) is further explained within the context of central island formation.

TECHNOLOGY PRINCIPLES

ENERGY BEAM PROFILE RELATIONSHIPS

There are multiple excimer laser systems. In order to better understand the technical and clinical features of each,

Pretreatment technique:
- The application of additional pulses to the central 2 to 3 mm of cornea beyond the full refractive treatment
- Compensates for corneal hydration
- Prevents central island formation
- Improves qualitative vision

it is important to further understand the relationship that exists between the energy beam profile and clinical profile. Each excimer laser has a unique energy beam configuration, which is characteristic of that particular laser system.

As discussed earlier, the energy beam profile (see Figure 1-4) can be gaussian with greatest energy density centrally, homogeneous (flat) with equal energy distribution throughout the beam, or reverse gaussian with lowest energy density centrally. The specific energy beam profile for each laser system will determine the clinical profile for that laser system, including refractive predictability and stability, as well as the incidence of some complications such as central island formation. Therefore, through a better understanding of each excimer laser delivery system and beam profile, one is able to predict certain features with regards to the clinical outcome.

It is important to understand that the original Summit ExciMed (Figure 1-22) and the more recently introduced Summit OmniMed series differ in their energy beam profile

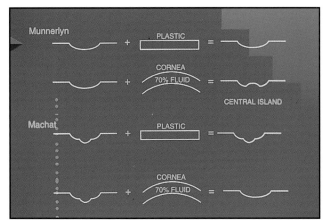

Figure 1-21.
Pretreatment applies additional pulses to the stromal surface beyond what is required to ablate a theoretical lenticular curve in order to compensate for the hydrated status (70% H_2O) of the cornea.

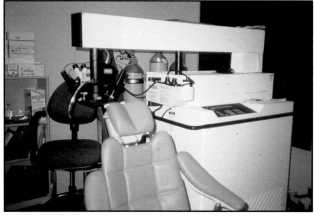

Figure 1-22.
Summit ExciMed UV 200 excimer laser system.

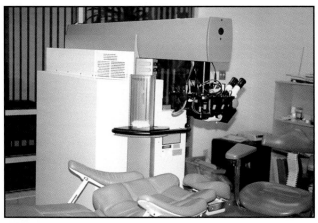

Figure 1-23a.
Summit OmniMed I excimer laser system.

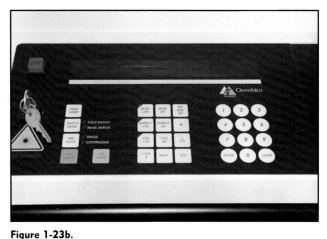

Figure 1-23b.
Summit OmniMed keyboard and internal computer with fixed microchip.

patterns and therefore differ in their clinical profiles. The Summit OmniMed has a flatter, more homogeneous energy beam profile than the ExciMed, although the OmniMed beam profile is still somewhat gaussian in nature. Summit developed its excimer laser specifically as an ophthalmic excimer laser. The power output of the ExciMed laser head was created to obtain good beam quality at a 3- to 4-mm optical zone in the late 1980s. The Summit ExciMed UV 200 did not produce adequate beam homogeneity for an optical zone greater than 5 mm, thus a more powerful laser head was designed and the evolution of the OmniMed series began (Figures 1-23a and 1-23b). The larger optical zone size capability is able to reduce both night glare and myopic regression. With the development of the Summit Apex, the unit currently approved for sale in the United States, and the Summit SVS (Summit Vision Systems) Apex Plus, formerly Apogee,

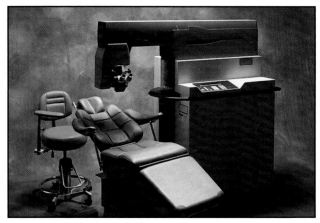

Figure 1-24.
Summit SVS Apex Plus excimer laser system.

Figure 1-25.
Biomicroscopic slit lamp photograph of RK incisions. Courtesy of Dr. Richard Baker.

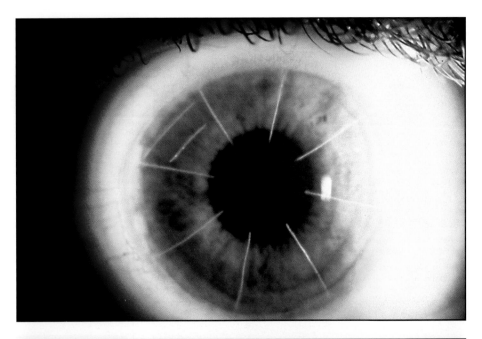

Figure 1-26.
Corneal videokeratography overview of RK demonstrating squared off central flattening and individual incisions on tangential view.

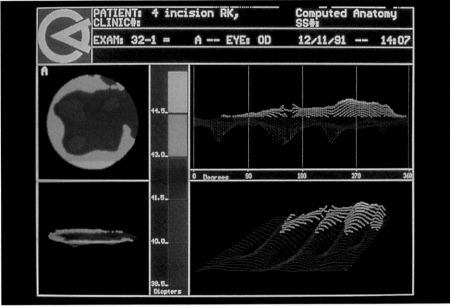

which incorporates the mask in optical rail system which is available for sale internationally, further beam refinements were made. The SVS Apex Plus beam (Figure 1-24) is quite homogeneous with a healing regression pattern.

In PRK it is important to understand that surgical optical zone is equivalent to the effective optical zone, in contrast with radial keratotomy (RK) where the effective optical zone exceeds the surgical optical zone. That is, if a 5.0-mm optical zone PRK is performed, the effective optical zone is equivalent at 5 mm. If a 3.0-mm RK is performed, the effec-

tive optical zone is greater at 5 to 6 mm (Figures 1-25 and 1-26). A pronounced form of spherical aberration is created with inadequate PRK optical zone size, producing disabling night glare. Also, although there is exponentially increased depth of ablation with larger optical zones, there is a lower rate of regression compared with smaller optical zones. The Summit OmniMed series has the capability of ablating a 6.5-mm optical zone. Conversely, the VisX 20/20 excimer laser system was essentially an industrial laser system concept toned down, rather than an ophthalmic laser beefed up,

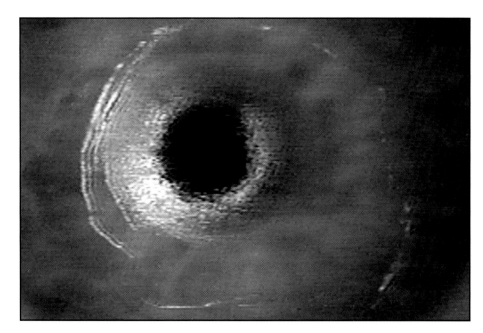

Figure 1-27.
Central translucency indicating increased hydration of central stroma during PRK photoablation. Central island formation related to differential hydration status of stroma intraoperatively.

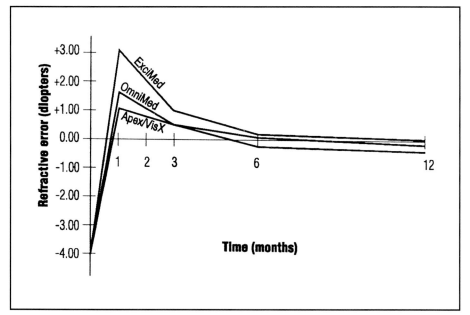

Figure 1-28.
Refractive change over 1 year for the Summit ExciMed, OmniMed, and VisX 20/20 series. Significant hyperopic overshoot with Summit ExciMed with slow stabilization noted. Minimal hyperopic overshoot observed with VisX 20/20. Intermediate refractive healing pattern experienced by patients treated with Summit OmniMed series.

thus having ample laser output to create a homogeneous 6- or even 7-mm optical zone. A 6.0-mm minimum optical zone is mandatory for PRK.

Fundamental to the understanding of energy beam profiles is that the clinical profile is altered both in terms of intraoperative and postoperative findings, as well as complications.

INTRAOPERATIVE CLINICAL FINDINGS

The small optical zone, gaussian beam profile Summit ExciMed created an evenly moist stromal surface during ablation, whereas the VisX 20/20 and Chiron Technolas lasers (Figure 1-27) resulted in a target pattern with increased translucency centrally. There are probably two reasons for this pattern: the acoustic shockwave of a flat energy beam profile (Machat) and the naturally increased hydration of the central stroma (Lin). The gaussian beam pattern of the Summit lasers counteract this by having greater energy density centrally. This is further discussed in Chapter 5.

TABLE 1-2

PHOTOREFRACTIVE DELIVERY SYSTEMS

Broad Beam (Wide Area Ablation)

Advantages	1. More forgiving of decentrations 2. Shorter procedure time 3. Lower repetition rate 4. No eyetracking necessary
Disadvantages	1. High output energy requirements 2. More complex delivery system (increased number of optics/homogenization system) 3. Higher maintenance 4. Higher beam uniformity required 5. Increased incidence of central islands 6. Limited ablation patterns (except with erodible mask) (eg, asymmetric astigmatism) 7. Greater acoustic shockwave

	SUMMIT ExciMed, OmniMed, Apex, SVS Apex Plus	VISX 20/20 Model B, 20/15 (Taunton), STAR	CHIRON TECHNOLAS Keracor 116	COHERENT-SCHWIND Keratom I/II	
Models					
Fluence (mJ/cm2)	180	160	130	Variable <250	
Pulse Frequency (Hz) [Maximum]	10	6 [30]	10 [40]	13	
Maximum Pulse Area	6.5 mm	8.0 mm	7.0 mm	8.0 mm	
Myopic Ablation Pattern	Iris diaphragm or erodible mask	Iris diaphragm	Iris diaphragm	Enlarging circular apertures	
Astigmatic Ablation Pattern	Emphasis erodible mask	Sequential and elliptical programs, iris diaphragm, rotatable slit	Linear scanning	Enlarging oval apertures	
Hyperopic Ablation Pattern	Emphasis erodible mask	Rotating scanning slit	Annular scanning spot	Annular apertures	
Eyetracker	None	None	Active	Passive	
Miscellaneous		Automated calibration	Oscillating beam joystick		

TABLE 1-2 (CONTINUED)
PHOTOREFRACTIVE DELIVERY SYSTEMS

Scanning	
Slit	**Spot**
1. Intermediate energy output requirements 2. Improved beam uniformity 3. No central islands 4. Reduced acoustic shockwave 5. Smoother ablative surfaces 6. No optical zone limitations for PRK/PTK	1. Small energy output requirements 2. More complex ablation patterns possible, including hyperopia 3. Lower beam homogeneity requirements 4. Lowest maintenance and fewest optics 5. No optical zone limitations for PRK/PTK 6. Reduced acoustic shockwave 7. No central islands
1. Eyetracker more important 2. Eye mask awkward 3. Slower procedure	1. Eyetracker necessary 2. Slowest procedure 3. Higher repetition rate necessary 4. Unknown/evolving algorithms

AESCULAP-MEDITEC MEL 60	NIDEK EC-5000	AUTONOMOUS TECHNOLOGIES CORPORATION (CIBA) Tracker-PRK	LASERSIGHT Compak-200 Mini-Excimer	CHIRON TECHNOLAS Keracor 117	NOVATEC LightBlade (non-excimer)
250	130	180	160 to 300	130	100
20	30 [46]	100	100	20 to 40	>200
1.5 x 10 mm	2 x 7 mm, optical zone 7.5 mm maximum, TZ 9.0 mm maximum	1 mm	<1 mm	1 to 2 mm	<0.3 mm
Rotating eye mask	Iris diaphragm, scanning slit rotates 120°/pass	Spiral scanning program	Rotating linear scanning spot	Spiral/random scanning spot	Spiral scanning spot
Rotating (variable) eye mask	Rotatable scanning slit beam	Meridional scanning	Meridional scanning	Meridional scanning	Elliptical scanning spot
Rotating (inverse) eye mask	Annular scanning slit beam	Annular scanning spot	Annular scanning spot	Annular scanning spot	Annular scanning spot
None	None	Active dual axis	Passive	Active	Active
		Laser radar= LADAR eyetracking			Solid-state tunable titanium sapphire

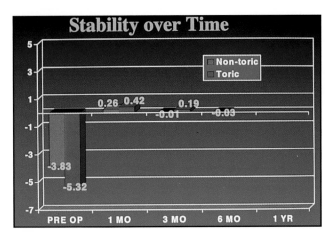

Figure 1-29.
Refractive healing pattern of Chiron Technolas Keracor 116 demonstrating rapid stabilization with no significant hyperopic overshoot.

POSTOPERATIVE CLINICAL FINDINGS

In the immediate postoperative period there is a distinct difference in clarity of vision dependent upon the laser system utilized. Patients treated with the Summit ExciMed series laser have significantly improved vision immediately upon sitting up, whereas most other flat energy beam profile lasers result in blurry vision immediately following the procedure. All patients become blurry during the epithelial phase for the first 3 days.

Some results indicate that the Summit ExciMed series laser has shown a greater rate of regression postoperatively related to the gaussian energy beam profile configuration and limited optical zone size. Refraction of a patient treated with the ExciMed gaussian beam was approximately +2.00 to +4.00 D at 10 days, regressing to plano to +1.00 D over 3 months, and reducing another +1.00 D over the next year. The Summit ExciMed algorithm was set higher to account for this regression of effect. That is, it is not the beam profile that produces hyperopia, but rather reduced stability which requires more initial treatment. The OmniMed, having a less gaussian beam and larger optical zone, creates better stability. Early data are favorable, with the initial hyperopic overshoot being reduced to +0.75 to +1.50 D. Patients treated with the Technolas, VisX, and the newest SVS Apex Plus are expected to regress about 1.00 D due to their flatter beam profiles and large treatment areas, therefore, initial overcorrection should be in that range (Figures 1-28 and 1-29).

The risk of central island formation is reduced with gaussian beam profile lasers independent of optical zone size, although all three are related. Of interest is that the Summit OmniMed laser at 5.0-mm optical zone size will produce greater hyperopic overshoot initially, and at 6.5-mm optical zone size, central islands have been reported particularly with LASIK since the deeper stroma is more hydrated. The pattern and incidence of haze formation is related to both macrohomogeneity and microhomogeneity. Focal areas of increased energy density are associated with a greater incidence of focal haze (Figure 1-30). Increased regression can result in diffuse haze formation, which is also associated with small optical zones.

PRINCIPLES OF A PHOTOABLATION SYSTEM

The most important consideration when evaluating and comparing various excimer lasers is the beam delivery system utilized (Table 1-2). To understand the importance of this consideration, one must first re-emphasize some basics concerning excimer lasers. The 193-nm far ultraviolet light energy beams emitted from excimer lasers are inherently nonhomogeneous. In addition, the greater the diameter of the beam the greater the degree of inhomogeneity. As the diameter of the excimer beam expands, the clinical effect is such that the central portion is less effective clinically. A useful analogy is a tent, whereby the tarp sags centrally as the tent poles are placed further apart. Once again, fluence represents the amount of energy within the ablative zone and homogeneity represents the pattern of energy distribution. Increased fluence improves homogeneity, the same as pushing the tent stakes further into the ground lessens the sagging of the covering tarp.

Broad beam systems are similar in concept to a projection system for 35-mm slides or a rear-projection television system, projecting the entire beam on the stromal surface and utilizing an iris diaphragm or variable aperture system to create the myopic ablation.

Scanning delivery systems utilize a slit beam or small spot to scan the surface of the cornea and alter the topography, imaging the surface similar to a television monitor produced by a picture tube. The advantages of scanning systems are the versatility for creating various topographical patterns: hyperopia, asymmetrical astigmatism including forme fruste keratoconus, and total surface ablations for PTK. Additionally, smaller beam size allows for a more easily created homogeneous beam, requiring fewer optics and a less powerful laser head. An eyetracking or eye coupling system is much more important due to the fact that these systems are much less forgiving of even small decentrations. Also, higher repetition rates are mandatory, requiring complex ablation patterns to allow thermal energy dissipation

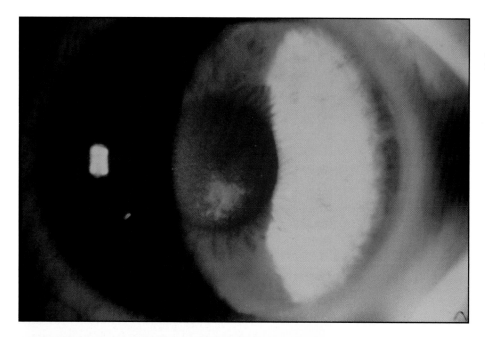

Figure 1-30.
Biomicroscopic slit lamp photograph of focal confluent haze following Summit ExciMed PRK.

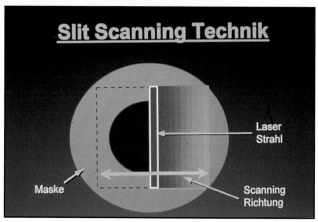

Figure 1-31.
Schematic diagram illustrating scanning slit delivery system of Aesculap-Meditec MEL 60.

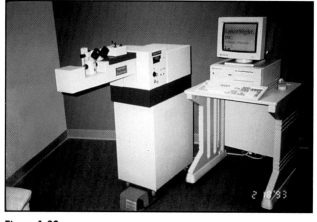

Figure 1-32.
LaserSight Compak-200 Mini-Excimer laser system.

between pulses at the same location.

The Chiron Technolas laser appears on both lists, indicating that it has a hybrid delivery system capable of utilizing one or a combination of modes to create the desired ablation pattern. It is software programmable.

Most photorefractive procedures worldwide have been performed with broad beam delivery systems utilizing a variable aperture system such as an iris diaphragm to control the pattern of ablation. Broad beam delivery systems are limited by their dependence upon producing an adequate beam diameter of sufficient homogeneity. Large ablative zones are essential for reducing night glare and myopic

regression. Scanning systems utilize a small beam to scan the surface of the cornea, with their chief advantage being a reduction in the beam homogeneity requirements. However, they require a method of locking onto the eye, either mechanically or through an eyetracking system. Scanning slit laser delivery systems (Aesculap-Meditec MEL 60 and Nidek EC-5000) apply a narrow band of 193-nm ultraviolet light to alter corneal topography (Figure 1-31). In addition, scanning systems require high pulse repetition rates to shorten prolonged procedure times, and nomogram development is still not as evolved. The ability to ablate complex and large diameter patterns with minimal acoustic shockwave and with a dramatically reduced requirement for exquisite beam homogeneity is fundamental to understanding why scanning lasers will dominate future excimer delivery system technology. The Technolas Keracor 116 is the only excimer laser with the capability to bridge the transition in technology with the Keracor 117 PlanoScan software design (see Clinical Note). The LaserSight Compak-200 Mini-Excimer laser (Figure 1-32) and CIBA–Autonomous Technologies Corporation Tracker-PRK laser have essentially made the transition with flying spot delivery systems. The Novatec LightBlade non-excimer solid-state photorefractive laser is a tunable crystal laser consisting of titanium sapphire in the 208- to 213-nm wavelength range which utilizes a scanning mode.

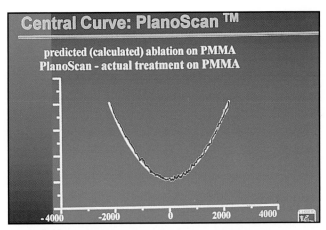

Figure 1-33.
Central curve PlanoScan.

Clinical Note

PlanoScan Program: Chiron Technolas Excimer Laser

The PlanoScan program of the Chiron Technolas laser is representative of newer, more sophisticated ablation profiles created by scanning delivery systems. Other scanning or flying spot delivery systems include the CIBA–Autonomous Technologies Corporation Tracker-PRK laser, LaserSight Compak-200 Mini-Excimer, and the non-excimer solid-state Novatec LightBlade system. These programs utilize a small beam diameter of 0.5 to 2 mm to scan the surface of the cornea at very high repetition rates ranging from 40 to over 100 Hz.

The PlanoScan program creates a more precise and smoother ablation profile when compared to the multizone contour (Figures 1-33 and 1-34). The advantage of scanning spot technology is that these delivery systems utilize the most homogeneous central portion of the excimer beam. In this way, sensitivity to beam homogeneity disturbances is dramatically reduced and variations with beam quality do not tend to have an impact on clinical results. The maintenance requirements for these lasers is therefore reduced, and the number of optics required for the homogenization process is similarly reduced since a large diameter beam of good homogeneity is not necessary. As depicted in Figure 1-35, the ablation profile is identical in all three ablations despite the fact that good homogeneity is only present in the first example. The second and third examples illustrate two asymmetrical fluence patterns which constitute unacceptable homogeneity patterns for wide field ablation: an astigmatic pattern and a sweeping pattern.

The smoothness of scanning technology easily exceeds that of broad beam delivery systems which utilize

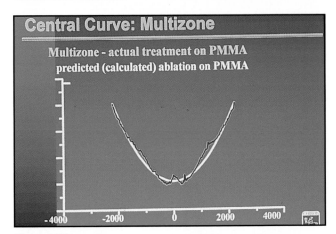

Figure 1-34.
Central curve multizone.

an iris diaphragm or variable-sized apertures which produce ablation ridges. Even with multi-multizone blending processes the smoothness of ablation even under high magnification is unparalleled (Figure 1-36), with perhaps the only exception being the erodible mask used in the Summit SVS Apex Plus system.

Excellent clinical results were achieved in very preliminary clinical trials performed by Maria Clara Arbelaez, MD, in Cali, Colombia, in September 1995 on 27 eyes treated with LASIK for -0.75 to -7.50 D with the PlanoScan program. There was minimal regression with rapid refractive stabilization (Figures 1-37 and 1-38). There also appeared to be rapid recovery of best corrected visual acuity with many patients actually gaining one line of best corrected vision by 4 weeks (Figure 1-39).

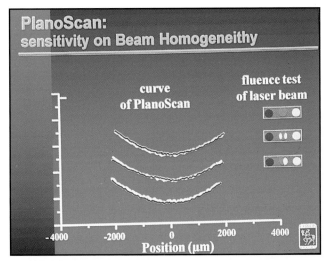

Figure 1-35.
PlanoScan sensitivity on beam homogeneity.

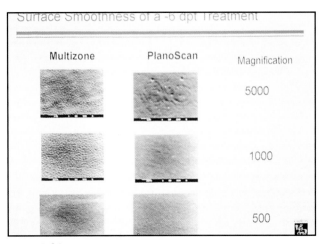

Figure 1-36.
Surface smoothness after excimer laser ablation on PMMA.

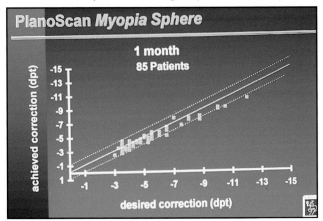

Figure 1-37.
Attempted vs. achieved corrections 1-month, post-LASIK with PlanoScan.

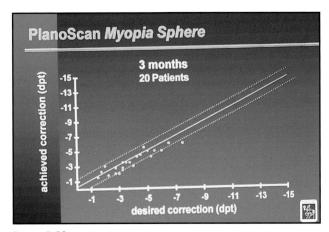

Figure 1-38.
Attempted vs. achieved corrections 3-months, post-LASIK with PlanoScan.

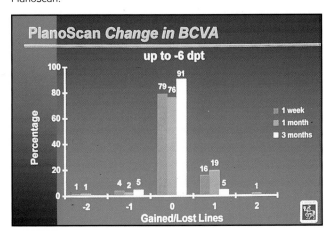

Figure 1-39.
Best corrected vision postoperatively following PlanoScan LASIK.

The LaserSight Compak-200 Mini-Excimer Laser

Craig Beyer, DO

HISTORY

The LaserSight Compak-200 Mini-Excimer laser utilizes the same wavelength of utraviolet light (193 nm) to photoablate corneal tissue for PRK as its predecessors. The original concept for the laser was developed by J.T. Lin, PhD. In 1990, Dr. Lin and others evaluated the idea of using a frequency-quintupled neodymium:YAG (Nd:YAG) solid-state laser that operated at 213 nm to perform PRK. A flashlamp-pumped, Q-switched Nd:YAG (1064 nm) laser operating at 10 Hz, 10 nanoseconds/pulse with an output energy of 50 mJ/pulse was used. The fundamental beam was focused into a non-linear optical crystal to obtain the second harmonic frequency of 532 nm. The fourth harmonic was obtained by frequency doubling the green (532 nm) radiation in a beryllium boroxylate (BBO) crystal. Finally, frequency mixing the fundamental (1064 nm) wavelength and the fourth harmonic (266 nm) in another BBO crystal resulted in the fifth ultraviolet harmonic (213 nm).

Prior to 1991, there were several problems which slowed the further development of the LaserSight solid-state 213-nm laser. After frequency quintupling, an output level of only 0.4 mJ/pulse was obtained. In order to perform wide area ablation PRK similar to the VisX or Summit lasers, much more energy would be required (at least 32 mJ/pulse). In 1991, LaserSight was able to obtain up to 5 mJ/pulse from the solid-state 213-nm LaserHarmonic laser, however, the energy remained too low for wide area ablation. In order to solve this problem, a paradigm shift was necessary regarding the delivery of laser energy to the cornea. By developing a computer-controlled galvanometric scanning delivery system that was capable of precisely and rapidly scanning a 0.5- to 1.0-mm diameter ultraviolet laser beam on the corneal surface, the LaserHarmonic achieved the same corneal fluence as its predecessors (160 to 180 mJ/cm²) and the laser achieved the same wide area effect.

Ren et al used the prototype solid-state LaserHarmonic, LaserSight laser (213 nm) with the computer-controlled scanning delivery system to perform in vitro and in vivo studies. The authors concluded that the laser was capable of reshaping the corneal surface with a smooth transition on human cadaver eyes. In rabbits, the LaserHarmonic resulted in a clinical course and histopathologic findings similar to the 193-nm excimer laser ablations. For a 3.00 D ablation over a 5-mm ablation zone, 1618 pulses at a repetition rate of 10 Hz required 162 seconds.

The advantages of a scanning spot delivery system became readily apparent. First, as mentioned above, significantly less energy is required from the laser head to attain ablative threshold at the corneal surface (nearly 10 times less). The resulting acoustic shockwave is also significantly less, which proportionally reduces the chance for corneal endothelial damage. Second, virtually any pattern can be scanned onto the corneal surface by merely making a change in the software; no hardware changes are necessary. Current software designs strive for spatially resolved, aspheric, customized ablations that optimize the quality of vision and decrease the chance of regression. Third, the scanning approach produces an extremely smooth corneal surface compared to wide area beams which tend to accentuate surface irregularites after each pulse. With a scanning delivery system, each scan layer can be oriented in such a way so that the peaks and valleys of the previous layer are smoothed out by the succeeding scan layer.

Fourth, with a scanning spot, laser beam homogeneity and corneal fluid dynamics are less important in determining the final surface ablation quality. For instance, wide beams must be extremely homogenous to prevent the production of iatrogenic surface irregularites. In addition, broad flat beams force corneal fluid centrally which decreases the ratio of the central ablation rate to the peripheral ablation rate, leading to central island formation. Finally, once corneal imaging techniques become sophisticated enough to provide real-time corneal topography and surface elevation, this information can be fed directly into the computer-controlled delivery system so that even the most highly irregular corneal surface can be made spherical with a customized ablation pattern.

Other problems continued to delay the commercialization of the LaserHarmonic system. The solid-state laser technology remained prohibitively expensive and the frequency ranging from 10 to 50 Hz was too slow; procedures would last minutes instead of seconds. Therefore, using the same scanning delivery system as the LaserHarmonic laser, the 193-nm Compak-200 Mini-Excimer laser was developed in 1992. The Mini-Excimer laser was significantly cheaper and operated at 10 times the frequency (100 Hz). In addition, due to the decreased energy requirements, the Mini-Excimer possessed the same advantages as the solid-state laser, which were decreased maintenance and decreased operating expenses. Finally, the Mini-Excimer operated at the same wavelength (193 nm) as previous lasers, and therefore, mutagenicity concerns were much less of an issue.

The Mini-Excimer completed Phase I FDA investigations under the direction of Dr. Asbell in 1994. Five Phase IIa investigators have been selected, and the clinical trials began in June 1995. Over 50 Mini-Excimer laser systems have been installed worldwide and over 5000 procedures have been performed. Over the past 4 years, solid-state laser technology has advanced. The new LaserHarmonic operates at 200 Hz, twice as fast as the Mini-Excimer.

THE DELIVERY SYSTEM

Because of the increased number of components within their delivery systems, typical, wide area ablation, ultraviolet lasers must rely upon high energy excimer lasers to achieve ablation threshold (120 to 180 mJ/cm^2) at the corneal surface. Utilizing a large diameter beam (5 mm or greater), over 350 mJ of energy may be required from the laser head in order to achieve 30 to 35 mJ at the corneal surface. This represents an energy efficiency of approximately 10%; the remaining 90% of the energy is absorbed by the laser's optics and other mechanical components of the delivery system which can decrease the overall lifetime of these systems.

As previously mentioned, decreased energy requirements, increased treatment flexibility, and increased surface smoothness are the prime advantages of the unique LaserSight scanning delivery system. The Mini-Excimer laser head produces a 193-nm beam with a maximum laser output energy of 5 mJ/pulse. The pulse duration is 2.5 nanoseconds and the maximum frequency is 100 Hz. The delivery system utilizes approximately a 1-mm diameter raw beam emitted from the laser head without incorporating numerous optics or any other mechanical beam shaping or beam homogenizing devices, such as iris apertures, slits, rotating dove prisms, optical integrators, telescopic zooms, etc. Instead, the Mini-Excimer delivery system relies upon four basic components to create a broad, smooth, ablative surface:

1. An energy attenuator
2. A condensing lens
3. A pair of computer-controlled galvanometric (x and y) scanning mirrors
4. A 45° mirror

The Mini-Excimer delivery system has an energy efficiency of 50%. For example, when 2 mJ of laser energy passses through the delivery system, 1 mJ emerges. Since the beam diameter is less than 1 mm, 1 mJ of energy at the corneal surface exceeds the corneal ablation threshold and is equivalent to the power density (160 to 180 mJ/cm^2) produced by other excimer lasers which utilize a 5-mm, 30 to 35 mJ, broad beam.

The first component of the Mini-Excimer delivery system is the attenuator. Immediately following a gas refill, the laser head operates near its maximum output of 5 mJ. Therefore, the attenuator decreases the beam energy from 5 to 2 mJ to maintain 1 mJ of energy at the corneal surface. As the laser output diminishes after several procedures, less attenuation is required. One important point for preservation: never expose the optics of the Mini-Excimer delivery system that follow the attenuator to more than 2 mJ of energy.

The condensing lens is the second component of the Mini-Excimer delivery system. It improves the gaussian beam profile and focuses the beam to a 0.85-mm diameter. The third components in the delivery pathway are the x and y mirrors driven by the computer-controlled galvanometric scanning motors. These serve to overlap the gaussian laser beam profile on the corneal surface by 30% to 50% in both x and y directions. A larger overlap increases the smoothness of the ablated surface, but also increases the duration of the procedure. The computer software not only determines the degree of beam overlap, but also can be programmed to ascribe nearly any pattern or sequence of ablative patterns on the corneal surface. The final component, the 45° mirror, changes the horizontal direction of the laser beam into a downward, vertical direction perpendicular to the patient's cornea.

Excimer lasers function at a fluence of 100 to 200 mJ/cm^2 and a pulse repetition rate of 5 to 10 Hz for non-scanning lasers. The broad beam laser systems utilize a computer-controlled iris diaphragm with variable capabilities from less than 300 steps to more than 1000 steps. The iris aperture expands from as little as 0.8 mm to as great as 7.0 mm. The unique delivery system of the Chiron Technolas Keracor 116 incorporates a scanning mode which is based around the scanner block. The scanner block houses the final polishing mirror optic, which is also computer controlled and software driven. The polishing mirror oscillates 50 microns about the point of fixation and therefore blends each pulse into previous pulses. Clinically, this oscillation effect may have three benefits:

1. Smoother ablation
2. Reduced regression
3. Reduced haze formation

The classic circular ridges commonly observed from

Figure 1-40a.
Immediate postoperative view of Chiron Technolas corneal ablation demonstrating smoothness of stromal bed under low magnification.

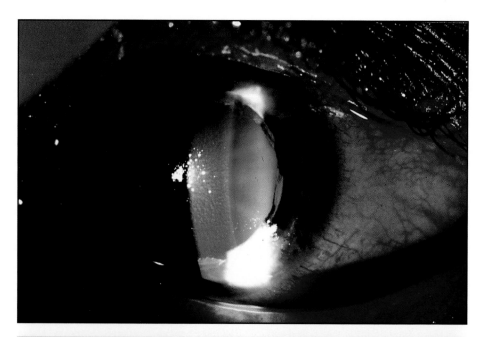

Figure 1-40b.
Immediate postoperative view of Chiron Technolas corneal ablation demonstrating smoothness of stromal bed under high magnification.

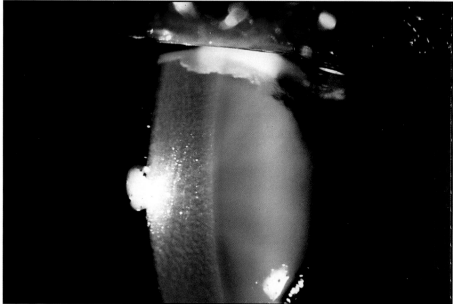

the expansion of the iris diaphragm during a myopic correction following broad beam photoablation are dramatically reduced (Figures 1-40a and 1-40b). The multi-multizone technology also reduces the ridges and smoothes the surface. The scanner block enables the system to perform a toric ablation pattern, a hyperopic ablation pattern, and both a scanning and broad beam myopic ablation pattern. The toric ablation pattern is produced by scanning across the minus cylinder axis with increasing diameter to create a 4 by 12 mm cylinder. The hyperopic pattern is created by scanning a midperipheral trough, which is blended central-

ly and peripherally to reduce regression and haze (Figures 1-41a and 1-41b). The Nidek EC-5000 system (Figure 1-42) uses a scanning slit which rotates 120° with each pass to blend each ablation into the previous ablation with a transition zone of 9.0 mm. The Aesculap-Meditec MEL 60 excimer laser is a scanning slit laser which does not rotate the slit, utilizing an eyecup device with a rotatable mask that allows myopic, hyperopic, toric, and even presbyopic ablation patterns to be performed (Figures 1-43a through 1-43c). The Summit OmniMed series is capable of utilizing an erodible mask (Figures 1-44a and 1-44b) which

The Novatec Laser

Casimir A. Swinger, MD, and Shui T. Lai, PhD

We developed a new laser technology, the Novatec LightBlade, for ophthalmic and corneal refractive surgery (Figure B-1). The Novatec laser is solid state, and addresses some current concerns with excimer laser technology—reliability, beam homogeneity, flexibility, and maintenance. The Novatec laser has the following operating parameters when used in the ultraviolet surface mode:

- Wavelength: 0.21 microns
- Fluence: 100 mJ/cm^2
- Delivery system: computerized scanning
- Spot size: 0.10 to 0.50 microns (typically 0.30 microns)
- Optic zone: unlimited
- Eyetracker: active (redirects the laser beam within ±5.00 mm)

The Novatec technology was developed to provide the refractive surgeon with the maximum of versatility while reducing ocular trauma. The low fluence and small spot size reduce the energy on the cornea by more than 500x at any instant when compared to excimer lasers, thus dramatically reducing acoustic shock. The variable spot size, unlimited optic zone, eyetracker, and computer-directed scanning delivery system allow any customized profile to be ablated, even asymmetric or irregular astigmatism, through software alone.

The laser is also capable of operating at a transmissive wavelength, near 1 micron. This allows surgery to be performed inside the cornea itself, for use in intrastromal cavitation, incisional keratectomy, or as a laser microkeratome.

The Novatec laser has been undergoing clinical trials (Tables B-1 and B-2) since June 1994. Surgery on 50 eyes for the US Phase IIa study of low to moderate myopia (1 to 6 D) was recently completed and follow-up is 3 months. Epithelialization of the cornea was rapid, with a mean closure time of 2.4 days and 12% by day 1. Visual recovery was also rapid, and at 1 month, 43% of patients have an uncorrected vision of 20/20 and 97% are 20/40 or better. At 3 months, 50% of eyes were within 0.50 D and 80% were within 1.00 D. These 50 eyes comprise the first sighted eye study in the world using this laser. The laser produces minimal hyperopic overshoot (approximately 0.30 D during the first 3 months). At 3 months, 10% of eyes gained two lines of vision but none lost two lines.

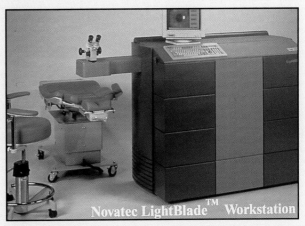

Figure B-1.
Novatec LightBlade.

Mean haze was trace (0.5) at 3 months. Corneal topography showed that the eyetracker provided excellent centration and no central islands were seen in this series of 50 eyes. We believe the scanning delivery system will not produce central islands.

In addition to myopic PRK, the Novatec laser has been evaluated for surface hyperopic PRK. Thus far, nine sighted eyes have been recruited in a Canadian study. The optical zone is 6 to 7 mm and the total ablation diameter is 9.5 mm. The laser has been used to correct overcorrected myopic PRKs, failed holmium LTK, and also overcorrected RK. The mean correction at 1 month in this series was 5.5 D at 1 month. At 1 month, 40% of eyes were <0.50 D and 80% were <1.00 D. There was only mild regression between months 1 and 3. Visual recovery appears to be slightly slower with hyperopic PRK than with myopic PRK, as 40% of the patients have not recovered their preoperative acuity at the 3-month examination. Haze, however, appears to be very minimal with a mean haze of 0.30 in the periphery.

The Novatec laser will undergo clinical trials for producing penetrating keratoplasty incisions using the UV surface mode, in addition to studies of toric ablations and LASIK. The intraocular modules will also begin clinical evaluation.

TABLE B-1

A COMPARISON OF NOVATEC AND EXCIMER LASERS

	Novatec	Summit	VisX	Chiron Technolas
Laser Characteristics				
Laser Medium	Crystal	Excimer gas	Excimer gas	Excimer gas
Wavelength (nm)	210	193	193	193
Pulse Repetition Rate (per second)	>200	10	5	10
Excimer Gas Consumption	None	Yes	Yes	Yes
Beam Characteristics				
Beam Diameter	0.3 mm	6.5 mm	6.0 mm	7.0 mm
Laser Beam	Single mode, fundamental	Multi-mode	Multi-mode	Multi-mode
Beam Homogenization Method	None required	Use expensive optics (UV damaged over time)	Use expensive optics (UV damaged over time)	Use expensive optics and beam wobble (UV damaged over time)
Beam Collimation	Collimated. Ablation characteristics not dependent on patient cornea height position.	Focused. Ablation characteristics sensitive to patient cornea height position.	Focused. Ablation characteristics sensitive to patient cornea height position.	Focused. Ablation characteristics sensitive to patient cornea height position.
Patient Fixation	Fixation beam, laser beam, and physician's line of sight, all three co-axial.	Fixation and laser beam co-axial. Physician's line of sight at 8°.	Fixation and laser beam co-axial. Physician's line of sight at 8°.	Fixation and laser beam co-axial. Physician's line of sight at 8°.
Centration of Ablation				
Automatic Tracking	Eyetracker locked on during procedure, maintaining centration	No eyetracker	No eyetracker	Active eyetracker
Response Time	Faster response time, follows all eye movement (10 times faster than Chiron)	None	None	Fast (10 million calculations/second)
Tracking Range	10-mm diameter area	None	None	3 mm
Clinical Applications				
Myopia (optic zone)	Yes (6 to 7 mm)	Yes (6.5 mm)	Yes (6 mm)	Yes (7 mm)
Astigmatism	Yes (5 to 7 mm)	Emphasis ablatable mask	Yes (4 to 5 mm)	Yes (4.5 mm)
Hyperopia	Yes (9.5 to 10 mm)	Emphasis ablatable mask	Rotating slit	Under development up to 9 D (9 to 10 mm)
Laser Trephination	Yes	No	No	No
PTK	Yes	Yes	Yes	Yes
Ablation Time (seconds), 5 D, 6 mm	60	25	45	25
Thermal Damage	Minimal	Minimal	Minimal	Minimal

TABLE B-1 (CONTINUED)
A COMPARISON OF NOVATEC AND EXCIMER LASERS

	Novatec	Summit	VisX	Chiron Technolas
Beam Delivery	Beam scanning	Iris diaphragm, ablatable mask	Iris Diaphragm	Iris diaphragm (Keracor 116), beam scanning (Keracor 117)
Optic Zone Size	Up to 10 mm	6.5 mm	6.0 mm (STAR 8.0 mm)	7.0 mm
Procedure Findings				
Alignment	Two crossing He-Ne for patient cornea height, rings in microscope ocular for horizontal positioning	Two crossing He-Ne only	Microscope focus and ocular rings	Microscope focus and two crossing He-Ne
Cornea Surface	Smooth	Step structure	Step structure	Smooth
Cornea Wet/Dry During Ablation	Not wet, not dry, consistent over entire area	Dry periphery, wet at center	Dry periphery, wet at center	Dry periphery, wet at center (117 consistent)
Tissue Smell During Procedure	Yes	Yes	Yes	Yes
Myopia Clinical Results (1 to 6 D)				
Regression at 3 Months	0.4 D	1.5 D	0.75 D	0.75 D
Haze at 3 Months	0 to 1.0	0 to 1.0	0 to 1.0	0 to 1.0
Epithelial Closure Time	2 to 3 days	3 days	3 days	3 days
Pain	First 18 hours, controllable with NSAIDs and contact lens	First 18 hours, controllable with NSAIDs and contact lens	First 18 hours, controllable with NSAIDs and contact lens	First 18 hours, controllable with NSAIDs and contact lens

TABLE B-2
NOVATEC MYOPIA CLINICAL RESULTS
(1 TO 6 D)

Refraction Accuracy	66% within ±0.5 D 98% within ±1.0 D (at 1 month)
Uncorrected Visual Acuity	>20/25 (0.8), 76% >20/40 (0.5), 100% (at 1 month)
Best Corrected Visual Acuity	90% within ± one line 10% gain two lines No loss of two lines (at 3 months)
Induced Astigmatism	None
Hyperopic Overshoot During 2 Weeks to 3 Months	Minimal, <0.2 D
Central Island	None
Acoustic Shock	Low shock (200 times less than excimer), no audible sound during ablation

Sources of the Clinical Data

The Novatec clinical data are based on the FDA Phase IIa trial in the United States.

The VisX clinical data are based on the FDA Phase III study, Myopic Photorefractive Keratectomy: The Experience in the United States with the VisX Excimer Laser *by Marguerite B. McDonald and Jonathan H. Talamo. Edited by James Salz and Peter McDonnell. Mosby; 1995.*

The Summit clinical data are based on Photorefractive Keratectomy with the Summit Excimer Laser: The Phase III US Results *by Keith P. Thompson, Roger F. Steinert, Jan Daniel, and R. Doyle Stulting. Edited by James Salz and Peter McDonnell. Mosby; 1995.*

The Chiron clinical data are based on the 6-month overall results of the Canadian users, reported by Jeffery J. Machat, MD.

Figure 1-41a.
Graphic of hyperopic ablation profile of Chiron Technolas system for low degrees of hyperopia.

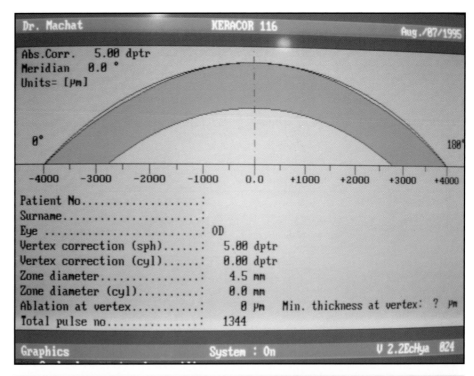

Figure 1-41b.
Graphic of hyperopic ablation profile of Chiron Technolas system for high degrees of hyperopia.

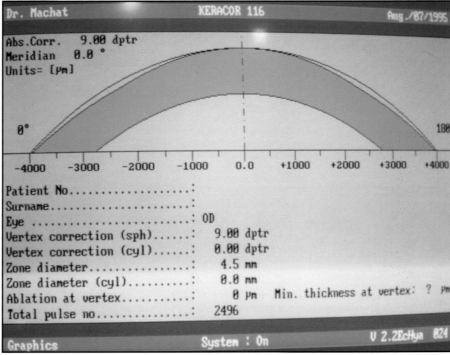

eliminates the circular ridges and potentially could provide a seamless blend over the entire ablation. The Emphasis erodible mask acts as a template, much like the mirror image of a contact lens, to create myopic, hyperopic, or toric ablation patterns. The mask is made of PMMA material on a quartz substrate for support as quartz, unlike plas-tic, is transparent to ultraviolet radiation. A myopic abla-tion pattern is created by varying the thickness of the PMMA, with the thinnest region being central and the thickest region peripheral. No iris diaphragm is necessary but can be used with the mask simply blending the diaphragmatic steps. The beam is transmitted through the

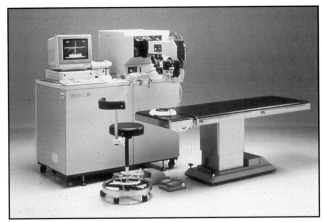

Figure 1-42.
Nidek EC-5000 excimer laser system.

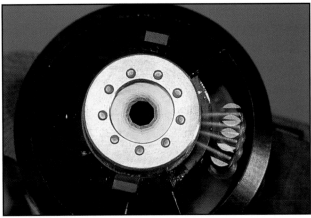

Figure 1-43a.
Aesculap-Meditec metallic rotatable mask for myopia.

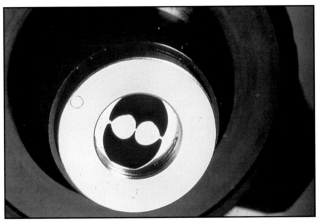

Figure 1-43b.
Aesculap-Meditec metallic rotatable mask for hyperopia.

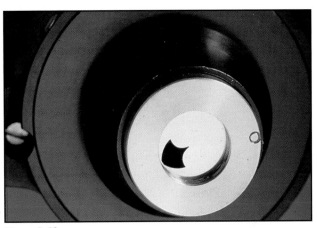

Figure 1-43c.
Aesculap-Meditec metallic rotatable mask for presbyopia.

Figure 1-44a.
Summit SVS Apex Plus
Emphasis erodible mask.

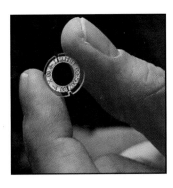

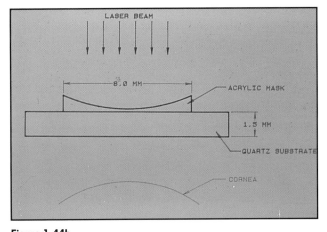

Figure 1-44b.
Schematic of Emphasis erodible mask composed of PMMA supported on quartz substrate. Erodible mask acts as a template for shape transfer process.

mask as it perforates the PMMA, centrally first for myopic ablations and peripherally first for hyperopic patterns. Complex, even asymmetric, ablation patterns based on topography can be formulated. The clinical potential of the Emphasis erodible mask remains enormous, but the clinical results to date have been variable. It is hoped that the future incorporation of the Emphasis erodible mask car-

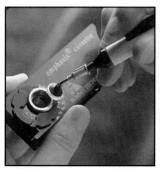

Figure 1-45a.
Summit SVS Apex Plus Emphasis cartridge which supports the mask and allows for astigmatism alignment.

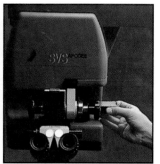

Figure 1-45b.
The laser disc or mask encoded with the refractive correction is inserted into the cassette and loaded into the Summit SVS Apex Plus system.

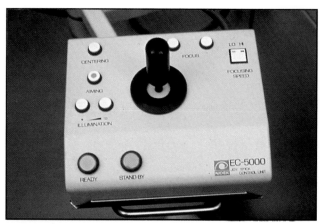

Figure 1-46a.
Joystick apparatus of the Nidek EC-5000.

tridge system within the optical rail of the Summit SVS Apex Plus system will improve refractive predictability (Figures 1-45a and 1-45b).

PTK control with a joystick (Figures 1-46a through 1-46c) has been introduced by Nidek EC-5000, Chiron Technolas, and VisX STAR, allowing localized ablation while the patient remains fixated upon the stationary red target LED. The joystick control obviates the need for controlling PTK with head movement which is quite rudimentary. The control of beam size and frequency remain important and essential elements of advanced PTK mode design. These systems allow for ablation of any size lesion to be carefully titrated both in size and depth, first at high, then later at low pulse repetition rates. Furthermore, the ablation can be blended into the surrounding stroma with gentle rotary motions of the joystick. The Aesculap-Meditec MEL 60 excimer laser is capable of scanning limbus to limbus and performing PTK without the usually associated hyperopic shift (Figure 1-47).

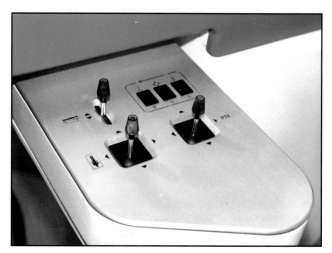

Figure 1-46b.
Joystick apparatus of the Chiron Technolas Keracor 116.

CIBA-Autonomous Technologies Corporation Tracker-PRK

The Autonomous Technologies Corporation developed their scanning excimer laser (Figure 1-48) based upon the fundamental and correct belief that wide area ablation has inherent problems with beam homogeneity. Their background with eyetracking technology designed for NASA and military defense purposes, the STAR WARS initiative, was a necessary prerequisite for the centration of scanned ablation profiles utilizing a small diam-

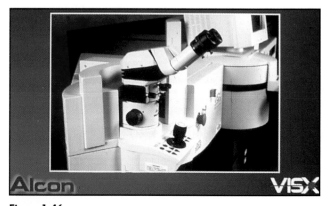

Figure 1-46c.
Joystick apparatus of the VisX STAR for axis alignment.

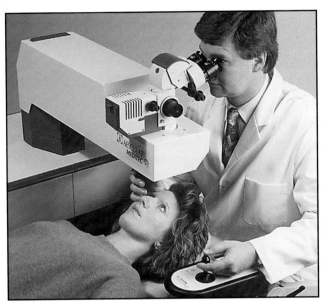

Figure 1-47.
PTK procedure technique with the Aesculap-Meditec MEL 60.

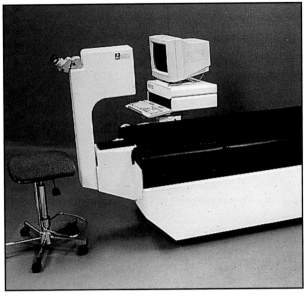

Figure 1-48.
CIBA Autonomous Technologies Corporation laser system.

eter beam; the assumption being that the eyetracker could stabilize the eye adequately to allow a small beam of high homogeneity to ablate the corneal surface in any desired pattern and with any optical and transition zone desired. The Autonomous Technologies Corporation eyetracker is the most sophisticated active eyetracker incorporated into an excimer laser delivery system and is capable of tracking even the most radical eye movements. Described as laser radar, or "LADAR", it utilizes an active dual axis tracking mechanism which is engaged immediately following epithelial debridement with a dilated pupil. The importance of the eyetracking system is emphasized by the trademarked procedure description, T-PRK, or tracker-assisted PRK. The menu of ablation profiles is considerable with the future capability of performing custom ablations based upon real-time corneal topography. The computer monitor from which the procedure is programmed and eyetracker engaged displays both the natural eye movement during fixation and the eyetracked image which appears stationary. The CIBA–Autonomous Technologies Corporation system is smaller with reduced gas and maintenance requirements because of the reduced beam homogenization process necessary.

The myopic ablation program utilizes a spiral-like program with a fluence of 180 mJ/cm^2 and a beam diameter less than 1.0 mm. Marguerite McDonald, MD, demonstrated superior histology and unparalleled smoothness with the scanning delivery system. Preliminary clinical

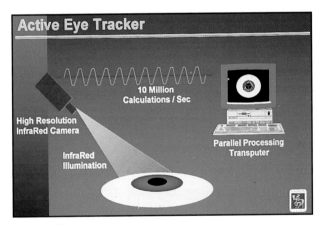

Figure 1-49.
Chiron Technolas eyetracking system, 50-micron resolution, 50 frame/second compensation.

results with 42 sighted eyes treated by Ioannis Pallikaris, MD, for spherical myopia between -3.00 and -6.00 D demonstrated excellent safety and efficacy. Despite an algorithm target of -0.75 D, almost three quarters were within 1.00 D of emmetropia, with 54% achieving 20/25 or better and 93% achieving 20/40 or better uncorrected visual acuity. There was approximately 0.35 D of myopic regression over the first 3 months with no initial hyperopic overshoot observed. There was no loss of best corrected vision recorded in any study patient.

Nidek EC-5000 Laser Features and Results

F. Linton Lavery, MCh, FRCSI, FRCS Ed DOMS

The Nidek EC-5000 has a rotating, scanning, overlapping delivery system. The small beam results in good homogeneity and the constantly moving slit eliminates any minor defects in the beam quality. The optical zone can be varied up to 6.5 mm, transition edge blend up to 9 mm. The large area of ablation with a finely tapered blend zone discourages epithelial hyperplasia. A smooth corneal surface present at the end of treatment speeds re-epithelialization (Figure C-1). Lasers using an iris diaphragm leave trenches in which new collagen is deposited. The large optical and transition zone reduces the possibility of halos at nighttime.

Hertz rate can be varied from 10 to 50 Hz. The microscope

and delivery system can be moved in an x/y direction, as well as up and down to focus. Indeed, it is the only excimer that has this facility (Figure C-2). The microscope uses a high quality operating Zeiss microscope, giving the surgeon excellent visualization, which is especially important when performing procedures such as LASIK. All treatments are entered and stored in a computer and the surgeon can view all the parameters before each surgery (eg, the ablation depth) (Figure C-3). Back vertex distance calculations are automatic and in the very near future this laser will feature an automatic recalibration on PMMA done by computer between each case. This laser is economical to use and can treat up to 40 cases on one gas fill. The Nidek

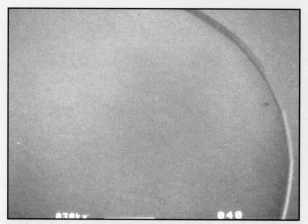

Figure C-1.
Smooth ablative surface of Nidek EC-5000.

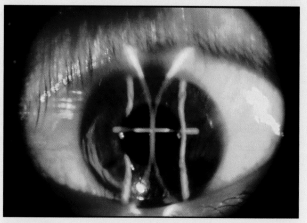

Figure C-2.
Alignment system of Nidek EC-5000.

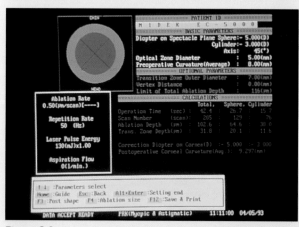

Figure C-3.
Treatment screen of Nidek EC-5000 demonstrating parameters and graphic illustration of optical and transition zones

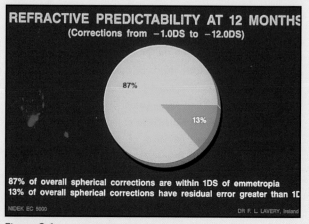

Figure C-4.
Refractive predictability at 12 months.

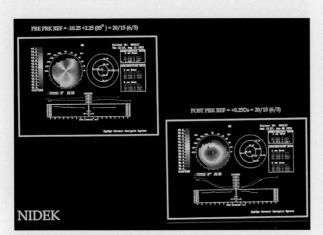

Figure C-5.
Pre- and postoperative corneal maps of Nidek high myopia and astigmatism correction.

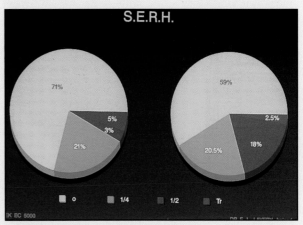

Figure C-6.
Comparing the degree of haze in PRK (on the right) and PARK (on the left), there is little difference. We have no grade 1 (mild) or grade 2 (moderate) haze. Bear in mind that steroids are not used for a sphere equivalent up to -8.0 D.

EC-5000 has the facility to correct myopia, hypermetropia, and astigmatism. Astigmatic correction is done by scanning along a slit which is at right angles to the steep axis. The slit opens to the preset diameter along the steep axis. In the correction of hypermetropia, the optical zone is 5.5 mm and the transition zone is 9 mm. Hertz rate is 46 Hz and the hyperopic treatment is very fast (eg, at +6.00 D takes 12 seconds).

When reviewing the following results, it is to be noted that topical steroids are not used in patients up to a spherical equivalent of -8 D. In 70% of spherical equivalents less than or equal to -6 D, refraction was within +0.5 D of the intended results. Twenty-five percent of these patients are between 0.5 and 1 D of their intended result, and 5% have a residual error greater than 1 D. In the group of all corrections up to -12 D, 87% are within 1 D of emmetropia (Figure C-4). Thirteen percent have

a residual error greater than 1 D.

Toric corrections are used for all patients with a cylinder above 0.5 D; the highest cylinder corrected to date is spherical 5.00 D (Figure C-5). Seventy-four percent of these cylindrical corrections are within 0.75 D of their full cylindrical correction. Ninety-five percent have a residual spherical equivalent of 1 D of their target. Sixty-five percent of cylindrical corrections are within 15° of the original axis. The axis does vary in the other 32% of cases where the visual outcome was good. The average change in axis is 13°. At 12 months, the mean residual cylindrical error was 0.67.

Haze is minimal and at 12 months, 68% of corneas are clear and 32% have trace haze (Figure C-6). There are no grade 1 or worse cases of haze. Hyperopic shift is maximal at 1 month, which is far less than with our old Summit laser.

Eyetracking systems are present on the LaserSight Mini-Excimer, the Chiron Technolas Keracor 116, and the CIBA–Autonomous Technologies Corporation Tracker-PRK laser, and are a prerequisite for complex scanning ablation patterns. The Novatec LightBlade non-excimer PRK laser system is also equipped with eyetracking capabilities. The Chiron Technolas system consists of an infrared camera which monitors the pupil-iris margin contrast difference and can be locked at any position (Figure 1-49). The eyetracking software actively follows the eye within a 3.0-mm triangulated area and deactivates the laser outside the 3-mm area.

The Technolas system monitors the eye position every 10 milliseconds, and adjusts and reacts to position changes every 20 milliseconds. The CIBA–Autonomous Technologies Corporation eyetracking system or laser radar is the most sophisticated system with remarkable precision and monitoring of the eye (Figures 1-50a and 1-50b).

EXCIMER LASER MAINTENANCE CONSIDERATIONS

All excimer lasers require continual maintenance and increased maintenance with increased volume of procedures. Another consideration is that all broad beam deliv-

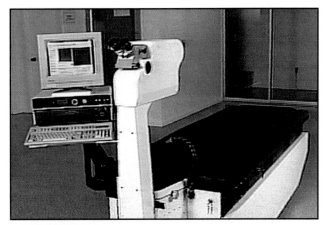

Figure 1-50a.
CIBA—Autonomous Technologies Corporation Tracker-PRK excimer laser system with advanced eyetracking capabilities.

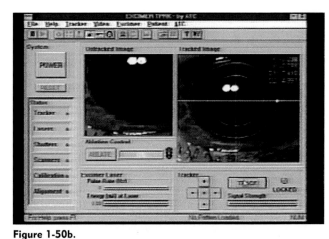

Figure 1-50b.
Eyetracking mode demonstrates real-time eye movement on left screen and fixed tracked eye on right screen, which is the stable image presented to the laser system. Pupil must be dilated for "laser radar" eyetracking program to be engaged.

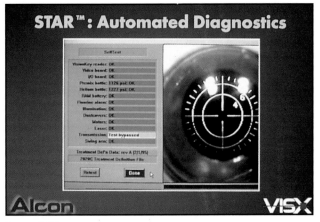

Figure 1-51.
VisX STAR automated diagnostics screen.

ery systems require greater maintenance than comparable scanning systems (Figure 1-51). Broad beam delivery systems have greater energy requirements in laser head design and a more complex optical pathway for beam homogenization, which both result in greater maintenance demands. Optic degradation is a natural event as the laser energy damages the lens and mirror coatings and decreases beam quality.

Scanning lasers have a reduced need for complex optics and are less affected by degraded beam quality relative to broad beam systems. Optics are replaced every 100 to 500 procedures depending on the optic coating and laser system. Although scanning spot lasers contain fewer optics, each procedure requires more pulses and may still lead to optic degradation and frequent turnover. All the optics require

replacement at variable intervals. Similarly, the volume of procedures performed per month and the efficiency of laser usage will determine the duration a gas cylinder will last. That is, it is more efficient to perform multiple procedures on any particular day rather than a few procedures on multiple days. Systems which lack the ability to examine the beam qualitatively will have a higher threshold for unscheduled maintenance and more undetected beam abnormalities. Clinical results are dependent upon the proper functioning of these highly sensitive lasers.

EXCIMER LASER RECALIBRATION

The recalibration system allows the surgeon to test the laser prior to each case to examine the beam energy output both quantitatively and qualitatively, making this the most important feature. I will be examining the concepts behind recalibration with respect to the Chiron Technolas but these are significant concepts to all lasers.

The recalibration system consists of a phototherapeutic or fixed 5-mm diameter ablation of a fluence test plate, which consists of a thin micron layer of foil glued onto a red test plastic. The fluence test plates are calibrated so that the foil and glue are fully ablated, revealing a homogeneous red endpoint pattern at the point at which a correct fluence of 130 mJ/cm^2 is achieved. The normal number of pulses required to reach the endpoint is 65. If a greater number of pulses is required to reach the endpoint, then the fluence (energy within each pulse) is too low. Conversely, if fewer than 65 pulses is required to reach the target endpoint then the fluence is greater than 130 mJ/cm^2. The flu-

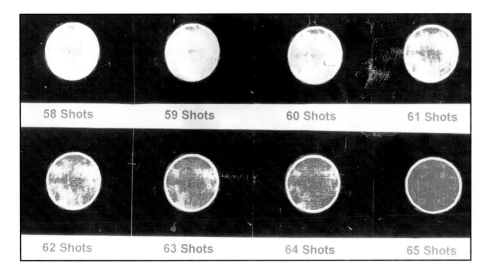

Figure 1-52.
Chiron Technolas excimer laser system calibration/fluence test, representative of acceptable shot profiles.

ence can be adjusted from the computer keyboard by altering the energy control bar which adjusts the voltage attenuator. The fluence test applies pulses at 10 Hz for the first 50 pulses, then at 2 Hz, and so the entire fluence test requires less than 15 seconds. Fluence adjustments can be made within seconds by depressing the right and left shift keys to increase and decrease the energy output, and the fluence test repeated to ensure that the precise fluence is maintained for each procedure (Figures 1-52 and 1-53). Since the energy from the laser head fluctuates, one source of over- and undercorrections can be significantly reduced. The fluence test also examines the energy output qualitatively as the pattern of ablation of the foil and glue accurately represents the beam homogeneity, both with respect to macrohomogeneity (overall energy beam profile) and microhomogeneity (local energy beam hot and cold spots). The degree of inhomogeneity can also be quantified with respect to the number of pulses required to reach the ablation endpoint from one point to the next. Alignment of the optical pathway and need to replace optics can be better evaluated and monitored.

There is no specific refractive check and PMMA plastic is a poor model to assess the ablative behavior of the beam upon the stroma. A collagen or gel model is necessary to properly evaluate this aspect of the calibration. The rapid recalibration technique and high sensitivity of this method to both quantitatively and qualitatively assess the energy beam output is mandatory for maximizing clinical results and safety. The VisX STAR and Coherent-Schwind Keratom excimer laser systems incorporate sophisticated auto-recalibration systems.

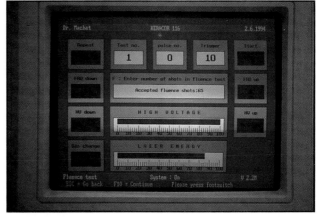

Figure 1-53.
Chiron Technolas Keracor 116 fluence calibration program. The surgeon activates the program by pressing the "S" key for Start and ablates the test foil calibration plate. The energy is then raised or lowered by adjusting the laser cavity voltage with the right and left "shift" keys based upon the test ablation results. A gas exchange "G" is performed if inadequate energy is achieved with maximum voltage in order to place fresh argon-fluoride premix gas within the laser cavity.

Clinical Note
VisX STAR

The STAR represents a significant redesign of the VisX 20/20 Model B, with a number of technological improvements (Figure 1-54). These improvements may not have a direct impact upon the clinical results but are innovative and helpful to the surgeon. The first change is the smaller size and footplate of the laser system, but the more important aspects of the redesign center around surgical performance of the procedure (Figure 1-55). The

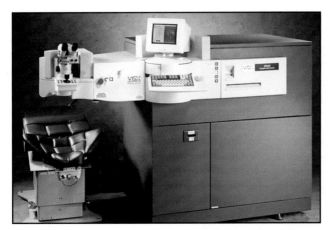

Figure 1-54.
VisX STAR excimer laser system.

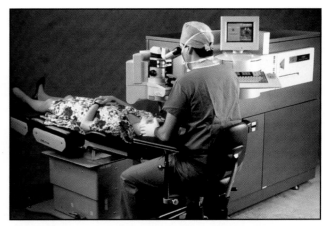

Figure 1-55.
PRK procedure with the VisX STAR excimer laser system demonstrating the incorporated computer terminal and small footplate size.

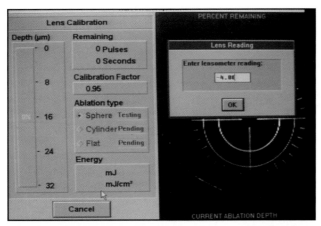

Figure 1-56.
VisX automated calibration program.

computer monitor is built into the laser with a Windows-based program. The 4.01 software incorporates anti-island ablation profile (following the pretreatment technique [Machat 1992]). The alignment and centration of the eye are enhanced through joystick control which allows for fine-tune focusing while a reticle is projected onto the surface of the cornea. There is a heads-up display in the microscope delineating the percentage of treatment remaining and current depth of ablation. An improved dual illumination system provides both a central ring as well as oblique lighting with independent control. Probably one of the most important developments concerns the advances with respect to the recalibration system, which is fully automated and performed prior to each treatment (Figure 1-56).

A number of serious maintenance and cost issues were identified with the VisX 20/20 Model B system which were addressed in the STAR. The optical pathway was redesigned, and the use of premix gas made more efficient. The gas cavity is smaller with no liquid nitrogen required. One of the most innovative developments allows for a partial gas exchange or gas boost to the laser cavity to complete a procedure, thus conserving premix.

The STAR is also designed to incorporate future developments with a standard pulse frequency of 6 Hz, which can be increased to 30 Hz, and an optical zone of 6.0 mm, which can be similarly increased to 8.0 mm. Hyperopic PRK corrections are in trial utilizing a rotating slit program.

Preliminary clinical results are superior to those achieved with the VisX 20/20 Model B, but long-term data are still required. The improvements in the alignment and calibration systems, physician interface, and cost-efficiencies in gas utilization are important steps forward for VisX.

Clinical Note
Coherent-Schwind Keratom

The Coherent-Schwind Keratom excimer laser system represents a substantial improvement over previous broad beam designs incorporating rotating apertures, such as the Taunton-VisX 20/15 (Figures 1-57a and 1-57b). The aperture system creates myopic, toric, and hyperopic ablation patterns with a peripheral transition zone to reduce regression of the refractive effect achieved (Figures 1-58a and 1-58b). The beam homogenization process incorporates a zoom optical delivery system to smooth beam irregularities. The optics are coated and optical pathway purged in nitrogen to promote optic longevity. The fluence is calibrated at the start of each day with a fluence sensor gener-

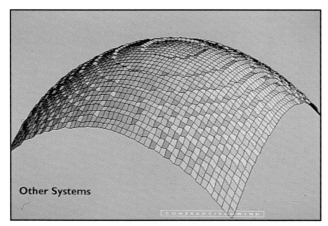

Figure 1-57a.
Ablation patterns with diaphragmatic systems and aperture systems previously created circular ridges with myopic ablation patterns.

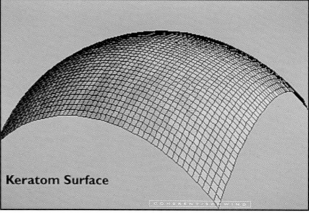

Figure 1-57b.
The ablation pattern with the Keratom is blended to create a smoother corneal surface.

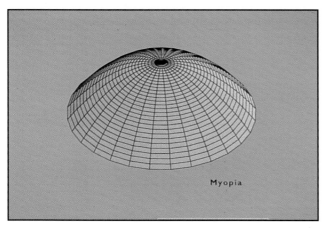

Figure 1-58a.
Coherent-Schwind Keratom myopic ablation patterns with peripheral transition zones to reduce regression.

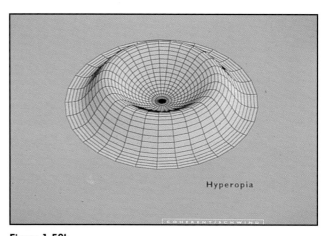

Figure 1-58b.
Coherent-Schwind Keratom hyperopic ablation patterns with peripheral transition zones to reduce regression.

ating a graphic computer assessment, then the sophisticated autocalibration system adjusts the beam energy automatically between procedures (Figure 1-59). An automatic gas refill system controls argon-fluoride premix utilization, with HaloPure, a halogen generator providing a weekly fluoride recharge, improving safety and gas purity. A back-up power system provides further safety.

A passive eyetracking system allows for autocentration, monitoring as little as 7 microns (Figure 1-60). The microscope has variable magnification ranging from 3.5 to 32 times, and the incorporated slit lamp is of great clinical value in monitoring progress during phototherapeutic procedures (Figures 1-61a and 1-61b). The laser working distance is compatible for LASIK (Figure 1-62). The computer monitor and software menu allow for a user-friendly interface with both calibration and programming (Figures

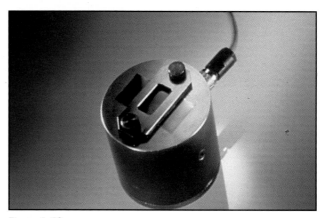

Figure 1-59.
Coherent-Schwind Keratom fluence sensor calibrates energy from beam and displays graphic analysis on monitor. The information gained is then used during automated recalibration throughout the day, precluding further manual recalibration.

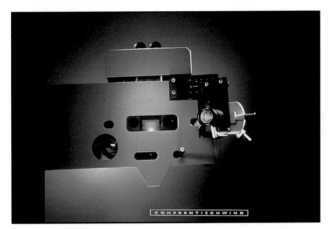

Figure 1-60.
The autocentration is performed through a fixation monitor which enables and disables the laser.

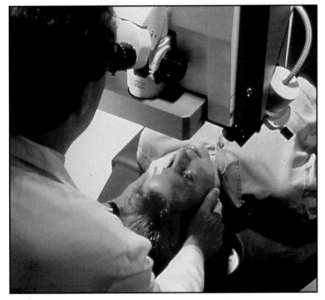

Figure 1-61b.
Surgeon view illustrating head position and alignment for microscope fixation system and slit lamp view.

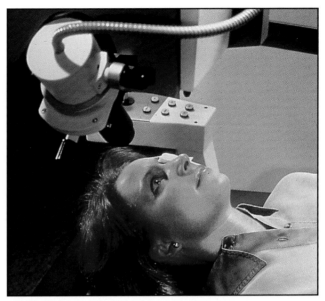

Figure 1-61a.
Side view illustrating head position and alignment for microscope fixation system and slit lamp view.

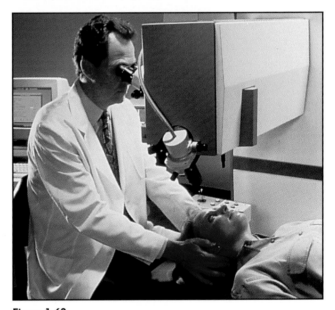

Figure 1-62.
Working distance has been extended to easily allow for lamellar procedures in concert with photoablation.

1-63a and 1-63b).

Keratom clinical study results for low to moderate myopia (<-7.25 D) with at least 6 months have demonstrated excellent refractive and visual results with complication rates similar to other advanced excimer systems.

- 88% 20/25 or better uncorrected visual acuity
- 98% 20/40 or better uncorrected visual acuity
- 88% within 1.00 D of emmetropia
- 68% within 0.5 D of emmetropia
- 3% confluent haze
- 0.7% loss of two or more lines of BCVA

SOFTWARE DESIGN FOR BROAD BEAM EXCIMER LASERS

The Technolas Keracor 116 is equipped with the pretreatment multi-multizone software program which appears clinically to be the best modality for myopic corrections with a homogeneous broad beam delivery system (Machat, August 1993). The software pretreatment applies additional

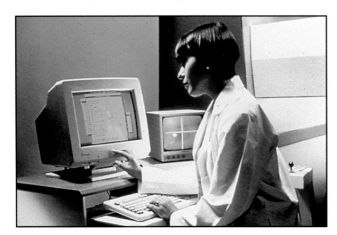

Figure 1-63a.
Coherent-Schwind computer monitor and eye display.

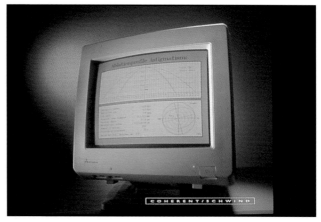

Figure 1-63b.
Coherent-Schwind schematic illustration of procedure ablation program.

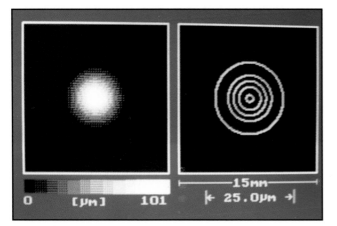

Figure 1-64a.
Graphic illustration of spherical profile of the Chiron Technolas Keracor 116.

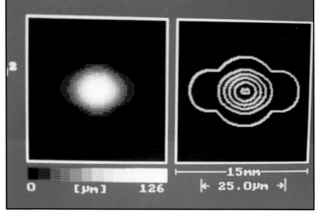

Figure 1-64b.
Graphic illustration of toric ablation profile of the Chiron Technolas Keracor 116.

pulses to the central 2.5 to 3.0 mm beyond the full refractive correction to prevent central island formation and improve qualitative vision (Machat, July 1992). The myopic ablation pattern (Figure 1-64a) is then applied in a multizone pattern, in several steps with increasing optical zones from 3.0 to 7.0 mm. Toric ablation patterns (Figure 1-64b) are introduced at the second step to allow the successive spherical component to blend the cylinder into the new anterior corneal curvature. Each successive zone is larger than the preceding zone and begins at fixation with a closed iris diaphragm. Therefore, this application pattern provides for maximum blending, with each pulse blending the previous pulse and each zone blending the previous zone. Another fundamental principle of surgical technique is that smaller zones should always precede larger zones to improve blending, whether for PRK or PTK. The scanner block also oscillates each pulse about the point of fixation to further improve blending.

> **Smaller zones should always precede larger zones to improve blending, whether for PRK or PTK.**

The primary benefit of the multi-multizone technique is that it allows for a 7.0-mm optical zone with a substantially reduced ablation depth (Table 1-3). The large optical zone is essential to reduce night glare and myopic regression. If the entire correction were applied in a single zone fashion, the depth of ablation would not only be far greater but the contour would be much less stable. For example, a -10.00 D correction with a single 7.0-mm optical zone penetrates to a depth over 160 microns, whereas the Technolas multi-multizone technique literally reduces the ablation depth by 40%, while still achieving the benefits of the large optical zone. The primary benefit of the Technolas pretreatment multi-multizone technique is that it provides for an exceptionally

TABLE 1-3

**COMPARISON OF ABLATION DEPTH:
SINGLE ZONE VS.
MULTI-MULTIZONE TECHNIQUE**

-10.00 D Myopic Correction		
Single Zone Technique		*Multi-Multizone Technique*
5.0-mm optical zone	83 microns	
6.0-mm optical zone	120 microns	7.0 mm multi-multizone 97 microns
7.0-mm optical zone	163 microns	

smooth recontouring process, reducing depth of ablation, haze, and regression through blending multiple zones. Future software developments center upon a scanning program designed to avoid the limitations of broad beam delivery systems, specifically central island formation, sensitivity to beam homogeneity, and asymmetrical ablation patterns.

The flexibility of the Chiron Technolas multi-multizone program allows the user to manipulate the optical zone parameters, such as the number, size, and dioptric distribution. Therefore, the user may alter the parameters for any specific case, such as increasing the dioptric correction at 7.0 mm for a patient with excessively large pupils and sensitivity to night glare. Similarly, the pretreatment may be increased to account for alterations in the energy beam profile or surgical technique which will counteract any increase in the incidence of central island formation. For example, an experienced surgeon using rapid mechanical debridement of the epithelium will require greater pretreatment to account for the increased degree of stromal hydration compared to either a slower novice surgeon or one experiencing the dehydrating effects of alcohol upon the stroma. The tremendous flexibility enables new multizone or continuous curve aspheric patterns to be quickly formulated for new procedures such as LASIK.

In summary, there are several essential features which enable the excimer laser to resculpt the cornea for refractive and therapeutic procedures. The most important of these is

that 193-nm ultraviolet light energy is capable of submicron precision with virtually no significant damage to the surrounding tissue. The lack of any significant thermal energy effect allows for a smooth ablative surface to be produced, thereby minimizing wound healing and preventing any significant loss of corneal transparency within the visual axis. However, despite phenomenal precision in tissue ablation, excimer laser PRK is still limited by its dependence upon wound healing. Wound healing depends upon a number of variables, including technique factors (ie, depth of ablation) and laser parameters (ie, beam quality). A permanent loss of transparency within the visual axis would make wide area surface photoablation encompassing the central cornea unsuitable for an elective refractive procedure. Insight into the laser and surgical parameters which preserve corneal transparency is essential.

The inherent nonhomogeneity of the excimer beam requires sophisticated optical delivery systems to improve beam quality and recalibration methods to measure the beam quality produced both quantitatively and qualitatively. Understanding excimer laser dynamics is the foundation upon which laser refractive surgery principles are based.

All excimer lasers are still evolving. As our understanding develops, the future will most likely move toward scanning technology with reduced concerns of beam homogeneity, greater clinical capabilities, and reduced maintenance requirements.

CHAPTER 2

Preoperative PRK Patient Evaluation

Refractive surgery is rapidly becoming not only an accepted subspecialty, but a viable option for many myopic patients. With the introduction of laser refractive surgery, the number of potential candidates will dramatically escalate. It is not unusual, however, for a patient to wait 6 to 12 months prior to proceeding with refractive surgery. The preoperative evaluation is part of an educational process that begins long before the initial consultation. Optometrists and ophthalmologists alike should routinely introduce the topic as a possible method for refractive error correction, just as they would suggest contact lenses. In this way, potential candidates will seek their opinion prior to considering refractive surgery and involve their personal doctor into their refractive surgery process. It is important, however, that all optometrists and ophthalmologists be educated with respect to refractive surgery in order to speak more accurately and confidently with their patients.

Photorefractive keratectomy (PRK) treats refractive errors by altering the anterior corneal curvature utilizing computer-controlled pulses of 193-nm ultraviolet light energy. The simplest way to explain PRK to patients is to state that the laser essentially reproduces the curvature of their contact lens or glasses prescription onto the front surface of their eye.

By early 1996, it is estimated that over 500,000 PRK procedures will have been performed in close to 50 countries on five continents worldwide. That number is expected to double within a year. However, as addressed earlier, despite the submicron precision of the excimer laser, clinical results and complications are dependent upon proper wound healing and therefore the consultative process remains a necessary and ever-present preoperative step.

CONSULTATIVE PROCESS

As with all refractive procedures, the aim of PRK is to reduce the functional dependence of the patient upon corrective lenses, with no guarantee that the procedure will eliminate their need. Although most refractive surgeons stress this basic insight, the mere fact that the procedure utilizes a laser appears to build unrealistic expectations. The consultative process (Figure 2-1) is directed at dealing with two fundamental elements: patient complications and patient expectations. The former may be important from a medical-legal perspective, but it is the latter that is essential to producing satisfied patients, as success is defined as meeting patient expectations rather than a visual goal. Patients must come away with the understanding that even good candidates may still require glasses for certain activities such as night driving or reading.

The consultative process is directed toward four critical issues of the potential candidate's agenda:

1. What is the best result the patient can hope for?
2. What is the worst possible outcome?
3. What are the financial costs involved?
4. What are the qualifications of the surgeon?

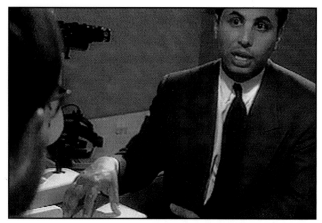

Figure 2-1.
Preoperatively, each patient must be evaluated and an informed consent conducted including consultation directly with the surgeon. Management of postoperative expectations is best handled preoperatively.

WHAT IS THE BEST RESULT THE PATIENT CAN HOPE FOR?

The first issue on the patient agenda is based on prior success of the procedure, both in general and in the hands of the specific surgeon. This question is usually answered on the basis of statistical success rates of achieving a given level of vision. However, success rates can be misleading

> **Two fundamental elements of the consultative process:**
> - Complications
> - Expectations

> **Meeting patient expectations defines success.**

since they usually are based on achieving legal driving vision of 20/40 uncorrected visual acuity, which is not satisfactory to many individuals. Typically, 20/25 or better uncorrected visual acuity is what most patients desire, and many patients who experienced 20/15 vision with their rigid gas permeable contact lenses may never be satisfied. It has been stated that all but the last diopter takes the focus of a patient to 1 m and it is the last diopter of myopic correction that takes the patient from 1 m to infinity. Thus, it is not surprising that patients with 1 D of residual myopia still desire further correction regardless of the severity of their preoperative refractive error.

Many surgeons demonstrate 20/40 vision or -1.00 D undercorrection utilizing trial lenses or a phoropter in an

effort to better enable patients to develop reasonable expectations. The most significant problem with this approach is that patients compare the -1.00 D undercorrection with their uncorrected vision preoperatively, however, postoperatively they compare the -1.00 D undercorrection with their best corrected vision. In my experience, even presbyopic myopic patients prefer to be rendered plano to +0.25 D, rather than be left -0.50 D, which is far more practical. Furthermore, the difficulty with all statistics is that preoperatively potential candidates do not believe that they will be in the 1% or 2% of patients who have complications and all believe, and most demand, that they will be in the percentage who achieve 20/20 uncorrected visual acuity no matter how small the percentage quoted.

A second problem that patients can encounter is that of qualitative visual loss rather than quantitative visual gain. That is, patients may achieve 20/20 vision yet be unsatisfied because of loss of qualitative vision, such as that which may occur with central islands or small optical zones producing night glare. This is far more difficult for patients to comprehend preoperatively. Needless to say, when asked even a satisfied patient will comment upon at least some aspect of his or her vision which is not quite optimal. The concept of optical performance of the cornea following all forms of refractive surgery has not been adequately addressed. Measurements of contrast sensitivity do not completely encompass this issue, but suffice to say that optical performance will be diminished in some manner in most patients, but that only a very small percentage will be severely hampered by that reduction. The optical performance issue is equally associated with patient expectations and patient complications.

WHAT IS THE WORST POSSIBLE OUTCOME?

The worst possible outcome with any form of eye surgery is blindness, although a few surgeons actually discuss possible death, which has occurred secondary to cardiac arrhythmias, within the realm of possibilities and so inform their patients. One of the best questions that I have ever been asked is, "What is the second worst possible outcome," to which I began to explain a loss of best corrected vision of greater than two lines. I explain that a loss of best corrected vision involves a loss of sharpness, crispness, or clarity of vision that glasses cannot even restore. I state that the loss is similar in nature to wearing glasses that are a couple of years out of date but that one is unable to purchase a new pair. I also elaborate that 100% of patients immediately following surgery experience a loss of qualitative vision and that 99% improve over 6 months, most within 2 to 4 weeks, but that 1% do not. Therefore, patients are aware that their vision may have a degree of blurriness immediately and that this is normal, and furthermore that it may require months to improve. Similarly, I explain that they will undoubtably experience night glare immediately, which also clears gradually over months in all but a small percentage, which is optical zone dependent. Further discussion of night visual disturbances can be found in Chapter 5.

WHAT ARE THE FINANCIAL COSTS INVOLVED?

The financial obligations are a significant consideration for many patients, because the cost of laser refractive surgery very likely will exceed that for radial keratotomy (RK). It is important that this issue be addressed appropriately and a variety of financing options be available. Patients who base their decision to proceed with refractive surgery upon the savings of never having to purchase corrective lenses again should either be dissuaded or must clearly understand that it is not a question of economics before proceeding with any refractive procedure.

Surprisingly, the majority of patients do not find the costs prohibitive so long as they recognize and perceive the procedure to add value to the quality of their life. I was very surprised by the fact that the majority of my initial patients were individuals who did not have a great deal of disposable income. Individuals who could readily afford the procedure appeared with increasing frequency later in my practice.

There are and will always be a number of individuals who will seek out the least costly vision correction modality or refractive center regardless of any other consideration. All doctors must evaluate for themselves what procedure fee structuring and financing they feel comfortable with, whether they are developing their own center, referring a patient, or determining what value the procedure has at a personal level.

WHAT ARE THE QUALIFICATIONS OF THE SURGEON?

The confidence that the surgeon instills in the patient is the most important factor in the patient decision-making process, even more so than success rates. Confidence is developed through the consultative process, not so much by what the surgeon says, but by the manner in which patient concerns are addressed. How the surgeon answers questions is fundamental to what the patient gains from the consultation. Those refractive surgeons who have gained considerable experience recognize that the consultation is not an

opportunity to sell the procedure, but to inform and build realistic expectations. Overselling the procedure is detrimental to the consultative process, and although it may gain the occasional patient, it will detract from the informed consent process, resulting in reduced patient satisfaction. Surgeons who are only beginning to add refractive surgery to their practices must realize and remember that most are created from word of mouth referrals. If reasonable expectations are set forth and procedure benefits are balanced with procedure limitations, patients with difficulties will be more easily managed and patient expectations more easily met.

The beginning refractive surgeon can usually offset surgical inexperience by investing time in self-education through courses and visiting other refractive surgeons both locally and abroad. The practical knowledge gained through these methods will serve any refractive surgeon well. Explaining to prospective candidates the extent of training completed is the first element in securing their confidence, and responding to their concerns knowledgeably is the second element.

Surgical experience and proficiency only add to surgeon credibility, as does the professionalism of staff members. The first level of endorsement, however, is derived from friends and family who may have had refractive surgery themselves or from the referring and comanaging doctor. Confidence is developed during the initial telephone contact with the refractive surgery facility—the crucial first step in building patient confidence. It is often the importance of this first contact with the refractive facility that centers underestimate and on which they expend few resources. The final step is dependent upon the interpersonal skills of the surgeon, the ability to communicate effectively, and foremost, the ability to answer questions without hesitation. It is very difficult at times to be blunt and address patient concerns directly, but patients are generally appreciative of an honest approach, and if complications do occur both the surgeon and the patient are in a better position to deal with them.

INFORMED CONSENT CONCEPTS

Refractive surgery helps many people in many ways. However, refractive surgery is not for everyone; it is a viable option for a defined group of individuals within the population. The potential market will vary with many factors such as cost and availability. The risks which are acceptable to one individual may not be acceptable to another. Everyone defines his or her own parameters of acceptability.

Many optometrists and ophthalmologists, when first dealing with refractive surgery candidates, feel that they are somehow responsible for the outcome and the decision of the patient to proceed. It is essential to know how to counsel the patient; however, the decision to proceed is solely the patient's personal choice. The surgeon should only offer an unbiased presentation of information for the patient to accept or decline. It is inappropriate for the referring doctor to make the decision for the patient to proceed or not to proceed. Both the doctor and the patient must never feel that the doctor is personally responsible for the decision made. The referring doctor should simply state, "From what I understand, you are a good candidate and I would expect you to do well but the decision to proceed is yours. I will be happy to care for you after the surgery if you do decide to proceed." The surgeon should go to great lengths to ensure the patient is well-informed but should never guarantee results, only his or her best efforts.

Consent Recommendations

- Patient should not sign consent form when dilated

- Patient should ideally receive and sign consent form (see Appendix A) prior to the day of surgery

- Patient should write in his or her own handwriting personal motivation for surgery

- Patient should write in his or her own handwriting possible need for corrective eyewear despite surgery

- Patient should write in his or her own handwriting significant risks of surgery

- Patient should be offered choice between and appreciate risks of unilateral versus bilateral simultaneous surgery

- Surgeon should be part of informed consent process and meet with patient and review risks personally prior to surgery

- Surgeon should avoid any form of explicit or implicit guarantees

- Surgeon should avoid any advertising stating procedure is safe without qualifiying such a statement

- Surgeon should avoid any advertising specifying throwing away glasses or implying permanent freedom from corrective eyewear

- Surgeon should inform patients about alternative techniques and future technology

The preoperative evaluation is based upon patient education, first by the staff and later by the doctor. All participants involved must be part of the education process. Potential candidates are simply seeking information. A good philosophy to maintain is that more information is better than less information. It is the risks, not the benefits, that the patient must understand and accept. The patient is actually less likely to consent to the procedure if he or she does not have a full understanding of the risks. Negatives add credibility to positives. Eliminating the fear of the unknown is of critical importance preoperatively. Lawsuits are less likely when communication is an integral part of the perioperative care process. Communication also results in happier patients.

Although the success rate for good candidates (<-6.00 D with mild astigmatism) is about 90% to 95% for 20/40 vision, only about half of these candidates achieve 20/20 vision. It is best to describe the outcome in terms of specific activities rather than an achieved level of visual acuity, such as vision that is good enough to play sports, watch television, and drive a car without correction. The vision that is achieved is typically good enough to be functionally independent of glasses for 90% of activities requiring good distance vision, but glasses for reading, night driving, or bad weather driving may be required at some time.

Success is not a visual goal.

IT IS NOT A VISUAL GOAL

Defining the goals and limitations of the procedure is one of the most important aspects of the preoperative consultative process. A patient must understand that 20/20 alone does not define success. Achieving the best vision possible in the safest, most conservative manner is the aim.

Patients must understand that the laser will not transform their eyes into emmetropic eyes, but simply myopic eyes that have a reduced dependence upon glasses. The need for continued annual dilated retinal examinations, especially in higher myopes, should be addressed. Many patients have the misconception that their risk of retinal tears and retinal detachments will be reduced or that their retinal potential will be improved. The latter is particularly important to address and document when treating any eye with reduced best corrected visual acuity.

Making statements such as "The procedure is permanent and safe without long-term complications" is unwise, as these facts have yet to be determined in absolute terms. However, one can state what is known and give personal opinions to address patient concerns (ie, "From everything we know to date the procedure appears to be safe," "The procedure has been performed thousands of times around the world in dozens of countries and no one has ever gone blind," and "The procedure was first performed in 1987 and the results appear to remain stable after the first 6 to 12 months)." The risk of a serious sight-threatening complication is much less than 1%. The long-term effects will not be known for decades, thus our opinion is based upon our understanding of the mechanism by which the laser works to improve vision. Thus, even in a few years the very long-term effects will not be known much beyond what is known today. The lack of thermal collateral damage, limited penetration depth, retained corneal stability, and safety to the endothelium provide ample evidence for long-term safety.

Clinical Note

Effect of PRK on Endothelium and Epithelium

The long-term concern of photoablation upon the epithelium and endothelium has been studied by several investigators and has failed to demonstrate any clinically significant alterations in these structures to date. Although very long-term effects are not known, there is no evidence to suggest that future concerns will surface.

Endothelial Studies

In vitro clinical studies demonstrated that no endothelial changes were induced unless the ultraviolet radiation penetrated to within 50 microns of the endothelium. The concern of endothelial damage secondary to acoustic shockwaves generated with surface ablation is of greater concern, especially with the prevalence of broad beam delivery systems and movement toward larger ablation zones.

In vivo studies by Amano et al examined central corneal endothelial cell densities at 1 month and 1 year postoperatively in 26 eyes of 20 patients and found no differences in mean cell density or the coefficient of variation of mean cell area compared with preoperative data. Carones and Brancato et al examined endothelial cell density, mean coefficient of cell area variation, and percentage of hexagonal cells at 3 months and 12 months in 76 eyes of 61 patients, treated for up to -13.50 D of correction at an estimated maximum cell depth of 113 microns. They found no endothelial damage following PRK and noted improvement in some indices they conjectured possibly

related to discontinuance of contact lens wear. Perez-Santonja confirmed these clinical findings in a 6-month prospective study on 14 eyes, demonstrating the mean cell density was unchanged and the degree of polymegathism was only minimally altered in contact lens wearers. Cennamo et al, reported another small short-term follow-up series of 19 patients concluding that myopic photoablation did not induce endothelial cell damage. These studies have failed to demonstrate any clinical significant endothelial changes associated with PRK.

Epithelial Studies

Another clinical study by Amano et al investigated corneal epithelial changes following the ablation of Bowman's layer and failed to demonstrate any reproducible morphological abnormalities of the superficial epithelium following PRK. Seiler and others have described central epithelial iron deposits which appear to have no clinical effects and appear to be related to a static pattern of tear flow. Busin and Meller, among others, have described epithelial map-dot type changes in the epithelium. Recurrent corneal erosion syndrome has been described following PRK but very rarely.

A number of epithelial clinical findings become apparent during PRK retreatment. First, mechanical debridement of epithelium prior to retreatment of clear corneas indicates that smooth ablation surfaces reduce epithelial adherence, as the epithelium is typically much easier to remove. It remains somewhat unclear the mechanism by which PTK is able to arrest recurrence of corneal erosions despite the fact that the epithelial adherence does not appear to be very strong with newer ablation techniques. The original Summit ExciMed UV 200 laser produced a more irregular surface ablation than current laser systems and was in fact associated with a clinically tighter bond when epithelial debridement for retreatment was attempted. Krueger and other investigators have described the continuity and smoothness of a pseudomembrane formed following surface ablation and the importance of intraoperative hydration and diaphragmatic blending in its structure and development. Second, during a transepithelial approach for retreatment, the epithelium in some cases of myopic regression is often very thick and ranges from 60 to as much as 100 microns. Delayed re-epithelialization is one of a number of factors which promotes haze formation. There have been no persistent epithelial abnormalities of clinical concern described to date.

TABLE 2-1
DR. RICHARD LINDSTROM'S CLINICAL OVERVIEW: PRK RESULTS AND COMPLICATIONS

Degrees of Myopia	Low to Moderate (<6.00 D)	Severe (-6.00 to -10.00 D)	Extreme (>-10.00 D)
Efficacy Visual Result (%)			
$\geq$20/40	90% ($\pm$10%)	75% ($\pm$10%)	60% ($\pm$10%)
$\geq$20/25	75% ($\pm$10%)	55% ($\pm$10%)	35% ($\pm$10%)
$\geq$20/20	60% ($\pm$10%)	30% ($\pm$10%)	10% ($\pm$10%)
Safety			
Loss of $\geq$two lines at 1 year	<5%	5% ($\pm$5%)	15% ($\pm$5%)
Severe loss $\leq$20/50	$\leq$0.2%	$\leq$5%	$\leq$10%
Major adverse reaction (eg, infection)	$\leq$0.1%	$\leq$0.1%	$\leq$0.1%
Stability			
>95% stability	6 to 12 months	1 to 2 years	2 to 3 years
Retreatments			
	10% ($\pm$5%)	25% ($\pm$10%)	40% ($\pm$10%)
Complications			
Undercorrections $\geq$1.00 D	10% ($\pm$5%)	25% ($\pm$10%)	40% ($\pm$10%)
Overcorrections $\geq$1.00 D	10% ($\pm$5%)	$\leq$5%	$\leq$5%
Induced regular astigmatism $\geq$1.00 D	$\leq$5%	$\leq$5%	$\leq$5%
Central islands early	$\leq$25%	$\leq$25%	$\leq$25%
1 year (less with new nomograms)	$\leq$5%	$\leq$5%	$\leq$5%
Decentration $\geq$1 mm	$\leq$5%	$\leq$5%	$\leq$5%
Corneal haze early	$\leq$0.5%	$\leq$5% ($\pm$5%)	$\leq$12% ($\pm$5%)
Late (1 year), persistent	$\leq$1%	$\leq$10%	$\leq$25%
Potential Severe Adverse Reactions			
Severe corneal scar	$\leq$0.2%	$\leq$0.5%	$\leq$10%
Infectious keratitis	$\leq$0.1%	$\leq$0.1%	$\leq$0.1%
Secondary glaucoma	$\leq$0.1%	$\leq$0.1%	$\leq$0.1%
Recurrent corneal erosion	$\leq$0.1%	$\leq$0.1%	$\leq$0.1%

CONSULTATIVE REVIEW OF PATIENT RISKS

It is important to recognize that patients are overwhelmed by the entire consultative process, and they will forget many of the complication and expectation issues raised and explained during their examination. It is important when reviewing the risks to first state, "These are the risks of the procedure", and to number the risks during the discussion. It is also important to discuss the risks in lay terms clearly and precisely. Documentation is as important as the discussion itself. An assistant taking notes during the consultation is invaluable.

1. **Infection** is probably the simplest risk for patients to appreciate, and the risk of an infectious infiltrate is approximately 1 in 500, with risk of a severe corneal ulcer being approximately 1 in 1000. Lid hygiene and broad spectrum antibiotic prophylaxis can reduce the incidence in half. The risk of infection is during the first 72 hours, and only during epithelial healing. The risk is for a superficial corneal infection, as it is with contact lenses. Infections are treated with topical antibiotics.

Patients are ideally checked daily during the first 72 hours to monitor for infection. Patients are given antibiotic medication before and after surgery as prophylaxis.

2. **Healing haze** is collagen protein produced in the cornea during the remodeling of the eye. It is almost never visible to the naked eye. It is not a fog or a blur. It usually develops after 1 to 2 weeks, just as patients note their vision is improving, although patients will often state the "haze" is clearing. The healing haze increases over the first 3 months, then decreases over the first year. Haze can rarely reduce best corrected vision. These cases appear to improve with time and with repeat laser surgery.

3. **Night glare** has been a problem with RK and with excimer laser PRK using smaller optical zones. Nonetheless, most patients improve with time and once both eyes have had surgery. Patients at greatest risk remain those with large pupils and moderate to severe myopia. Patients with night glare preoperatively will continue to have night glare postoperatively.

4. **Presbyopia** must be carefully explained to each candidate but especially to the pre-presbyopic group. Patients who participate in sports and social activities, drive, and watch television will benefit; however, avid readers and individuals who perform near work during the workday will have to balance any benefits achieved with clear distance vision against future need for reading. Presbyopia is the most difficult concept for patients to grasp unless they have already experienced the early symptoms.

5. **Regression** may be a problem in a small number of patients, especially those with severe myopia preoperatively. Therefore, the success rate is lower for these patients and thinner glasses may be the achieved outcome. Contacts are well tolerated after surgery. Repeat surgery may be performed. Most centers do not charge a fee for enhancement, which is best, but a policy will need to be established at each center. An unsatisfied patient who must pay additional fees for an enhancement is much more likely to be litigious.

6. **Postoperative pain** usually starts 30 to 90 minutes following surgery and is extremely variable. Medications are given to help patients sleep and avoid any discomfort. Pain is only a problem for the first 12 to 24 hours and I have found that some male patients seem to find this period the most difficult. Patients are then light sensitive for 3 to 4 days. Vision is quite blurry and patients need encouragement. The introduction of the bandage contact lens with a topical NSAID postoperatively has

dramatically improved patient comfort during epithelial healing.

7. **Steroid-induced complications** can occur during the first 3 to 4 months when patients are placed on topical steroid drops. Patients must be monitored for steroid-induced glaucoma. Occasionally, ptosis may develop related to topical steroid use.

8. Patients feel **unbalanced** during the first 1 to 2 weeks and will experience a loss of stereopsis. The treated eye will be hyperopic initially, and a plain lens in the patient's spectacles in front of the treated eye, or preferably, a contact lens in the fellow eye will ease the imbalance. For this and many other reasons, the second eye improves more quickly in most cases and is tolerated better. Night glare improves upon treatment of the fellow eye.

9. **Overcorrections** which fail to regress are likely the most troublesome and difficult patient management problem (see Chapter 5). Depending upon the nomogram and excimer laser system utilized, this usually occurs in 2% to 3% of patients. Undercorrections are easily managed with PRK retreatment after 6 months once stability is established.

10. **Loss of best corrected visual acuity**, discussed earlier, remains the most significant complication observed. Incidence varies with technique, laser system, and degree of preoperative myopia.

PRK Procedure Summary of Risk and Expectation Management

- Glasses may still be required
- Readers/presbyopia
- Overcorrections
- Undercorrections
- Repeat surgery
- Delayed visual recovery
- Regression
- Infection
- Pain
- Night glare
- Haze/scar tissue
- Induced regular/irregular astigmatism
- Loss of best corrected visual acuity
- Qualitative visual loss: ghost images, monocular diplopia
- Steroid induced side effects: cataracts, glaucoma, ptosis

In summary, PRK is not a perfect, complication-free procedure but it is probably the safest, most predictable procedure available for mild to moderate myopes, and the number of procedures will only continue to escalate over the next several years as public awareness increases. PRK will only increase in demand not because of visual results but because of patient perception, physician perception, availability, and marketability. Competition and the high cost associated with the technology will lead to surgeon desire to reduce patient barriers to the procedure; many will minimize risks while overpromising results. This recipe will only serve to undermine the physician-patient relationship, increasing medical-legal complaints while decreasing patient satisfaction and word of mouth referrals. PRK is still a procedure in evolution and borderline candidates should be persuaded to wait until technology has improved sufficiently. The consultative process is an essential element in proper patient preparation which serves us all well (Tables 2-1 and 2-2).

TABLE 2-2

DR. RICHARD LINDSTROM'S PRK RESULTS AND COMPLICATIONS

FDA

Summit	91%≥20/40	
	76% ≤1.00 D of emmetropia	
VisX	86%≥20/40	
	79% ≤1.00 D of emmetropia	
Approvable	50%≥20/20	
	70%≥20/25	
	90%≥20/40	
	≤5% lose two lines or more	
	≤0.2% lose five lines (serious adverse reaction)	

Lindstrom Personal PRK Results at 1 Year

99%≥20/40
85%≥20/25
-1.00 to -8.00 D

Night Glare

Common	≤5-mm optical zone	
	≥ 20%	
Rare	≥6-mm optical zone	
	≤3%	
	≤30% incidence	

Steroid Ocular Hypertension

Varies with steroid potency/duration
3% to 28% incidence
Three cases visual field loss
One required ALT
One required trabeculectomy

Clinical Note

Keloid Formers

I have performed PRK on patients known to form keloid scars. The first such case was a 28-year-old woman treated for a -4.00 D refractive error with a single zone technique in early 1992 with a Summit ExciMed UV 200 excimer laser with a 5.0-mm optical zone. Upon preoperative discussion with the patient, she specifically denied any healing problems for fear that it would have excluded her from the clinical study. Postoperatively, she developed severe confluent haze in a rather horseshoe configuration (Figures 2-2a and 2-2b). The haze pattern reflects steep edges related to a poor wound edge configuration common with single zone techniques, which act as a nidus for haze formation in predisposed patients. I had examined roughly 1000 Summit ExciMed patients at that time and had never observed such a severe degree of haze developing in such a low myope. After relating this to the patient, she went on to explain that her family has a strong history of keloid formation dating back at least three generations and notable in her two young children as well. In fact, she went on to tell to me a story of a small benign mole her dermatologist had excised on her back with a simple elliptical excision pattern which scarred so severely that he attempted to inject the scar with steroids but the needle broke. Remarkably, she maintained 20/30 uncorrected visual acuity as the visual axis was clear, but lost one line of best corrected visual acuity due to irregular astigmatism and distorted topography. Her corneal appearance and uncorrected visual acuity have remained unchanged for the past 4 years. No retreatment was ever performed as she has remained functional, happy, and stable. In other words, clinically significant haze in itself does not mean retreatment is indicated.

After 2 years of avoiding keloid formers, I treated a few with PRK for corrections up to -9.00 D without inciting clinically significant haze by ensuring that certain

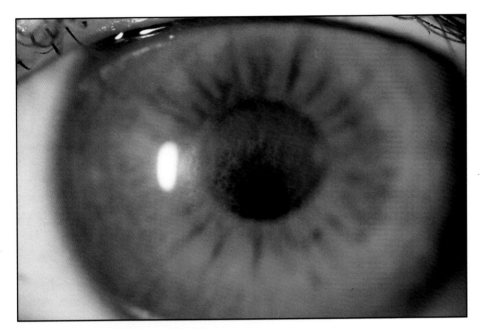

Figure 2-2a.
Peripheral confluent haze in horseshoe pattern in keloid former.

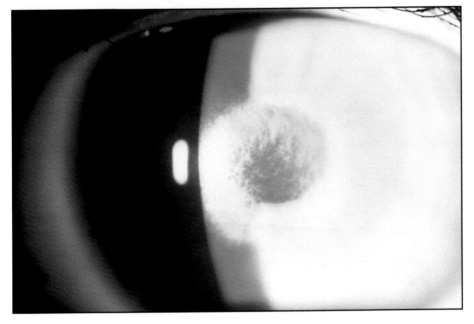

Figure 2-2b.
Patient was not retreated despite haze because of good uncorrected visual acuity through unaffected central cornea giving 20/30 unaided vision.

fundamental principles were maintained and patients were carefully informed. Three main principles were maintained: slight undercorrections were targeted to allow for prolonged steroid usage postoperatively, a well-hydrated stroma intraoperatively, and a pretreatment multizone technique to blend all wound edges. Currently, all such candidates are treated with LASIK without exception.

Range for PRK correction:
- -1.00 to -9.00 D of sphere, ideally <-6.00 D
- -0.50 to -6.00 D of cylinder, ideally <-3.00 D

Patients who are the best candidates have mild to moderate myopia (<-6.00 D) with less than 1.00 D of cylinder.

CANDIDATE SELECTION

The most ideal candidates for PRK are those with mild to moderate myopia up to -6.00 D, although PRK has been effective at treating up to -20.00 D of myopia and cylindrical errors up to 6.00 D. At these pathological ranges, the risk of wound healing abnormalities manifesting as haze and regression are much more evident. In general, the excimer laser can be programmed to perform toric ablations to correct astigmatism, however, the correction of myopia is still more predictable. Although PRK can also correct astigmatism, the ideal candidate will have less than - 0.75 D of cylinder. That is, the patient should have 20/30 or better vision with his or her spherical equivalent, or wear soft contacts with good vision.

PATIENT DEMOGRAPHICS

Candidates should be ideally over 21 years of age and have a relatively stable prescription, with no greater than 0.25 to 0.50 D change within the past year. Mean patient age is usually 35 years, with an acceptable range of 18 to 60 years. Young patients usually do not have a stable refraction and older patients are better suited for cataract extraction.

There is actually a trimodal age distribution in patients seeking PRK. The first peak occurs in young males 20 to 25 years old seeking a career opportunity such as law enforcement or those heavily involved in sports activities. The second peak occurs in the thirty-something crowd, those with disposable income, usually with an equal gender distribution. Their primary motivation is either contact lens difficulties, or more commonly, they are simply fed up of corrective lens dependence. It is with this group that refractive surgery first becomes more of a quality of life issue. The third group consists mainly of females over 40 years who are usually more severely myopic and are seeking a substantial change in their lifestyle.

There is a very slight preponderance of men overall, due primarily to career and sports requirements. Also, women generally feel more comfortable with using contact lenses and therefore have fewer limitations.

I have found that those patients who are not financially secure and desire the procedure will make the sacrifices necessary. This fact emphasizes the importance of payment plans and the acceptance of credit cards. More affluent patients, business people, and professionals tend to rationalize, intellectualize, and remain skeptical. As the procedure becomes more accepted and widespread, these latter patients will gravitate toward the procedure.

LOW MYOPIA CORRECTION

For low myopes, the uncorrected visual acuity must be sufficiently reduced to ensure that the risk-benefit ratio is reasonable. The uncorrected visual acuity should be below 20/40 vision in all cases and ideally less than 20/50. The basis for this is that legal driving vision in most places is 20/40. The patient must demonstrate good insight and have reasonable motivation, with increased career options being the most ideal. The other important consideration is patient age, since the presbyopic and pre-presbyopic candidates are ideal candidates for monovision.

MODERATE MYOPIA CORRECTION

Moderate myopes not only do particularly well with PRK, but achieve the best risk-benefit ratio with PRK compared to other forms of refractive surgery. RK is less effective for most moderate myopes, especially young females who exhibit greater regression. Laser in situ keratomileusis (LASIK) and automated lamellar keratoplasty (ALK) are both viable options but have a slightly greater associated procedure risk compared to PRK in the -4.00 to -6.00 D range. PRK continues to remain quite effective up to -8.00 D without a significant increase in the complication rate. Depending upon surgeon skill, techniques, and experience, LASIK may be the procedure of choice even in the mild myopia range.

HIGH MYOPIA CORRECTION

Although still very effective, PRK predictability begins to fall off somewhat with a greater rate of retreatment and haze formation. LASIK is the preferred procedure above -9.00 D, and, as stated, depending upon the level of surgeon experience, LASIK is the procedure of choice above -6.00 D. The degree of myopia at which the surgeon finds the clinical results and complication rates for LASIK and PRK interchangeable is directly related to the surgical experience of the surgeon with lamellar surgery.

Noncandidate:
+0.50 -2.00 x 180; Spherical Equivalent -0.50 D

Borderline candidate:
plano -2.00 x 180; Spherical Equivalent -1.00 D

Good candidate:
-0.50 -2.00 x 180; Spherical Equivalent -1.50 D

Best candidate:
-3.00 -2.00 x 180; Spherical Equivalent -4.00 D

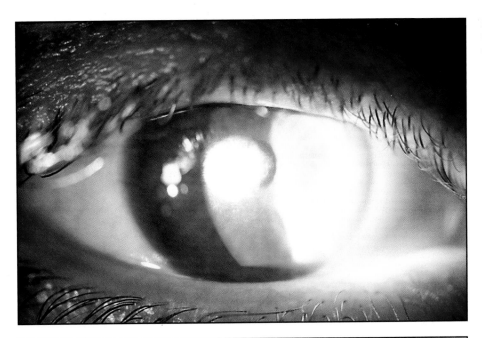

Figure 2-3a.
Depressed corneal scar. Contraindicated for PTK/PRK.

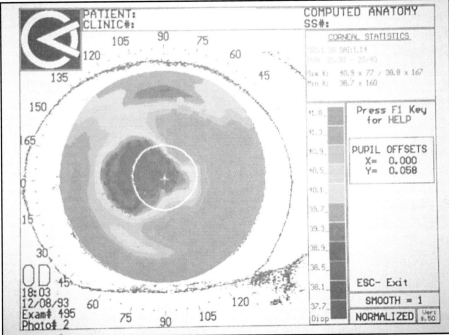

Figure 2-3b.
Accompanying topography of depressed corneal scar.

ASTIGMATISM CORRECTION

Patients with astigmatism must have net myopia to be candidates for PRK; that is, in the minus cylinder form, the sphere must be myopic. The refraction should always be assessed in the minus cylinder form when evaluating and planning a toric ablation, with respect to both candidacy and axis correction. PRK, or more accurately PARK (photoastigmatic refractive keratectomy), treats along the minus cylinder or flat axis, which is in direct contradiction to astig-matic keratotomy (AK), which involves a transverse incision along the plus or steep axis. Each pulse of the excimer laser corrects myopia as the cylinder is ablated. Mixed astigmatism is best treated with AK. Even if the spherical equivalent is myopic, the sphere must still be minus when the refraction is evaluated in the minus cylinder form. Spherical equivalent is defined as half the cylinder added algebraically to the sphere. The greater the sphere component, the greater the ability to blend the toric ablation into the anterior corneal curvature. Patients with a high degree of astigmatism should be informed of a higher incidence of residual cylinder requiring addtional surgery, in the form of PARK or AK. AK is a useful adjunct to achieve the best visual result, in cases of residual mixed astigmatism or cylinder which appears refractory to PARK.

CONTRAINDICATIONS

OCULAR HEALTH

No significant ocular pathology is acceptable. Numerous patients with a myriad of retinal, optic nerve, and hereditary conditions will inquire about the procedure. Patients with clinical keratoconus with corneal thinning or depressed corneal scars (Figures 2-3a and 2-3b) are contraindicated, although experimental treatment protocols have been attempted by a handful of investigators with some short-term success. Patients with amblyopic eyes represent a specific subset of patients. If the amblyopia is secondary to anisometropia with a myopic or astigmatic refraction, and only a mildly reduced best corrected visual acuity, the patient is still a candidate. The surgery will balance the patient and improve his or her uncorrected vision. Patients must be warned that they will not achieve vision better than their best corrected preoperative vision. Some amblyopic patients do improve their best corrected preoperative vision by one to two lines, but this should not be anticipated. These patients are usually happy postoperatively anyway because they can see with their bad eye and their relative risk was low since they did not use this eye before. Risk-benefit is an important concept to maintain. One-eyed patients are always contraindicated, and this includes the fellow eyes of patients with a dense amblyopia. Best corrected vision as a general rule should be better than 20/40 in both eyes.

Relative ocular contraindications:
- HSV keratitis history
- Previous ocular surgery
- Any active/residual/recurrent ocular disease
- Unstable/progressive myopia
- Irregular astigmatism
- Depressed corneal scars
- Forme fruste keratoconus (topographical changes)

Absolute ocular contraindications:
- Clinical keratoconus (or young forme fruste keratoconus)
- Monocular patients (actual/functionally)
- Severe dry eye with epithelial breakdown
- Exposure keratopathy (paralytic/non-paralytic)
- Herpes zoster ophthalmicus

Clinical Note

Keratoconus and Forme Fruste Keratoconus

I have treated two patients with clinical keratoconus in one eye, diagnosed both by corneal topography and anterior segment examination. Both patients were over 35 years of age, with one patient in his late 50s. Both had a stable refraction for over 5 years with pachymetry of greater than 500 microns at the cone. Both patients had become contact lens intolerant. Both patients had less than 50 microns of treatment. Both patients were fully informed that the procedure could worsen their condition and possibly increase their need for a corneal transplant. Both patients did exceptionally well with better than 20/30 uncorrected vision 1 year postoperatively and no loss of best corrected vision. Although there are a handful of small studies of keratoconus patients responding well to PRK, the concept of performing a thinning procedure on a cornea with a progressive, thinning disease continues to make clinical keratoconus generally contraindicated. Apical scarring preventing comfortable contact lens wear responds well to phototherapeutic keratectomy (PTK), but I will no longer perform PRK on patients with clinical keratoconus despite having had good success.

Keratoconus suspects comprise a subset of patients with no clinical signs of keratoconus on ocular examination, but topography findings demonstrating significant inferior, or less commonly superior, steepening. Occasionally, corneal warpage from contact lens wear is responsible and may clear over months. These patients should be considered to have keratoconus unless over 35 years of age with pachymetry greater than 500 microns. Young patients with suspicious maps should be avoided or be clearly informed of the unknown and possibly significant risks. There are, however, many patients with asymmetrical astigmatism and no disease. These patients respond better to PRK than RK, and perhaps even better to LASIK than surface ablation. If there is any question with

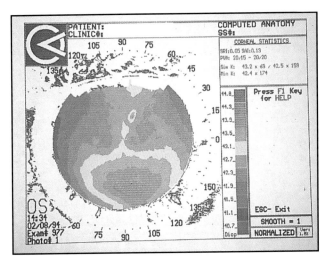

Figure 2-4a.
Preoperative corneal videokeratography map of forme fruste keratoconus.

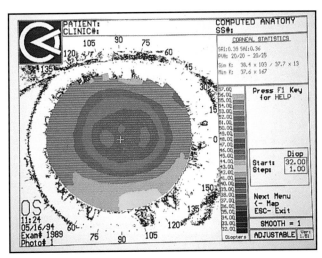

Figure 2-4b.
Postoperative corneal videokeratography map of forme fruste keratoconus treated with double pretreatment technique. Excellent central flattening noted with good subjective qualitative vision. Refractive treatment was centered, however, several microns of additional pretreatment were applied to the inferior steep area for topographical correction, prior to the refractive correction.

respect to the corneal thickness or possible progression, PRK remains the procedure of choice.

Corrective uphill decentration (CUD) is a useful technique to improve the induced surface topography. Developed by Mihai Pop, MD, this procedure deliberately decenters a portion of the procedure to apply several microns over the area of greatest steepening. CUD, however, may help specifically in more severe cases to improve visual outcome. In general, I use a double pretreatment technique in cases of forme fruste keratoconus where a significant amount of steepening occurs, and I perform two pretreatments, one over the steepest area and a second one centrally, with the remaining correction used to blend both into the cornea (Figures 2-4a through 2-4c).

Keratometry mires are the best method for identifying irregular astigmatism and continue to have their own role.

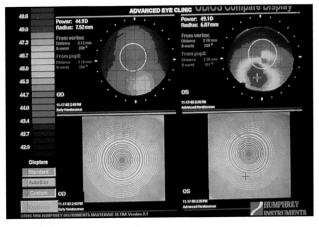

Figure 2-4c.
Humphrey MasterVue Ultra. OD/OS comparison display demonstrating clinical keratoconus, more marked OS.

General Health

Patients must be in good health and have a normal ocular examination. Since PRK is dependent upon proper wound healing, any systemic condition which may potentially be detrimental to the healing process of the eye should be a contraindication.

Relative general contraindications:
- Diabetes mellitus (Types I and II)
- Atopy if clinically significant
- Pregnancy/lactating mother

Absolute general contraindications:
- Autoimmune diseases: rheumatoid arthritis, lupus
- Immunosuppressed/immunocompromised patient
- Systemic illnesses which affect wound healing

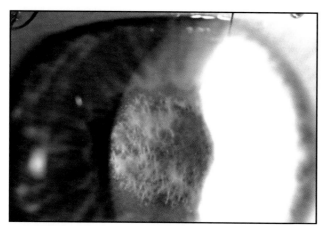

Figure 2-5a.
Dense confluent haze at 16x magnification associated with pregnancy 3 months following the PRK procedure. Only trace haze detectable 1 month following PRK with rapid progression of haze formation noted in association with significant hormonal changes of first trimester.

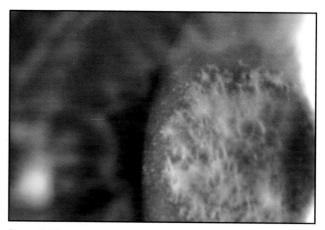

Figure 2-5b.
Dense confluent haze at 25x magnification associated with pregnancy 3 months following the PRK procedure. Only trace haze detectable 1 month following PRK with rapid progression of haze formation noted in association with significant hormonal changes of first trimester.

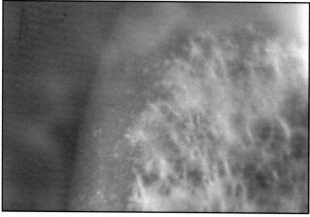

Figure 2-5c.
Dense confluent haze at 40x magnification associated with pregnancy 3 months following the PRK procedure. Only trace haze detectable 1 month following PRK with rapid progression of haze formation noted in association with significant hormonal changes of first trimester.

Clinical Note
Diabetes Mellitus

I have treated a number of diabetic patients with both PRK and LASIK, surprisingly none of whom have developed any related or even unrelated complication. The criteria utilized initially was the non-insulin dependent variety with no systemic or ocular manifestations of diabetes mellitus. Later, insulin-dependent diabetics were treated but once again limited only to those who did not demonstrate retinopathy, nephropathy, neuropathy, or other systemic clinical findings, nor any epithelial or other general wound healing problems. All diabetic patients are well aware that they may not heal typically, however, following PRK all patients to date (perhaps a dozen or more) have healed equally well to non-diabetics.

Clinical Note
Hormones and Pregnancy

Hormonal imbalance in female patients such as that associated with pregnancy and abnormal menstrual cycles or medications used in their treatment may interfere with the normal wound healing pattern following surface photoablation. Clinically significant haze may develop in association with hormonal fluxes, specifically when pregnancy ensues within the first 3 to 6 months following PRK. The relationship between pregnancy, even breastfeeding, and PRK wound healing appears to be directly related to hormone surges. I have treated seven female patients who became pregnant within weeks of their procedure. One patient had one eye treated several months after her first because of financial constraints but became pregnant soon after the fellow eye was treated. She developed dense confluent diffuse haze only in the eye most recently treated with the first eye remaining clear and stable (Figures 2-5a through 2-5c). After delivering the baby the eye was retreated and restored to 20/25 uncorrected vision with trace haze. Thus, there truly does appear to be a window within which pregnancy should be avoided, ideally 6 months.

The remaining six women who became pregnant help illustrate a second point: the greater the hormonal imbalance, the greater the effect generated upon wound healing. Two of the remaining women experienced severe morning sickness and had a difficult pregnancy; they similarly were observed to develop the most clinically significant haze. Two women had a relatively easy pregnancy in their own words, with virtually no morning sickness and continued to work until they delivered. Both of these women failed to demonstrate any degree of myopic regression and retained clear corneas. The final two women as predicted were intermediate in both their wound healing pattern and their hormonal fluxes associated with pregnancy.

As a result, some physicians feel that all women of child-bearing age have a negative pregnancy test prior to undergoing PRK and use adequate birth control. However, haze is treatable and therefore I personally do not go to such lengths. All patients who become pregnant complicate their postoperative course further because of the unknown effects of utilizing any medications during pregnancy.

Another issue to be considered is that the degree of myopia may increase somewhat, temporarily, or permanently in association with pregnancy or hormone alterations. One patient was stable for an entire year after being treated for -6.00 D correction with a VisX 20/20 excimer laser achieving 20/20 uncorrected visual acuity, plano refraction with clear corneas. She regressed to -1.00 D each time she underwent hormone therapy for her menstrual cycle. She was prescribed -1.00 D glasses to use as needed. Prior refractions should be checked and stability should be sought for all cases.

I have treated two patients in the early stages of pregnancy with LASIK. Needless to say, there was a long preoperative discussion outlining the experience with PRK and pregnancy, the unknown relationship of LASIK and pregnancy and other unrelated potential complications. Both patients had proven identical refractions from the previous year. Neither patient was given any preoperative sedation or perioperative medication other than topical anesthetic with a soaked surgical spear directly to the conjunctiva. Both patients were extremely myopic at -10.00 and -12.00 D. Fortunately, both patients did extremely well, with better than 20/40 uncorrected vision and less than 1 D of residual myopia, which was conservatively targeted. Since the degree of wound healing required with LASIK is considerably less, the effects of an altered hormonal balance would likely also be considerably less, as

these two cases may possibly illustrate. The need for postoperative medication both oral narcotic and non-narcotic analgesics and topical steroid preparations are also virtually eliminated. In general, pregnancy is still a contraindication, although it may represent a relative contraindication for LASIK and an absolute contraindication for PRK.

PREOPERATIVE EXAMINATION

Most of the essential aspects of candidate selection and informed consent have been covered under the previous section. This section will only summarize the specific aspects of the preoperative examination.

UNCORRECTED VISUAL ACUITY

It is important to document uncorrected vision preoperatively, especially in cases of mild myopia where a patient may be a borderline candidate. As we all know, a patient with -1.00 D of myopia may read 20/40 to 20/100 uncorrected. The level of visual disability preoperatively thereby becomes an important aspect as to whether the patient actually is a good candidate or not.

BEST CORRECTED VISUAL ACUITY

More importantly, best corrected visual acuity must be documented in order to assess for any loss of best corrected visual acuity postoperatively. Many myopic patients, especially those that are severely myopic, may not be able to read 20/20 or even 20/25 preoperatively and therefore should not expect to achieve this level of visual acuity postoperatively.

REFRACTION

Refracting a patient for surgery clearly has added significance, since any error may result in an over- or undercorrection and serious consequences. A cycloplegic refraction is important to ensure a significant accommodative component is not evident; however, many surgeons base their surgeries on a manifest (dry) refraction. It is essential to plan surgery the same way each time. That is, if the manifest refraction is usually -0.25 to -0.50 D greater than the cycloplegic refraction, the surgeon will typically get overcorrections and compensate for this in his or her personal nomogram.

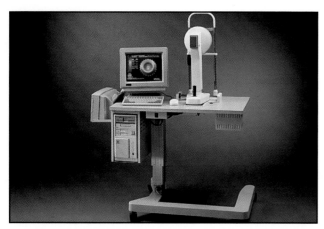

Figure 2-6a.
Humphrey Instruments MasterView Ultra corneal topography system.

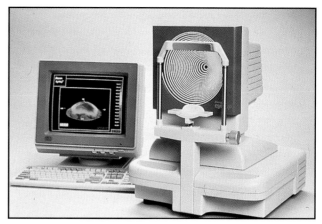

Figure 2-6b.
Alcon EyeMap corneal topography system.

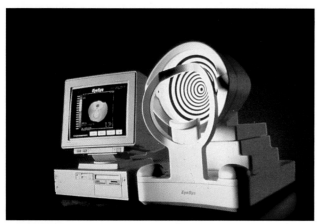

Figure 2-6c.
EyeSys System 2000 corneal topography unit.

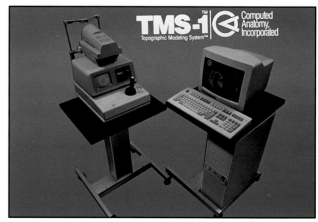

Figure 2-6d.
Tomey TMS-1 corneal videokeratography unit.

Clinical Note

Need for Cycloplegic Examination

A 35-year-old female patient was referred for LASIK with a cycloplegic refraction performed by her referring ophthalmologist of approximately -8.00 D. However, the patient had a 2-year-old pair of spectacles of -11.00 D. Autorefraction measured -12.00 D and manifest refraction utilizing a fogging technique corrected the patient to 20/20 with -11.00 D. The right eye of the patient was treated for -11.00 D, vertex distance corrected. One week postoperatively the patient measured 20/50 uncorrected with a manifest refraction of -1.00 D but a cycloplegic refraction that same day of +3.00 D. Fortunately, the patient regressed to +1.25 D and reads 20/15 uncorrected with no presbyopic symptoms. The fellow eye was treated for -8.00 D to correct the anisometropia and achieved 20/20 uncorrected vision with a plano refraction. Although this is the first patient I have documented to have such tremendous accommodation, all patients are currently cyclopleged with cyclopentolate 1%.

Refractions for refractive surgery are also different than those for glasses or contacts in that a fogging technique should be utilized to minimize the myopic sphere as much as possible to just achieve best corrected vision. The cylinder, however, should be maximized. As much cylinder as the patient will accept without reducing best corrected visual acuity should be dialed in. Minimum sphere and maximum cylinder (corresponding to the map) increase the odds of achieving emmetropia.

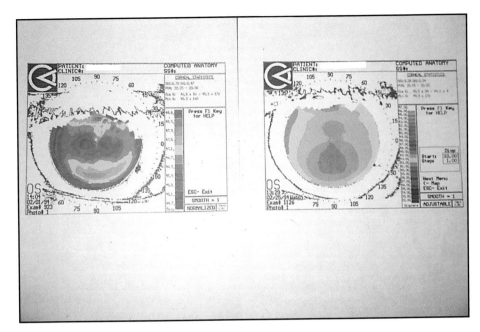

Figure 2-7.
Serial videokeratography immediately upon removal of rigid gas permeable lens demonstrating persistent central flattening and resolution of corneal warpage following several weeks of spectacle wear. Topographical steepening associated with increased myopia. These maps demonstrate the importance of removing rigid gas permeable lenses for several weeks prior to refractive surgery. Stability of refraction and topography are required prior to scheduling PRK.

ANTERIOR SEGMENT EXAMINATION

Anterior segment assessment preoperatively is essential to rule out preexisting pathology. Lids and lashes must be assessed for uncontrolled blepharitis which should be treated preoperatively. Corneal clarity should be evaluated, previous scars, neovascularization from contact lens use, evidence of keratoconus (apical thinning and scarring, iron ring, Vogt lines), hereditary dystrophies, and endothelial changes should all be noted. Lens changes are important to both document and discuss with the patient, as are other abnormalities no matter how benign, to ensure the patient is aware of them preoperatively.

Preoperative corneal topography is currently the standard of practice and should be performed prior to any refractive surgery.

Pupil size in dim light is another important consideration since degree of myopia and pupillary size remain the most important risk factors in night visual disturbances (ie, glare, starbursting, halos). Patients with larger pupils and high corrections must have at least a 6-mm optical zone treated and preferably a 7-mm zone. Patients should be informed accordingly.

Intraocular pressure should be documented preoperatively as a baseline prior to topical steroid use and to identify preexisting pathology.

RETINAL EXAMINATION

This patient population is at higher risk for retinal pathology. Not only must a dilated retinal examination be performed, the patient must understand that the risk of detachment does not decrease simply because his or her dependence on glasses decreases. Annual examinations are still required. Both myopic degeneration and peripheral retinal pathology should be documented and discussed with the patient.

CORNEAL TOPOGRAPHY

One must understand how topography works to read a map effectively, as it is based upon reflections from the tear film with color codes indicating changes in curvature. Better systems based upon different technology will eventually replace current technology (Figures 2-6a through 2-6d).

Preoperative topography is important in planning refractive surgery, and has clearly become the accepted standard of care. It helps us not only plan surgery, but also to identify what changes we have created postoperatively. It is effective in identifying early keratoconus and forme fruste varieties. It also allows us to understand a number of postoperative surgical parameters and problems, from why a patient does not achieve qualitatively good vision to how well centered the ablation is. There are various clinical features for identifying keratoconus, keratoconus suspects, and variants. Corneal topography may well be the gold standard for diagnosing keratoconus. There are two primary features

Figure 2-8.
Corneal videokeratography example of contact lens induced corneal warpage.

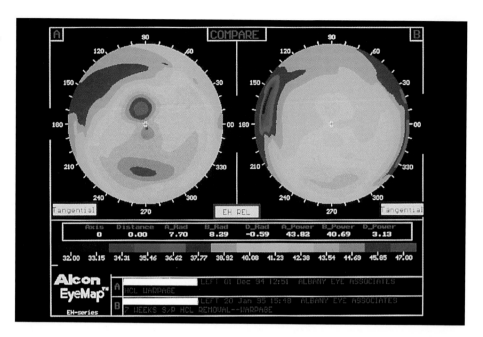

Figure 2-9.
Corneal videokeratography example of contact lens induced corneal warpage.

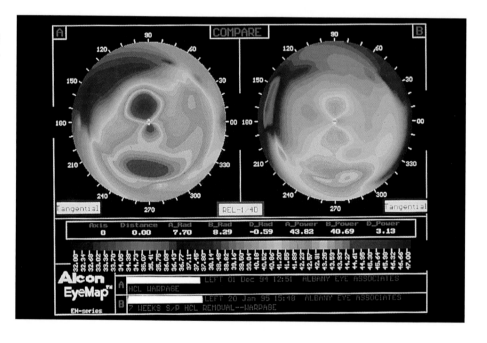

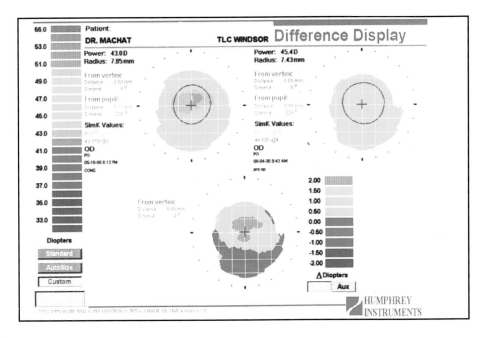

Figure 2-10.
Humphrey MasterVue difference display demonstrating corneal change upon discontinuation of RGP contact lens wear.

observed with keratoconus: corneal steepening and asymmetry. Corneal steepening of 47.00 D or greater is commonly observed, asymmetry not only between the superior and inferior aspects of the same cornea, but asymmetry between the two eyes is also observed.

CANDIDATE PREPARATION

Once candidates have completed the consultative process and preoperative examination, there are three specific issues to address:
1. Contact lens wear
2. Timing of the second eye
3. Factors that determine which eye to treat first

CONTACT LENS WEAR

It is important to ensure that the patient has discontinued contact lens wear with sufficient time preoperatively so as to allow the natural contour of the cornea to be re-established. It is more essential for the cornea to recover prior to PRK than LASIK, and more essential to allow a lengthier period for recovery in hard contact lens users, especially if they have a long history of usage (Figure 2-7). Soft daily contact lenses usually only require 48 to 72 hours, however some patients require much longer (Figures 2-8 and 2-9). If possible a period of 1 to 2 weeks without soft lenses is more suitable and it remains mandatory for those patients that utilize extended wear lenses and sleep in them. Hard lens users

require 4 to 6 weeks minimum without their contact lenses for adequate recovery (Figure 2-10). Although spectacles during the interim are preferable, soft disposable contact lenses are acceptable until 1 week prior to re-evaluation. The benefit of disposable lenses is that the refraction typically changes weekly and many high myopes refuse to wear spectacles for any length of time. Even with moderate amounts of astigmatism, fitting on the spherical equivalent works very well and helps the patient to prepare more realistic postoperative expectations.

It is important to examine and repeat corneal topography in hard lens wearers to ensure corneal warpage has resolved preoperatively. If areas of flattening and steepening consistent with contact lens wear still persist, surgery should be postponed and the patient re-evaluated every 2 to 4 weeks until stabilization. It can take as long as 6 months for full recovery in some cases. Add 4 weeks for every decade that the rigid gas permeable lens is worn, and in the case of PMMA lenses, add 6 weeks to the standard recommendation for a recovery time estimate.

TIMING OF THE SECOND EYE

The second eye is usually treated after 1 month (range: 2 to 6 weeks), but there is no true upper limit on when the patient should have the second eye treated. Many patients seek bilateral simultaneous surgery, and the risks and benefits should be conservatively evaluated for each patient. The benefits are convenience and least disruption of work and lifestyle for the most part, however, it is true that anxiety is reduced and side effects related to night glare and anisometropia are minimized. The risks are based upon the degree of myopia and the refractive predictability and complication rate for that group. Since patients never believe they will incur a complication, they readily accept the risk of bilateral infections, haze, or other healing problems. A more significant problem involves improper correction, specifically overcorrections rather than undercorrections, which are more difficult to manage. The most practical consideration is blurred vision bilaterally with an inability to drive and perhaps work for 1 to 2 weeks. For young myopes under 6.00 D with mild astigmatism, bilateral treatment is becoming the standard of care, with LASIK indicated for more severe myopes and astigmats desiring bilateral surgery with faster visual recovery.

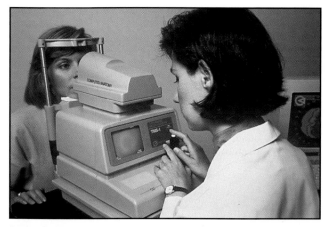

Figure 2-11a.
Preoperative corneal videokeratography evaluation of prospective candidate for refractive surgery with Computed Anatomy TMS-1 system demonstrating joystick alignment control.

Bilateral Simultaneous Surgery

Disadvantages:
- Bilateral complications: infections, haze
- Bilateral overcorrections
- Bilateral undercorrections
- Unable to compensate nomogram for improper refractive outcome with second eye
- Delayed visual recovery with inability to drive or work
- Bilateral loss of best corrected vision
- Bilateral need for retreatment

Advantages:
- Improved patient convenience
- Improved subjective vision (unable to compare to contact lens)
- Possibly reduced anxiety since not required to return for second eye
- Balance restored more rapidly
- Night glare improves more rapidly

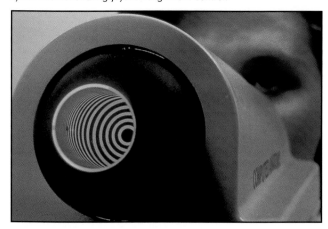

Figure 2-11b.
Placido disc cone projected on corneal surface of patient.

Patients who are candidates for monovision should be encouraged to wait as long as possible before treating their non-dominant eye. This is usually done after 2 months, but sometimes as long as 6 months is required to become accustomed to the change. The maximum tolerable difference between eyes is likely 3.00 D.

FACTORS THAT DETERMINE WHICH EYE TO TREAT FIRST

The final consideration is which eye to treat first if unilateral surgery is being performed. In general, I perform surgery on the non-dominant eye unless one of the three pro-

visions in the following boxed aside exists. The basis for performing PRK on the non-dominant eye is that the healing pattern for the patient can be determined and the more important dominant eye more accurately treated. The patient can function better in the interim focusing with his or her corrected dominant eye. Many patients feel more comfortable with having their non-dominant eye treated first when no contraindications are evident.

The non-dominant eye is treated first unless:
- The dominant eye tolerates a contact lens less.
- The dominant eye has the more severe prescription, greater astigmatism, worse best corrected vision, and/or uncorrected vision.
- Monovision is planned or considered or if there is a very significant delay planned before treating fellow eye.

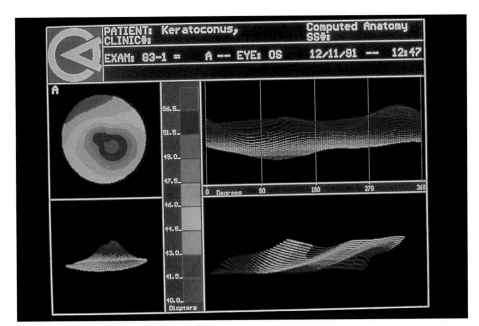

Figure 2-12.
Corneal videokeratography overview of clinical keratoconus.

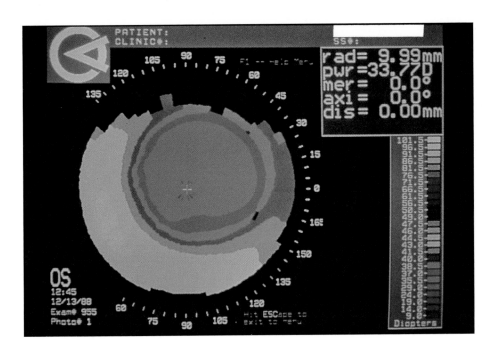

Figure 2-13.
Corneal videokeratography of mildly decentered PRK ablation.

Figure 2-14.
Humphrey corneal power map demonstrating poor qualitative vision is secondary to decentered PRK ablation with induced cylinder.

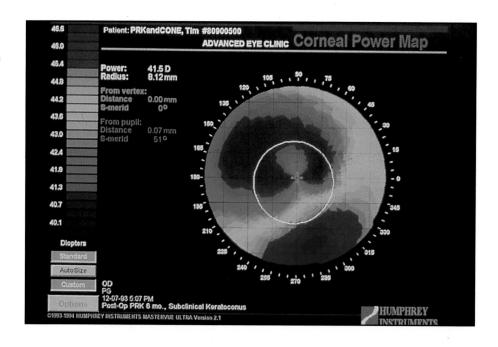

Figure 2-15.
Humphrey corneal topography difference display illustrating preoperative map in upper left, postoperative map in upper right, and effective ablation in difference map below with central island formation.

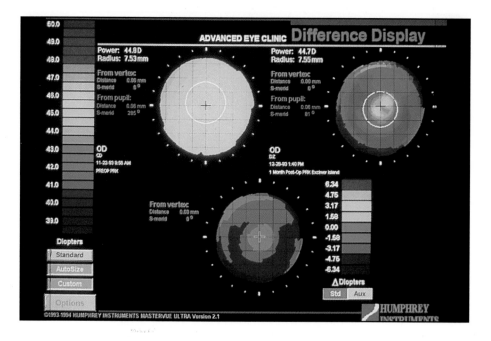

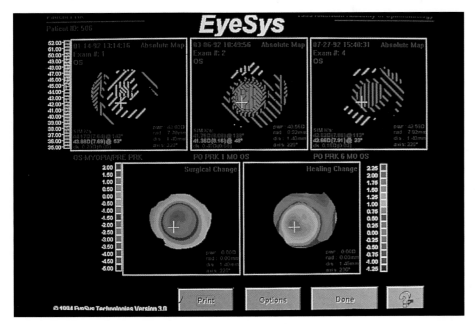

Figure 2-16.
STARS display of EyeSys 2000 system demonstrating preoperative and postoperative serial topographies over 1 year. The upper maps from left to right represent the preoperative, 1-month, and 12-month postoperative maps. The lower maps represent the difference maps, with the lower left demonstrating the surgical change between the preoperative and 1-month maps and the lower right representing the wound healing change between 1 month and 1 year.

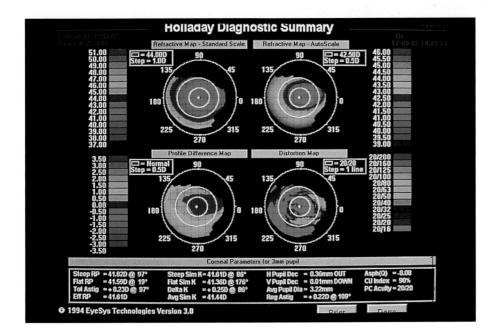

Figure 2-17.
Holladay Diagnostic Summary of a PRK patient. The software provides refractive maps set to both absolute and relative scales. A Profile Difference map compares the shape of the patient's actual cornea to the normal aspheric cornea (green), with red colors indicating corneal points which are steeper than the normal aspheric cornea, and blue colors indicating flatter areas. The Profile Difference map is used to detect overall corneal distortion (such as with keratoconus) and correlates well with the appearance of the retinoscopic reflex. The Distortion map looks at the optical quality of the corneal surface at every point. The distortion is mapped based upon the predicted level of Snellen visual acuity with green designated as 20/20, red 20/200, and blue 20/16 vision. The Distortion map is useful in correlating visual performance with corneal irregularities. There are also 15 corneal parameters and indices calculated evaluating factors such as procedure centration and irregular astigmatism.

Figure 2-18.
Contact lens fitting software developed by EyeSys.

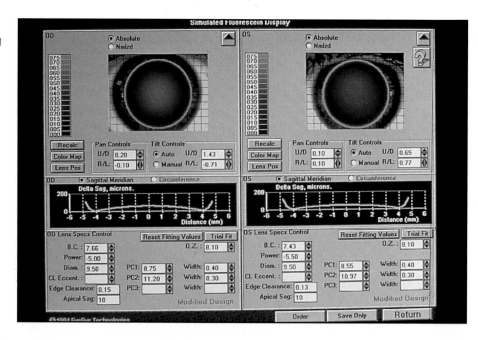

Figure 2-19.
RK planning software developed for EyeSys.

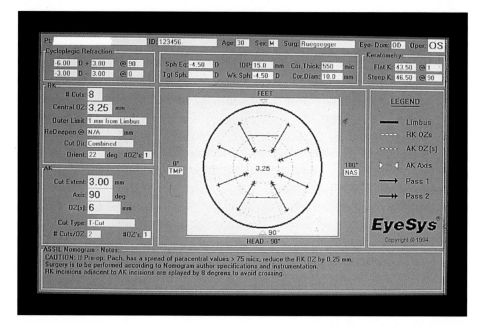

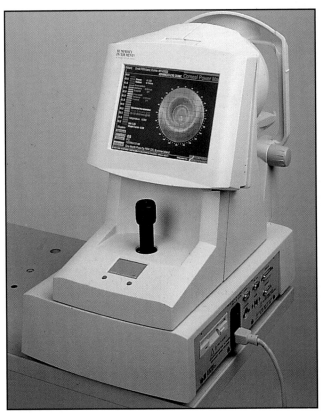

Figure 2-20.
Photograph of the ergonomically designed Humphrey Atlas Corneal
Topography System Model 990.

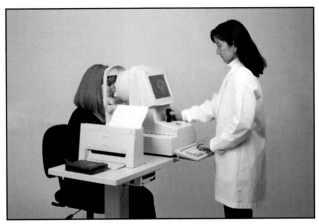

Figure 2-21.
Photograph of the self-contained Humphrey Model 990 unit
combining the monitor, computer, and capture system with the small
footplate, joystick alignment, mobile monitor screen with attached
keyboard, and printer.

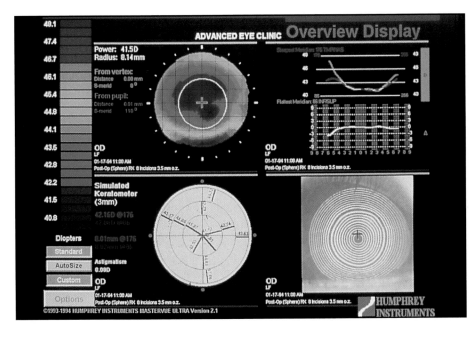

Figure 2-22.
Overview display of the Humphrey
MasterVue software demonstrating
corneal power map, simulated
keratometry, and Placido disc image.

Figure 2-23.
Display demonstrating contact lens fitting software available from Humphrey Instruments on MasterVue Ultra and Model 990 systems.

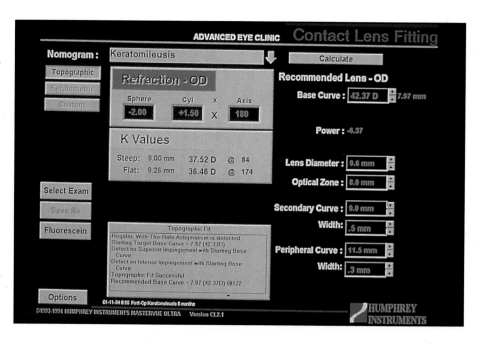

Figure 2-24.
PAR corneal topography system mounted on a slit lamp biomicroscope.

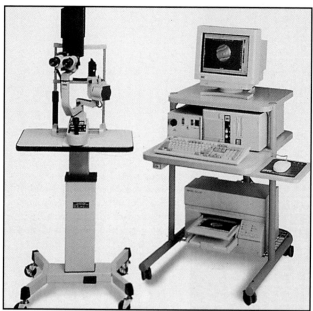

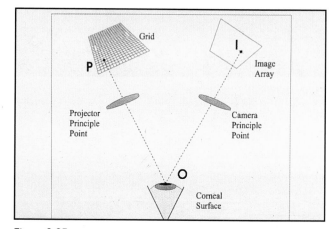

Figure 2-25.
A schematic diagram of the PAR CTS projection and imaging systems demonstrating the triangulation technique used for elevation calculations.

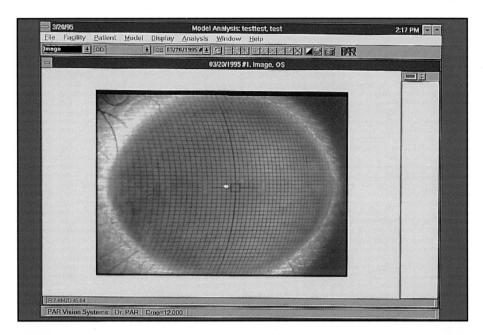

Figure 2-26.
PAR CTS grid projected onto a fluorescein-stained cornea for image capture.

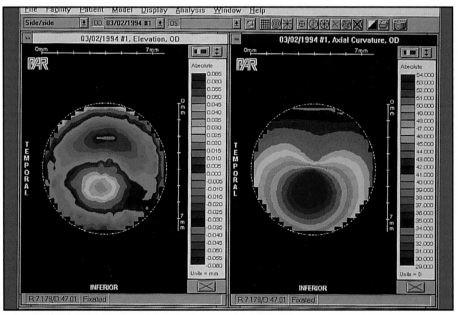

Figure 2-27.
PAR CTS display of clinical keratoconus illustrating corneal surface elevations. The left image depicts the actual extent of the cone, whereas the right image presents a more traditional axial curvature view of the same cornea.

Clinical Note

Perioperative Corneal Assessment
Corneal Topography

There are certain trends which not only become apparent in the evolution of both refractive surgery procedure techniques and technology, but also in the methods by which we assess them perioperatively. Pioneered by Stephen Klyce, PhD, and a handful of others over the past decade, corneal videokeratography has now become the standard of care in refractive surgery both during preoper-

ative evaluation of potential candidates and postoperative assessment of treated patients (Figures 2-11a and 2-11b). Preoperatively, corneal videokeratography has become paramount in the diagnosis of clinical and subclinical forms of keratoconus (Figure 2-12), as well as assessing the resolution of contact lens-induced corneal warpage. Its use has been instrumental in improving our understanding of both the positive and negative effects produced by refractive surgery. Corneal videokeratography is often the first clue as to why a patient expresses dissatisfaction post-

Figure 2-28.
PAR CTS Difference map of a LASIK patient demonstrating surgical change based upon elevation maps. The top left image is the preoperative cornea, the bottom left is the postoperative cornea, with the right image calculated from an elevation based subtraction of the two maps. The location and the amount of the intrastromal ablation can be determined. Courtesy of Dr. George Rozakis and PAR Technology.

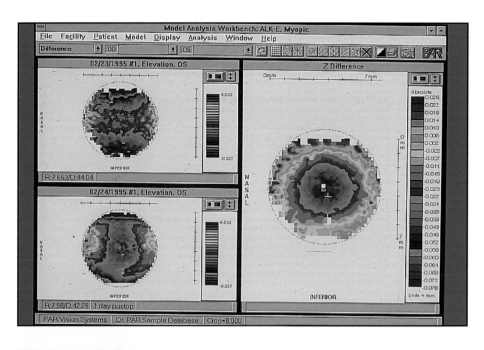

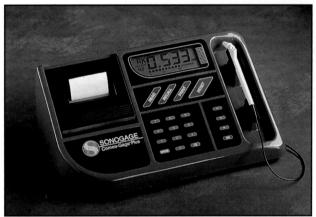

Figure 2-29.
Corneo-gage Plus 2 Ultrasonic Pachymeter from Sonogage with 50 MHz transducer for both epithelial-specific and total corneal thickness measurements.

operatively despite excellent quantitative visual acuity, why qualitative vision may be hampered as evidenced by an inadequate or decentered optical zone (Figure 2-13), or one of a variety of described topographical abnormalities (Figure 2-14). The triad of clinical symptoms of monocular diplopia, ghosting of images, and reduced best corrected vision were difficult to understand, treat, and finally prevent until one observed central island formation on corneal videokeratography (Figure 2-15).

Newer software packages introduced by Tomey and other manufacturers are able to provide predictability measures for keratoconus in prospective candidates. Other

software programs provide a new level of sophistication for the refractive surgeon with respect to data presentation and analysis, such as the Durrie STARS display and Holladay Diagnostic Summary introduced by EyeSys. The STARS display provides serial difference maps, demonstrating postoperative and wound healing corneal changes (Figure 2-16), while the Holladay display provides a true refractive map, aspheric profile difference map, and surface distortion map, as well as various corneal indices (Figure 2-17). It examines the cornea with respect to refractive power, shape, and optical quality. Other programs such as contact lens fitting programs (Figure 2-18) and RK planning systems (Figure 2-19) are available by a number of manufacturers.

Hardware advances within the realm of corneal videokeratography are also quite notable as systems become smaller, more economical, and easier to use. Humphrey Instruments has just unveiled the Humphrey Atlas Corneal Topography System Model 990 (Figure 2-20). This unit is unique in packaging as it provides the user with a complete, full-featured topographical system within a compact yet ergonomically designed unit with only a 1 by 3 foot footplate (Figure 2-21). The mobile screen can flip and rotate into the patient's view for demonstration and explanation purposes. The MasterVue software (Figure 2-22) and contact lens fitting software (Figure 2-23), as well as Refractive Surgery Services (RSS) and Slade-Machat Data Analysis software packages are available.

Other forms of corneal mapping based upon elevation

rather than corneal curvature and Placido disc imagery are under development. PAR Corneal Topography Systems (CTS) are based upon close range raster photogrammetry to measure and produce a topographical map of the corneal surface (Figure 2-24). The PAR CTS projects a grid onto the corneal surface and measures elevation relative to a reference plane (Figures 2-25 and 2-26). The advantage of the PAR CTS revolves around the fact that a true topographic map is produced based upon elevation which does not require a smooth reflective corneal surface for computer imaging (Figure 2-27). The primary clinical application of such a system would be the potential for real-time topographic assessment during photoablation, both during the primary procedure and during retreatment of patients with topographical abnormalities. The PAR CTS can even determine the amount of tissue removed with ALK or LASIK from an elevation subtraction or difference map, referred to as a Delta Z map (Figure 2-28). Theoretically, a scanning delivery system utilizing flying spot technology could be harnessed to an imaging system such as the PAR CTS to accurately ablate and create an ideal refractive outcome.

Corneal Pachymetry

Another area of development in properly assessing refractive surgery patients preoperatively and postoperatively is that of ultrasonic corneal pachymetry. Corneal pachymetry, both of the entire cornea and of the epithelium alone, is important in that the thickness of the cornea preoperatively affects the clinical response to procedures such as holmium laser thermokeratoplasty, and postoperatively, epithelial hyperplasia is associated with myopic regression following PRK and alters retreatment strategies. Sonogage has recently introduced the Corneo-gage Plus 2, with a 50 MHz transducer which is capable of measuring epithelial thickness (Figure 2-29). The unit provides automatic calibration, continuous read, and incorporates a dot-matrix printer.

Wound healing occurs at two levels with PRK and likely with RK and LASIK as well: first, at the level of the stroma and second, at the level of the epithelium. After utilizing a transepithelial approach on a number of RK patients for residual myopia, I observed that some of these patients had epithelium which measured 70 to 80 microns rather than 50 to 60 microns as would have been expected. Similarly, highly myopic PRK treated patients that have demonstrated significant regression with clear corneas typically have epithelium measuring 70 to 100 microns in thickness, and do poorly with retreatment for low levels of myopia, regressing repeatedly. The role of the epithelium in LASIK wound healing, although limited, has yet to be well defined.

Corneal pachymetry is mandatory during surgical planning for LASIK and ALK, as the maximum amount of stromal tissue that can be safely removed is directly related to the preoperative corneal thickness. Various rules of thumb exist, including an anticipated residual stromal bed no less than 250 microns, a total corneal thickness of greater than 300 microns, and the total depth of ablation (corneal flap plus ablation depth) limited so as not to exceed 50% of the total corneal thickness. I personally target a residual corneal thickness of at least 400 microns after one or more procedures; since the thinnest corneal flap I use is 160 microns, this leaves a residual stromal bed of 240 microns or more (see LASIK section).

It is clear that both corneal topography and corneal pachymetry are important elements in assessing the refractive surgery patient both preoperatively and postoperatively. These methods of evaluation provide important insight into not only selecting ideal candidates and guiding surgical technique, but also understanding the effects of the refractive procedure and wound healing upon qualitative vision.

CHAPTER 3

PRK Procedure

Although there are only a few steps to excimer laser photorefractive keratectomy (PRK), there are as many approaches as there are surgeons. PRK has a relatively uncomplicated learning curve, filled with few technical challenges and governed by a handful of fundamental principles. Despite the fact that many surgeons feel comfortable performing PRK without a thorough understanding of excimer laser technology and are able to achieve more than satisfactory results, developing an understanding of the nuances of PRK requires an understanding of the laser itself. Much in the same way that surgeons performing high volume phacoemulsification understand their units, so must the laser refractive surgeon if he or she is not only to be qualified but skilled and proficient as well. Management of complicated cases and altering ablation patterns based upon laser functioning can only be properly handled with understanding and insight into the technology.

PATIENT PREPARATION

It is first important to recognize that each step of the patient education process helps prepare the patient for the procedure and for postoperative recovery (Figure 3-1). Preoperative examination and consultation extends beyond informed consent and refraction, as virtually all patients are apprenhensive prior to any form of surgery, but particularly ocular surgery. Despite the fact that the surgeon may deem laser refractive surgery as a simple, minimally invasive pro-

cedure with low risk, it must be remembered that patients do not. They are filled with a mixture of nervous apprehension and eager anticipation. It is important to let patients know that these emotions are natural. Some patients are in fact more anxious with their second eye treatment for fear that it will not achieve the same result.

The following instructions should be given to the patient preoperatively:

1. There are no restrictions on eating, drinking, or taking medication prior to surgery, other than avoiding alcohol and medication that may produce drowsiness.

2. Patients should wear comfortable clothing.

3. No eye make-up is permitted the day of surgery and residual eye make-up should be carefully removed.

Before surgery, the following points should be confirmed and issues settled:

1. Ensure that the patient has in fact removed his or her contact lens as instructed. Patients wearing rigid gas permeable lenses will require repeat corneal topography and cycloplegic refraction to confirm stability has been achieved.

2. Confirm that the patient has arranged a driver or other transportation.

3. Confirm that the patient has arranged time for recovery.

4. Confirm that patient has arranged appropriate follow-up.

5. Confirm any known allergies.

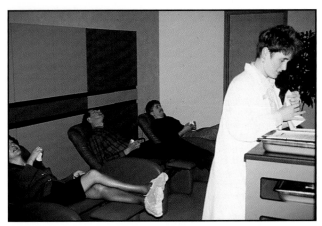

Figure 3-1.
Installation of preoperative topical medications in preparation area prior to PRK.

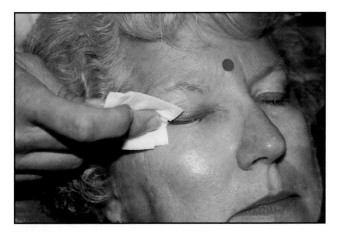

Figure 3-2.
Preoperative lid hygiene for PRK includes lid scrubs followed by antibiotic ointment to eyelashes.

PREOPERATIVE EYELID HYGIENE

The eyelashes and eyelids of each patient should be cleaned preoperatively as the eyelashes represent the single most important site of bacteria in the operative field and the most likely source from which a bacterial infection would arise (Figure 3-2). Even if no discernible blepharitis is apparent, lid scrubs preoperatively have a dramatic effect on decreasing the incidence of infection. Upon the implementation of lid scrubs and the application of polymyxin B sulfate and gramicidin (Polysporin, Warner Wellcome) ointment our incidence of bacterial corneal ulceration with PRK reduced from 1 in 1000 to zero in over 2500 cases.

PREOPERATIVE MEDICATIONS

Each surgeon uses his or her own regimen, but in general four topical agents are utilized:
1. Topical anesthetic
2. Topical non-steroidal anti-inflammatory drug (NSAID)
3. Topical antibiotic
4. Topical steroid preparation

Most surgeons no longer utilize any oral narcotic or sedative preoperatively, as it may impair target fixation intraoperatively. It is actually better for the patient to be slightly anxious rather than slightly sedated as centration is enhanced. The most important factor in controlling patient anxiety is to continually speak and reassure the patient. Despite the fact that the entire procedure is only a few minutes in duration and the laser application 15 to 60 seconds, patients perceive a much longer time. Although the patient is required to stare at a target fixation light, the patient is often unsure as to whether he or she is fixating properly. From the surgeon's perspective the role and responsibility of the patient appears simple, but patients are actually overwhelmed at times by the entire procedure. The speed of the procedure can be both a blessing and a nightmare, in that both the surgeon and the patient have a very brief period of time in which to perform the procedure properly. The beginning surgeon may prefer an excimer laser which operates at 5 Hz, while an experienced surgeon will prefer a laser with a pulse frequency of 10 Hz. Once the epithelium is removed, a limited amount of time may pass before the stroma becomes excessively dehydrated and the procedure predictability detrimentally affected.

TOPICAL ANESTHETIC

There are a variety of topical anesthetics which can be utilized, the most common of which include tetracaine 0.5%, proparacaine 0.5%, and xylocaine 2% to 4%. Tetracaine is available in minums for sterility and is more epitheliotoxic, which may aid epithelial debridement. Xylocaine has slower onset but may have prolonged action. Proparacaine is our standard topical anesthetic as it is less painful than tetracaine upon instillation and tolerated well by patients who seemingly require copious amounts of topical anesthesia preoperatively both for comfort and reassurance.

TOPICAL NSAIDS

Diclofenac sodium 0.1% (Voltaren, CIBA) and ketorolac tromethamine 0.5% (Acular, Allergan) are the two most commonly utilized topical NSAIDs. These appear to be equivalent in alleviating postoperative PRK pain, although diclofenac may have an additional topical anesthetic effect. These med-

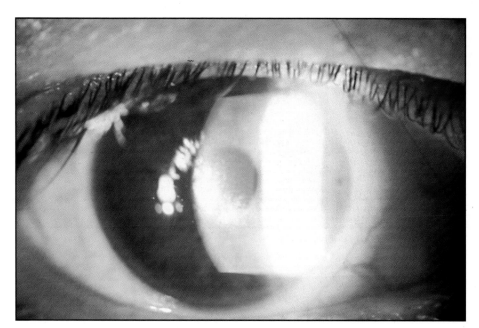

Figure 3-3a.
Decentered PRK ablation with arcuate confluent haze. Uncorrected vision measures 20/20-1, however, qualitative vision is disturbed with asymmetric night glare.

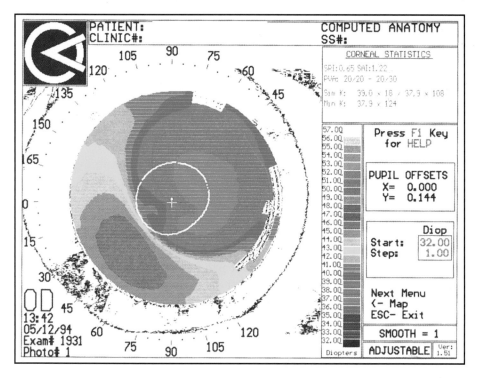

Figure 3-3b.
Corneal videokeratography of Figure 3-3a demonstrating the decentered stromal ablation. The degree of decentration appears greater on corneal videokeratography than is clinically apparent because the arcuate haze itself produces a local steepening effect.

ications are instilled both pre- and postoperatively, but excessive use may result in toxicity and delay epithelial healing. Other serious adverse reactions such as sterile infiltrates and stromal melts have also been reported related to NSAID usage. An important note is that a topical steroid should be used in combination with the non-steroidal anti-inflammatory preparation to reduce the incidence of sterile infiltrates observed, the pathology of which is explained in Chapter 5.

TOPICAL ANTIBIOTICS

There are a variety of topical antibiotics which can be used for prophylaxis. A combination antibiotic-steroid preparation such as TobraDex (Alcon) is commonly used. The disadvantage of tobramycin is the reduced effectiveness against streptococcal bacteria, although there is excellent staphylococcal and pseudomonal coverage. Aminoglycosides are also known to be epitheliotoxic; however,

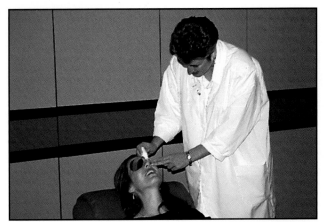

Figure 3-4.
Preoperative instillation of topical agents prior to PRK procedure. Standard regimen includes broad spectrum antibiotics: tobramycin 0.3%-dexamethasone 0.1% (TobraDex, Alcon), ofloxacin 0.3% (Ocuflox, Allergan); anti-inflammatory non-steroidal agent: diclofenac 0.1% (Voltaren, CIBA Vision Ophthalmics); and topical anesthetic agent: proparacaine 0.5% (Alcaine, Alcon).

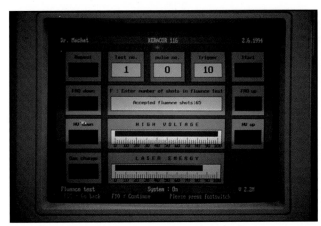

Figure 3-6.
Chiron Technolas Keracor 116 fluence calibration program. The surgeon activates the program by pressing the "S" key for Start and ablates the test foil calibration plate. The energy is then raised or lowered by adjusting the laser cavity voltage with the right and left "shift" keys based upon the test ablation results. A gas exchange "G" is performed if inadequate energy is achieved with maximum voltage in order to place fresh argon-fluoride premix gas within the laser cavity.

tobramycin is the least epitheliotoxic of all the aminoglycosides. With the introduction of fluoroquinolones with increased broad spectrum coverage and low toxicity, a separate fluoroquinolone antibiotic and a topical steroid preparation are recommended. Some surgeons use double antibiotic coverage with both an aminoglycoside and fluoroquinolone. The fluoroquinolones (see Clinical Note in Chapter 4) primarily used are Ciloxan (Alcon) and Ocuflox (Allergan). Both provide excellent antibiotic coverage, how-

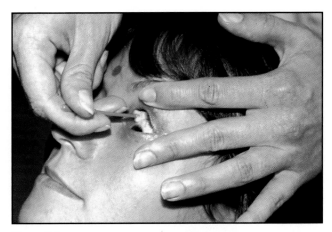

Figure 3-5.
Topical anesthesia is applied beneath the upper lid with a surgical spear soaked with lidocaine HCl (Xylocaine 4%, Astra).

ever, Ciloxan use may be complicated by crystallization of precipitates (see Chapter 5).

TOPICAL STEROIDS

Topical steroids were not initially utilized with PRK during the epithelial healing phases. Topical steroids preoperatively are optional, but postoperatively are recommended in concert with usage of a topical NSAID preparation to reduce sterile infiltrate formation. Topical steroids help reduce the degree of inflammation observed in the immediate postoperative period and may possibly reduce the associated discomfort. The clinical appearance of the eye is more quiet during the epithelial healing phase and the bandage contact lens is much better tolerated with the introduction of topical steroids into the perioperative regimen. The choice of topical steroids is at the discretion of the surgeon, with the range in potency extending from fluorometholone 0.1% to a full-strength topical steroid such as dexamethasone 0.1%, which is more commonly used.

Clinical Note
Preoperative Sedation and Decentration

I have consulted on two patients with clinically significant decentrations who received 20 mg of diazepam preoperatively. Neither patient could actually recall any aspect of the procedure. Neither patient had the fellow eye treated. Although one patient achieved 20/20 uncorrected visual acuity in his treated eye, his symptoms of decentration significantly impacted his visual quality and he sought legal recourse. The patient also developed arcuate confluent haze and mild induced cylinder (Figures 3-3a and 3-3b). The importance of these clinical histories are two-

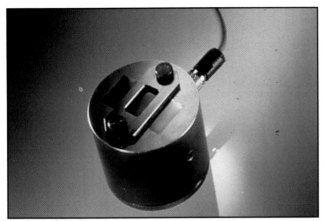

Figure 3-7.
Coherent-Schwind fluence sensor used in the calibration of the Keratom excimer laser system.

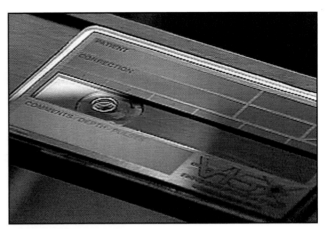

Figure 3-8a.
VisX STAR automated recalibration system calibration plate.

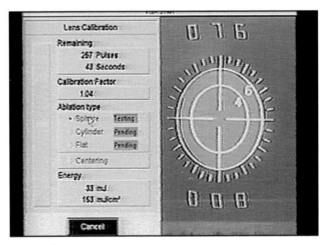

Figure 3-8b.
VisX STAR automated recalibration system monitor.

fold: first, with respect to avoiding preoperative sedation, and second, with respect to the impact poor centration can have upon vision outcome.

OTHER PREOPERATIVE MEDICATIONS

The use of a miotic preoperatively is at the discretion of the surgeon and varies with the laser alignment system. Pilocarpine 1% is part of the Summit preoperative medication protocol, as the alignment system requires a constricted pupil to verify centration. A miotic is not part of the VisX or Chiron Technolas recommended protocols because of the different alignment systems in place. There are advantages and disadvantages to instilling a miotic preoperatively. The benefit of constricting the pupil is that it reduces microscope glare for the patient which may improve not only patient comfort but self-fixation. The primary disadvantage with greatest clinical significance is that pilocarpine can produce a shift in the pupil of up to 2 mm supernasally. I no longer instill a miotic routinely (Figure 3-4).

APPLICATION OF TOPICAL MEDICATIONS

Preoperative drops are instilled at 5- to 10-minute intervals starting approximately 15 to 30 minutes prior to the procedure. Each patient will receive at least three sets of topical medications. Topical anesthesia is also applied directly to the superior fornix by means of an anesthetic-soaked surgical spear (Figure 3-5). Since most of the drops instilled accumulate in the lower fornix, anesthesia of the upper lid and fornix is best achieved in this fashion. Speculum dis-

comfort is reduced dramatically in this manner and patient cooperation improved. It is also useful to instill a few drops of topical anesthetic into the fellow eye to reduce blepharospasm and further improve patient cooperation and fixation. Each patient is assigned his or her own set of antibiotic, steroid, and non-steroidal bottles which are given following the procedure to reduce cross-contamination.

LASER CALIBRATION AND TESTING

Each laser has a series of steps which the operator or technician must adhere to in order to ensure proper calibration. As discussed in Chapter 1, fluence defines the amount of energy, whereas homogeneity represents the pattern of distribution of that energy. Each laser must be evaluated pre-

Figure 3-9.
Chiron Technolas excimer laser system calibration/fluence test, representative of acceptable shot profiles.

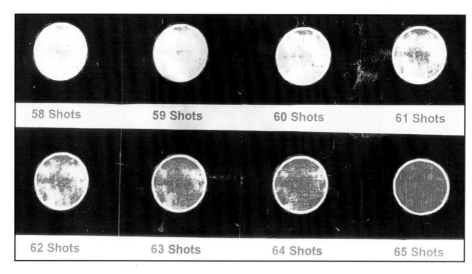

| 58 Shots | **59 Shots** | 60 Shots | 61 Shots |
| 62 Shots | 63 Shots | 64 Shots | 65 Shots |

operatively both quantitatively to ensure the correct fluence and qualitatively to ensure adequate beam homogeneity prior to use (Figure 3-6). In fact, excimer laser energy output is variable and should ideally be re-evaluated for each case. The software within each laser system is programmed to apply a specified number of pulses in a given pattern for each dioptric correction. The laser itself may have internal monitoring controls to ensure that adequate fluence is maintained within narrow guidelines; however, an external verification must be performed to set the fluence initially in all systems (Figures 3-7 through 3-8b). Results are dependent upon the laser system functioning properly. Therefore, the accuracy and predictability of PRK is entirely based upon the assumption that each pulse delivered is of specified energy and homogeneity. Fluence determines the ablation rate and improper fluence will result in reduced refractive predictability with over- and undercorrections.

Beam homogeneity is of equal importance to the final result, as irregularities in beam output will be compounded with higher corrections. There are two beam homogeneity problems which can arise: those related to microhomogeneity and those related to macrohomogeneity. Microhomogeneity represents localized energy irregularities, or hot and cold spots, which may incite focal haze formation or irregular or even regular astigmatism in high myopia correction. Macrohomogeneity represents the overall energy beam pattern or profile. Symmetrical and asymmetrical patterns can be observed. One example of a symmetrical pattern is the reverse gaussian pattern, where the beam is hotter peripherally than centrally, which increases the risk of central undercorrection and therefore central island formation. Understanding the effects of a reverse gaussian pattern would invite an experienced surgeon to increase the amount of treatment applied centrally, that is, increase the pretreatment amount programmed (see Chapter 5). The cause of this pattern is typically optic degradation, which tends to first occur centrally. Asymmetrical patterns, where the beam is hotter in one quadrant or one sector, will induce cylinder, and significant visual distortion can be produced. The procedure should be postponed until realignment of the laser optical system can be completed, as there is no effective method by which to compensate for this abnormal pattern. Understanding and evaluating beam homogeneity is an essential component of the procedure in order to achieve optimal results.

FLUENCE AND BEAM HOMOGENEITY TESTING

There are two primary factors which control the energy or fluence: voltage and gas. Increasing the voltage increases the energy density or fluence achieved from the laser head by creating more unstable argon-fluoride dimers from the gas premix within the laser head cavity. If increased voltage is not accompanied by an increase in the energy output, the gas may have been essentially expended requiring the gas within the cavity to be exchanged. Fresh gas has more argon-fluoride dimers available to be raised to a higher energy level.

If increased voltage and gas exchange are unable to achieve adequate energy density, then an optical pathway problem, such as a degraded optic, exists and a technician is required. The Chiron Technolas method of recalibration will be used to explain the principles of recalibration. The Chiron Technolas Keracor 116 recalibration system is based upon ablation of a specialized fluence test plate. The fluence plates consist of red PMMA plastic coated with a thin layer of glue and covered with foil. The fluence test plate is ablat-

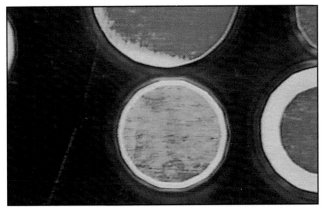

Figure 3-10a.
Homogeneous ablation pattern. The concept of breakthrough represents the "hottest" portion of the beam which first reaches the red endpoint. The point of breakthrough is noted inferiorly at the 6 o'clock position where the red endpoint pattern is discernible.

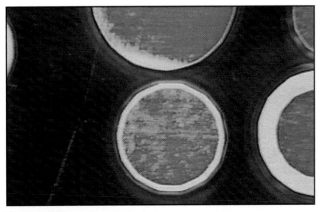

Figure 3-10b.
After an additional pulse, multiple areas of breakthrough become evident, signifying excellent beam homogeneity.

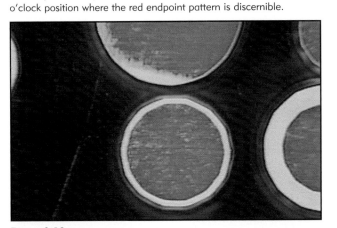

Figure 3-10c.
When virtually all the white test material has been ablated with one additional pulse, endpoint will have been reached. A three to four pulse difference between breakthrough and endpoint represents less than a 1-micron ablation difference and also represents superior beam quality.

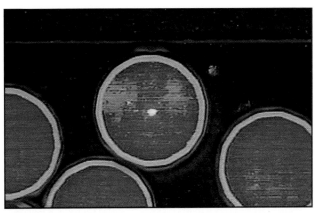

Figure 3-11.
Small beam abnormalities do not affect LASIK clinical results because of corneal flap masking, and are most detrimental to surface PRK high myopia results, as surface epithelium interaction produces focal haze and distortion. Four pulse elimination of cold spots within beam indicates clinically insignificant for all but PTK and high myopia PRK.

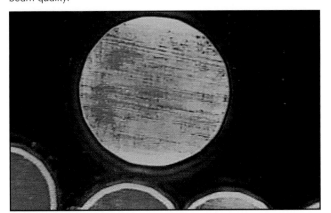

Figure 3-12.
Mild asymmetrical ablation test pattern at 7 mm. Larger test area increases sensitivity of homogeneity testing. Pattern is borderline for surgery as sweeping pattern demonstrated energy difference between left and right sides of below 5%. Low myopia correction or intrastromal LASIK would clinically be without topographical distortion, but high myopia surface ablation would result in poor qualitative vision.

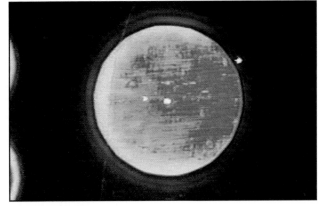

Figure 3-13.
Severe asymmetrical ablation test pattern at 7 mm. Pattern is unacceptable for surgery, as sweeping pattern demonstrated energy difference between left and right sides of test plate greater than 20%.

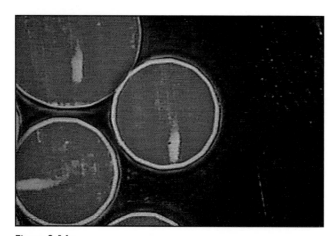

Figure 3-14a.
Focal beam abnormality with fixed cold spot in test pattern which is discernible at 5-mm homogeneity testing and remains consistent even with rotation of fluence test plate, which eliminates the calibration plate as a potential cause. Etiology of the abnormality was focal damage to an optic.

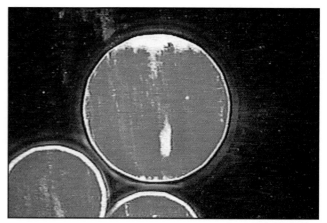

Figure 3-14b.
Focal beam abnormality with fixed cold spot in test pattern which is discernible at 7-mm homogeneity testing more centrally. Etiology of the abnormality was focal damage to an optic.

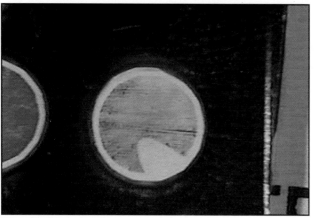

Figure 3-15.
Dense focal beam abnormality usually related to optical pathway abnormality. Unacceptable for surface PRK or LASIK, although much less clinically significant with LASIK. Number of pulses required to disappear beyond surrounding test plate determines density and clinical significance. Two to three pulse differences clinically insignificant with excellent beam homogeneity. Four to six pulse difference, clinically acceptable for all but PRK high myopia and transepithelial treatments. Greater than seven pulse difference (>10%) clinically unacceptable; expect topographical distortion unless small optical zone LASIK.

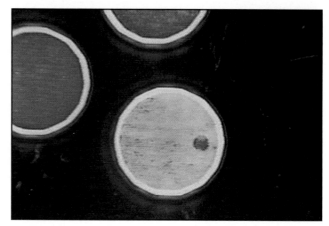

Figure 3-16.
Focal hot spot at 3 o'clock on 5-mm fluence test plate. Test pattern indicates small area of increased energy beam density usually related to energy beam pattern output of laser cavity. Number of pulses between focal area reaching endpoint and remaining test plate reaching endpoint determines clinical significance. Minimal clinical significance for LASIK, increased clinical significance for haze formation for high myopia surface ablation.

ed with the photorefractive keratectomy (PTK) mode at 5 mm, and the number of pulses required to penetrate the foil and glue determines the fluence. The fluence of the Chiron Technolas laser is 130 mJ/cm^2 which equates with 65 pulses to completely ablate the foil and white glue and achieve an even red test pattern. If more than 65 pulses are required, the fluence is too low; if less than 65, the fluence is too high. In reality, a range of 64 to 66 pulses is acceptable and some surgeons will accept a range as great as 62 to 68. The test-

ing requires about 15 seconds to complete (Figure 3-9). If the fluence is too low the voltage must be increased, and if increasing the voltage fails to achieve the required fluence of 130 mJ/cm^2 for which the ablation nomogram has been calibrated, a gas exchange is performed. This requires several minutes. As explained, if neither the voltage increase nor the gas exchange are able to achieve the desired fluence, that is, the fluence plate continues to require more than 66 pulses for complete ablation, an optical pathway problem exists

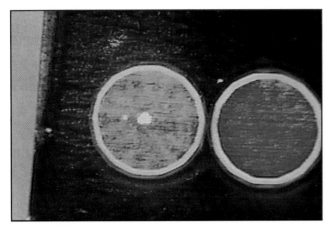

Figure 3-17a.
Excellent homogeneous energy beam profile with symmetrical, even ablation of test plate.

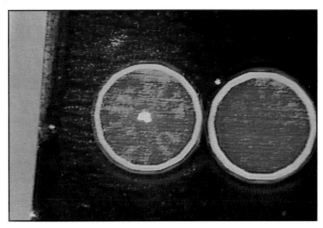

Figure 3-17b.
Entire plate achieves endpoint within two to three pulses. Excellent for transepithelial approach PRK, high myopia PRK and PTK, which all require a higher degree of beam homogeneity for good results.

and a technician is necessary. Often a surgeon or technician will observe that greater and greater voltage is required after a gas exchange to achieve the desired fluence, which indicates that the coating of an optic is likely deteriorating, requiring optic replacement at which time preventive maintenance can be performed.

The pattern of the ablation reflects the beam homogeneity. This recalibration method evaluates the beam both quantitatively, with respect to the number of pulses required to ablate the foil, and qualitatively, with respect to the homogeneity of the ablation pattern. Recalibration is performed between every case and is both rapid and accurate (Figures 3-10a through 3-17b).

The pattern of ablation which is indicative of the pattern of energy distribution or beam homogeneity is of equal importance to successful visual results as achieving proper fluence. With the Chiron Technolas recalibration system, the fluence test plates are very sensitive to both microhomogeneity and macrohomogeneity problems (Figure 3-18). As the white glue is ablated, the red PMMA becomes visible beneath, indicating areas of greatest energy density or hottest spots first within the beam. The coldest spots or areas of lowest energy density remain white the longest. A measure of homogeneity, therefore, is the number of pulses required from breakthrough (the first spot fully ablated and red) to the endpoint (the entire 5-mm area ablated and red). Each pulse removes 0.25 microns, therefore, a difference of four pulses from breakthrough to endpoint is about 1 micron. The maximum acceptable difference determined clinically is about six pulses or 1.5 microns, on a 5-mm test area. Greater inhomogeneities are apparent at larger diameters. Hot and cold spots would be representative of the

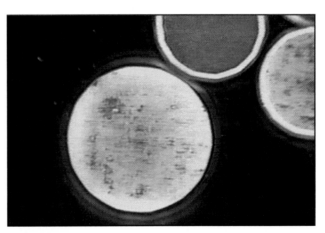

Figure 3-18.
Homogeneity evaluation with 7-mm beam diameter increasing sensitivity. Central 4 to 5 mm clearing slightly more rapidly, but with a clinically acceptable symmetrical pattern. Homogeneity testing is a dynamic process, meaning that to properly assess the beam quality, the pattern of ablation must be observed throughout the process.

microhomogeneity of the beam, and macrohomogeneity is determined by examining the overall pattern. Macrohomogeneity represents the energy beam profile, categorized as symmetrical and asymmetrical. Symmetrical patterns are gaussian, reverse gaussian, and homogeneous (Figures 3-19 and 3-20). Asymmetrical patterns, both sweeping and focal, are unacceptable for patient treatment (Figure 3-21).

That is, if a left to right sweeping pattern (Figure 3-22) was observed, this asymmetrical beam pattern would indicate that the energy density is highest on the left, perhaps ablating at 60 pulses, and lowest on the right, perhaps ablating at 70 pulses. The central area would have achieved the

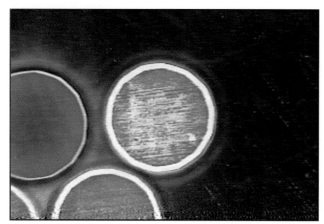

Figure 3-19.
Reverse gaussian energy beam profile with complete ablation of peripheral white test material, while residual test material is still observed centrally. The beam energy density is greatest peripherally and "coolest" centrally. This pattern is commonly observed during wide field PTK and transepithelial ablation, even with good beam homogeneity owing to ablation parameters and hydration factors, thereby requiring central pretreatment to avoid central islands.

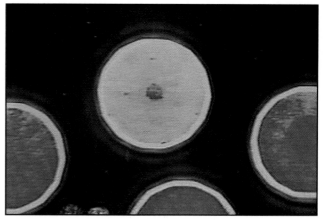

Figure 3-20.
Demonstration of a gaussian beam profile with greatest energy density centrally in PTK mode.

desired fluence at 65 pulses, but the pattern would be unacceptable. A laser with such an ablation pattern would produce an asymmetrical ablation pattern, treating the left side of the ablation zone at a greater ablation rate and removing more tissue than the right, resulting in a grossly abnormal corneal topography of apparent decentration and induced cylinder with poor qualitative vision. The larger the optical zone utilized, the greater the induced abnormality (Figures

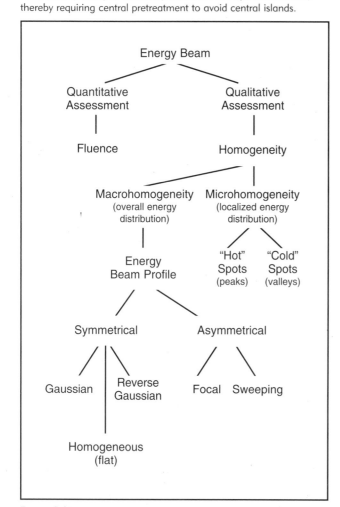

Figure 3-21.
Diagram of energy beam homogeneity test patterns.

Setting Fluence Analogy: Building a Staircase
If a staircase is built for a six story building, it is determined that it would require 100 steps to reach the top floor if each step were 10 inches, each floor requiring 20 steps. However, if the height of each step was miscalculated and made 10.5 inches, the error reached at the first level would be 10 inches or one stair height, but by the sixth floor the error would be 50 inches or the height of five steps. That is, the laser knows how many steps for each level of myopia to correct, but the size of each step is vital to the result of the overall outcome. If the fluence is too high, a small overcorrection will be produced in small treatments and a large overcorrection in higher attempted corrections. An analogy for homogeneity would be whether or not the stair is built evenly. If the left portion of the step is 10 inches, but the right portion is 10.5 inches, there would be a 10-inch difference between the left and right sides at the first floor, equal to one stair height. By the sixth floor it would be a 50-inch difference (or five stairs) between the two sides. From this example, it becomes clear that excellent homogeneity as well as proper fluence is required, especially for high myopia treatment.

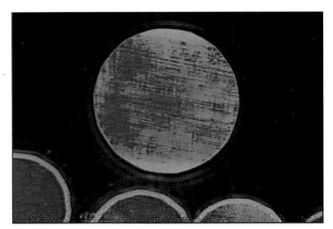

Figure 3-22.
Asymmetrical ablation test pattern demonstrating poor homogeneity with left to right sweeping pattern, as left portion of beam is ablating faster due to higher energy density. The left portion of the test plate has already achieved endpoint, whereas the right portion has only just reached the breakthrough point.

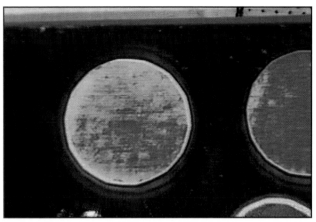

Figure 3-23a.
Asymmetrical ablation test pattern at 7-mm beam diameter with diffuse hot area inferiorly. Larger beam diameter is used after questionable 5 mm test result to better assess beam homogeneity pattern, which is always better for smaller beam diameters. Since the evolution has been toward larger beam diameters, we must assess the laser at larger diameters to know what effects we may produce.

3-23a and 3-23b). This is an important concept to understand, in that larger optical zone treatments with broad beam excimer lasers are more susceptible to beam abnormalities. If a small optical zone with such a sweeping pattern is used, less of the sweep is observed, and fewer pulses are required for any given dioptric correction, thus minimizing the beam abnormalities. The central area of the sweeping beam had a fluence of 130 mJ/cm^2 and therefore would achieve more predictable results with fewer topographical abnormalites than a large diameter ablation with the same ablation profile. The smaller zone would not be without problems, as it would have an increased tendency toward regression with haze formation and night glare depending upon the degree of correction attempted. This example of the impact of an asymmetrical beam pattern illustrates the clinical impact of improper or inadequate calibration and assessment of the beam output of an excimer laser.

OTHER SYSTEMS

Summit uses a gelatin wratten filter and polymethylmethacrylate (PMMA) block. Based upon the pattern and number of pulses required to penetrate the gel filter, the laser function is deemed acceptable or unacceptable. The laser is monitored internally and fluence adjusted between cases. The PMMA block is forwarded to the manufacturer for scanning.

The VisX 20/20 Model B utilizes PMMA test plastics (see Figure 3-8a). Fluence is adjusted by defocusing the microscope on black paper and reading the fluence off of the computer monitor. The pulse energy is increased if the fluence is low. The primary method for calibration is performed on PMMA blocks preoperatively for each case by

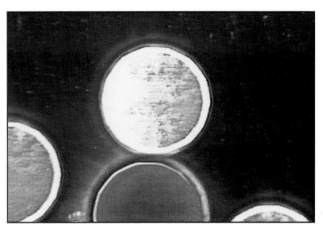

Figure 3-23b.
Asymmetrical ablation test pattern 5 mm. Pattern is unacceptable for surgery as sweeping pattern demonstrates energy difference between left and right sides of test plate of several pulses (>10%).

ablating a -4.00 D PRK correction. The achieved correction is read on a lensometer subjectively. The test plastic is also examined with a magnifier for ablation quality. This process can be difficult and time consuming if the fluence requires adjustment. The ablation rate or depth of cut per pulse is also adjusted based upon the degree of preoperative myopia correction targeted from a nomogram. The VisX STAR has a more sophisticated and automated calibration system which eliminates many of the concerns of the earlier system.

The important message to be gained is that these lasers must be recalibrated between cases, since results depend upon their functioning and gas excimer lasers have variable energy output.

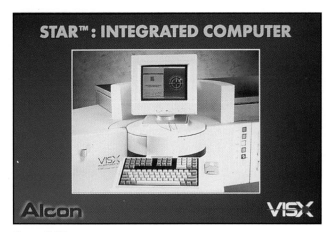

Figure 3-24.
VisX STAR integrated computer monitor and keyboard which can be positioned for surgeon or technician.

OPERATIVE STEPS AND PRINCIPLES

PROGRAMMING THE LASER

Once the patient is prepared and the laser calibrated, the planned treatment must be programmed. The cycloplegic refraction is corrected for vertex distance and entered into the computer (Figure 3-24). Some surgeons have found their laser system requires a fudge factor to improve refractive predictability. In particular, some surgeons using the Summit ExciMed and OmniMed systems input as little as 70% of the target correction to avoid overcorrections and achieve improved refractive efficacy. Other surgeons routinely use their fogged manifest refraction. It is important with all nomograms to minimize the degree of myopia, as undercorrections are far more easily managed than overcorrections. Cylinder magnitude is usually maximized by the refractionist, as it is typically undercorrected by most laser systems. Cylinder magnitude and axis should reflect not only the cycloplegic refraction, but it must be balanced with the corneal topography, manifest refraction, and spectacles worn.

COMMON OUTCOMES

The method by which the surgeon achieves the attempted correction is not as important as the fact that the surgery is repeated the same way for each patient so that the nomogram can be adjusted. That is, if a surgeon always discovers that he or she achieves a slight undercorrection he or she may be pleased or may increase his or her target correction slightly. More importantly, overcorrections can be similarly adjusted for by decreasing the attempted correction. Most patients prefer to be plano, even those over 40 years of age.

Example 1:

Cycloplegic refraction	-6.00 -1.25 x 180 20/20
Manifest refraction	-6.25 -1.75 x 170 20/20
Spectacle Rx	-6.00 -1.00 x 170 20/30 + 1.5 years old
Corneal topography	2.00 D of minus cylinder at 170
Attempted correction	-6.00 -1.75 x 170

Attempted correction reflects the least minus sphere from the cycloplegic refraction, the greater cylinder magnitude on manifest refraction and topography leads us to utilize the greater cylinder magnitude measured and the axis of 170 is consistent with not only the corneal topography but the manifest and spectacle refraction.

Example 2:

Cycloplegic refraction	-6.00 -1.25 x 180 20/20
Manifest refraction	-6.25 -1.75 x 170 20/20
Spectacle Rx	-6.00 -1.00 x 170 20/30 + 1.5 years old
Corneal topography	1.00 D of minus cylinder at 180
Attempted correction	-6.00 -1.25 x 180

The attempted correction reflects the cycloplegic refraction directly, as it remains the most consistent with the topography cylinder magnitude and axis, and provides us with the least spherical target correction.

Example 3:

Cycloplegic refraction	-6.00 -1.25 x 180 20/20
Manifest refraction	-6.25 -1.75 x 170 20/20
Spectacle Rx	-6.00 -1.00 x 170 20/30 + 1.5 years old
Corneal topography	spherical cornea
Attempted correction	-6.00 -1.00 x 175

Once again, the least minus sphere is attempted, while the cylinder magnitude reflects the spherical cornea. Despite the spherical cornea, one still corrects the cylinder as it is clinically evident both in the spectacles and upon refraction. Although the anterior corneal curvature may be spherical, posterior corneal or lenticular cylinder must be present and requires correction. The axis planned is intermediate between the manifest and cycloplegic refraction, as the spectacle refraction tends to concur with the manifest refraction.

Example 4:

Cycloplegic refraction	-6.00 D 20/20
Manifest refraction	-6.25 D 20/20
Spectacle Rx	-5.50 D 20/30 +
	2.5 years old
Corneal topography	1.00 D of minus cylinder
	at 180
Attempted correction	-6.00 D

The cycloplegic refraction is treated, as the corneal topography is merely one of three factors in the net manifest cylinder. Be aware, however, that postoperative with-the-rule cylinder may be manifest.

When looking at a skyline, one cannot perceive the small buildings, however, if the skyscrapers are demolished, the small buildings are readily apparent. In much the same way, cylinder can be seen to manifest once myopia is reduced or eliminated.

Example 5:

Cycloplegic refraction	-6.00 -0.50 x 180 20/20
Manifest refraction	-6.25 -0.25 x 180 20/20
Spectacle Rx	-5.75 D 20/30
	+ 2.5 years old
Corneal topography	1.00 D of minus cylinder
	at 180
Attempted correction	-6.00 -0.50 x 180 D

The small amount of cylinder is treated in this example, as the axis is consistent with the corneal topographical map.

Example 6:

Cycloplegic refraction	-6.00 -0.50 x 180 20/20
Manifest refraction	-6.25 -0.25 x 180 20/20
Spectacle Rx	-5.75 D 20/30
	+ 2.5 years old
Corneal topography	1.00 D of minus cylinder
	at 90
Attempted correction	-6.25 D

The small amount of cylinder is not treated, as the axis is inconsistent with the topographical map.

However, overcorrections in presbyopic individuals are not well tolerated and a more conservative approach is always warranted for these individuals.

Monovision should be discussed and planned for accordingly whenever possible. The amount of monovision targeted should be conservative, as most myopic patients primarily desire excellent distance acuity. Accordingly, 1.50 D or less of monovision is optimal with most preferring 0.75 or 1.00 D undercorrection. Monovision undercorrection should be performed in the non-dominant eye.

Age is another factor which must be considered in programming the attempted correction, as not only are presbyopic individuals less tolerant of an overcorrection, but they may experience less myopic regression than expected. That is, the ablation performed for any given correction compensates for the normal amount of regression that occurs during the healing process by performing a slight overcorrection, and older patients may experience less regression than younger myopes. In patients over 50 years, many surgeons typically target -0.50 D undercorrection. Depending upon the laser system, a greater undercorrection may be targeted at an even younger age. Gaussian energy beam profile laser systems like the Summit ExciMed, and to a lesser degree the OmniMed series, are more likely to produce an overcorrection in a older patient.

ALGORITHM PRINCIPLES

The ablation software for broad beam excimer lasers no longer use a single zone spherical correction for myopia but rather a multizone or aspheric approach. Scanning excimer laser systems which remove tissue with a less than 2-mm spot size do not have the same limitations with respect to ablation profile or beam homogeneity and central island formation. The advantage of broad beam lasers relative to scanning lasers are that they are more forgiving of minor decentrations and do not require an eyetracking system or eyecup fixation device. Scanning lasers also require a very high repetition rate. Broad beam excimer laser systems do require that certain principles must be applied to maximize clinical results.

Compensation for Central Island Formation: Pretreatment Technique

In general, homogeneous broad beam lasers will all produce a central undercorrection or central island if the optical zone utilized is 6 mm or larger and the cornea is not dehydrated. The diameter and depth or height of the central island is proportional to the amount of treatment attempted with single zone techniques. Therefore, the ablation pattern used must compensate for central island formation. Gaussian beam profile lasers which have a greater energy density centrally are less likely to produce an island (see Chapter 5).

An aspheric program which applies more treatment centrally and tapers out peripherally will compensate for the central undercorrection; however, single zone techniques require some additional central treatment, also known as pretreatment. Pretreatment is the application of additional pulses to the central cornea in addition to the full refractive correction which is based upon a theoretical lenticular curve, to compensate for the hydrated nature of the cornea.

> **Pretreatment is the application of additional pulses to the central cornea in addition to the full refractive correction, which is based upon a theoretical lenticular curve, to compensate for the hydrated nature of the cornea.**

Multizone techniques reduce the need for pretreatment. The amount of pretreatment required is based upon multiple factors outlined below.

Pretreatment should be performed at 2.5 mm for 6-mm optical zones and 3.0 mm for 7.0-mm optical zones. The amount of pretreatment is approximately 1 micron per diopter of attempted correction plus or minus a factor based upon the parameters listed. Pretreatment can occur at any point within the procedure, not just immediately preoperatively as the name implies. The advantage of performing pretreatment immediately prior to the refractive treatment is that it will be blended into the entire treatment and the hydration status of the stroma will be more uniform.

> **Ten Factors Defining the Amount of Pretreatment**
> 1. Single zone vs. multizone vs. aspheric
> 2. Size of optical zone(s) utilized
> 3. Total dioptric correction
> 4. Amount of dioptric correction 6.0 mm or greater
> 5. Technique of epithelial removal
> 6. Amount of cylinder correction
> 7. Presence of plume vacuum or blowing device
> 8. Use of intraoperative wiping or drying technique
> 9. Duration of procedure
> 10. Energy beam profile or macrohomogeneity of laser system

Pretreatment not only prevents central islands but improves qualitative vision. The pretreatment step does not have a refractive effect unless it is excessive.

Multizone Technique Parameters

Multizone techniques divide the refractive error into multiple steps, thereby reducing the total depth of ablation and maximizing the optical zone size provided. A single optical zone of 6.0 to 6.5 mm can be utilized for corrections up to -1.50 D, as the depth of ablation is small and the incidence of night glare low. Multiple zones should be utilized for all prescriptions above -1.50 D. The multizone technique is one which provides specific advantages for broad beam delivery system lasers. The ablation effect of the aspheric or one-step multizone technique is greater centrally than calculated, as the iris diaphragm remains small longer centrally, creating a drying effect and increasing its effectiveness centrally, preventing central islands. The advantage to multizone over an aspheric program, which also concentrates the treatment centrally with a peripheral transition curve, is the application of the multiple zones which blend one zone into the next to improve wound contour and smoothness. The optical zones should be treated in order of increasing size so

> **Multizones for myopia correction and multicylinder techniques improve wound contour and blending, reducing haze and regression.**

as to blend the preceding zone and improve the wound edge profile. Therefore, not only does each pulse blend the preceding smaller diameter pulse within the same zone, but each zone blends the preceding zone.

In terms of myopia correction, so long as the central portion is treated greater than the peripheral cornea, myopia correction will occur. However, a contracting iris diaphragm delivery system or treating the central zone last will result in ridges or steps on the stromal surface because of a lack of blending. This non-uniformity invites haze formation and regression. Hence, an important principle in understanding nomogram development is to improve blending and wound contour, and therefore always expand the treatment areas.

The multi-multizone technique I developed for the Chiron Technolas, introduced to North America in Summer 1993, is similar in concept to the multipass/multizone technique introduced a little later by another experienced Canadian ophthalomogist, Mihai Pop, MD, with his VisX 20/20 laser system. Dr. Pop is also the innovator for the corrective uphill decentration (CUD) technique to treat asymmetric astigmatism. The multi-multizone technique involved treating several zones of increasing size starting with a 3.0-mm pretreatment zone and ending with a 7.0-mm blend zone. A typical moderate myope would be treated with 3.0-, 4.0-, 5.0-, 6.0-, and 7.0-mm zones in increasing order. Higher myopes and toric ablations involved as many as nine zones. Both techniques provide identical blending, with each zone reblending the contour. That is, the dioptric correction is similarly divided into multiple zones, with zones of increasing size. The multipass/multizone technique pioneered by Dr. Pop also involved performing larger zones at the same size as previous zones to improve blending.

Multi-Multizone Machat	Multipass/Multizone Pop
• Multiple zones	• Multiple zones
• Zones of increasing size	• Zones of increasing and equal size
• Maximal blending	• Maximal blending
• Maximal optical zone size	• Maximal optical zone size
• Submaximal glare reduction	• Maximal glare reduction
• Minimal depth of ablation	• Increased depth of ablation
• Maximally blended wound edge	• Submaximally blended wound edge

For example, a -6.00 D patient may be treated with the multipass/multizone technique by ablating -2.00 D at 4 mm, -1.50 D at 5 mm, -1.50 D at 6 mm, followed by another -1.00 D at 6 mm. The repetition of two passes at the same optical zone invites two theoretical problems with this approach, although clinically they appear equivalent. The first theoretical problem is that the objective of the multizone approach is to limit the depth of ablation while maximizing the diameter of the optical zone. The treatment of two zones of equal size fails to reduce the depth of ablation, as a greater proportion of treatment is performed at a large optical zone. The second theoretical problem is that the wound edge profile is less blended since the final optical zone merely overlaps the preceding zone. If the second last zone were to be slightly smaller than the maximum optical zone diameter, 5.5 mm even, the depth of ablation would be reduced by several microns and the final zone would blend the wound edge contour better. The importance of the smoothness of the wound edge profile is the prevention of arcuate haze. The primary distinct advantage of repeating

the largest optical zone is improved night vision by maximizing the effectiveness of the largest optical zone, which may in itself be a valuable tool in patients with larger pupils.

The important conclusion to be drawn is that there is an understanding that is heightened with the performance of PRK, and that understanding can help develop innovative techniques and software to improve wound contour and clincal results. Similarly, newer techniques and software seem to identify and evolve in one direction even without a coordinated effort as certain principles become identified. The similarities between the multi-multizone and multipass/multizone techniques are of greater importance than the differences in identifying the fundamental wound edge contour principles upon which both are based. Dr. Don Johnson currently utilizes a transepithelial approach combined with the multipass/multizone technique with his VisX laser system with improved clinical outcomes.

Treatment Steps

The dioptric input for each zone should be based upon obtaining an equivalent depth of ablation (ie, each depth per zone). That is, we tend to think in diopters rather than in microns, which may possess greater meaning to the cornea. The cornea in effect needs to be resculpted with the desired contour as smoothly as possible to reduce the effects of wound healing. We are attempting to achieve a new curvature; the dioptric correction programmed merely provides us a means of defining that new curvature. We must address the correction in terms of the number of microns we must remove from each point, much the same way that future scanning delivery systems will.

It appears clinically that the ideal depth per step is about 15 microns. If greater than 20 microns is removed per zone, there appears to be increased regression as the smoothness of the contour is reduced; that is, the steps are too big. Conversely, if less than 10 microns is removed with each zone of multizone ablation, the effect is partially lost—the step is too small to have a significant clinical impact on the resultant contour. This is observed particularly at larger diameters which fail peripherally to impact the corneal topography, resulting in increased night glare. It must be recognized that with myopic ablations, the depth of ablation defined is that centrally, and the peripheral depth of ablation is far less. It appears that a certain depth is required to overcome the hydration effects of the cornea, which is particularly evident when ablating intrastromally where the cornea is more hydrated.

Other techniques can be used for controlling the hydra-

The Multipass/Multizone PRK Technique to Correct Myopia and Astigmatism

Mihai Pop, MD

Undesirable effects, such as haze, regression, and poor quality of ablation, have always been challenges to good corrections for all levels of myopia and astigmatism, especially when myopia exceeds 6 D. Some investigators in the area of high myopia have concluded that PRK was not the best approach to effectively correct vision with the types of lasers and software available.

Two discoveries in the meantime have challenged this assumption. First, a multizone technique was developed to decrease the ablation depth for lasers treating surfaces of diameter larger than 5 mm. Second, it was noted that the smoothness of the ablation tended to decrease the production of scar tissue.

The way the VisX 20/20 produces the ablation still leaves a surface rigged with a series of small concentric steps (Figure A-1A). Scar tissue can thus be deposited in those microscopic ridges and produce a visible corneal haze. In 1993, we developed new algorithms to address this issue. By dividing the treatment into a series of mini-treatments of 10 to 20 seconds duration at different ablation diameters, a technique we call multipass/multizone, we are able to smooth the surface (Figures A-1B and A-1C).

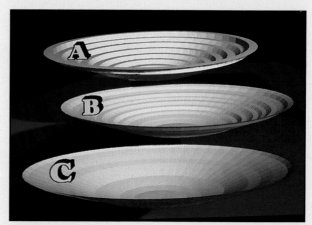

Figure A-1.
A represents single zone, single pass with diaphragmatic ridges. **B** and **C** illustrate smoothing with multiple passes.

INTENDED CORRECTION				
% of Eyes at 6 Months				
Groups	**± 2D**	**± 1D**	**± 0.5D**	**Number of Eyes**
Low myopia	100%	95.5%	84.8%	145
Moderate myopia	91.3%	84.8%	65.2%	92
High myopia	78.4%	59.5%	37.9%	37

Mihai Pop, M.D.   V.50616

Table A-1.
Comparison of results obtained of good correction at ± 1 D at 6 months.

An analysis of our 315 first eyes done using the MP-PRK technique shows that there is a minimal amount of haze produced. One month after surgery, the mean haze was at trace level, 0.5 on a scale from 0 to 4, and was not significantly different between low, moderate, and high myopia. The only difference was in the rate of disappearance, which is slower for high myopia.

A comparison between our results of good correction at ±1 D at 6 months and results obtained in other centers demonstrates that our patients have between 10% and 20% more chance of being in the right range of the intended correction in myopia exceeding 6 D (Table A-1).

Further research is being done to evaluate long-term effects. But present results challenge the assumption that other techniques, such as LASIK, are more appropriate for high myopia; PRK can be a less demanding method, resulting in fewer complications.

tion status of the cornea, such as wiping with a spatula during PRK (Figure 3-25) or air drying during laser in situ keratomileusis (LASIK). The ideal central depth of ablation per zone for PRK is in the range of 15 to 20 microns. The number of zones utilized should be such that each zone removes 15 to 20 microns. A 60 micron ablation for the correction of moderate myopia can have three to four zones, divided equally from the 2.5- to 3.0-mm pretreatment zone to the 6.0- to 7.0-mm blend zone.

Advanced Treatment Options: Patients With Large Pupils

Understanding that patients with large pupils are at higher risk for night visual disturbances enables us to reformulate our treatment parameters with certain laser systems. It is beneficial to increase the treatment at the largest optical zone diameter in an attempt to minimize night glare, despite the fact that the overall depth of ablation will be greater. That is, increasing the 6.0-mm zone from 15 micron depth to perhaps 20 micron depth. A second option is not merely to alter the dioptric distribution, increasing the treatment performed at 6.0 mm or greater, but to alter the zone distribution. That is, if each zone step remains at 15 microns, but instead of evenly distributing the same six zones every 0.6 mm at 3.0, 3.6, 4.2, 4.8, 5.4, and 6.0 mm, applying them at 3.0, 4.2, 5.4, 5.6, 5.8, and 6.0 mm. In this manner, the induced topographical change will demonstrate effective flattening for 6.0 mm, which is usually more than adequate to limit the development of any night glare. It is important to remember that as large optical zone ablation is increased with broad beam excimer laser systems, the amount of pretreatment or central correction should be increased accordingly to avoid central island formation.

Clinical Note

Double Pretreatment Application for the Management of Forme Fruste Keratoconus

Decentering the entire treatment or portions of it, as in the corrective uphill decentration (CUD) technique proposed by Mihai Pop, is said to be quite effective for the management of forme fruste keratoconus, but risks side effects associated with decentration. The CUD technique treats the patient based upon a curvature map derived from videokeratography. Despite the fact that these patients have an asymmetric videokeratographic picture of their cylinder, they are typically corrected to 20/20 with normal, well-centered spectacles, suggesting that treatment should perhaps still be applied centrally and not decentered.

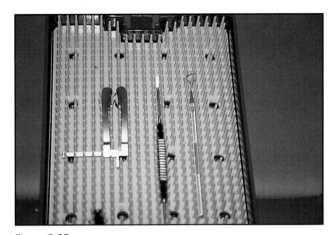

Figure 3-25.
PRK basic instrument tray includes 6-mm optical zone marker, blunt paton spatula, and solid blade eyelid speculum.

The technique I developed for treating forme fruste keratoconus is a variation of my pretreatment technique for central island prevention. In cases of asymmetrical astigmatism where there is inferior steepening (Figure 3-26), I apply a pretreatment application of pulses to the peak of the "cone", followed by the standard pretreatment application centrally. The steep area is treated first to allow blending of that area by the remaining application of pulses. The remaining treatment is unchanged and is not decentered. The amount of pretreatment applied is proportional to the intended dioptric correction and is the same inferiorly and centrally. That is, the standard procedure and pretreatment is applied centrally but is preceded by an additional pretreatment which is first applied over the steepest area denoted on preoperative videokeratography. I found this double pretreatment technique to be effective in improving qualitative vision and postoperative videokeratography (Figure 3-27). No side effects or complications have been associated. In this manner, the treatment remains well-centered, but the asymmetry of the videokeratography is still addressed.

PATIENT POSITIONING AND PREPARATION

Once the laser is programmed, the patient can be brought into the laser suite. Minimizing the actual time the patient is beneath the laser helps alleviate anxiety, thus all preparation of the laser should be performed prior to the arrival of each patient. The first routine check should be to confirm patient name and operative eye. If the non-dominant eye is to be treated on a presbyopic patient, the question of

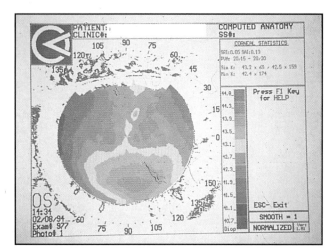

Figure 3-26.
Preoperative corneal videokeratography map of forme fruste keratoconus.

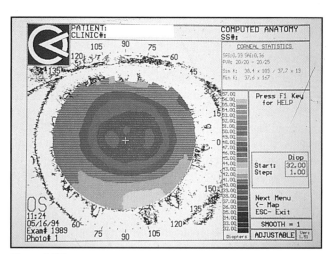

Figure 3-27.
Post-operative corneal videokeratography map of forme fruste keratoconus treated with double pretreatment technique.

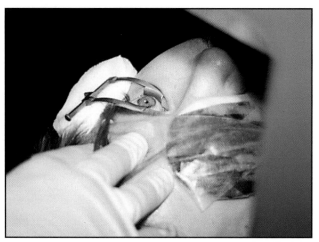

Figure 3-28.
Operative preparation for left eye PRK procedure with eyelid speculum, taped eyelid pad and right eye covered with opaque eyeshield.

targeting monovision or not should be verified.

The head should be aligned and eye perpendicular to the path of the laser beam. We have discovered that the beam output is more stable if the room is maintained at a lower ambient temperature of about 60°F or 18°C. It is helpful to have a blanket for the patient available, both for warmth and security. We also encourage one family member to enter the laser suite and accompany the patient to reduce severe anxiety. Although this presents other problems with respect to efficiency and sterility, it has been instrumental in many difficult cases. Each facility must develop a policy.

The fellow eye should be covered, ideally with a solid eye shield instead of a pressure patch. This allows the patient to keep both eyes open during the procedure to avoid

a Bell's phenomenon in the operative eye. The first step is to instill additional anesthetic, particularly to the upper fornix where the least amount of anesthetic is received. The fear of pain is the greatest concern to patients at this time and creates the most anxiety, so addressing this concern immediately helps to improve cooperation. An anesthetic-soaked surgical spear (see Figure 3-5) placed beneath the upper eyelid as the patient is requested to look down is of greatest benefit as it is the upper blade of the eyelid speculum that most patients sense when not fully anesthetized. Topical anesthetic in the fellow eye is useful in cases of blepharospasm.

Eyelid Speculum

Once the patient is positioned beneath the laser and the operative eye aligned, an eyelid speculum should be inserted (Figure 3-28). It is preferable to use a rigid and adjustable eyelid speculum rather than wire to prevent the patient from squeezing against it, resulting in the operating eye rolling up. A solid blade is also best to keep eyelashes away from the operative field. The patient should be instructed to look above his or her head toward the surgeon when inserting the lower blade and toward his or her feet and when inserting the upper blade beneath the upper lid. If the patient complains of discomfort, anesthetize the fornices once again with a surgical spear soaked in topical anesthetic for a few seconds. It is important to minimize any discomfort as patients who squeeze against the eyelid speculum will roll their eyes and affect not only centration but allow tears to contact the denuded stroma. The alteration of the the hydration status of the ablative surface will reduce refractive pre-

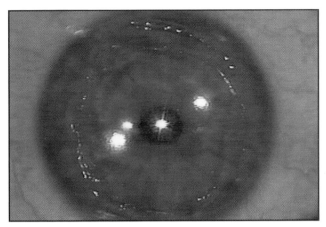

Figure 3-29.
Intraoperative view of cornea during alignment of PRK procedure. The central red reflex represents the pupil center, which coincides in this patient with the visual axis. A brighter reflex is achieved with proper alignment for both the patient and surgeon. The Chiron Technolas alignment system directs a green helium-neon light from the right side which intersects the well-aligned red fixation light at the corneal plane and transmits through to the iris plane, which is visible to the left of the visual axis. The dual microscope lights illuminate the eye from the nasal and temporal aspects, producing the two other white corneal light reflexes.

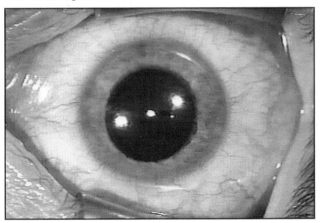

Figure 3-30b.
Proper alignment of the eye under medium magnification demonstrating perpendicular alignment of the eye and head.

dictability, producing undercorrections, and create abnormal topography if the surface is irregularly hydrated.

Marking the Optical Zone

There is a continuing controversy as to whether PRK should be centered about the unconstricted pupil or the visual axis (Figures 3-29 through 3-30e). I believe that the unconstricted pupil is probably a wiser choice; however, if there is a great disparity between the two, a slight shift toward the visual axis is best. The reason for the pupillary entrance being best is that unlike the multifocal topography

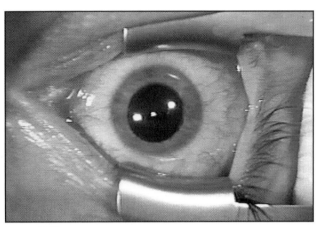

Figure 3-30a.
Alignment of the eye is one of the few critical components of the PRK procedure. Proper alignment of the eye under low magnification demonstrating perpendicular alignment of the eye and head. Note the equal amounts of sclera exposed above and below the cornea from the surgeon's perspective.

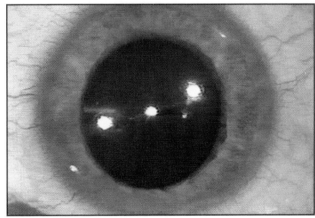

Figure 3-30c.
Proper alignment of the eye under high magnification demonstrating perpendicular alignment of the eye and head.

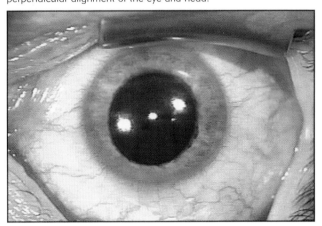

Figure 3-30d.
Occasionally, a patient will elevate his or her chin and become misaligned. A small amount of pressure on the patient's forehead helps stabilize the head in the proper position.

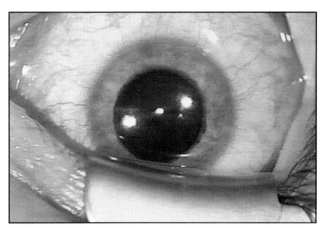

Figure 3-30e.
More commonly, a patient will depress his or her chin and become misaligned. Again, a small amount of pressure on the patient's forehead helps stabilize the head in the proper position.

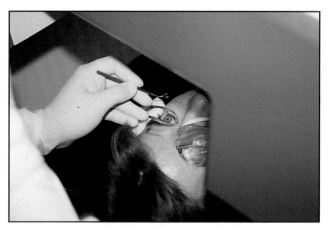

Figure 3-31.
Marking of optical zone during left eye PRK procedure.

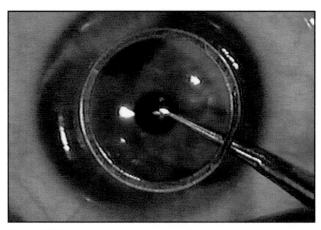

Figure 3-32a.
Demarcation of the optical zone during PRK

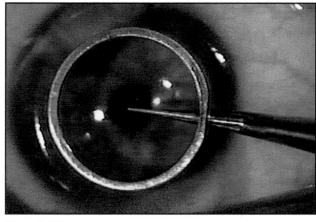

Figure 3-32b.
Initial rotation of the optical zone marker clockwise in a cookie-cutter fashion to incise the epithelium and provide a smoother edge for both debridement and re-epithelialization.

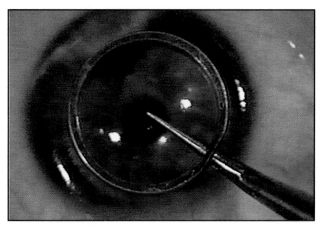

Figure 3-32c.
Final rotation of the optical zone marker counter-clockwise in a cookie-cutter fashion to incise the epithelium and provide a smoother edge for both debridement and re-epithelialization.

of radial keratotomy (RK), PRK ideally creates a large homogenous circular ablation pattern so that small shifts in decentration are clinically insignificant. A pupil that expands beyond the ablative zone will create halos if symmetric, crescents of glare if asymmetric, and if significant, monocular diplopia can be created. Therefore, it becomes more significant to center around the pupil than the visual axis for PRK.

One trick for efficient and rapid epithelial debridement is to aggressively incise the cornea with the optical zone marker (Figure 3-31); that is, a cookie cutter rotation of the optical zone marker while providing firm pressure (Figures 3-32a through 3-32c). This creates sharp epithelial edges for more efficient removal and faster re-epithelialization. The

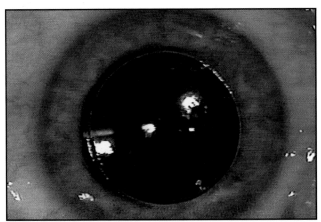

Figure 3-33.
Optical zone demarcation at 6 mm, equal to largest ablation diameter. Epithelium is incised with optical zone marker to create smooth edges.

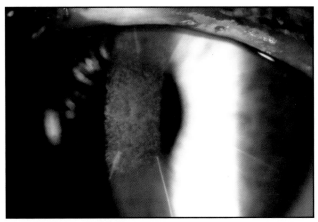

Figure 3-34.
Uncomplicated PRK performed for residual myopia following eight-incision RK, subsequently developing central confluent haze. Courtesy of Dr. R. Bruce Grene.

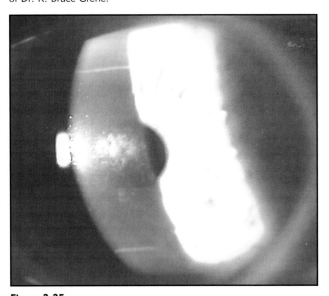

Figure 3-35.
Combined AK and PRK treatment of compound myopic astigmatism. Patient was treated with AK 1 month prior to spherical PRK. Patient developed focal area of dense confluent haze postoperatively.

optical zone marker itself should be equal to the largest optical zone size ablated, and not 0.5 to 1.0 mm larger as is sometimes recommended. This principle is based on the fact that recurrent corneal erosions can be produced in any area that is mechanically debrided and not ablated. Also discussed in Chapter 5, corneal erosions post-PRK tend to occur within a 1.0-mm ring outside the area of ablation but within the area of epithelial debridement. Photoablation is an excellent therapeutic modality for the treatment of recurrent corneal erosions, therefore, the surgeon should avoid creating a larger surgical abrasion than that which is ablated.

Removal of the Epithelium

There are many methods by which the epithelium may be removed, including mechanical, laser, and chemical means as listed below. Mechanical debridement (Figure 3-33) may be sharp or blunt debridement, performed with either a surgical blade or spatula. Laser removal of the epithelial layer or a transepithelial PTK approach may be performed. The transepithelial approach may be used to remove the entire 50 to 55 micron depth of the epithelial layer or partial depth of about 40 microns with the last 10 microns or so removed mechanically. Therefore, a transepithelial approach may be referred to as either with or without mechanical debridement. The final option involves chemical debridement or assist, using 5% to 25% alcohol or even 4% cocaine.

My personal preference is for blunt mechanical debridement for primary procedures and repeat PRK for residual myopia correction without clinically significant haze. A transepithelial approach for repeat PRK to correct residual

> **Methods of Epithelial Removal**
> - Mechanical debridement: blunt or sharp
> - Transepithelial removal: with or without epithelial debridement
> - Chemical debridement: alcohol 5% to 25% or cocaine 4%

myopia associated with clinically significant haze is preferable. Epithelial debridment following RK presents additional challenges and care must be taken to avoid opening healed RK incisions (see Clinical Note).

Figure 3-36.
Mild reticular haze with area of confluence observed along superotemporal RK incisions following PRK treatment of residual myopic astigmatism.

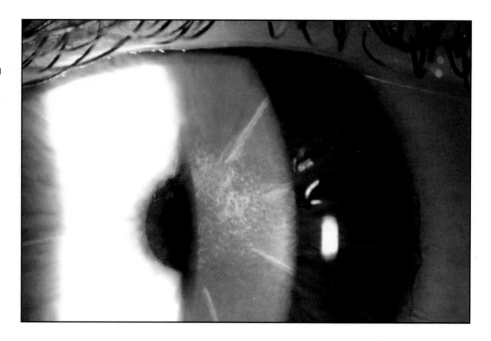

PRK and RK

I have performed about 180 RK enhancements with PRK, including 57 eyes that required one or more retreatments, 12 required two retreatments, five required three retreatments, and one required four retreatments for regression with confluent haze. The incidence of clinically significant haze ranged from 5% to 8% depending upon the technique and laser system utilized (Figures 3-34 through 3-36). This incidence is surprisingly high considering that the overwhelming majority of these patients had a residual myopic refractive error of less than 3.00 D. The incidence of haze and need for retreatment were reduced as technique improved. Loss of best corrected vision of two or more lines was approximately 2% and was secondary to dense haze and irregular astigmatism (Figures 3-37a through 3-38). Collagen plaque formation was amenable to treatment with a 70% to 80% success rate as indicated above. Irregular astigmatism following RK was not amenable to PRK with any technique.

RK patients with smaller optical zones and a greater number of incisions represented a unique subset of RK patients and experienced a higher incidence of confluent haze, regression, irregular astigmatism, and poor refractive predictability (Figure 3-39). I had one patient referred to me with a 16-incision RK and 2.25-mm optical zone with an original refractive error of -11.00 D who required five PRK procedures for recurrent haze and regression.

I had two presbyopic female RK patients treated only once who became measurably hyperopic in the range of 2.00 to 3.00 D, despite targeting an undercorrection. Topical steroids were discontinued to produce regression of effect, but haze formation ensued, reducing qualitative and best corrected vision. This situation of hyperopia, haze, and RK incisions remains the most difficult challenge as treatment of the haze requires further surface ablation and produces increased hyperopia. Procedures for hyperopia management in these cases are difficult as holmium laser thermokeratoplasty (LTK) may potentially open the RK incisions and produce irregular and regular astigmatism. Automated lamellar keratoplasty (ALK) for hyperopia is less predictable post-RK and post-PRK since it would have to be performed on a thinner cornea as well. The Grene Lasso, developed by R. Bruce Grene, MD, could potentially be performed following surface ablation to clear the haze, however, this would be a temporary measure while the suture remained in place. Future hyperopic PRK techniques may be long-term solutions but haze recurrence is likely. PTK techniques which could remove haze while not producing increased hyperopia are possible by scanning limbus to limbus and removing an equal amount of tissue from the entire surface (Paolo Vinciguerra, Aesculap-Meditec). Hyperopic LASIK software is under development and refinement and shows great promise in reversing hyperopia in these challenging cases, as well in virgin corneas.

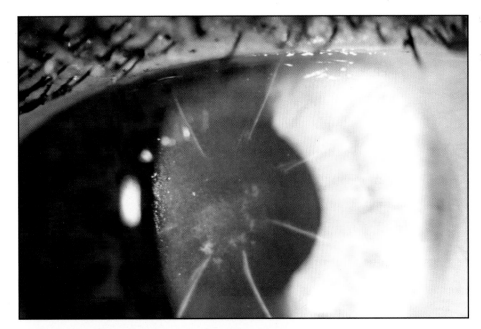

Figure 3-37a.
Focal 2-mm area of confluent central haze under medium magnification observed 6 months post-PRK for the treatment of residual myopia following RK.

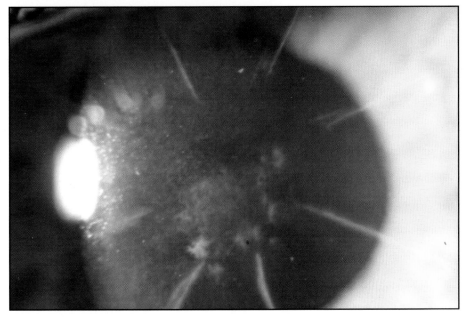

Figure 3-37b.
Focal 2-mm area of confluent central haze under high magnification observed 6 months post-PRK for the treatment of residual myopia following RK.

In both hyperopic RK cases, I re-instituted topical flu-orometholone 0.1% once or twice daily and titrated steroids carefully over 2 to 3 months to stabilize the regression pattern with as little as one drop per week. Once stabilized, although the qualitative vision was still poor, the natural course of confluent haze is to clear gradually over 1 to 3 years. It has been over 1 year and both patients have improved considerably from 3+ haze to 1+ haze. Best corrected visual acuity is reduced by two lines in each patient and uncorrected vision is similar at 20/50 and 20/60.

Important aspects of treating patients for residual refractive errors post-RK are to counsel and select candidates carefully. Intraoperatively, a transepithelial approach or gentle blunt debridement is acceptable. Do not be surprised if the epithelium is unusually thick centrally, as epithelial hyperplasia can occur following RK in response to corneal flattening. Be careful not to ablate too deep peripherally; stroma is encountered peripherally first with a transepithelial approach, as this will incite crescentic haze formation. Mechanical debridement must avoid opening healed RK incisions and the blunt spatula should

Figure 3-38.
Confluent areas of haze developing post-PRK treatment of undercorrected RK upon withdrawal of topical steroids. Once confluent haze develops, reinstitution of steroids will not reverse this process. Rapid refractive shift toward emmetropia, in association with increasing reticular haze, should be managed with a much more gradual steroid taper over 6 months.

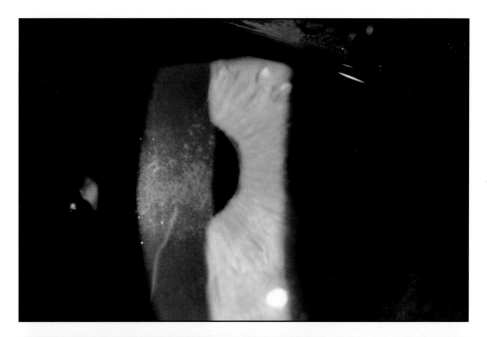

Figure 3-39.
Dense confluent haze developing in patient with 16-incision RK following PRK treatment of residual myopia. Note the healing of the RK incisions and small optical zone, both risk factors for confluent haze development.

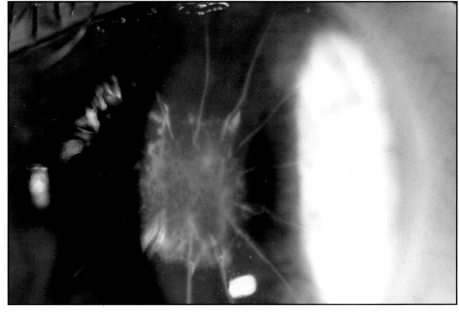

be maintained parallel to the incisions. I typically start to debride centrally within the clear optical zone in patients with RK and then extend the defect between the RK incisions. Lastly, I will attempt to clear the intervening epithelium from along the incisions but I much prefer to leave a little epithelium than to disturb the incisions. It is important to have a relatively moist stroma intraoperatively, as a dehydrated stroma also incites haze formation. A 6.0-mm or larger optical zone is recommended, as is a multizone approach to improve blending. An undercorrection should

always be targeted and the surgery based upon an early morning cycloplegic refraction. Postoperatively, never discontinue topical steroids abruptly as haze will ensue. Should significant hyperopia be evident, it may be related to a thinner epithelial layer in the early postoperative period, and tapering steroids rapidly to even once daily may be sufficient. Monitor very closely, and once regression to +1.00 D occurs, increase steroids to bid or more to restabilize the healing process. It should also be remembered that irregular astigmatism in the immediate postoperative

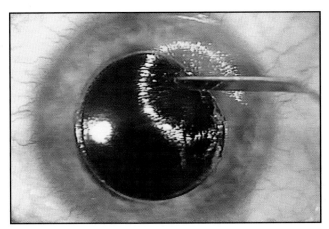

Figure 3-40a.
Technique of blunt mechanical epithelial debridement demonstrating initial starting point along optical zone mark.

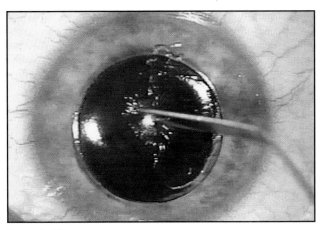

Figure 3-40b.
Blunt spatula is held at an acute angle, roughly 70°, during epithelial removal.

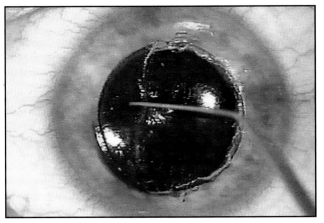

Figure 3-40c.
Rapid vertical strokes across optical zone along leading edge of debrided epithelium speeds removal.

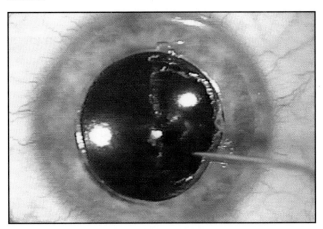

Figure 3-40d.
Careful removal of epithelium circumferentially along optical zone mark with special care taken to avoid removal of epithelium outside of demarcated area.

period results in a hyperopic refraction and ciliary spasm or a central island produces a myopic refraction, with all three clearing over time.

RK patients typically achieve improved uncorrected vision, reduced night glare, and many patients have even commented upon reduced fluctuation following PRK treatment of their residual refractive errors. The reduction of their residual refractive error is responsible for most of their subjective improvement, but reduced fluctuation may also be related to a hyperplastic epithelium increasing corneal stability. Overall, patient satisfaction is high, and with improved techniques and careful postoperative monitoring over 90% of RK patients with one or more procedures will achieve 20/40 or better visual acuity.

Blunt Debridement

Blunt debridement is recommended because of less trauma to Bowman's layer compared to sharp debridement. Sharp instrumentation has been shown to leave less residual epithelial debris and tends to be faster for inexperienced surgeons. Epithelial debridement, although not difficult, is more technique-oriented than is immediately apparent. The angle of the blunt paton spatula is important in the speed of removal. The epithelium along the edge of the incised optical zone provides a useful starting point. There is no benefit clinically in removing the central epithelium last, as this will if anything keep the central stroma more hydrated and increase the potential for central islands. Starting at the edge of the incised optical zone, rapidly debride the epithelium with vertical strokes across the visual axis. For a right-handed surgeon, debriding from right to left (Figure 3-40a) is

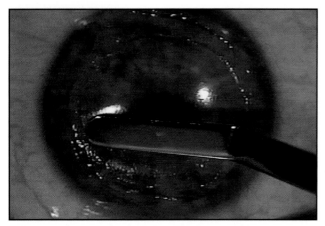

Figure 3-40e.
Following epithelium removal, the blunt spatula is passed parallel to the stromal surface in even strokes to provide a more even level of stromal hydration and to remove any residual epithelium.

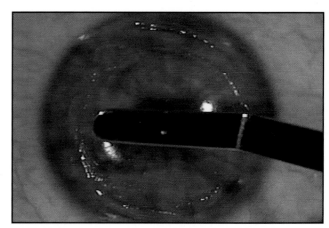

Figure 3-40f.
Following each stroke or pass, the spatula is cleaned with sterile gauze to avoid re-implantation of epithelial debris within the ablative zone.

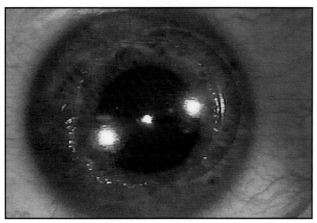

Figure 3-41.
Epithelial debridement should leave a smooth stromal surface with no epithelial remnants or damage to Bowman's layer, as the laser will accurately reproduce the presented surface. Note the crisp light reflex indicating a good preoperative surface for PRK. The stromal hydration status of the stroma should also be homogeneous.

most convenient, and conversely from left to right for left-handed surgeons. The spatula should be angled acutely at about 70° (Figure 3-40b) for this step and should be passed specifically along the advancing epithelial edge (Figure 3-40c). Controlled rapid passes are most efficient and a finger from the opposite hand can be used to better control the spatula. Once all the epithelium is removed, the spatula must be supported more horizontally, parallel to the stromal surface, to wipe the remaining debris out of the ablative region with even strokes. In this manner, corneal hydration is more evenly controlled and the ablative area smoothed. Epithelium remaining within the marked optical zone along the edges should be debrided carefully (Figures 3-40d

through 3-40f) to avoid enlarging the optical zone. Peripheral epithelial debris can be removed with a surgical spear. A dry surgical spear should not be used on the denuded stromal surface as it will create scratches which will be reproduced with submicron precision by the excimer laser. A blunt spatula is preferable for this reason.

It is important to continue to reassure the patient throughout the debridement procedure (Figure 3-41) as this is the most disconcerting portion of the procedure. Specifically, informing patients that the fixation light will become blurred and move around creating a "kaleidoscope effect" or "laser light show" is very helpful.

It is not unusual for epithelial removal to take several minutes for an inexperienced surgeon and less than 1 minute for an experienced PRK surgeon. Clearly, the amount of time required for epithelial removal will affect the hydration status of the stroma and increase the incidence of overcorrections while decreasing that of central islands. If the stromal surface becomes excessively dry, rehydrating the stroma may be indicated. In general, the application of any fluid such as balanced salt solution (BSS), artificial tears, topical anesthetic, or even a wet surgical spear is not recommended as it will alter the stromal hydration and alter the intended outcome.

There is tremendous variability of the integrity and adherence pattern of the epithelium. The problems in debriding highly adherent epithelium revolve around leaving epithelial remnants and developing an excessively dehydrated stroma. The concerns with an eye with loosely adherent epithelium are a slower re-epithelialization process and an increased incidence of recurrent corneal erosions. It is

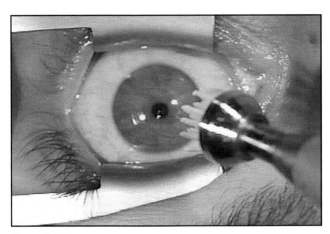

Figure 3-42a.
Pallikaris epithelial brush.

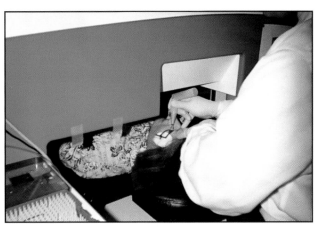

Figure 3-42b.
Epithelial removal with Pallikaris epithelial brush.

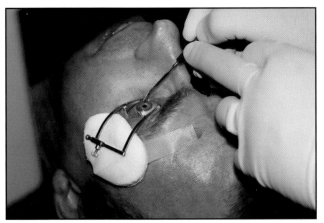

Figure 3-42c.
Intraoperative clinical appearance of epithelial removal technique demonstrating hand positions and instrument alignment. Mechanical debridement of epithelium with blunt spatula at acute 70° angle.

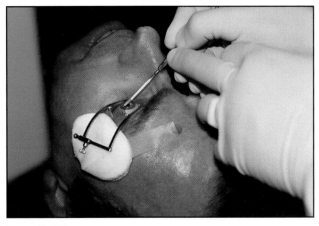

Figure 3-42d.
Removal of residual epithelial cells, smoothing of surface stroma, and controlling of stromal hydration. Note use of second hand to support spatula.

important to have deeply incised the epithelium with the optical zone marker in these loosely adherent cases, as this will help prevent a sheet of epithelium from detaching and create a smoother edge for re-epithelialization.

A mechanical epithelial brush (Figures 3-42a through 3-42e) is a method that a number of surgeons including myself have spent considerable time investigating to rapidly and efficiently debride the epithelium, leaving a smooth stromal surface for photoablation.

Transepithelial Approach

A transepithelial approach is easier for the patient but the endpoint is more difficult to define for the surgeon. The most important factor in defining the endpoint is to ensure that the room lights and microscope light are as dark as pos-

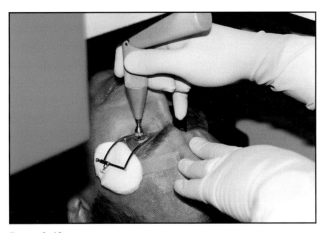

Figure 3-42e.
Perpendicular application of Pallikaris epithelial brush. Note support of hands on head with all three techniques and control of head movements with second hand.

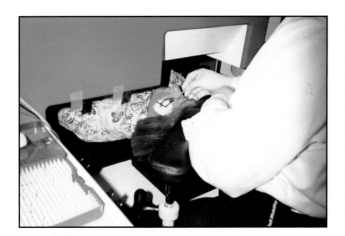

Figure 3-43.
Epithelial removal using 10% ethyl alcohol placed within optical zone marker with micropipette for 15 seconds. A surgical spear is used to soak up the alcohol at the end of the time interval and the epithelial surface then irrigated with BSS. Excessive stromal drying and keratocyte toxicity can result from prolonged application. The loosened epithelium can then be easily debrided mechanically with a spatula or surgical spear. An epithelial capsulorhexis technique can also be utilized.

sible. The pseudofluorescence produced during epithelial ablation creates a green glow to the ablative region which ceases upon reaching the stroma, which appears black. The most important aspects with respect to patient instructions are to warn the patient about the very loud snapping sound produced when ablating epithelium and the "burnt-hair" odor produced from the ablative by-products.

As will be discussed, a pretreatment should be performed on the surface of the epithelium for the central 2.5 to 3.0 mm whenever a transepithelial approach is performed if not combined with epithelial debridement. This pretreatment does not alter the need for a stromal pretreatment. Once again, a larger stromal pretreatment could be performed rather than two pretreatments but it is more simplistic to separate treatment of the epithelium and stroma. The amount of pretreatment required is 5 to 10 microns using the PRK modality, approximately 1 to 2 microns for each 10 microns of PTK. The VisX 20/20 transepithelial program is adjusted to compensate for central undercorrection in the software. The Chiron Technolas technology does not, whereas the Summit is at a lower risk because of the hotter central beam.

One or two brief tests utilizing a couple of pulses then stopping should be performed to allow the patient to become familiar with the sound. Informing the patient that you expect him or her to be startled is useful. The larger the optical zone and drier the corneal epithelium, the louder the

sound. As the epithelium is ablated, the pseudofluorescence will become evident. The room and the microscope lights should be dim and, once started, extinguished to accentuate the pattern. If the surface epithelium appears irregular, a slightly moistened surgical spear should be passed across the epithelium to even the moisture. Once stroma is reached, after approximately 200 pulses or 50 microns, the ablation should be stopped. The stromal endpoint is when the surface just starts to become black. It is important to recognize that the epithelium will disappear at the periphery first, then break up into islands, clearing centrally last. It is always best to stop early than late to avoid overcorrections and the peripheral clearing should signal the endpoint.

There are four important considerations when performing a transepithelial approach which may make blunt epithelial debridement preferable. First, that PTK alone will produce a central island resulting in peripheral clearing foremost, and therefore an additional pretreatment step is required. Second, that any beam abnormalities will be transmitted and exacerbated through the 200 pulses required to ablate the epithelium. Therefore, the beam must be qualitatively excellent with superior beam homogeneity.

Third, the epithelium is not uniform. Removal of the epithelium entirely with the laser will leave areas of epithelium and areas of ablated stroma at the commencement of the PRK. In particular, the peripheral clearing will create a peripheral trough of variable depth which may induce peripheral arcuate haze if deep. In the treatment of abnormal topography this fact is beneficial, as it will help blend regions together by utilizing the epithelium itself as a PTK blocking agent, much in the same way as methylcellulose is used. The fourth and final consideration is that the ablation nomogram is based upon calculations from the surface of Bowman's layer and not the surface of the epithelium. Therefore, an additional component of refractive predictability error is introduced, especially if the stromal surface endpoint is not correctly identified.

Clinical Note

Potential Complications of Transepithelial Approach

A transepithelial approach was performed on a patient requiring a -1.00 D correction. An undetected beam abnormality related to the output of a new laser head resulted in 4.00 D of induced with-the-rule cylinder. Astigmatic keratotomy (AK) was performed twice, a superior and an inferior 60° arc, in an attempt to treat the induced cylinder but only achieved a 50% reduction in cylinder. Corneal clarity remained excellent. Best corrected visual acuity remained

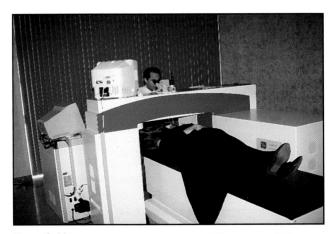

Figure 3-44.
A 34-year-old Russian nun treated bilaterally with Chiron Technolas laser for -4.00 -1.00 x 180 OU. Patient was highly uncooperative intraoperatively with multiple fixation losses requiring multiple interruptions in the procedure for realignment and refixation. Despite operative difficulties, patient remarkably achieved 20/20 uncorrected vision OU by day 5 and has remained stable over 2 years.

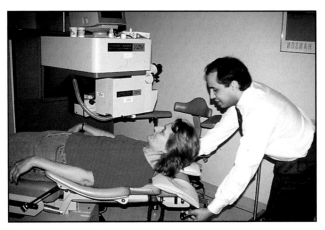

Figure 3-45.
Clinical case of author's mother-in-law who was treated for -2.75 D OD for monovision correction with VisX 20/20 excimer laser system. Numerous arrests in procedure were required for loss of fixation despite brief nature of procedure. Patient still achieved 20/15 uncorrected vision which has remained stable over 3 years. Case illustrates that loss of fixation, if managed appropriately, will not result in a compromised outcome.

at 20/15-1 with -0.75 +2.00 x 67 but a reduction of qualitative vision was subjectively appreciated by the patient. The patient was fitted with a rigid gas permeable lens with the hope that future surface or intrastromal ablation of the residual cylinder would be able to achieve emmetropia. The important observation to be drawn is that blunt epithelial debridement would have prevented this problem from developing in such a mild myope.

Transepithelial approach with epithelial debridement avoids many of the difficulties encountered with PTK alone such as defining the stromal surface endpoint. Central islands and abnormal topography related to beam abnormalities are also not problematic as the stroma remains unaffected. A smooth wound edge is created, promoting rapid re-epithelialization. The only other clinical note is that the residual 10 microns of epithelium can be difficult to remove at times as it appears to be almost compressed. This technique is recommended.

Many surgeons utilize a transpithelial approach without epithelial debridement and achieve excellent results, as they have adjusted their personal nomogram and are experienced in performing the technique well. The advantages of the transepithelial approach are threefold. First, the "no-touch laser" approach has appeal to both patients and surgeons in that it is both more rapid and less disconcerting to

patients. Second, some surgeons believe that a transepithelial approach helps preserve corneal clarity and reduces haze formation. Third, re-epithelialization is more rapid, and there is a reduced incidence of recurrent corneal erosions. This technique is only recommended for experienced PRK surgeons and only when excellent beam homogeneity has been confirmed. Don Johnson, MD, of Vancouver utilizes this technique combined with the multipass/multizone technique.

Chemical Debridement
Using alcohol to remove the epithelium is efficient but alters the stromal hydration pattern (Figure 3-43). Alcohol reduces the incidence of central islands but appears to increase haze and regression, and may have detrimental effects on keratocytes. Concentrations of 5% to 25% for 10 to 20 seconds are advocated, with the lowest concentration for the least duration preferred. A typical regimen is 20% ethyl alcohol for 15 seconds, but 10% is likely more than adequate. The duration of contact should be accurately timed for nomogram development and the avoidance of excessive dehydration. A couple drops of alcohol are placed within the optical zone marker, then a surgical spear is used to soak up the alcohol, and BSS is used to irrigate the eye. Alternatively, a circular 6- or 7-mm disc-shaped sponge can be immersed in the alcohol and centered on the epithelium for 15 seconds, then removed. A spear or spatula is then used to wipe away the loose epithelium. The process is very

The Eye Fixation Speculum: A New Instrument to Immobilize the Eye During Refractive Surgery

Neal A. Sher, MD, FACS, Thomas Burba, BA, and Andrew Bergin, BS

For refractive surgical techniques to be accurate, predictable, and safe, the eye should be safely and comfortably immobilized. Misalignment or movement of the eye during excimer laser PRK can result in decentered ablations with induced astigmatism, degraded images, night glare, monocular diplopia, and undercorrection. These decentered ablations cannot be easily remedied with retreatment or contact lens fitting. Furthermore, saccadic eye movement during excimer PRK can also result in an undesirable surgical outcome.

Ophthalmologists have used hand-held instruments to stabilize the eye, including a variety of forceps and ring-type designs (ie, Thornton ring), but all these instruments have drawbacks that make them unsuitable for use during excimer laser procedures. These shortcomings include pain, which increases patient anxiety, and subconjunctival hemorrhage. Another disadvantage is incyclo- or excyclotorsion of the globe that occurs when the patient attempts to move an eye held by single-point fixation. Depending on the varying amount of pressure exerted by the surgeon on any hand-held instrument, IOP can fluctuate greatly. Also, forceps and ring-type instruments are easily applied to the eye at different angles and with uneven force, causing corneal distortion during the refractive surgery. These devices also occupy one of the surgeon's hands, which prevents holding other instruments or securing the patient's head. Obviously, these fixation devices are less than satisfactory.

Currently surgeons rely on patient self-fixation during excimer PRK, but this method, too, has serious drawbacks. Steady fixation by the patient is made difficult if not impossible by the hazing of the dried, ablated surface of the cornea during PRK. It also assumes a cooperative patient who is not distracted by the noise of the laser pulse striking the cornea or startled by other room noises. Finally, with self-fixation, patients cannot prevent the small, very quick saccadic eye movements. In addition, the Bell's phenomenon causes some patients to have an upward eye movement with attempted lid closure. This results in significant wetting of the superior portion of the cornea and ablation zone. Uneven ablations can then occur because of the excimer laser's decreased ablation rate on hydrated cornea tissue as compared to dehydrated cornea tissue.

Recently published research by Ludwig et al[1] examined the effects of decentration and saccadic movement during excimer ablation. Ludwig created a computer simulation of the eye undergoing excimer PRK. A Landolt ring target was used to measure retinal contrast. The image of the Landolt ring on the retina was assigned a value of 1.0 to indicate an ideal optical system. The unoperated normal human eye had a value of 0.94. In simulated excimer PRK, the retinal contrast was reduced to 0.53. Decentration up to 1.0 mm did not significantly affect the retinal image contrast during simulated PRK. However, when saccadic eye movements and epithelial healing were also factored into the simulated PRK procedure, the retinal contrast image was significantly reduced to 0.38.

When performing excimer PRK for astigmatism, the alignment of the eye will be critical and require even more precise fixation. When the patient is supine or sedated there is a tendency for the eye to incyclo- or excyclotort. During excimer PRK to correct astigmatism, an axis misalignment of even 5° can result in a 15% to 20% loss of effectiveness. Furthermore, the total laser time to correct astigmatism and higher myopia with the newer multizone and multipass techniques will only increase and this longer procedure time diminishes any reliability of patient self-fixation.

To immobilize the eye without the problems encountered when using existing fixation methods, eyeFix Inc. has developed the Eye Fixation Speculum. This inexpensive, sterile, and disposable device is designed to be used during a variety of refractive surgical procedures. Made of several types of plastic materials, the device consists of a speculum for holding the patient's eyelid open and a luminescent, low-profile scleral vacuum fixation ring with axis markings. The fixation ring comfortably adheres to the episcleral tissue and is permanently attached to the speculum with an arm and locking mechanism.

In use, the speculum is first inserted into the eyelid margin and seated against the bony orbit. The speculum has been designed to give wide exposure and be more comfortable by modifying the lid retractors which insert under the lid. With the lid speculum in place, the surgeon has the patient look directly at a target to properly align the eye. Then the vacuum fixation ring is placed concentrically around the limbus and the ring is secured to the episcleral with vacuum provided by a 3 cc syringe. This locks the ring in place, preventing the eye from moving. The arm that attaches the fixation ring to the speculum is designed to restrict patient eye movement while allowing the eye and ring to be easily moved by the surgeon if any final adjustments are needed. A removable bubble level can be placed on top of the vacuum ring to assist the surgeon in adjusting the eye. With the ring positioned concentrically to the limbus and the patient supine, the level will indicate if the iris plane is exactly horizontal. Once the device is in place and the eye is correctly positioned, both of the surgeon's hands are free to be used for other tasks such as holding the patient's head. The top portion of the fixation ring is luminescent and this will assist the surgeon to visualize the eye with the microscope and room lights dimmed or off during epithelial removal with the excimer laser.

When applied to the patient, the Eye Fixation Speculum results in only a minimal increase in IOP. Preliminary studies indicate an increase of 10 to 15 mmHg. The rise in IOP is predictable and uniform. Most importantly, there is no corneal distortion because the vacuum is evenly distributed throughout the ring. Topographical maps of a cornea before and after the Eye Fixation Speculum is applied demonstrate no significant difference between before and after instrument application. This is in contrast to the distortion produced from forceps and other methods of external fixation.

In clinical trials, during which some of the procedures lasted up to 6 minutes due to multipass and multizone techniques, the Eye Fixation Speculum was proven to be comfortable and the eye was firmly secured. No complications occurred. The patients commented very favorably on the device, with the majority of patients indicating they were less anxious during the procedure because they did not have to worry about keeping their eye immobilized.

Eyetracking devices have been proposed and prototypes are under development which will keep the laser beam correctly aimed on the cornea. These aiming devices are expensive and may further complicate the already complex delivery system of excimer lasers. The tracking may also alter the angle of the incoming laser energy from perpendicular to some unknown angle, depending upon the angle of deviation of the eye. Eyetracking devices cannot compensate for a change in the rate of ablation caused by corneal wetness, should the patient move the eye under the lid. These tracking systems would be more efficient when used in conjunction with the Eye Fixation Speculum.

References

1. Ludwig K, Schafer P, Gross H, Lasser TH. Influence of decentration and saccadic eye movements during photorefractive keratectomy (PRK) on the retinal image contrast. *Invest Ophth Vis Sci.* 1994;35(4):2019.

efficient and leaves a smooth, somewhat dehydrated stromal surface. The use of cocaine 4% is effective at debriding the epithelium but is not advocated because of toxicity.

ALIGNMENT DURING PRK

One of the most important principles of performing the PRK procedure is stopping. Lifting your foot from the foot pedal may sound simple, but it is often very difficult for the beginning PRK surgeon. Patients frequently lose fixation briefly (Figure 3-44) or begin to slowly drift. Stopping to allow the patient to regain fixation is essential. Continuing the procedure because there are only a few pulses left, following the eye, or torquing the eye back into position with forceps are unacceptable solutions. So long as each pulse is placed centrally, multiple interruptions in the procedure are preferable to the application of decentered pulses. Stopping is recommended, however, if the cornea dries excessively,

the risk of hyperopia becomes real.

Clinical Note

Intraoperative Loss of Fixation

Some surgeries may even require stopping every few seconds for the entire procedure, but the result will be a well-centered ablation and excellent vision. One such case was my mother-in-law, who achieved 20/15 uncorrected visual acuity following -2.75 D correction. The procedure was complicated by continual loss of fixation, which required stopping the procedure 15 times in 25 seconds. The only important element was placement of the pulses once refixation was achieved (Figure 3-45).

Patients have a tendency to depress their chin in an effort to move away from the surgeon; it is important to ensure the eye remains perpendicular and well fixated. Patients rarely

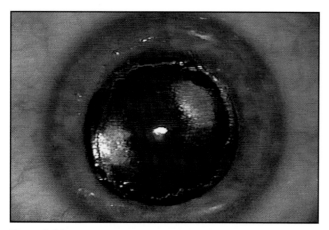

Figure 3-46.
Central translucency indicating increased hydration of central stroma during PRK photoablation. Central island formation related to differential hydration status of stroma intraoperatively.

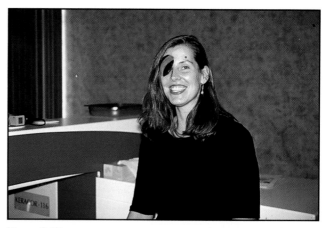

Figure 3-47a.
PRK patient immediately following unilateral surgery for -3.75 D treated with Chiron Technolas excimer laser with multizone blending techniques and oscillating beam. Vision at this point remains blurry at approximately 20/100.

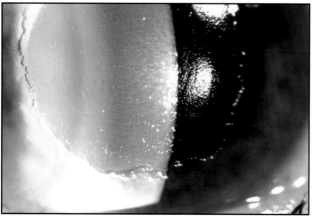

Figure 3-47b.
Despite blurred vision, high magnification view of treated eye demonstrates very smooth refractive surface. By Day 13 patient was 20/25 uncorrected in the treated eye.

Ten Important Procedure Points
1. Stop at the first sign of eye drift
2. Self-fixation is best
3. Maintain the eye and head perpendicularly
4. Do not torque the eye to maintain fixation
5. Reduce the microscope light intensity if tearing or poor fixation occur
6. Keep both eyes open to prevent Bell's phenomenon
7. Use topical anesthetic in non-operative eye to prevent blepharospasm
8. Avoid preoperative sedation
9. Center upon the unconstricted pupil with slight adjustment for the visual axis if a large angle kappa exists
10. Reassure the patient frequently

move their eyes abruptly, but rather drift slowly, and it is this gradual drift which must be watched. As stated earlier, preoperative sedation, although comforting for patients, may result in loss of fixation. Patients having a great deal of difficulty maintaining fixation should be reminded to keep both eyes open to reduce the Bell's phenomenon response. The microscope lights should be dimmed to reduce glare, as this is often the cause of excessive tearing and eye movement intraoperatively. Fixation should be centered around the pupil center. Reassurance is important throughout the procedure, as this will improve fixation.

The procedure should be divided into multiple steps. Throughout the procedure, the surgical assistant should call out the time remaining to help inform and comfort the patient.

Controlling Stromal Hydration Status

During the PRK procedure with a homogeneous broad beam delivery system, circular ablation patterns of increasing diameter become clinically evident. As the ablation diameter expands, fluid begins to accumulate centrally (Figure 3-46). The differential pattern of hydration is important, as it will result in a central undercorrection. The overall hydration pattern of the stroma is also of importance, as it will alter the refractive predictability. One technique to help control both the overall hydration status and the differential hydration status to create a more uniform and standardized level of hydration is to wipe the stromal surface with a blunt spatula. Wiping once or twice for each zone with the flat side of the spatula parallel to the surface of the cornea provides for more homogeneous hydration of the ablative region. If the stroma is very moist, the blunt spatula can be used to wipe fluid away more frequently, to both reduce the risk of undercorrection and central island formation. If the stroma is excessively dry, no wiping is performed. Excessive drying promotes overcorrections, increases haze and irregular astigmatism, and worsens self-fixation. No wiping is required with scanning excimer laser delivery systems, such as the Nidek EC-5000 or Technolas PlanoScan program, as no central island formation is observed.

There are many nuances to performing PRK founded not only on surgical principles and procedure technique but insight into the technology (Figures 3-47a and 3-47b). Understanding the excimer laser is as much a part of performing PRK as the actual procedure. PRK is far more than inputting the refractive error and depressing the foot pedal. Superior clinical results can be achieved and complications both avoided and managed better when an understanding of the corneal-laser interaction is gained.

CHAPTER 4

Postoperative PRK Patient Management

Postoperative care following excimer laser photorefractive keratectomy (PRK) is as important to the clinical outcome as the performance of the procedure itself. Although postoperative care is important for all forms of refractive surgery, it is especially true for PRK more than any other procedure.

IMMEDIATE POSTOPERATIVE CARE

Immediately following PRK, the patient receives an almost identical series of topical medications as he or she received preoperatively. Each surgeon, however, uses his or her own regimen which typically includes a topical antibiotic, a topical steroid, a topical non-steroidal anti-inflammatory agent, and possibly additional topical anesthetic (Figure 4-1).

Although not required, additional topical anesthesia may help with both bandage contact lens insertion and improved comfort as the lens settles. A recent prospective, randomized, double-masked British study conducted by Verma, Corbett, and Marshall challenged conventional thinking and found improved comfort without impaired re-epithelialization with continued use of tetracaine during epithelial healing. The topical antibiotic and topical steroid or combination preparation is repeated postoperatively. The instillation of the non-steroidal agent is important in achieving prolonged comfort. The importance of non-steroidals in the immediate postoperative period cannot be overstated, as it reduces the degree of inflammation and specifically the formation of prostaglandins, which appear to mediate the pain. Some surgeons even soak the bandage contact lens in the non-steroidal preparation in an attempt to alleviate postoperative pain; however, the efficacy does not appear to be enhanced and re-epithelialization may be slowed. As discussed in the preoperative preparation and medication section of Chapter 3, the choice of agents is at the discretion of the surgeon.

Postoperative Regimen
- Topical antibiotic
- Topical steroid
- Topical non-steroidal
- Bandage contact lens

A typical postoperative regimen during the first few days of epithelial healing would include an antibiotic such as tobramycin, ofloxacin, or Polytrim. Use a topical steroid such as fluorometholone 0.1% or 0.25%, or more commonly dexamethasone 0.1%, or a combination antibiotic-steroid preparation for patient convenience and compliance. The choice of non-steroidal preparation may be ketorolac tromethamine 0.5% (Acular, Allergan) or diclofenac sodium 0.1% (Voltaren, CIBA). There appears to be no decisive clinical advantage to either agent, although diclofenac may have dual activity with prostaglandin inhibition and topical anesthetic effects. My primary NSAID agent has been Voltaren

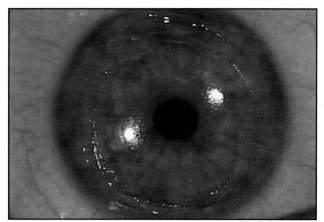

Figure 4-1.
Immediate postoperative clinical appearance following multi-multizone PRK ablation with Chiron Technolas Keracor 116 for -4.75 D. Note the smooth ablative surface and absence of mechanical iris diaphragm ridges.

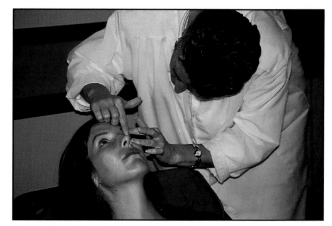

Figure 4-2.
Bandage contact lens insertion following PRK to help reduce postoperative discomfort. Our standard contact lens (CIBA NewVue base curve 8.4) is inserted manually by a trained staff member utilizing sterile technique rather than with forceps by the surgeon. There does not appear to be a clinical difference in the incidence of postoperative infection.

(CIBA) and primary antibiotic-steroid preparation TobraDex (Alcon), although recently Ocuflox (Allergan) is my antibiotic preference alone or in combination with TobraDex. Other postoperative medication options are available.

Lubrication is recommended with preservative-free sterile minums, however, patients must be instructed not to dilute their other medications by inserting them at the same time. The eye should be closed for 15 seconds after instillation to ensure that the bandage contact lens will not be accidently lost. Cycloplegia may be achieved with cyclopentolate 1%, tropicamide 1%, or homatropine 2% or 5%. There appears, however, to be questionable benefit to these agents. Surprisingly, unlike traumatic corneal abrasions, these agents seem to increase photophobia rather than simply relieve ciliary spasm. Some surgeons have found benefit and include these agents in their immediate postoperative regimen but only immediately following surgery.

BANDAGE CONTACT LENS

The use of a bandage contact lens in combination with a topical non-steroidal has had a dramatic impact upon the acceptability of the PRK procedure, as the control of postoperative pain had been a major impediment. Although certain patients will be unable to tolerate or maintain a contact lens in their eye and will require pressure patching, the majority will be fitted with a therapeutic contact lens (Figure 4-2). The bandage contact lens may be soaked in the antibiotic or non-steroidal agent prior to insertion, although this is not my standard routine; a disposable contact lens is typi-

cally used as the therapeutic bandage lens. The base curve of the disposable contact lens is somewhat controversial in that many surgeons feel that the flattest base curve should be fitted. However, if the bandage contact lens moves excessively, not only will patient discomfort be greater but re-epithelialization will be slowed. Ideally, the bandage contact lens should fit snugly with little movement as patient comfort and the re-epithelialization rate are improved. If the lens is too tight, stromal edema will be evident clinically the following day and epithelial healing will be impaired.

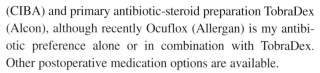

Specific Postoperative Regimen
- TobraDex qid
- Ocuflox qid
- Voltaren bid
- CIBA NewVue (base curve 8.4, -0.50 D)

Refractive power of the bandage contact lens is unimportant, but is typically +0.50 D, -0.50 D, or plano. Some surgeons prefer +0.50 D as slight overcorrection is common, some prefer -0.50 D as ciliary spasm is common. I typically fit a CIBA NewVue base curve 8.4, -0.50 D contact lens which has served my patients well, although CIBA has recently developed a PRK-specific therapeutic contact lens, the Protek contact lens, with Marguerite B. McDonald, MD. In drier climates, a flatter base curve is routinely required.

Postoperative Oral Medications

- Narcotic: Demerol
- Anti-emetic: Phenergan
- Sedative: Lorazepam

IMMEDIATE POSTOPERATIVE ORAL MEDICATIONS

Despite the introduction of topical non-steroidals and bandage contact lenses, approximately 5% to 10% of patients continue to experience moderate to severe pain requiring oral narcotic agents. Prior to the current therapeutic lens-topical medication regimen, 50% of patients experienced moderate to severe pain despite pressure patching and cycloplegia. These patients required oral narcotics including Demerol (meperidine), Percocet (oxycodone hydrochloride-acetominophen), codeine, and morphine sulfate. Current oral analgesic requirements are usually non-narcotic, but Demerol is prescribed for patients experiencing severe pain. The amount and potency of narcotic agents has reduced dramatically.

Despite the epithelial defect healing gradually over 3 days, pain usually peaks the first day. Phenergan (promethazine hydrochloride, Rhone-Poulenc Rorer) or Gravol (dihydraminate) is also prescribed to control nausea and promote sleep. A benzodiazepine, either Valium (diazepam) or Ativan (lorazepam), a shorter-acting agent, is recommended as sleep is beneficial. Patients often try to alleviate eye irritation with narcotic agents and become ill. Instructions for use must be specific and quantities limited. It is always best to recommend an anti-emetic or sedative prior to a narcotic agent as sleep will speed recovery and avoid the accompanying nausea of narcotics.

Clinical Note

Identical Female Twins and PRK Postoperative Regimens

A double-blind identical twin study was performed to determine two aspects of postoperative care:

1. Importance of an anti-inflammatory non-steroidal drop in pain relief post-PRK
2. Importance of topical steroid potency in refractive outcome in the management of high myopia

The identical twins both measured -16.00 and -13.50 D of preoperative myopia but in contralateral eyes (Figure 4-3a). Twin A (the first born) recorded better preoperative visual acuity by one line in one eye. All other clinical find-

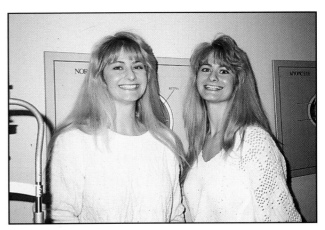

Figure 4-3a.
Female identical twins treated for extreme myopia with VisX 20/20 Model B excimer laser system.

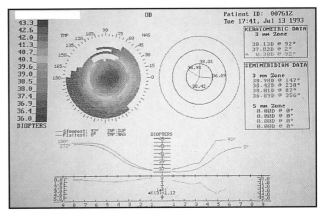

Figure 4-3b.
Corneal videokeratography of Twin A demonstrating significant central flattening postoperatively.

ings preoperatively were identical, including occupation.

In the first double-blind study, both twins were treated with multizone PRK with the VisX 20/20 Model B in early 1992, utilizing a no-blow technique and patient self-fixation. A three-zone treatment was performed following a 2.5-mm pretreatment, at 4.0 (50%), 5.0 (30%), and 6.0 mm (20%). There were no intraoperative complications. The -16.00 D eye of each twin was treated first. Postoperatively, both twins received Polytrim (trimethoprim sulfate and polymyxin B sulfate) antibiotic prophylaxis and an AcuVue (Johnson & Johnson) -0.50 D disposable contact lens was inserted. Each twin was provided with an unlabeled bottle (A or B) that contained either artificial tears or Voltaren (diclofenac sodium 0.1%, CIBA). Patients had received two drops 30 and 15 minutes preoperatively and two drops 5 minutes postoperatively. Each twin then instilled both drops qid, 5 minutes

The Management of Postoperative Pain After Excimer PRK

Neal A. Sher, MD, FACS

If not properly handled, patients may experience moderate to severe eye pain after excimer PRK. This pain usually begins within 30 to 60 minutes after the procedure and becomes severe within 4 to 6 hours despite preoperative counseling and treatment with oral narcotics, cycloplegics, and ice packs. In the early clinical trials of the excimer laser in 1989, a number of surgeons found the pain to be one of the major drawbacks to performing the surgery and a significant clinical challenge. Some patients had to be given large doses of narcotics and frequently would return to the clinic or office nauseated and ill.

The pain after PRK is much more severe and is akin to the pain of a severe corneal abrasion, erosion, or ultraviolet keratitis. Patients usually describe the pain as severe, sometimes throbbing in nature. It is usually associated with a burning, stinging sensation as well as tearing and nasal congestion. Some have characterized this pain as the worst they ever experienced.

There may be a number of reasons for the intense pain after excimer PRK. The primary cause may be the mechanical disruption of the epithelium and the complex of corneal nerve endings over a wide area (36 to 49 mm^2) of ablated cornea. Other physical effects of the excimer include ultraviolet keratitis, thermal effects, and acoustic shockwave damage. Ultraviolet radiation exposure of the cornea produces a ultraviolet keratitis with tearing, stippling, hyperemia, haze, discharge, photophobia, blepharospasm, and pain. Thermal effects and acoustic shockwaves may also damage tissue and contribute to pain. These physical stimuli which disrupt cell membranes may release a number of chemical factors, such as prostaglandins, substance P, histamine, epithelial neurotropic factors, and other chemicals. Some of these chemical mediators have been shown to produce pain in a variety of tissues.

In 1991, an ophthalmic NSAID formulation, diclofenac sodium 0.1% ophthalmic (Voltaren, CIBA) was introduced in the United States for the treatment of postoperative inflammation following cataract surgery. Sher[1] first suggested that topical diclofenac, when used with a bandage soft contact lens, could reduce the severe postoperative pain of excimer PRK. This lead to a retrospective review of 70 patients' charts, half of whom received topical diclofenac immediately after myopic PRK and then qid. In a survey of postoperative pain conducted

24 hours after PRK, the diclofenac group rarely indicated more than mild pain, whereas the untreated control group of patients had pain which was frequently described as moderate or severe.[2] To determine the efficacy and safety of diclofenac sodium ophthalmic solution for the attenuation of postoperative ocular pain following excimer PRK, a prospective two-center, randomized, double-masked, parallel group, placebo-controlled comparison was performed.[3]

In this study, the diclofenac was applied immediately postoperatively, 5 minutes postoperatively and then four times a day until the epithelium healed. Patients were all admitted overnight to the hospital and a number of subjective questionnaires given frequently. The results were clear-cut and striking. Sixty percent of the diclofenac-treated patients described no pain vs. 25% of the placebo vehicle group. The pain peaked at 4 hours in the placebo group. Close to one third (31.3%) of the placebo group vs. 6.3% of the diclofenac group experienced moderate pain. The time course of the development of pain is shown in Figure A-1. The pain in the placebo group began within 1 hour and increased in intensity until 4 hours after the procedure. The pain experienced by the diclofenac group peaked at 1 hour and remained at an average "mild level" for the next 12 hours and then gradually declined until 24 hours. The more intense pain experienced by the placebo group did not decline to the level of the diclofenac group until after 72 hours. There was a statistically significant difference between the diclofenac and placebo group beginning at 2 hours ($p<0.01$) and continuing through 36 hours, except at hour 10 ($p<0.066$) and hour 18 ($p<0.061$). Seventy-five percent of the patients receiving diclofenac did not require any supplemental oral narcotic, whereas 31.3% of placebo patients required supplemental narcotic and medication.

A number of other surgeons have confirmed this work in other studies, including Jeffrey Robin, MD, Marguerite B. McDonald, MD, Peter McDonnell, MD, Steve Arshinoff, MD, and Jim Salz, MD. Similar studies were done by Raymond Stein, MD, Harold Stein, MD, and Al Cheskes, MD, on topical ketorolac (Acular, Allergan) with similar results.[4]

It has recently been suggested that there may not be a need for postoperative corticosteroids after PRK.[5] These authors found no significant effect from corticosteroids on long-term corneal haze or refractive error, but did not comment on the effects of postoperative pain. Caution should be used in eliminating corticosteroid usage with replacement by a topical cyclo-oxygenase inhibitor such as diclofenac or ketorolac. In a survey of 58 Canadian surgeons performing PRK, Patricia Teal, MD, found that surgeons using non-steroidals and a bandage lens without steroids observed a sterile corneal infiltrate in one of 200 to 250 eyes. When topical steroids were added to the regimen, Teal found the incidence of infiltrates to be much less.[6] It is postulated that some of the analgesic effect of topical NSAIDs may be related to the inhibition of cyclo-oxygenase and the reduction in the transformation of arachidonic acid to prostaglandins such as Prostaglandin E2. Diclofenac may have some limited effect on the lipoxygenase pathway which leads to the formation of leukotrienes and other mediators which lead to the influx of inflammatory cells, but the clinical effect on this pathway may not be significant. Topical corticosteroids also inhibit prostaglandin biosynthesis at a more preliminary location in the pathway by inhibiting phospholipase A2, which blocks arachidonic acid from the phospholipase pool.

Excimer PRK and PTK produce considerable inflammation in the cornea from the mechanical injury to the epithelium and ultraviolet keratitis. In an experimental PRK model in rabbits, polymorphonuclear (PMN) cell infiltration is seen as early as 8 to 10 hours.[7] These same authors demonstrated that diclofenac treatment alone, while reducing PGE2 levels in the cornea, actually increased the infiltration of PMN into the cornea. They postulate that by blocking the cyclo-oxygenase pathway with these types of drugs, an increased amount of arachidonic acid may be shunted to the lipo-oxygenase pathway and lead to the production of leukotrienes, which stimulate the migration of leukocytes into the cornea. Topical corticosteroid, while only having a modest effect on PGE2 levels, markedly reduced the PMN infiltration.

From our clinical observations and some of the experimental evidence presented here, we strongly suggest that topical corticosteroids be used during the acute postoperative period in conjunction with topical diclofenac or ketorolac. It is not known how long the topical corticosteroids are needed. Clinical observations indicate that diclofenac or ketorolac are only needed for several days for pain control. It would seem reasonable for the topical corticosteroids to be used intensively at the time of surgery and in a tapering dose regimen for the first week or two after surgery.

Our current postoperative regimen includes a bandage soft contact lens and diclofenac or ketorolac immediately postop-

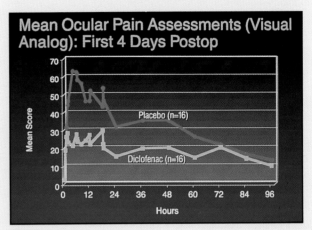

Figure A-1.
Patient assessment of pain, visual analog scale. Time course of pain to 96 hours after surgery in the diclofenac-treated and vehicle control groups. All patients in both groups were given soft contact lenses, topical steroids, and antibiotics. All points represent mean of 16 patients in each group. Extended bars represent SE.

eratively and three or four times a day until re-epithelialization is complete (usually by day 3). In addition, a topical corticosteroid antibiotic mixture such as TobraDex is used at least qid until the epithelium is intact. This is then discontinued and replaced with fluorometholone 0.1% alcohol (FML or Fluor-op) in a tapering regimen for up to 4 months. Ciprofloxacin should be avoided because of the possibility of crystalline precipitates on the ablation bed. Patients should be examined daily until re-epithelialization is complete. The bandage soft contact lens should be replaced if there is excessive movement. A somewhat tight lens is desirable and probably speeds epithelial resurfacing.

Rapid re-epithelialization after excimer PRK is desirable for a number of reasons, including the elimination of pain and discomfort, the reduced risk of infection, and the more rapid improvement of visual acuity. Eyes with persistent epithelial defects post PRK have greater haze and scarring. It is not known which postoperative regimen (ie, bandage contact lenses, patching) aids in achieving the quickest re-epithelialization. NSAIDs and topical corticosteroids probably inhibit re-epithelialization to some degree and should be used in the minimal effective doses and for the shortest amount of time. The optimal dosage of both diclofenac and the topical corticosteroid is not known and less frequent dosing should be investigated. Reduction of potential corneal toxicity from the multiplicity of drops used postoperatively may be possible with the use of non-preserved formulations of these drugs.

The use of a bandage soft contact lens may predispose the eye to a higher risk of bacterial keratitis and delayed healing. This risk may be offset by the more frequent application and higher concentration of antibiotics which can be achieved in a non-patched eye with a bandage soft contact lens, as well as increased patient comfort and improved vision. The main disadvantage of a bandage soft contact lens is the difficulty in fitting the ablated cornea. The lenses are frequently tight when seen the next day and it is not unusual to see mild striate folds in the cornea. If the lens is too tight or has significant deposits, it should be replaced or discontinued. Patients should be strictly cautioned against replacing the lens themselves at home if it is displaced; this is the probable source of the infiltrates in two of these patients. In over 1000 cases of PRK and PTK at the Phillips Eye Institute, there has been one other case of bacterial keratitis, possibly caused by the patient's use of a contaminated contact lens solution at home. The best way to reduce healing complications is to follow patients daily until the epithelium heals.

References

1. Sher NA, Barak M, Daya S, et al. Excimer laser photorefractive keratectomy in high myopia. *Arch Ophthalmol.* 1992;110:935-943.

2. Eiferman RA, Hoffman RS, Sher NA. Topical diclofenac reduces pain following photorefractive keratectomy. *Arch Ophthalmol.* 1993;111:1022. Letter.

3. Sher NA, Frantz JM, Talley A, et al. Topical diclofenac in the treatment of ocular pain after excimer photorefractive keratectomy. *J Refract Corneal Surg.* 1993;9:425-436.

4. Stein R, Stein HA, Cheskes A, et al. Photorefractive keratectomy and postoperative pain. *Am J Ophthalmol.* 1994;117:403-405. Letter.

5. Gartry DS, Kerr Muir MG, Lohmann CP, Marshall J. The effect of topical corticosteroids on refractive outcome and corneal haze after photorefractive keratectomy: a prospective, randomized double blind trial. *Arch Ophthalmol.* 1992;110:944-952.

6. Sher NA, Krueger RR, Teal P, Jans RG, Edmison D. Role of topical corticosteroids and nonsteroidal antiinflammatory drugs in the etiology of stromal infiltrates after excimer photorefractive keratectomy. *J Refract Corneal Surg.* 1994;10:588. Letter.

7. Moreira H, McDonnell PJ, Fasano AP, Silverman DL, Coates TD, Sevanian. Treatment of experimental pseudomonas keratitis with cyclo-oxygenase and lipoxygenase inhibitors. *Ophthalmology.* 1991;96:1693-1697.

apart. The study was to continue for 3 days until re-epithelialization was complete, however, Twin B complained of severe postoperative pain while Twin A remained completely comfortable and required no oral analgesics. After several hours of persistent pain, preventing sleep and requiring 100 mg of Demerol (meperidine) and 50 mg of Gravol (dihydraminate) twice in 8 hours, Twin B literally stole her sister's drop À at 2:00 am. Furthermore, after instillation of the masked drop A, Twin B stated that she experienced sudden and dramatic clinical improvement with complete resolution of her pain. Although the study was not completed as designed, the concomitant use of Voltaren with a bandage contact lens was dramatically effective in controlling postoperative PRK pain. The treatment of identical twins with identical techniques and medications in a double-blind fashion clearly demonstrates Voltaren as an effective adjunct in the management of postoperative PRK pain.

The second part of the double-blind clinical study was initiated following re-epithelialization and was designed to examine the role of topical steroid potency in postoperative management following PRK for extreme myopia. Both patients received masked bottles of topical corticosteroids, containing either FML 0.1% (fluorometholone, Allergan) or FML Forte 0.25% (fluorometholone, Allergan). Both patients were instructed to use the drops qid for the first month, tapering monthly over 4 months.

The pattern of refractive and visual stabilization did not demonstrate any significant clinical differences between the full-strength and the low-strength corticosteroid (Figure 4-3b). The final refractive and visual outcome was similar at 6 months. Although both patients did well at 6 months, they continued to demonstrate long-term myopic regression without haze requiring retreatment. During the first enhancement procedure performed with a transepithelial approach in Twin A and mechanical debridement in the Twin B, significant epithelial thickening was observed in the range of 70 microns and as much as 90 microns with the second enhancement of the same eye over 1 year later.

Three years postoperatively, neither twin has lost best corrected vision in either eye and one twin gained one line of best corrected vision in one eye. Both twins required two PRK retreatments in their -16.50 D eye and are pending further enhancement of their -13.00 D eye. Neither twin developed confluent haze at any time.

Immediate Postoperative Patient Instructions

- Patients should be instructed to rest as much as possible for the first 3 days during epithelial healing.
- Medication and postoperative follow-up compliance is emphasized. Eye drops should be instilled as instructed. Lubrication as desired between prescribed topical medication.
- Common patient symptoms should be reviewed with particular emphasis on the expected visual recovery.
- Showers, baths, and hairwashing are permitted but care should be taken to keep the eyes closed and avoid shampoo entering the eyes.
- Handwashing is important and hands should be kept away from the eyes.
- No swimming, whirlpools, or make-up for 5 to 7 days.
- Exertional activities are not prohibited but rest is encouraged to speed epithelial healing.
- Patients should be instructed not to drive until further notice—minimum 3 days if one eye was treated, and usually 1 to 2 weeks if simultaneous bilateral surgery was performed. Blurred vision and loss of stereopsis make driving more hazardous, especially at night. Oral medication may also produce drowsiness and impair reflexes.
- Patients should be forewarned that their depth perception will be affected and care should be taken when pouring hot coffee, hammering a nail, or driving in the initial stages of healing.
- Patients should be instructed not to remove the bandage contact lens and that if it is accidently lost, the lens should not be replaced but the eye closed and patched until a new contact lens is reinserted by the doctor.
- Although not prohibited, prolonged reading or watching television may result in drying of the contact lens and increased discomfort.
- Patients traveling great distances postoperatively should be instructed to keep their eyes closed in a car or airplane, as forced dry eye will increase discomfort as the contact lens dries. Humidification may improve comfort during epithelial healing.
- Sunglasses are helpful to improve comfort. A cool compress over the eyes in a dark room is helpful in reducing eye discomfort.

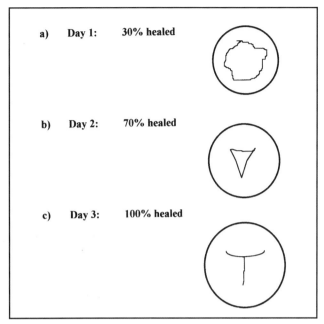

Figure 4-4.
Schematic diagram of Day 1 epithelial healing with approximately 30% closure of epithelial defect observed (a). Schematic diagram of Day 2 epithelial healing with approximately 70% closure of epithelial defect observed (b). Schematic diagram depicting closure of epithelial defect on Day 3 with classic Y-healing pattern (c).

Ten Most Common Immediate Postoperative Symptoms
1. Photophobia
2. Epiphora
3. Runny nose
4. Eye irritation with foreign body or "eyelash" sensation
5. Eye redness and swelling
6. Eyelid swelling or puffiness
7. Increased night glare
8. Unbalanced feeling and loss of depth perception if unilateral treated (symptoms related to loss of stereopsis and anisometropia)
9. Difficulty reading
10. Blurred vision

Analogy for Patients: Be Conservative
Like golf, the aim is to get the ball on the green while avoiding the sand trap just beyond, with the anticipation that one can be more accurate putting the ball in the cup at that reduced distance.

Figure 4-5.
Postoperative eye following PRK with therapeutic contact lens in position.

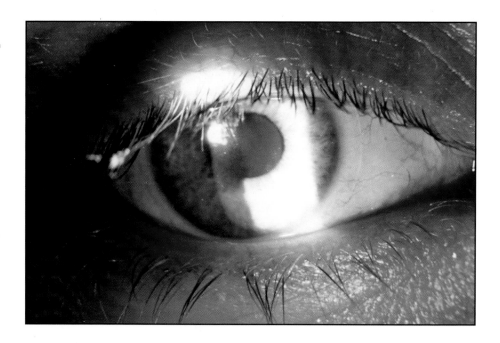

Figure 4-6.
Day 1 PRK treated eye with bandage contact lens. Common clinical findings postoperatively include conjunctival injection and eyelid edema.

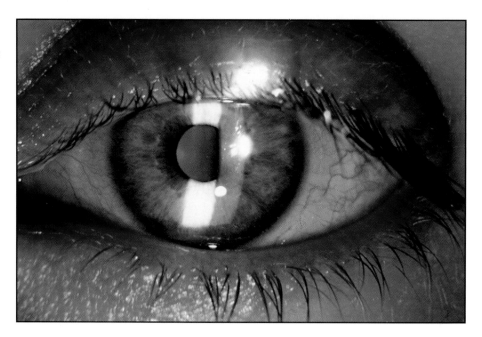

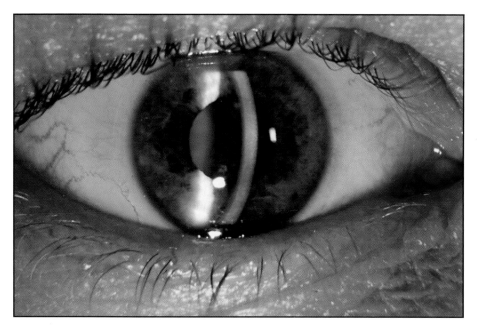

Figure 4-7a.
Day 1 PRK treated eye with trace corneal edema often misinterpreted as corneal haze. Very little inflammation is evident.

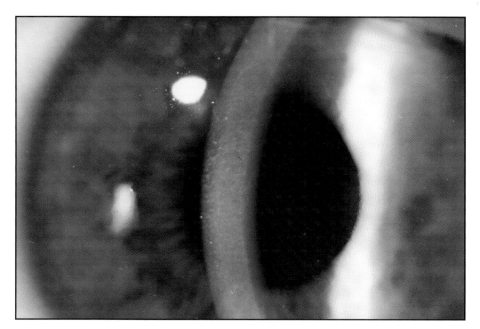

Figure 4-7b.
High magnification of stromal edema in Figure 4-7a.

Figure 4-8.
Epithelial defect less than 24 hours postoperatively demonstrating denuded central stroma and advancing epithelial edge. No stromal edema evident.

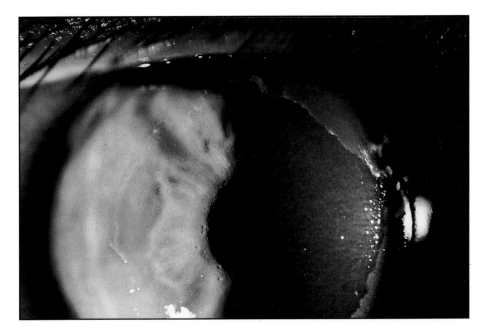

Figure 4-9.
Increased inflammation following loss of bandage contact lens on first postoperative day. Conjunctival injection and corneal edema evident.

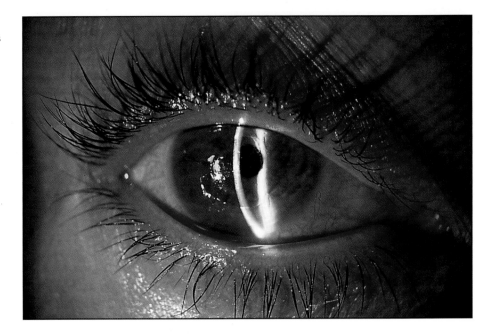

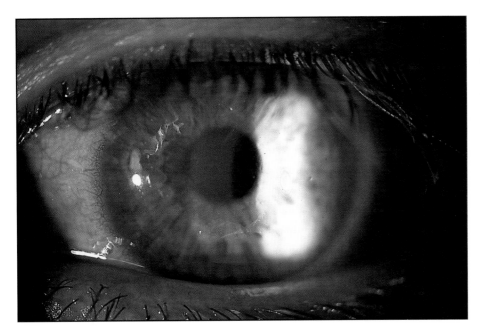

Figure 4-10.
Mild inflammation with no corneal edema observed following loss of therapeutic contact lens on first postoperative day of PRK treated eye. Approximately 25% epithelial healing noted.

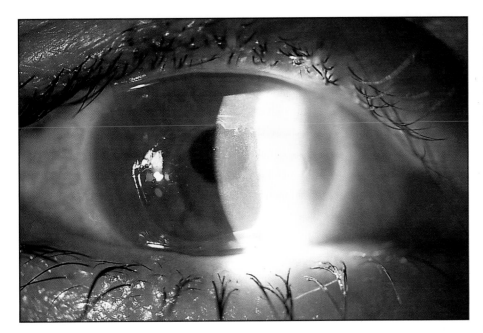

Figure 4-11.
Traumatic loss of bandage contact lens on second postoperative day of PRK treated eye with enlargement of epithelial defect inferiorally. Rolled inferior margin of epithelium will delay re-epithelialization and may require pressure patching.

Figure 4-12.
Rapid re-epithelialization with 90% closure of epithelial defect observed 48 hours following PRK treatment. Well-defined epithelial margins commonly associated with rapid healing pattern.

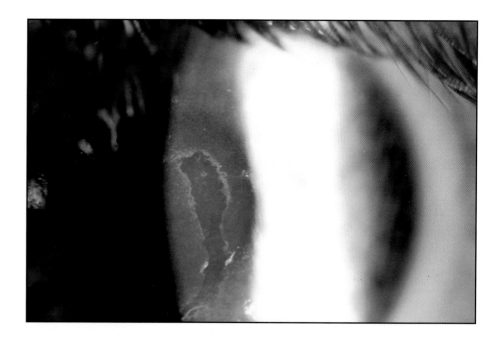

Figure 4-13.
Clinical appearance on second postoperative day following PRK with poorly adherent epithelium beneath bandage contact lens giving the clinical appearance of debris. Premature removal or manipulation of the bandage contact lens will dislodge epithelial cells. The contact lens should remain in position until the epithelial cells have become adherent. A patch is indicated if the surface still appears irregular after removal of the contact lens at 72 to 96 hours.

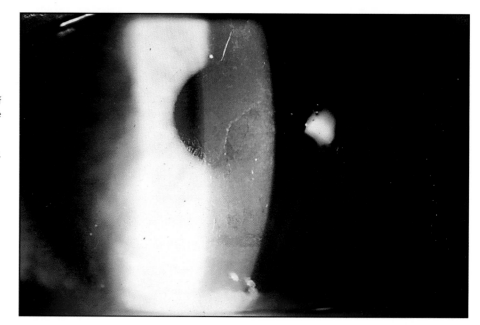

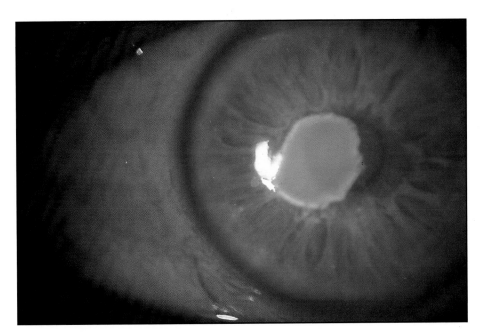

Figure 4-14.
Day 2 epithelial healing post-PRK stained with fluorescein to better demonstrate epithelial defect remaining. Bandage contact lens need not be removed to examine eye until healed.

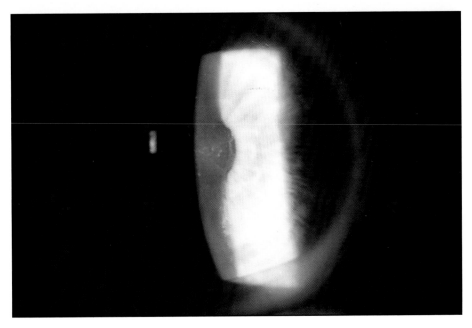

Figure 4-15.
Day 3 1-mm triangular epithelial defect evident.

Figure 4-16.
Clinically significant stromal edema with 3+ folds in Descemet's membrane following uncomplicated PRK. A tight bandage contact lens is the most likely etiology for the edema noted.

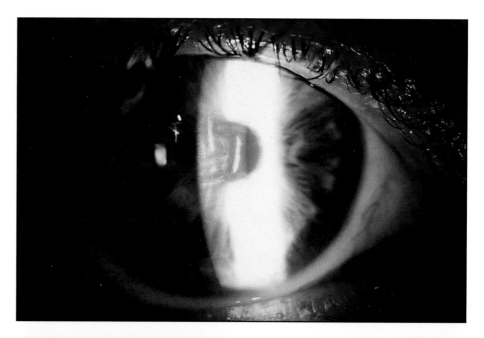

Figure 4-17.
Medium magnification view of PRK treated eye with significant stromal edema secondary to tight contact lens syndrome. Epithelial defect approximately 80% closed, however, degree of swelling will often delay re-epithelialization.

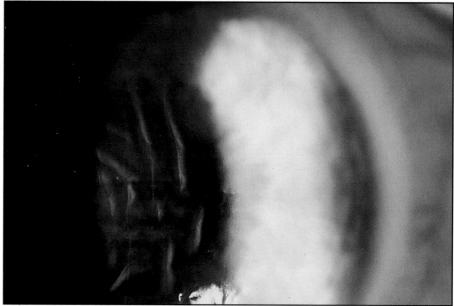

VISUAL RECOVERY

It is important to explain to patients that their vision will be blurry immediately postoperatively so that they do not expect restoration of sight immediately, as they may have heard from friends who had radial keratotomy (RK). It is also important to explain that the vision will fluctuate and generally worsens over the first 3 days, followed by improvement within 48 hours of epithelial closure. Vision can be quite good the first postoperative day, varying from 20/30 to 20/200 with 20/70 being most typical. As the epithelial healing pattern encroaches upon the central axis, vision diminishes. Once the epithelium is intact, the central healing pattern smooths over 1 to 2 days and vision improves rapidly.

EARLY POSTOPERATIVE CARE

EPITHELIAL HEALING

The absence of an intact epithelium during the first few days of PRK healing comprises the period of greatest risk for the operative eye, as the cornea remains vulnerable for

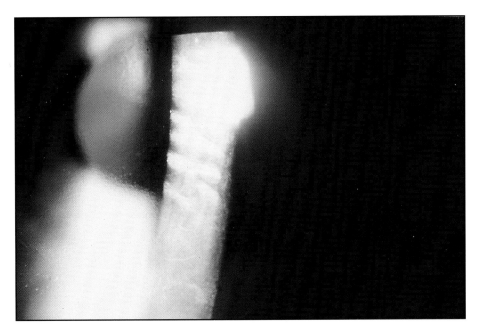

Figure 4-18.
Moderate stromal edema following PRK. Management involves frequent full-strength topical steroids and refitting with flatter base curve contact lens. In cases associated with significant inflammation, discontinue contact lens use with patching.

infection throughout this period. Daily clinical observation during epithelial healing is required to ensure optimal safety (Figure 4-4). A prolonged epithelial healing time not only increases the risk period for infection but promotes haze formation. The epithelial healing phase may also be rarely complicated by a stromal melt in conjunction with either a systemic vasculitic disorder or topical non-steroidal anti-inflammatory agent.

Postoperative Days 1, 2, 3
Clinical

Patient comfort with a topical NSAID-bandage contact lens regimen is remarkably good for most patients (Figure 4-5). Severe pain, when it does occur, usually strikes the first night. Increased discomfort and irritation also occur during the last 12 hours of epithelial healing (Figures 4-6 through 4-7b). Visual recovery during epithelial healing is variable and not indicative of the final visual and refractive outcome. Subjective vision usually falls as the epithelial healing edge encroaches upon the visual axis. The epithelium is usually only about 30% healed on the first postoperative day (Figures 4-8 through 4-11), with roughly 1 to 2 mm of peripheral epithelial growth observed. The second day (Figures 4-12 and 4-14) is the day of greatest progression as an additional 3 to 4 mm of epithelial growth is observed providing about 70% to 80% coverage in most cases. The third day a typical Y-epithelial healing pattern is observed. The epithelium remains somewhat irregular centrally, producing visual distortion; however, comfort dramatically improves.

Epithelial healing occurs more rapidly superiorly and less rapidly inferiorly as is observed with traumatic epithelial abrasions. The more smooth and defined the edges of the epithelium, the more rapid re-epithelialization occurs. Patients who had loosely adherent epithelium (Figure 4-15) noted on mechanical debridement will tend to have irregular edges. Most patients have mild conjunctival injection associated, although a few will have mild eyelid swelling and conjunctival chemosis associated. Corneal edema (Figures 4-16 through 4-18) is surprisingly absent with most patients; however, trace, mild, and even moderate stromal edema with Descemet's folds may be observed. The concern with corneal edema is that the bandage contact lens may be excessively tight, especially if associated with perilimbal injection. Re-epithelialization proceeds more slowly once corneal edema is evident. Corneal infiltrates are not usually evident on the first day, whether infectious or sterile, but classically on the second day.

Management

Three specific aspects of healing are evaluated daily during epithelial healing. First, the extent of epithelial healing is monitored to ensure a normal or satisfactory rate of progression. Second, the presence and fit of the bandage contact lens is assessed. Occasionally, a bandage contact lens is lost during instillation of topical medications or lubrication. Excessive contact lens movement is equally if not more detrimental to the epithelial healing rate than an excessively tight lens and is more painful. It is best that the contact lens fit somewhat steeply without producing perilimbal conjunctival injection or corneal edema. Typically, about 0.5 mm of contact lens movement with blinking is recommended. Topical steroids help control corneal edema and ocular inflammation in most cases with a somewhat tight therapeutic lens. Third, it is important to examine for the presence and features of corneal infiltrates. Each visit during the epithelial healing phase should require no more than a few minutes. Reassurance is an important element during this acute recovery. Informing patients that they are healing in a typical manner is all that most patients require to alleviate their anxiety with respect to their pain and visual blurring.

IOP Monitoring Post-PRK

- IOP must be monitored at least monthly while patient is on topical steroid therapy.
- More frequent monitoring is required if IOP is elevated by 5 to 8 mmHg but still within normal range.
- IOP measurement may be underestimated with flat corneas post-PRK.

Clinical Note

Fluoroquinolones

Ofloxacin 0.3% solution (Ocuflox, Allergan) and ciprofloxacin HCL solution (Ciloxan, Alcon) are both members of the fluoroquinolone family with broad spectrum antibiotic coverage. Both are bactericidal and act through inhibition of DNA gyrase. A third fluoroquinolone, Norfloxacin, appears to have less overall activity. Both gram positive and gram negative bacteria are susceptible to these agents with Ciloxan possessing greater pseudomonas coverage. Ciloxan and more recently Ocuflox have been proven in clinical study to be effective as single agent therapy in the treatment of corneal ulcers. Of limited clinical significance is the occurrence of crystalline precipitates in 18.8% of 154 patients when treated with Ciloxan aggressively for corneal ulcer therapy. All precipitates were noted between 1 to 7 days and cleared spontaneously over 1 to 13 days. As discussed, Ciloxan may rarely produce precipitates with qid prophylactic dosing and interfere with re-epithelialization. Delayed re-epithelialization is one of the known etiologic factors in confluent haze formation. Crystalline precipitates have not been described with Ocuflox. In light of the fact that staphylococcal and streptococcal species (likely related to untreated blepharitis) are the primary bacterial causes of postoperative PRK infec-

tions, fluoroquinolones are preferential to tobramycin which has reduced streptococcal efficacy.

Gram positive bacterial coverage:

- *Staphylococcus aureus*
- *Staphylococcus epidermidis*
- *Streptococcus pneumoniae*

Gram negative bacterial coverage:

- *Haemophilus influenzae*
- *Pseudomonas aeruginosa* (Ciloxan)

Our current prophylactic PRK regimen includes Ocuflox (Allergan) and TobraDex (Alcon) qid. Our preference for Ocuflox was based upon our observation of crystalline precipitates with Ciloxan. Dual coverage was preferred because of our desire to have improved *pseudomonal* coverage with bandage contact lens use. The dexamethasone steroid preparation with tobramycin is required to help prevent sterile infiltrates related to our concomitant use of Voltaren (diclofenac sodium 0.1%, CIBA) bid for postoperative pain control.

Postoperative PRK medications:

- Ocuflox—one to two drops qid until re-epithelialization is complete
- TobraDex—one to two drops qid until re-epithelialization is complete
- Voltaren—one to two drops bid maximum 3 days

Epithelial healing usually requires 3 days to complete, but many patients require 4 days and some as long as 1 week. Conversely, patients treated with a transepithelial approach or small optical zone or those who sleep continuously may

---

Management of Tight Contact Lens Syndrome

- Remove bandage contact lens
- Insert flatter bandage contact lens and increase topical steroids if no significant edema
- Pressure patch with antibiotic-steroid ointment if significant edema

---

Postoperative PRK medications:

- Ocuflox—one to two drops qid until re-epithelialization is complete
- TobraDex—one to two drops qid until re-epithelialization is complete
- Voltaren—one to two drops bid maximum 3 days

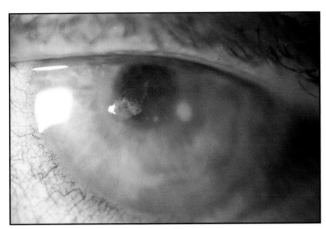

Figure 4-19a.
Pneumococcal corneal ulcer with focal central infiltrate and peripheral arcuate infiltrate. Denuded central epithelium with significant conjunctival injection.

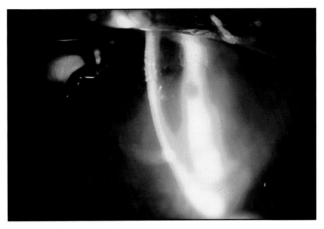

Figure 4-19b.
Infectious arcuate infiltrate first observed on second postoperative day, the most common day infectious and sterile infiltrates are observed. Patient experiencing severe pain clinically, which does not distinguish infectious nature. Epithelial defect typical of infectious infiltrates but can also be seen with non-infectious reactions. Arcuate nature more typical of sterile immune ring, but this case represents a gram positive infection. This clinical example illustrates the need for culture and sensitivity studies in all indeterminate cases, with the institution of fortified antibiotics pending microbiology results.

heal in 2 days. If epithelial healing is not completed by 3 days and the eye is inflamed, the bandage contact lens should be removed and the eye pressure patched with antibiotic-steroid ointment. Delayed epithelial healing beyond 4 days even with a quiet eye should be managed by removal of the therapeutic contact lens and pressure patching.

Pressure patching with antibiotic-steroid ointment should also be instituted in cases of tight contact lenses with

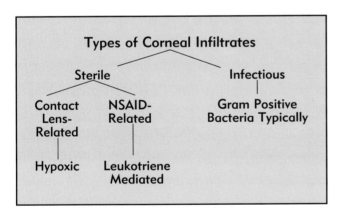

Types of Corneal Infiltrates

- Sterile
  - Contact Lens-Related
    - Hypoxic
  - NSAID-Related
    - Leukotriene Mediated
- Infectious
  - Gram Positive Bacteria Typically

Features of Infectious Infiltrates
- Typically central or paracentral
- Variable size from 0.5 to 2.0 mm initially
- Indistinct margins with central density
- Typically round or oval, can be arcuate
- Epithelium denuded over infiltrate
- Associated with ocular inflammation
- Possible anterior chamber reaction
- Increased pain and photophobia

corneal edema and non-progressive epithelial healing. A tight but comfortable contact lens with normal re-epithelialization and without stromal edema should be left in place and watched closely. Topical NSAID should be tapered or more preferably discontinued in any case of retarded re-epithelialization even at 2 days, especially if the eye is comfortable. A tight, comfortable contact lens with slow re-epithelialization but no corneal edema or inflammation requires refitting with a flatter base curve or patching.

Excessive contact lens movement if associated with discomfort or slow re-epithelialization should also be managed by contact lens exchange for a steeper base curve or simply with patching. It is always preferable if clinically unclear to remove the bandage contact lens and pressure patch the eye. The patient should always be forewarned that contact lens exchange or pressure patching will result in increased pain acutely related to the manipulation of the eye. Patching in general is less comfortable than a bandage contact lens independent of the use of NSAIDs.

The presence of corneal infiltrates demands clinical identification of the infiltrate as sterile or infectious. If infectious, management of corneal infiltrates following PRK is very much the same as that related to contact lens use. The contact lens must be removed and the infiltrated stroma cultured if the epithelium is denuded over the infiltrate (Figures 4-19a and 4-19b).

Figure 4-20.
Single peripheral, flat, well-demarcated sterile infiltrate related to contact lens-induced corneal hypoxia.

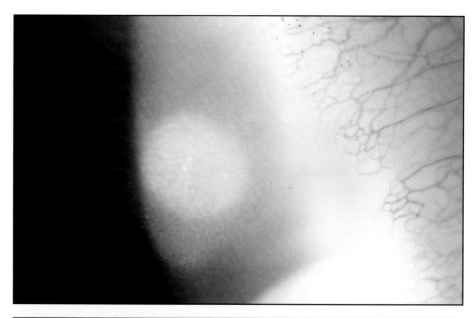

Figure 4-21.
Multiple sterile infiltrates secondary to use of topical anti-inflammatory non-steroidal agents without adequate topical steroid coverage. This particular case involved bilateral infiltrates as the patient had undergone bilateral simultaneous PRK.

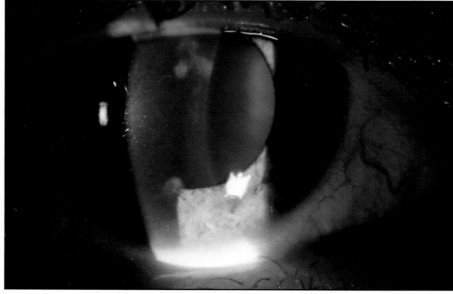

If the epithelium is intact and the infiltrate is peripheral, flat, and well-defined (Figure 4-20), it is likely sterile and

Features of Contact Lens-Related Sterile Corneal Infiltrate
- Peripheral most common, beneath upper lid
- Small, less than 1.0 mm usually
- Well-defined or slightly indistinct margins
- Round or oval, may be multiple
- Epithelium typically intact
- Mild to moderate ocular inflammation
- Rarely any anterior chamber reaction
- Mild pain or discomfort common

may be treated conservatively by removing the lens and treating with a broad spectrum fluoroquinolone used hourly while awake. Small, possibly multiple infiltrates typically located superiorly beneath the upper eyelid are often related to hypoxia induced by overnight contact lens wear. Untreated, the epithelium may break down and lead to an infectious corneal ulcer. A topical steroid-antibiotic combination is highly effective at improving and resolving contact lens related infiltrates, but infection must be ruled out.

A more difficult clinical differential diagnosis to resolve on occasion is that of NSAID-related corneal infiltrates, which most commonly are observed paracentrally, often in an area where the epithelium is not intact. These infiltrates can be large and multiple, but are typically flat and well-cir-

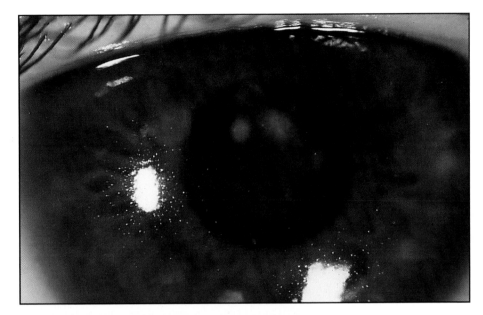

Figure 4-22.
Two paracentral sterile infiltrates, well demarcated, with intact epithelium related to topical non-steroidal anti-inflammatory use.

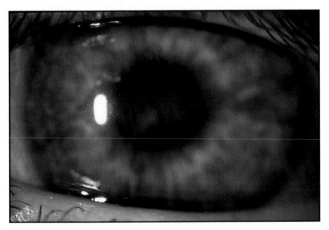

Figure 4-23a.
Residual central scarring following PRK secondary to previous stromal infiltration from topical NSAID use.

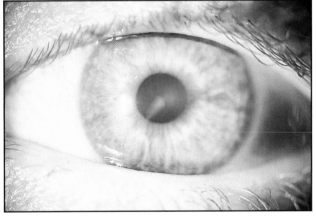

Figure 4-23b.
Central scarring associated with minimal, visually insignificant, stromal melt.

cumscribed with distinct margins (Figures 4-21 and 4-22). Similarly treated, the removal of the contact lens and discontinuation of the topical NSAID is essential. Despite the sterile nature of NSAID-related infiltrate, a localized stromal melt can be induced and intensive topical steroid therapy is definitely indicated once infection has been ruled out. Further described in Chapter 5, it is believed that NSAIDs, while decreasing the production of prostaglandins responsible for much of the PRK pain, increase the production of leukotrienes resulting in white blood cell chemotaxis and stromal infiltration. The incidence of these infiltrates is about 0.5% but the concomitant use of topical steroids drastically reduces their formation to less than 0.1% (Figures 4-23a and 4-23b).

Features of NSAID-Related Corneal Infiltrate

- Paracentral most common
- Typically larger, 1.0 to 3.0 mm
- Well-defined margins typical
- Round and flat appearance
- Epithelium intact or denuded
- Minimal ocular inflammation
- No anterior chamber reaction
- Mild if any discomfort

NSAID-Infiltrates and Immune Ring

A 26-year-old male patient underwent bilateral PRK for -3.75 +0.50 x 62 OD and -3.50 +1.25 x 101 OS. Preoperative best corrected vision was 20/20 in both eyes. There were no intraoperative complications. Postoperatively, the patient developed severe pain and photophobia in his left eye on the third postoperative day. On clinical examination, there were multiple paracentral infiltrates in a circular pattern forming an immune ring (Figure 4-24). The epithelium was intact. The topical non-steroidal anti-inflammatory agent prescribed, Voltaren (diclofenac sodium 0.1%, CIBA), was immediately discontinued. The patient was cyclopleged and placed on hourly Predforte (prednisolone acetate 1%, Allergan). The bandage contact lens was removed and Ocuflox (ofloxacin, Allergan) was initially continued every 2 hours while awake by the comanaging ophthalmologist as the correct differential diagnosis was an infectious etiology. A fungal etiology can also be entertained with this corneal presentaion.

The patient was followed daily. After 1 week, the inflammation was reduced significantly with no corneal edema or anterior chamber reaction noted. The stromal infiltrate penetrated one third the corneal depth and produced considerable irregular astigmatism preventing adequate refraction at 1 week. Uncorrected visual acuity at 1 week was 20/80 but gradually improved to 20/20-1 after 3 months. The stromal opacities decreased in intensity over the first month but residual scarring remained even after several months (Figures 4-25a and 4-25b). Predforte had been discontinued after 1 week and a mild topical corticosteroid, fluorometholone 0.1%, re-instituted with the standard 4-month tapering regimen. The fellow eye had an uneventful course and achieved 20/20+ uncorrected visual acuity.

The important aspect to successful management of immune and other NSAID-induced reactions is prompt discontinuation of the offending agent, consideration of an infectious etiology, and frequent instillation of a full-strength topical corticosteroid. Antibiotic prophylaxis is recommended and patients should be closely monitored every 12 to 24 hours. An epithelial defect increases suspicion of a microbial keratitis and management involves culture and instillation of standard corneal ulcer therapy pending microbiology results and clinical response. Potent topical steroids such as prednisolone acetate 1% and dexamethasone 0.1% remain the mainstay of NSAID-related inflammatory and immune reactions.

Management of Suspected Infectious Corneal Infiltrates

- Remove bandage contact lens independent of cause
- Discontinue NSAID use
- Culture if epithelium not intact
- Start hourly broad spectrum antibiotics
    Fluoroquinolone first choice of antibiotics: Ocuflox or Ciloxan
- Add hourly fortified antibiotics if corneal ulcer clinically evident or culture positive
    Choice of fortified antibiotics: cefazolin 50 mg/cc and tobramycin 14 mg/cc for triple coverage
    Alternative choice of fortified antibiotics: vancomycin 1 mg/cc and amkacin 20 mg/cc
- Cycloplegia recommended
- Re-examine in 12 to 24 hours, then daily to reassess progression
- Oral narcotics usually required for pain
- No pressure patching unless confirmed sterile
- Subconjunctival antibiotics and hospital admission if unresponsive

Occasionally, it is impossible to discern clinically whether a corneal infiltrate is infectious or sterile, and as such two important principles govern care of the patient. First, it must be assumed that the infiltrate represents an infectious clinical entity and is treated as such pending culture results. Second, the patient must be monitored closely to assess progression or resolution on topical antibiotics. Clinically, the presence of intact epithelium overlying the infiltrate is the most reliable, although not absolute, objective sign that an infiltrate is sterile. Subjectively, pain may or may not be associated with sterile infiltrates, but disproportionate or severe pain is more common with infectious corneal ulcers. The resolution or improvement of pain and clinical symptoms after 24 hours of topical antibiotics, despite little change in the clinical appearance, is highly suggestive of an infectious etiology being controlled. Often, the epithelial defect will remain unchanged, yet the symptoms and discomfort experienced have significantly subsided.

Removal of Therapeutic Contact Lens

The technique for removal of the contact lens is important as improper removal may result in another epithelial

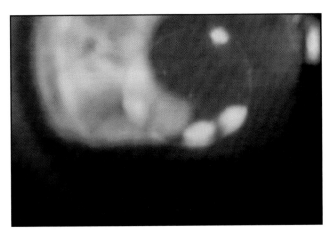

Figure 4-24.
NSAID-related immune ring with focal areas of infiltration.

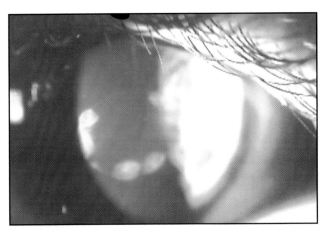

Figure 4-25a.
Corneal scarring secondary to NSAID-related immune ring and infiltrates.

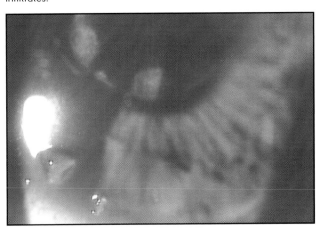

Figure 4-25b.
Corneal irregularity secondary to NSAID-related reaction.

defect. The most fundamental principle for removal is to lubricate the contact lens with copious artificial tears or topical anesthetic to literally float the contact lens prior to removal (Figures 4-26a through 4-26c). The use of topical anesthetic is disputed by some doctors who prefer to evaluate the comfort level of the patient immediately following lens removal and like to avoid any epitheliotoxic agent. The benefit of topical anesthesia, however, is facilitation of lens removal, resulting in a more atraumatic maneuver with less risk to the epithelium. Placing the patient in a semi-recumbent position, the contact may be removed by gently pulling down the lower eyelid while the patient directs his gaze upward, and after drawing the lens down, grasping the contact with the thumb and forefinger. More ideally, the inferior portion of the contact lens is grasped with non-toothed forceps preferably at a slit lamp under direct observation. The contact lens is pulled inferiorly and away from the eye. This technique is remarkably comfortable for patients, gentle on the epithelium, and simple to perform even in patients with blepharospasm.

> ## Technique for Bandage Contact Lens Removal
> - Lubricate eye copiously to float contact lens
> - Ensure adequate topical anesthesia
> - Direct patient to gaze superiorly
> - Grasp inferior aspect of lens with non-toothed forceps
> - Pull contact lens inferiorly and away from the eye

The same technique may be used if foreign matter or excessive epithelial debris is trapped beneath the bandage lens, especially if it appears to be retarding epithelial healing. In general, a small amount of debris is not uncommon or harmful and removal of the bandage lens and replacement with a new contact will not only be painful for a short while but may result in a larger epithelial defect. Nonetheless, if any concern is present with regard to trapped foreign particles, epithelial debris, or rolled epithelial edges, the lens should be replaced and the patient alerted to expect increased discomfort.

Occasionally after 3 days, the cornea does not demonstrate a smooth epithelial surface with the classic central Y-epithelial healing pattern indicative of an intact epithelium, but rather a localized area of boggy epithelium. This clinical picture is suggestive of non-adherent epithelium. As long as the eye is not inflamed, the contact lens should be left undisturbed for an additional day for the epithelium to solidify. The topical NSAID should be withdrawn in all cases where epithelial healing is incomplete by 3 days or the rate of progression even at 2 days is less than anticipated. If the contact lens is removed, it is typical for the boggy

Review of Postoperative Care for Epithelial Healing

- Epithelial healing should be complete by 3 days.
- The patient has been fitted with a bandage contact lens and placed on topical antibiotic, topical steroid, and topical NSAID.
- The patient should be assessed daily for epithelial healing progress, tight contact lens syndrome, and corneal infiltrates.
- Do not remove the contact to examine the eye. If none of these findings are evident, the contact should be left in and removed at 72 hours. Trace or mild edema is normal.
- If the epithelium is not healed at 72 hours, patch with antibiotic-steroid ointment or antibiotic daily until healed.
- Copious amounts of topical anesthetic or artificial tears should be instilled prior to removal of the contact lens to literally float the contact and simplify removal.
- Patients will experience irritation and blurring for an additional 1 to 2 days with gradual visual improvement.
- Should epithelium breakdown occur again, simply repatch for 24 hours.

Postoperative PRK Regimen During Epithelial Healing

- Antibiotic: tobramycin 0.3% or ofloxacin 0.3% two drops qid until healed
- Steroid: dexamethasone 0.1% or fluorometholone 0.1%/0.25% two drops qid until healed
- Non-steroidal anti-inflammatory drugs: diclofenac sodium 0.1% or ketorolac tromethamine 0.5% two drops bid to qid for 3 days maximum
- Bandage contact lens, fit snugly

Postoperative PRK Regimen After Epithelial Healing

Fluorometholone 0.1% x 4 to 5 months

qid x 1st month

tid x 2nd month

bid x 3rd month

QAM x 4th month

q 2 days x 5th month

epithelium to leave a denuded area locally, producing acute pain and requiring pressure patching. If the contact lens is removed and the epithelium remains intact but irregular and somewhat edematous focally, the eye should be similarly patched at least for 6 to 12 hours for the surface to become better adherent.

Topical Agents After Epithelial Healing

Once the epithelium is healed, start a 4-month tapering regimen of fluorometholone 0.1%:

- qid x 1 month
- tid x 1 month
- bid x 1 month
- QAM x 1 month

If not stable, fluorometholone 0.1% can be continued every 1 to 2 days for the fifth month. Never continue steroids indefinitely; the maximum is 6 months. It is safer to retreat for regression. It is best to measure intraocular pressure (IOP) at least monthly while the patient is on topical steroids.

Clinical Note

Steroid Management of Elevated IOP

Management of an IOP of 30 mmHg while the patient is on fluorometholone 0.1% qid would involve the addition of a topical beta-blocking agent.

1. If the IOP falls below 20 mmHg within 1 to 2 days, the steroid regimen can be continued and then re-evaluated in 2 weeks.
2. If the IOP remains elevated above 20 mmHg, the frequency of the topical steroid must be reduced to bid dosing and the pressure re-evaluated within a few days. If the IOP continues to remain elevated, the steroid frequency is reduced to daily and then finally discontinued altogether. If still elevated, attempts are made to re-institute it every other day only once the IOP is controlled.
3. If the patient had been on a more potent topical steroid initially, the first aspect of management would have been to reduce the potency of the topical steroid to fluorometholone 0.1%.

Stromal Wound Healing

The fundamental principle governing PRK healing is that it occurs at two levels, first at the level of the epithelium and then at the level of the stroma. Therefore, regression occurs at these two levels, with epithelial hyperplasia and stromal haze. More importantly, it is the epithelial-stromal

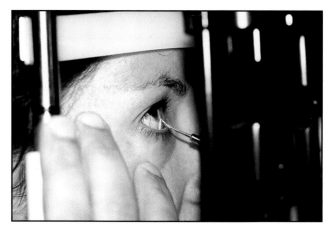

Figure 4-26a.
Removal of bandage contact lens. Patient gaze directed superiorly.

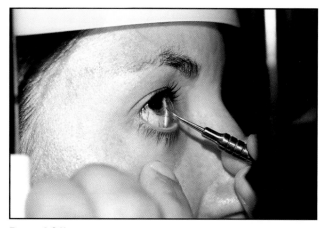

Figure 4-26b.
Removal of bandage contact lens. Fine non-toothed forceps used to grasp inferior aspect.

interaction that guides these two levels of healing. The epithelium becomes hyperplastic in response mostly to contour alterations of the stroma, and the stroma produces haze in response to some poorly understood interaction between these layers. It appears that the epithelium reacts to certain types of irregularities and disturbances of the newly fash-

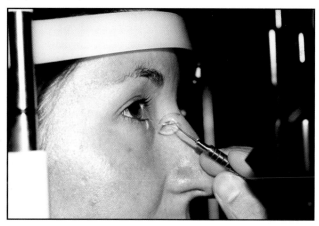

Figure 4-26c.
Removal of bandage contact lens. Contact lens pulled down and away from eye.

Postoperative Examination Schedule for PRK Patients

Days 1, 2, 3:
- Monitor epithelial healing progress
- Ensure proper bandage contact lens fit
- Monitor for infection

Note: Monitor daily until epithelium intact.

Day 14:
- Fogged manifest refraction
- Record uncorrected and best corrected visual acuity
- Measure IOP
- Grade corneal clarity

Months 1, 2, 3, and 4:
- Fogged manifest refraction
- Record uncorrected and best corrected visual acuity
- Measure IOP
- Grade corneal clarity

Months 6 and 12:
- Cycloplegic refraction
- Record uncorrected and best corrected visual acuity
- Grade corneal clarity
- Assess for enhancement at 6 months (minimum 5 months) when refraction and topography stable

ioned superficial stroma, resulting in the formation of subepithelial haze formation. With respect to the epithelium and epithelial-stromal interaction, it is not simply how much tissue that is removed but how it is removed with respect to contour and other inciting factors (ie, smoothness or thermal energy damage).

Laser in situ keratomileusis (LASIK) avoids these two levels of wound healing, leaving the epithelium and surface stroma undisturbed to potentially conquer refractive predictability. LASIK introduces new limitations of altered, deeper stroma hydration and creation of the flap itself.

Durrie and other surgeons have described three distinct types of healing patterns observed after surgery: normal healers, aggressive healers, and non-healers. In actuality, there appears to be a bell curve (Figure 4-27) continuum upon which patient healing patterns lie. The majority of patients fall into the center with a normal healing pattern,

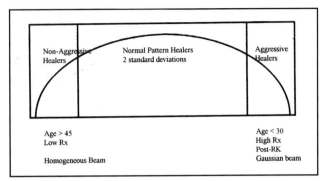

Figure 4-27.
Machat bell curve classification of healing patterns.

producing trace amounts of reticular haze and experiencing mild regression as predicted to overcome their initial hyperopic overshoot to achieve near-emmetropic results.

A subset of patients to the right of the curve are aggressive healers with an increased tendency toward myopic regression with clinically significant or confluent haze formation. Aggressive healers require greater steroid use to control their healing pattern for the first few months. Aggressive healing patterns are more frequently observed in young patients, especially those with higher refractive errors.

Non-healers are another subset of patients, usually over 40 years of age, on the left end of the bell curve continuum who seemingly stabilize immediately and fail to experience

---

Daniel Durrie Classification Healing Types

Group I: Normal healers
- Normal healing pattern with predictable refractive outcome
- Standard topical steroid regimen

Group II: Non-healers
- Underhealers with minimal to no haze
- Little regression, less than expected
- Hyperopic refractive outcome
- Rapid steroid taper or early discontinuation of steroids
- Increased need for holmium LTK

Group III: Aggressive healers
- Overhealers with significant haze formation
- Significant regression, more than expected
- Myopic refractive outcome
- Increased steroid requirements
- Increased need for PRK retreatment

---

even minor regression to overcome the planned initial overcorrection. These patients remain hyperopic with clear corneas and are unresponsive to steroid withdrawal.

These three types of healing patterns are much more clinically apparent with gaussian beam lasers utilizing smaller treatment zones because they broaden the curve or shift it to the right. Corneas ablated with gaussian beams and small optical zone treatments are more subject to myopic regression and more responsive to steroid titration with manipulation of the refractive outcome possible. Scanning lasers and multizone blending techniques utilizing large treatment areas shift the curve to the left. The left shift results in reduced myopic regression and less hyperopic overshoot being necessary in compensation; therefore, clearer corneas with more stable refractive and rapid visual outcomes are achieved. Retreatment of previous RK shifts the curve to the right. For higher degrees of myopia correction with surface ablation the curve also appears to be shifted to the right. In summary, patients are not defined in absolute terms as good healers and bad healers, but rather relative terms as a point along the bell curve which can be shifted somewhat by changing factors, such as technique and laser system utilized.

POSTOPERATIVE MEDICATIONS

After epithelial healing, the topical antibiotic and topical NSAID are discontinued and the topical steroid regimen commenced. Surgeons differ widely in their use of topical steroids from intensive 6-month or longer regimens to no postoperative topical steroids. In general, topical steroids are beneficial in reducing the development of postoperative stromal haze and improving refractive stability. Since topical steroids are associated with potentially serious side effects and PRK is an elective procedure, a conservative approach with careful monitoring is advocated during the first 3 to 4 months when stromal wound activity is maximal. Although stromal healing at the cellular level occurs over the first 12 to 18 months, the greatest activity is within the first 6 months. Steroid control, or suppression of wound healing, is an important aspect in preserving corneal clarity and achieving optimal refractive results. In essence, topical steroid use maintains the healing pattern curve to the left, reducing regression and haze formation. However, topical steroids are analogous to oral narcotics requiring gradual withdrawal to avoid a deleterious rebound effect, resulting occasionally in profound regression with haze formation.

Fluorometholone 0.1% is a mild topical steroid which

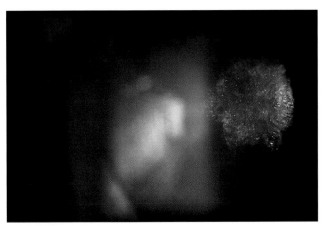

Figure 4-28.
Posterior subcapsular cataract formation secondary to topical dexamethasone 0.1% regimen following PRK. Steroid-induced cataracts observed in four patients, each treated with dexamethasone 0.1%, ranging in dosing from every 2 hours for 9 months to qid for only 3 months.

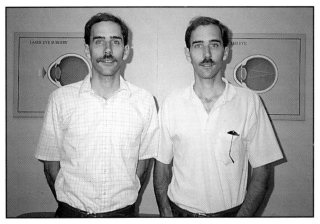

Figure 4-29.
Male identical twins treated with PRK for low myopia. Various postoperative anti-inflammatory regimens were evaluated in a prospective manner with 20/15 vision achieved OU for both twins.

appears to be advocated by most surgeons performing PRK. More potent topical steroids, such as dexamethasone phosphate 0.1%, prednisolone acetate 1%, and to a lesser extent fluorometholone 0.25% are associated with increased risk of steroid-induced rises in IOP and cataract formation, but may have a limited role in the postoperative management of PRK. Historically, more potent topical steroids were required to control wound healing, but improvements in technology and contouring techniques have reduced this need.

Gartry et al performed well-conducted, double-blind randomized studies to evaluate the long-term benefit of steroids and concluded that although beneficial short-term, there was no prolonged effect. Limitations of such a clinical study revolve around the use of a gaussian beam laser with limited optical zone and ablation algorithm capabilities. A large standard deviation of patient responses indicates steroid titration is an important element in such an evaluation, with prolonged use and gradual withdrawal necessary in certain individuals. At the other extreme, some surgeons continue to utilize long-term potent steroids which enable these surgeons to achieve superior clinical results, preserving corneal clarity and preventing regression. The risk of irreversible steroid complications such as glaucomatous visual field loss and cataract formation is elevated with these aggressive regimens and such complications have been reported (Figure 4-28). A more conservative approach with a gradually tapering mild corticosteroid is one that is advocated in light of the elective nature of this procedure, accepting a higher retreatment rate but inviting less serious adverse reactions.

Clinical Note

Postoperative Regimens in Identical Male Twins for Low Myopia

A double-blind prospective study was developed to examine the role of various postoperative regimens on both the refractive outcome and corneal clarity in identical twins (Figure 4-29). Both twins were treated with the Summit ExciMed UV 200 excimer laser system. Neither twin had a history of contact lens use and each twin measured upon cycloplegic refraction -3.00 D OS and -2.25 D OD. The left eye of each twin was treated first. Each twin was placed on a masked drop of either Maxidex (dexamethasone 0.1%, Alcon), our standard regimen in early 1992, or FML (fluorometholone 0.1%, Allergan). The topical agents were used qid for the first month and tapered monthly over 4 months. The medication regimen code was not revealed until the conclusion of the clinical trial 1 month after all topical steroids were discontinued. The twin who had been prescribed the low potency fluorometholone 0.1% healed more rapidly but both patients achieved 20/15 uncorrected visual acuity with no significant residual refractive error and absolutely clear corneas (Figure 4-30).

The right eye was treated 3 months after the first eye, as was our standard protocol at the time. Each twin was randomized into either postoperative treatment with artificial tears alone or Voltaren (diclofenac sodium 0.1%, CIBA), a non-steroidal anti-inflammatory agent. The medication bottles were masked to both patient and examiner.

Postoperative Corticosteroids Following PRK: Literature Review

Louis E. Probst V, MD

The value of topical corticosteroids following PRK continues to be controversial. Postoperative steroids were used in the early primate and blind eye studies[1,2] after they were shown to reduce the synthesis of new collagen and the associated stromal haze in the rabbit cornea following PRK.[3] Studies of PRK under the Phases IIb and III FDA trials generally used low potency postoperative steroids on a 4-month tapering schedule.[4] Because topical steroids have been associated with a number of complications following PRK, including elevated IOP, posterior subcapsular cataracts, ptosis, superficial keratopathy, and reactivation of herpes simplex keratitis,[5] investigators have attempted to define the minimal adequate dose of topical steroids after PRK.

Tengroth and coworkers found that topical dexamethasone reduced myopic regression of at least 0.50 D at 3 months postoperatively in 20% of the group treated for 3 months, compared to 47% of the myopic regression in the group treated for 5 weeks after PRK with the Summit laser.[6] This group also noted significant regression in 86% of their patients who did not receive any postoperative topical steroids,[7] which was reversible if the steroids were initiated within 3 months of the PRK.[8] The refractive results of patients whose first PRK eye was treated with steroids after surgery, and whose second eye was not, demonstrated significantly more regression in the untreated eyes with an average refractive difference of over 1.50 D.[7] Corneal topography has demonstrated the ability of dexamethasone to cause corneal flattening with a resultant hyperopic shift 3 to 8 months after the original steroids were discontinued,[9] which can correct late myopic regression in up to 30% of cases.[6,10]

Double-masked clinical trials comparing the refractive results and corneal haze following PRK in groups with and without steroids have been unable to confirm the efficacy of postoperative topical steroids. Gartry and coworkers found only a transient reduction in the myopic regression in their steroid group with no significant difference in the stromal haze.[11] In a prospective, randomized, observer-masked study of 86 patients with 1-year follow-up, O'Brart and coworkers found that corticosteroids maintained the hyperopic shift during their administration; however, this effect was reversed on cessation of treatment.[12] Both studies found no significant reduction in the corneal haze in the steroid groups.[11,12] In a randomized Korean trial, Baek and coworkers found a significantly greater hyperopic shift in the high myopia steroid group which became insignificant with treatment cessation.[13] All the other variables in this study, including visual acuity results, refractive changes in the low and moderate myopic groups, and stromal haze, were not significantly different between the steroid and the no-steroid groups.[13]

Corbett and coworkers[14] have recently provided an extensive review of the current experience with topical corticosteroids following PRK. The decrease in haze and collagen synthesis in rabbit and monkey studies investigating the use of postoperative corticosteroids has been inconsistent with the experience in human eyes. Reasons for this dichotomy may include:

- The absence of Bowman's membrane in rabbit cornea
- Animal studies were conducted on growing corneas
- Stromal healing in animal studies primarily involves collagen deposition, while human cornea healing involves glycosaminoglycan deposition

Since the refractive effect of topical corticosteroids can occur within days and wound healing after PRK can take up to 18 months, it is unlikely that they induced their refractive effect by modification of keratocyte activity or collagen synthesis. This group has proposed that corticosteroids induce a transient central corneal dehydration of the epithelial or subepithelial glycosaminoglycans, which causes a reversible flattening of the central cornea and a hyperopic shift. They concluded that there is no justification for the routine use of topical corticosteroids following PRK for low or moderate myopia. In accordance with these conclusions, McDonald and coworkers have recently reported that they are no longer using postoperative corticosteroids following PRK because no beneficial effect was found in their own comparative clinical trials.[15]

Despite these considerations, most surgeons still use postoperative topical corticosteroids. Concerns regarding the complications of postoperative corticosteroid therapy and the questions regarding their efficacy have resulted in most surgeons prescribing topical steroids with the minimal potency and concentration. A double-masked steroid trial in identical twins with low myopia found no difference in the visual acuity results or the corneal clarity between postoperative topical dexamethasone or fluorometholone 0.1%.[16] Most surgeons now use fluorometholone 0.1% on a tapering schedule of qid for the first month, tid for the second month, bid for the third month, and once a day for the fourth month.[4,17,18] Sher and coworkers have suggested that the use of a bandage contact lens and topical non-steroidal anti-inflammatory agents after PRK in the absence of topical corticosteroids may lead to inflammatory corneal infiltration.[19]

Recently, frequent postoperative topical corticosteroids have been suggested by Shaninian and Lin as a method of modulating the postoperative refraction and controlling haze and regression in patients with severe myopia undergoing PRK; however, they were felt to be far less important in patients with low to moderate myopia.[20] This group uses a multiple zone technique followed by dexamethasone qid for the first week, fluorometholone 0.25% six times a day and dexamethasone once a day for 2 weeks, and then fluorometholone 0.25% five times a day for 4 weeks, qid for 4 weeks, tid for 4 weeks, bid for 4 weeks, and one time per day for 4 weeks. This is then switched to fluorometholone 0.1% once per day for 4 weeks.

References

1. McDonald MB, Frantz JM, Klyce SD, et al. One-year results of photorefractive keratectomy for myopia in the nonhuman primate cornea. *Arch Ophthalmol.* 1990;108:40-47.

2. McDonald MB, Liu JC, Byrd RJ, et al. Central photorefractive keratectomy for myopia: partially sighted and normally sighted eyes. *Ophthalmology.* 1991;98:1327-1337.

3. Tuft SJ, Zabel RW, Marshall J. Corneal repair following keratectomy. A comparison between conventional surgery and laser photoablation. *Invest Ophthalmol Vis Sci.* 1989;30:1769-1777.

4. Salz JJ, Maguen E, Nesburn AB, et al. A two year experience with excimer laser photorefractive keratectomy for myopia. *Ophthalmology.* 1993;100:873-882.

5. Maguen E, Machat JJ. Complications of photorefractive keratectomy, primarily with the VisX excimer laser. In: Salz JJ, McDonnell PJ, McDonald MB, eds. *Corneal Laser Surgery.* St. Louis, Mo: Mosby; 1995.

6. Tengroth B, Epstein D, Fagerholm P, et al. Excimer laser photorefractive keratectomy for myopia. Clinical results in sighted eyes. *Ophthalmology.* 1993;100(5):739-745.

7. Fagerholm P, Hamberg-Nystrom H, Tengroth B, Epstein D. Effect of postoperative steroids on the refractive outcome of photorefractive keratectomy for myopia with the Summit excimer laser. *J Cataract Refract Surg.* 1994;20(Suppl):212.

8. Tengroth B, Fagerholm P, Soderberg P, et al. Effect of corticosteroids in postoperative care following photorefractive keratectomies. *Refract Corneal Surg.* 1993;9(Suppl):S61-S64.

9. Fitzsimmons TD, Fagerholm P, Tengroth B. Steroid treatment of myopic regression: acute refractive and topographic changes in excimer photorefractive keratectomy patients. *Cornea.* 1993;12:358-361.

10. Carones F, Brancato R, Venturi E, et al. Efficacy of corticosteroids in reversing regression after myopic photorefractive keratectomy. *Refract Corneal Surg.* 1993;9(Suppl):S52-S60.

11. Gartry DS, Kerr Muir MG, Lohmann CP, et al. The effect of topical corticosteroids on refractive outcome and corneal haze after phototherapeutic keratectomy. *Arch Ophthalmol.* 1992;110:944-952.

12. O'Brart DPS, Lohmann CP, Klonos G, et al. The effects of topical corticosteroids and plasmin inhibitors on refractive outcome, haze, and visual performance after photorefractive keratectomy. A prospective, randomized, observer masked study. *Ophthalmology.* 1994;101(9):1565-1574.

13. Baek SH, Kim WJ, Chang JH, Lee JH. The effect of topical corticosteroids on refractive outcome and corneal haze after excimer laser photorefractive keratectomy: comparison of the effects on low-to-moderate and high myopia groups. *Invest Ophthalmol Vis Sci.* 1995;36(4):S713.

14. Corbett MC, O'Brart DPS, Marshall J. Do topical corticosteroids have a role following excimer laser photorefractive keratectomy? *J Refract Surg.* 1995;11(5):380-387.

15. McDonald MB, Talamo JH. Myopic photorefractive keratectomy: the experience in the United States with the VisX excimer laser. In: Salz JJ, McDonnell PJ, McDonald MB, eds. *Corneal Laser Surgery.* St. Louis, Mo: Mosby; 1995.

16. Machat JJ. Double-blind corticosteroid trial in identical twins following photorefractive keratectomy. *Refract Corneal Surg.* 1993;9(Suppl):S105-S107.

17. Talley AR, Hardten DR, Sher NA, et al. Results one year after using the 193-nm excimer laser for photorefractive keratectomy in mild to moderate myopia. *Am J Ophthalmol.* 1994;118(3):304-311.

18. Maguen E, Salz JJ, Nesburn AB, et al. Results of excimer laser photorefractive keratectomy for the correction of myopia. *Ophthalmology.* 1994;101:1548-1557.

19. Sher NA, Krueger R, Teal P, Jans R. Are steroids necessary after excimer photorefractive keratectomy? ISRK Pre-American Academy of Ophthalmology; October 28-29, 1994.

20. Shaninian L, Lin DTC. Clinical analysis of excimer laser photorefractive keratectomy using a multiple zone technique for severe myopia. *Am J Ophthalmol.* 1995;120(4):546-547. Letter.

Figure 4-30.
Excellent preservation of corneal clarity observed with twin A following PRK for -3.00 D with standard steroid regimen.

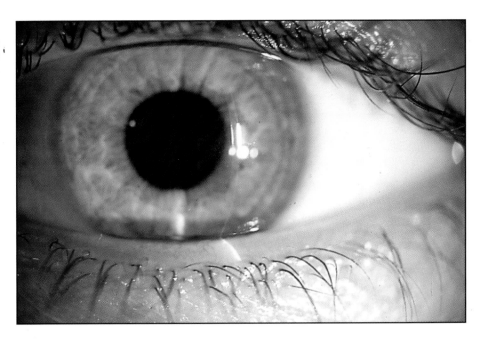

Both twins once again achieved excellent final refractive and visual outcomes with a plano refraction at 6 months that has remained stable. Voltaren in 1992 in Canada contained thimerosal as a preservative and resulted in a superficial toxic keratitis. Since 1993, sorbic acid has been the preservative used in the formulation of Voltaren in Canada, as in the United States. There was a slight degree of clinically discernible haze initially in the Voltaren-treated eye, otherwise the clinical outcome was identical.

After more than 3 years, both twins remain stable with 20/15 OU uncorrected vision and clear corneas. The conclusion with respect to postoperative management is not a general one with broad implications, but that topical steroids do not provide any long-term refractive benefit in cases of low myopia. These clinical findings and conclusions are also specific to the Summit ExciMed UV 200 laser and may also be specific to patients with excellent innate wound healing capabilities.

A further issue concerning the use of NSAIDs in place of topical steroids in the postoperative management of PRK is questioned by this identical twin study. Another young female patient treated at the same time with the Summit ExciMed laser for -4.00 D OU experienced topical steroid-induced ptosis with her first eye and was treated with Voltaren postoperatively with her second eye. She did not develop a clinically significant superficial keratitis but did develop trace haze which subsequently cleared. No ptosis was associated with Voltaren use. The increased haze was observed in several other patients treated with

NSAIDs, both with Acular (ketorolac tromethamine 0.5%, Allergan) and Voltaren without thimerosal. Increased haze was also observed in a number of other patients who developed a postoperative keratitis not associated with NSAID use.

It appears that NSAIDs may be associated with increased haze formation, and possibly increased myopic regression in my clinical experience, when used beyond the first few days for refractive outcome management. Furthermore, superficial keratitis from any cause may produce haze and myopic regression as well.

Topical steroids are not required in all patients, but clearly in some patients. A number of patients, especially those with low myopia, will do well regardless of the postoperative regimen used. The innate wound healing capabilities of the patient may dramatically alter outcome regardless of steroid regimen, as evidenced by the clinical photos of dense confluent haze in Figures 2-2a and 2-2b of a -4.00 D patient with a strong personal and family history of keloid formation. As it is impossible to predetermine at present which patients have aggressive wound healing characteristics, conservative overtreatment appears to be the rule. That is, treating all patients with a very low potency tapering regimen of fluorometholone 0.1% or learning the art of titration of topical steroids with closer monitoring of all patients. With improvements in PRK technique and excimer laser system technology, there continues to be a reduced need for topical steroid use.

TABLE 4-1

INTRAOCULAR PRESSURE

<22 mmHg <8 mmHg Rise	≥22 mmHg ≥8 mmHg Rise	≥30 mmHg	≥40 mmHg
1. Continue to monitor IOP. 2. Same topical steroid regimen.	1. Add beta-blocking agent if no respiratory or cardiac contraindications. 2. Reassess at 1 week. 3. If controlled, continue topical steroid regimen. 4. Monitor at least biweekly.	1. Reduce topical steroid dose by 50%. 2. Add beta-blocking agent if no respiratory or cardiac contraindications. 3. Reassess daily until IOP controlled. 4. If controlled, maintain lower steroid dose for full duration then taper off. 5. If uncontrolled, add topical carbonic anhydrase inhibitor (CAI) if no sulfonamide allergy. 6. If still uncontrolled, discontinue topical steroids until controlled, then attempt to reintroduce topical steroids (fluorometholone) at once daily while maintaining IOP controlling agents. 7. Oral CAI not recommended.	1. Discontinue topical steroids. 2. Start topical beta-blocking agent if no respiratory or cardiac contraindications. 3. Add topical CAI if no sulfonamide allergy or other contraindications. 4. Monitor IOP daily. 5. Once IOP controlled, may attempt to reintroduce topical steroids (fluorometholone) once every 2 to 3 days while maintaining other IOP agents. 6. LASIK for fellow eye. 7. Instruct patient of higher risk of glaucoma development in future.

Once a patient has initiated topical corticosteroid use, it is important to monitor the patient carefully for elevation of IOP. As stated, topical steroids should always be gradually withdrawn with a tapering regimen over several weeks. Abrupt discontinuation of steroids may result in increased myopic regression often associated with haze formation. There are only two indications for rapid steroid withdrawal: significantly increased IOPs, whereby the addition of a topical beta-blocking agent is either contraindicated or inadequate, and significant overcorrections. Low potency topical steroids are usually re-instituted at a lower frequency once the desired improvement has been achieved to restabilize wound healing.

It is important to maintain the patient on the lowest frequency and potency possible during the first 3 to 4 months to prevent severe myopic regression and haze formation once the IOP has been controlled. If the patient must be retreated for haze and regression, the vicious cycle will begin once again as topical steroids will be required (Table 4-1).

TABLE 4-2

REFRACTION AT 1 MONTH
FLUOROMETHOLONE 0.1% QID X 1 MONTH

<-1.00 D	Plano	+1.00 D
1. Consider unplanned monovision.	1. Expect further regression of 0.50 to 1.00 D until stable. Consider unplanned monovision.	1. Ideal refraction at 1 month.
2. Represents true undercorrection rather than regression.	2. If emmetropia is desired, maintain fluorometholone 0.1% qid for additional month, then taper more gradually over 6 months total.	2. Continue standard regimen.
3. Most patients will desire retreatment.	3. Maximum steroid regimen duration is 6 months.	
4. Do not withdraw topical steroids abruptly; must taper off gradually to avoid haze formation.	4. Maximum steroid potency is fluorometholone 0.25% qid for 4 weeks maximum.	
5. Once initiated, steroids must be tapered always, but can do so over 6 to 8 weeks instead of 12 weeks if desired, or finish standard regimen.	5. Always better to retreat when stable, then continue steroids indefinitely with low or high potency agents. Risk of steroid-induced complications contraindicate this form of management.	
6. Increased steroid frequency and potency may reverse regression, but usually inadequate at this point if >1.00 D undercorrected.	6. Prolonged low potency topical steroid regimen may reduce regression to <-0.50 D and avoid need for retreatment with second course of topical steroids.	
7. Do not retreat early. Must achieve new refractive level of stability. Early retreatment will result in undercorrection since full extent of regression is not known. In general, wait a minimum of 1 month, but preferably 3 months off topical steroids prior to retreatment.	7. If a presbyopic patient, refractive result will be ideal. If a younger patient, he or she will likely complain. Night driving glasses are better than retreatment.	
8. If a presbyopic patient, undercorrection is best. If a younger patient, expect to retreat in several months.		

POSTOPERATIVE VISUAL RECOVERY

Most mild to moderate myopes are able to achieve functional vision in the 20/40 range within the first 1 to 2 weeks, and their best uncorrected vision within 1 to 3 months. Each laser system has its own pattern of healing. It is important for patients to realize that there is a gradual return of vision but that they may return to work once their epithelium has healed, typically in 3 days. Patients over 40 years of age appear to heal more slowly but eventually achieve the same clinical results. Presbyopic patients experience slower visual recovery as they are unable to accommodate sufficiently to overcome the early overcorrection experienced. Healing occurs at the microscopic level during the first 6 to 18 months. The overwhelming majority of patients who have achieved a good refractive and visual result at 6 months appear to remain stable. Best corrected vision may be

TABLE 4-2 (CONTINUED)
REFRACTION AT 1 MONTH
FLUOROMETHOLONE 0.1% QID X 1 MONTH

+1.50 D	+2.00 D	>+2.00 D
1. Ideal refraction for young patient, likely will yield 20/20 uncorrected vision.	1. Reduce fluorometholone 0.1% to bid then recheck in 2 weeks.	1. Discontinue topical steroids and monitor weekly.
2. May yield slight overcorrection in presbyopic patient. Recheck in 2 weeks to enure regression continues.	2. If still ≥+1.50 D, reduce fluorometholone 0.1% to QAM and reassess in 2 weeks.	2. Must re-institute topical steroids to prevent rapid myopic regression with haze.
3. If no regression on fluorometholone 0.1% at 6 weeks, 2 weeks after tid dosing initiated, reduce to bid and recheck in 2 weeks. Reduce dose every 2 weeks if no regression.	3. At 2 months if still hyperopia ≥+1.50 D, discontinue topical steroids.	3. Monitor rate of regression as well as refractive error at each visit.
4. Continue standard regimen if regression noted, typically longer healing pattern, with full regression requiring 6 to 9 months.	4. At 2 months if <+1.50 D but >+1.00 D, continue drops once daily.	4. Once refraction reaches +1.00 D, restart fluorometholone 0.1% bid if rapid rate of regression over 2 to 4 weeks, or QAM if slow rate of regression over 4 to 12 weeks. Taper slowly over months until stable to prevent further regression with haze.
	5. Once refraction decreases to +1.00 D, patient should be placed on fluorometholone 0.1% once daily.	
	6. If rate of regression (and haze) increases, increase topical steroids to bid to slow recovery.	
	7. These patients must be monitored at least biweekly during 4-month active healing phase.	
	8. These patients must have topical steroids re-instituted when they reach +0.50 to +1.00 D to fine tune regression toward plano. If not, regression will continue and haze formation will increase.	

reduced by one to two lines for the first few weeks, but generally recovers by 3 to 4 weeks in most patients. Prolonged reduction of best corrected vision may be observed in patients treated for severe and extreme myopia.

POSTOPERATIVE REFRACTIVE MANAGEMENT

Refractive error management postoperatively in PRK is both pharmacological and surgical. Indications include both hyperopic overcorrection and myopic undercorrection or regression. Myopic regression can be both early and late. Both early and late myopic regression can be with or without haze formation (Table 4-2).

Myopic Undercorrection or Regression

Early undercorrection is evident immediately, whereas myopic regression signifies an achieved result which is lost.

The end result of both is residual myopia or astigmatism which must be addressed.

Treatment can be pharmacological, surgical, or none. No treatment may be indicated in presbyopic patients who achieve unplanned monovision. Patients who are observed to regress in the early postoperative period can be managed pharmacologically by increasing steroid potency and/or their frequency of application. The risk of steroid-related complications increases and these patients must be followed more closely with particular emphasis on frequent IOP measurements. If the degree of myopic regression increases beyond -1.00 D, the need for surgical retreatment is

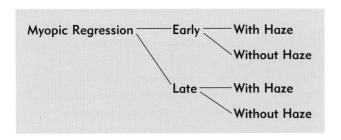

increased and the topical steroids should be tapered to avoid any cumulative cataractogenic effects. In general, if the rate of regression is greater than anticipated, such as in a patient who is -0.25 D within the first month, increasing topical steroid use is most effective. Increased topical steroids during the first 3 to 6 months will help reduce the rate of regression and promote stabilization during the most active period of stromal wound healing. Once a patient has regressed excessively, steroids are of limited benefit. That is, although topical steroids have been demonstrated to reverse regression, usually only 1 D of effect can be achieved maximally.

Myopic regression with and without clinically significant haze requires different approaches. The hallmark of clinically significant haze as described in the next section is the presence of confluence. Once confluent haze (Figure 4-31) is present, the use of topical steroids to control regression becomes controversial. Topical steroids control but do not eliminate haze. Patients who develop significant subepithelial haze regress dramatically (Figures 4-32a through 4-32c). Topical steroids reduce the induced myopia and improve vision quantitatively, although vision remains poor

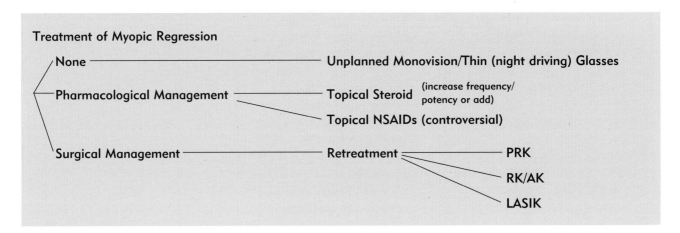

qualitatively. Retreatment is indicated for these patients after a minimum of 3 months and preferably 6 months. Patients should be stable and off medication for 1 month. Stability is defined as two refractive readings 1 month apart within 0.25 D with stable corneal topography. In many cases, however, haze formation is progressive and no defined stability is observed.

The most common period for myopic regression to occur is immediately upon cessation of topical steroids. It is surprising that even fluorometholone 0.1% used once daily can prevent myopic regression. In fact, once a week use has controlled some patients despite the fact that the drug half-

Surgical Retreatment Approach

Mechanical Debridement
   Regression without haze
   Central island

Transepithelial Approach
   Regression with haze
   Complex/asymmetric topographical
      abnormalities

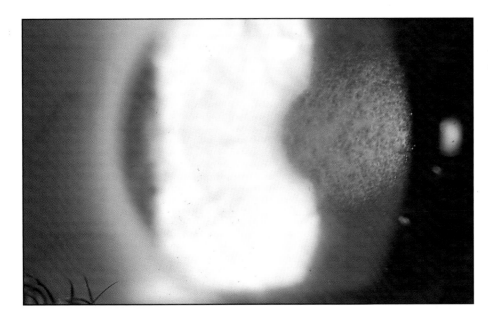

Figure 4-31.
Diffuse confluent haze following PRK for moderately severe myopia correction.

life has been exceeded. Re-institution of topical steroids at once a day or once every other day for 1 to 2 months has been highly effective at promoting stabilization and permitting total steroid withdrawal. If the patient has been off topical steroids for a couple of weeks prior to being re-evaluated and is determined to be -1.00 D, topical steroids will likely have to be re-instituted at a higher frequency. Usually fluorometholone 0.1% qid tapered weekly is effective, with the patient remaining on once daily drops for an additional 3 to 4 weeks. If the extent of myopic regression exceeds -1.00 D, fluorometholone 0.25% may be required. In general, rapid myopic regression greater than -1.00 D will require retreatment once restabilized. Disposable contact lenses can be fitted in the interim but removed well in advance of the scheduled retreatment.

Clinical Note
Myopic Regression With Haze

A 34-year-old woman treated for 8.00 D of myopia develops a dense central plaque of collagen, resulting in 4 D of regression. Topical steroids will shrink the collagen plaque by removing water from the glycosaminoglycans within the subepithelial plaque and therefore reduce the residual myopia to -1.00 D. The patient experiences improved uncorrected vision, the doctor measures less myopia, and both are happy. The topical steroids are withdrawn after a few months and the myopia once again increases with the patient and the doctor both becoming disillusioned. The topical steroids are restarted often with increased steroid frequency and potency with almost immediate clinical improvement. The cycle continues over years or until a cataract or other sight-threatening complication occurs.

Clinical Note
Myopic Regression Without Haze

A 38-year-old man treated for -5.00 D of myopia measures +0.25 D at 4 weeks in his right eye and reads 20/20 uncorrected. Corneal clarity is excellent and the patient is on fluorometholone 0.1% qid with an IOP of 10 mmHg. He is about to taper to fluorometholone 0.1% tid for his second month of postoperative medication. Based upon these clinical findings it is anticipated that the patient will regress to -1.00 D or less. Since his right eye is his dominant eye, monovision is not an option. Management involves the continuation of topical steroids at a minimum of qid. Consideration is made to increase the fluorometholone 0.1% frequency to every 3 hours or potency to 0.25% at the same qid frequency for 1 month, then taper gradually. The IOP is reassessed after 2 weeks to ensure the IOP is not significantly elevated. If the IOP is elevated to 18 mmHg after 2 weeks, a topical beta-blocker can be instituted and the steroid tapered earlier to 0.25% tid or 0.1% back to qid. The topical steroids should be gradually withdrawn over 5 months. If the refractive error continues to regress despite the increased steroid use, the drops should be tapered and retreatment planned once stabilization has occurred.

Figure 4-32a.
Thirty-one-year-old man had uncomplicated PRK for -7.25 D in April 1994. In May 1994, patient was 20/20 uncorrected with a clear cornea with +0.75 D hyperopia. Patient regressed with confluent central cornea haze over several months.

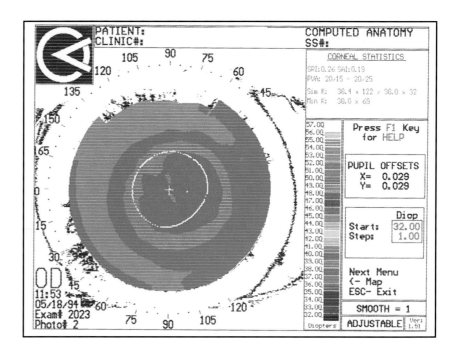

Late myopic regression may occur even after 1 year or longer following PRK. Although highly unusual, some patients will suddenly regress several months after appearing to be stable off topical steroids. The most frequent clinical indication that a patient will experience late myopic regression is the presence of focal confluent haze (Figure 4-33).

The natural history of haze is gradual resolution over many months or years, but occasionally haze can be reactivated. The factors that can reactivate haze are poorly understood but include hormonal alterations, such as those which occur with pregnancy, and excessive ultraviolet radiation from sunlight. Anecdotal stories of patients who after being stable for several months experienced significant myopic regression following skiing and tropical vacations lend support to sunlight as a factor. Other patients with clear corneas have been known to regress 1 D or more even 2 years postoperatively without any identifiable inciting factors. Management of late myopic regression consists not only of surgical retreatment but pharmacological manipulation. Surprisingly, topical steroids can be re-instituted even 1 year later with about a 50% chance of reversing the regression and re-establishing stability. Although some surgeons advocate longer regimens with more potent steroids, the recommended steroid regimen is a 2-month tapering schedule of fluorometholone 0.1%:

- qid x 2 weeks
- tid x 2weeks
- bid x 2 weeks
- QAM x 2 weeks

If effective, continue QAM for 4 to 6 weeks. Surgical retreatment may be performed after the patient is off topical steroids for a minimum of 1 month and stable.

Hyperopic Overcorrection

There are a number of variables that determine the amount of hyperopic overcorrection which is acceptable following surface photoablation. These variables include the time period elapsed since PRK was performed, the degree of preoperative myopia, the age of the patient, the laser beam profile utilized, and the target endpoint desired. In general, for most broad beam and scanning laser systems expect a maximum of +1.25 D of hyperopia at the initial 2 to 4 week refraction. Gaussian beam profile lasers which are associated with greater regression of effect may well have a greater acceptable degree of hyperopia. A patient with a lesser or greater degree of hyperopia regardless of laser system utilized may still achieve the desired refractive outcome simply because of the healing response of the individual patient. Conversely, even if the patient refracts precisely as anticipated at the 3-week interval, the patient may stabilize prematurely or regress aggressively despite proper postoperative management. Each specific excimer laser produced by any manufacturer will also have a particular beam profile and healing pattern associated, giving it a unique "personality" that each surgeon will identify through trial and error usage. Some surgeons routinely target a 30% undercorrection with their excimer laser unit to achieve emmetropic refractive results because of the unique gaussian profile of

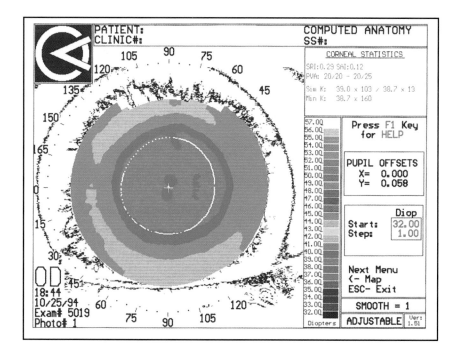

Figure 4-32b.
Thirty-one-year-old man had uncomplicated PRK for -7.25 D in April 1994. Patient regressed with confluent central cornea haze over several months. Corneal videokeratography in October 1994 demonstrates central corneal steepening consistent with clinical findings.

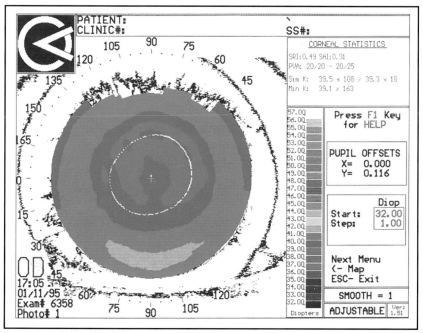

Figure 4-32c.
Corneal videokeratography demonstrates central corneal steepening consistent with increasing central haze.

their beam. The combination of surgeon technique and unique laser parameters must be identified through careful clinical observation when first beginning to learn the personality of the laser system. Complicating this issue further is that a new surgeon will be much slower in mechanical epithelial removal, resulting in increased stromal dehydration and greater risk of overcorrections independent of the laser system. The new laser refractive surgeon should always begin by targeting undercorrections, which can always be more easily managed than overcorrections. A

conservative approach is once again preferred.

Even with the same excimer laser system, surgeons with differing PRK techniques can produce diverse clinical results with different rates of regression. For example, utilizing ethyl alcohol to remove the epithelium or small single optical zone techniques will result in greater degrees of regression and haze formation. Each surgeon must develop a personal nomogram based upon personal clinical experience. Alterations in personal technique may be accompanied with profound alterations in refractive predictability

Figure 4-33.
Focal confluent haze.

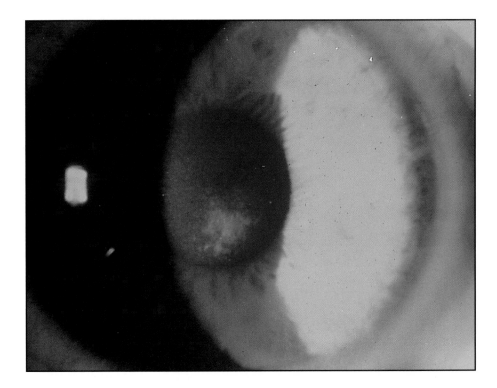

and should be anticipated and possible overcorrections specifically avoided.

Hyperopic overcorrections of greater than +1.50 D within the first month, in patients who are not treated for severe myopia or who are in the presbyopic age group, are initially managed pharmacologically. Topical corticosteroids are discontinued if measured refractions are above +2.00 D and tapered more rapidly, usually weekly or biweekly, if between +1.50 to +2.00 D. The topical corticosteroid should be restarted once or twice daily as outlined earlier once the refraction has regressed to +1.00 D. It is important to monitor these patients closely during steroid withdrawal, usually weekly or biweekly, as haze formation and abrupt regression may occur.

If the patient remains hyperopic and stable after steroid withdrawal there are limited options prior to additional refractive surgery to reverse hyperopia. These corneas usually maintain excellent corneal clarity which is characteristic of non-healers (Figures 4-34a through 4-34c). Durrie advocates the use of contact lenses for both functional and therapeutic benefit. The mechanism by which contact lens wear may reverse hyperopia is hypoxia restimulating the wound healing process. A second technique recommended by Durrie is mechanical debridement of the epithelium, which may also reactivate the wound healing process signified by minimal haze formation.

Current Holmium Sunrise Nomogram:

- No patients over 2.50 D of hyperopia unless post-PRK or LASIK
- All patients over 40 years of age unless post-PRK or LASIK
- Corneal pachymetry <560 microns

Energy: 220 to 240 mJ/spots
Seven to eight pulses per ring
One ring at 6.0 mm +1.00 D
One ring at 6.5 mm +1.25 D
One ring at 7.0 mm +1.50 D
Two rings at 6.0 and 7.0 mm +2.00 D
Three rings at 6.0, 6.75, and 7.5 mm +2.50 D
Holmium LTK retreatment: Same as above with second session after 6 to 9 months.

Post-PRK or LASIK can reduce number of pulses from eight to five and energy 220 to 240 mJ/ring with one ring maximum per session at 6.0- to 7.0-mm optical zone size.
6.0 mm +1.50 to +2.00 D
6.5 mm +1.50 to +2.50 D
7.0 mm +1.50 to +3.00 D

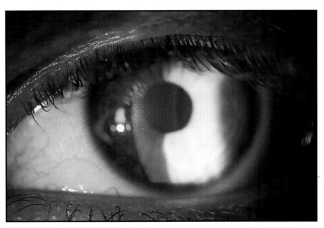

Figure 4-34a.
Clinical example of clear to trace corneal haze grades following PRK treatment of low to moderate myopia.

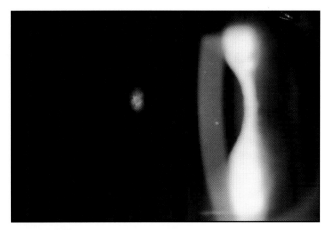

Figure 4-34b.
Clinical example of clear to trace corneal haze grades following PRK treatment of low to moderate myopia.

Surgical correction of hyperopic overcorrections post-PRK centers upon the holmium laser, as hyperopic PRK nomograms, hexagonal keratotomy, and automated lamellar keratoplasty (ALK) for hyperopia are not recommended. Hyperopic LASIK programs will be advocated in the near future in hyperopia correction, especially for hyperopia correction above +3.00 D. Hyperopic PRK programs are still developing with the Aesculap-Meditec MEL 60 scanning slit laser, which is the industry leader in this area at present. Hyperopic PRK will be a preferred technique to manage overcorrected RK once more adequately developed. Currently, the Grene Lasso is advocated.

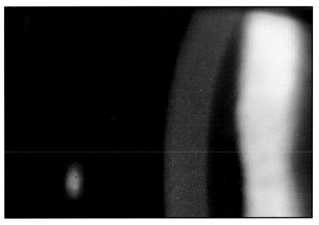

Figure 4-34c.
Clinical example of clear to trace corneal haze grades following PRK treatment of low to moderate myopia.

Clinical Note

Steroid Management of Significant Overcorrection

Abrupt cessation of topical steroids is indicated in a patient with a measured refractive error of +2.25 D at 2 weeks. The reading is far less concerning and requires no intervention if the initial refractive error had been -12.00 D in a 24-year-old woman who not only is able to accommodate well, but will likely increase her refractive error with age. The degree of myopic regression will likely leave the patient only minimally hyperopic by 3 months. The same hyperopic reading is very disconcerting in a 47-year-old man who was treated for -4.00 D. Steroids should be withdrawn and the patient monitored monthly for refractive improvement and clinical haze formation. Once the patient has regressed to +1.00 D, topical steroids should be re-instituted at once or twice daily depending on the rate of recovery. Some patients will rapidly regress once steroids are discontinued and others will either improve slowly or remain stable. If the rate of regression is rapid over a few weeks, bid dosing is appropriate to slow down the final diopter of regression; if over months, once daily dosing is sufficient. If steroids are not re-instituted, regression continues, resulting in residual myopia typically with haze. Steroids must be used to stabilize the refractive error as the target refractive error is approached. Re-instituting steroids once the target refractive error has been reached will be too late for proper stabilization. If no regression occurs, a hyperopic refractive procedure is indicated, the procedure of choice for which is LTK. (See section on postoperative refractive management.)

Holmium: YAG LTK With a Fiber-Optic Delivery System

Vance Thompson, MD

INTRODUCTION

Lanz suggested in the late 1800s that localized heating of the cornea could induce corneal power changes. Since then, various modalities have been investigated to heat corneal collagen to induce corneal curvature changes. The most popular technique for performing collagen shrinkage procedures in the past has been the Fyodorov technique of radial thermokeratoplasty. Various problems, including a lack of predictability and a high incidence of regression, have accompanied this procedure. It is believed that the holmium:YAG laser represents an advancement in the field of corneal collagen shrinkage.

THE PHYSIOLOGY OF COLLAGEN SHRINKAGE

When mammalian collagen is subjected to the proper amount of heat, the collagen fibrils will shrink to approximately one-third of their initial length. The temperature at which this phenomenon occurs is approximately 55° to 60°C. It has also been shown that as soon as the temperature of the collagen is increased above 65° to 70°C, it starts to relax. Even higher temperatures will cause necrosis of the collagen fibrils. Thus, it is important when performing collagen shrinkage procedures not to heat the collagen too much, or one will cause relaxation of the collagen, even necrosis.

In the Fyodorov technique of radial thermokeratoplasty, a wire probe is penetrated to approximately 90% of the corneal

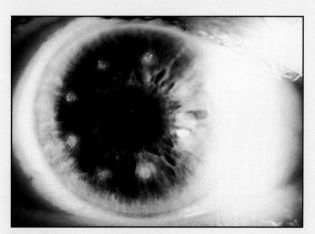

Figure B-1.

depth and heated 600°C. The coagulations are made in a radial fashion, with a typical procedure consisting of eight rows of three or four applications each. It appears that one of the primary reasons that radial thermokeratoplasty showed a lack of predictability was the high temperatures that the collagen was being subjected to, causing necrosis and relation with some areas experiencing collagen shrinkage. This rather extreme variation in heat exposure may be one of the reasons that problems with significant regression and lack of predictability has led researchers to evaluate other technologies for collagen shrinkage.

THE SUMMIT TECHNOLOGY FIBER-OPTIC DELIVERY SYSTEM FOR PERFORMING HOLMIUM:YAG LASER

This solid-state laser emits radiation in the infrared region of the electromagnetic spectrum at 2.06 microns. At this wavelength, the cornea exhibits efficient absorption characteristics capable of increasing the temperature of the corneal water, which in turn causes heat-induced shrinkage of collagen fibrils. This wavelength is ideal because the penetration depth of infrared radiation at this wavelength is comparable to the corneal thickness, which is ideal for achieving deep, consistent collagen shrinkage zones in a controlled fashion.

The holmium:YAG laser energy is delivered along a 600-micron core quartz fiber-optic handpiece and then focused with a specially designed sapphire tip with a cone angle of 120°. This tip is applied to the corneal surface and helps focus the laser energy to form a reproducible wedge-shaped collagen shrinkage zone. This wedge has an angle of approximately 90°. The diameter of the cone at the corneal surface is approximately 700 microns, and the apex is approximately 450 microns in depth, thus maintaining a safe distance from the corneal endothelium. The repetition rate is 15 Hz, and the energy delivered per pulse is approximately 19 mJ. Each treatment location receives approximately 25 pulses, which raises the temperature of the collagen in that location to a maximum of approximately 60°C, which effectively shrinks the collagen in that location. This system for collagen shrinkage thus minimizes any collagen relaxation phenomenon or stromal necrosis by preventing higher temperatures from occurring.

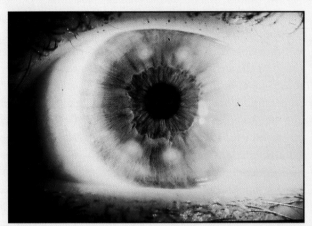

Figure B-2.
Postoperative clinical appearance of Summit contact LTK.

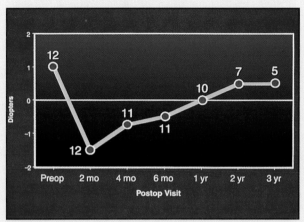

Figure B-3.
Graph depicting refractive stability over time following contact LTK. Initial myopic overcorrection with gradual stabilization at 1 year and slight regression over 2 years.

SURGICAL TECHNIQUE

Preoperatively, the patient receives topical anesthesia and a topical antibiotic. The patient is positioned under the laser and a lid speculum is placed. With the patient fixating on the fixation light in the laser, the central cornea is marked with a 3.0-mm optical zone marker. For a purely hyperopic procedure, one or two rings of eight treatment locations are placed at variable optical zones ranging from 6.0 to 9.0 mm in diameter, depending on the amount of treatment desired. After the marks have been placed, the focusing tip, which is attached to the laser handpiece, is placed in contact with the cornea at the marked treatment site, the foot pedal depressed, and the laser energy delivered over an approximately 1.9-second period. Surgeon variables that need to be concentrated on include keeping the sapphire tip perpendicular to the corneal surface with a slight amount of pressure to nullify any other surgeon's tremor. After all eight or 16 treatment spots have been placed, the epithelium that has been coagulated is gently rubbed off with a cotton-tipped applicator. Antibiotic ointment is instilled, the eye patched, and the patient sent home with instructions to use his or her antibiotic ointment three times a day. The vast majority of patients are re-epithelialized by day 1. Pain is typically minimal and pain medications are not routinely prescribed.

For patients with hyperopic astigmatism, the only difference in technique is the marker utilized. Since the holmium laser causes a rather dramatic flattening at the treatment site accompanied by a central steepening, astigmatism is treated by placing the coagulation spots in the flat axis. Marks are thus placed in the flat axis of astigmatism, and the treatment spots are placed.

Two or four spots are placed on either side of the variable optical zone, ranging from 6 to 9 mm in diameter. It is of note that in addition to steepening the flat axis there is an overall myopic shift in spherical equivalent so that patients who are ideal for this type of treatment are those who have a hyperopic spherical equivalent along with their visually significant astigmatism.

CLINICAL RESULTS

Phases I and II of the hyperopia clinical trials have led to observations that the ideal age for shrinking collagen is greater than 40 years. There also appears to be an upper limit of collagen shrinkage with this system that is probably around 2 D of hyperopia. For the hyperopic astigmatism procedure, it appears that the upper limits of treating astigmatism are approximately 3 D. Again, the patients who have responded the most favorably to this procedure with hyperopic astigmatism have been older than 40 years. Both the hyperopia and hyperopic astigmatism clinical trials are currently in Phase III.

CONCLUSION

The holmium:YAG laser appears to show promise for the treatment of low hyperopia in the range of 2 D and under. Also in the area of hyperopic astigmatism, it has shown some promise for 3 D and under of hyperopic astigmatism. Age appears to be an important factor and patients who appear to benefit the most from this procedure are patients older than 40 years. Further studies are important in helping to define the true significance of utilizing the holmium laser for the treatment of hyperopia and hyperopic astigmatism.

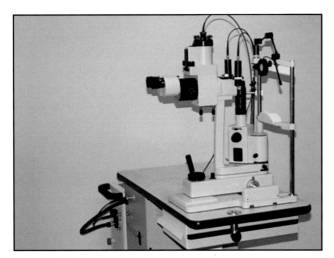

Figure 4-35.
Sunrise holmium.

Holmium Laser for Overcorrected PRK

The holmium laser is a mid-infrared solid-state laser used to perform laser thermokeratoplasty (LTK). There are two types of holmium delivery systems: contact and non-contact. The Summit holmium delivery system, as part of its OmniMed series refractive workstation, is an example of a contact system, utilizing a sapphire crystal tipped probe to deliver the thermal energy at one spot at a time. The Sunrise system (Figure 4-35) is an example of a non-contact design consisting of two components: a laser source and a delivery system. The delivery system is comprised of a Nikon bio-microscopic slit lamp with a faceted crystal which splits the beam into eight equal beams. LTK with the Summit contact method results in a conical or wedge-shaped burn, wide at the corneal surface and tapered at Descemet's membrane. The Sunrise non-contact system results in a cylindrical burn penetrating approximately two thirds to three quarters corneal depth. The laser source is a holmium-doped YAG (yttrium-aluminum-garnet) crystal within a mirrored cavity which generates the 2100-nm wavelength beam. A single strand quartz fiber connects the delivery system to the laser console. The LTK mode produces 100 to 300 mJ/pulse, with the standard setting of 240 mJ divided into eight spots providing 30 mJ at each spot. The laser ring has an adjustable optical zone of 3 to 8 mm with 6 to 7 mm standard ring sizes. The pulse frequency is 5 Hz, with 5 to 10 pulses required at each spot over 1 to 2 seconds. Each ring of holmium LTK typically corrects +1.00 to +1.50 D of hyperopia with a mean of +1.25 D. Hyperopic cylinder correction occurs by blocking four of the eight spots and aligning the four along the minus cylinder axis.

The Sunrise LTK procedure takes approximately 1 to 3 minutes to perform. A wire nonadjustable eyelid speculum is typically inserted and the tear film can dry naturally over 1 to 2 minutes or have compressed air applied. The patient is seated at the delivery slit-lamp and the intersecting green helium-neon beams converge at the pupil center when the proper distance is achieved. Eight red alignment beams indicate the placement sites for the LTK spots. A cobalt blue filter can be used to increase contrast and reduce microscope glare (Figures 4-36a and 4-36b). In general, one to three rings consisting of eight spots each are used to treat hyperopia, with each ring 0.5 to 1.0 mm larger. Cylinder correction is usually performed at the smallest optical zone first when hyperopic astigmatism correction is attempted (Figures 4-37a and 4-37b). It may be more predictable, however, to treat cylinder in the first of two sessions, followed by the hyperopia correction in a later treatment session once stabilization at 3 months or longer has been achieved.

Clinical Note
Overcorrected PRK

Although other laser refractive surgeons have achieved variable success with contact lenses and mechanical debridement, I have attempted both these techniques on a handful of overcorrected PRK patients with poor success. One 37-year-old man treated for -3.50 D upon initial release of the VisX central island factor (CIF) software measured +1.00 D and remained stable despite steroid withdrawal, contact lens fitting, and mechanical debridement. The patient was treated successfully with the Sunrise holmium laser for +1.00 D after 9 months. He was treated with a single LTK ring of five pulses at 240 mJ/pulse at 6.0 mm. He measured -0.25 D after 3-month stabilization with resolution of his presbyopic symptoms and with much improved procedure satisfaction.

Topical anesthesia is all that is required preoperatively, although a topical non-steroidal anti-inflammatory preparation and antibiotic are recommended. Immediately postoperatively, topical NSAID use and lubrication are beneficial at maintaining patient comfort. The use of topical steroids is unclear as reports of postoperative steroids producing regression of effect have been reported. Short-term use of topical antibiotics and steroids for 4 to 7 days is typically recommended. Epithelium is usually intact following Sunrise non-contact LTK, although it is usually necrotic

Correction of Hyperopia by Non-Contact LTK

Mahmoud M. Ismail, MD, and Jorge L. Alió, MD, PhD

For the correction of hyperopia, LTK with holmium laser was proposed as a safe and predictable technique.[1,2] The process consists of the application of laser spots to shrink the peripheral corneal stroma at 6, 6+7, or 6+7+8 mm of the fixation point. This tightens a girdle in the periphery, increasing the central curvature.

We have applied the non-contact technique using the Sunrise Technologies gLase 210 model (Figure C-1). We have performed more than 500 cases with this technique. Our clini-

cally controlled study of 18 months includes 86 eyes of 52 hypermetropic patients.[3,4] Preoperative refraction ranged from +1.5 to +5 D (mean: 3.8 ± 1.2 D). The energy used varied between 215 to 255 mJ. No sight-threatening ocular complications were recorded during the postoperative period even with repeated treatment. Recovery of the preoperative best corrected visual acuity took from 2 to 6 weeks after LTK treatment (Figures C-2a through C-2d). A regression of the LTK effect was evident in all cases. This regression was virtually total in 14

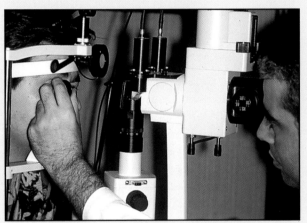

Figure C-1.
Photograph illustrating surgical technique of laser thermokeratoplasty with Sunrise holmium laser system.

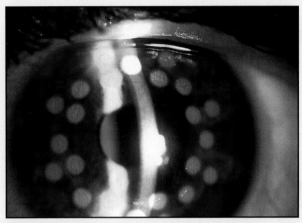

Figure C-2a.
Immediate postoperative view of Sunrise holmium LTK demonstrating a combined double radial ring and single skewed ring of spots.

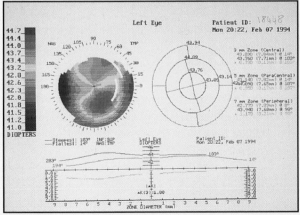

Figure C-2b.
Serial corneal videokeratography of Figure C-2a demonstrating preoperative congenital hyperopic astigmatism.

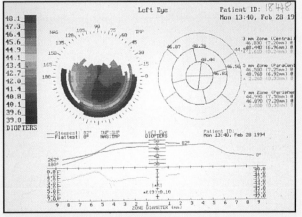

Figure C-2c.
Serial corneal videokeratography of C-2a demonstrating postoperative steepening at 1 month following LTK.

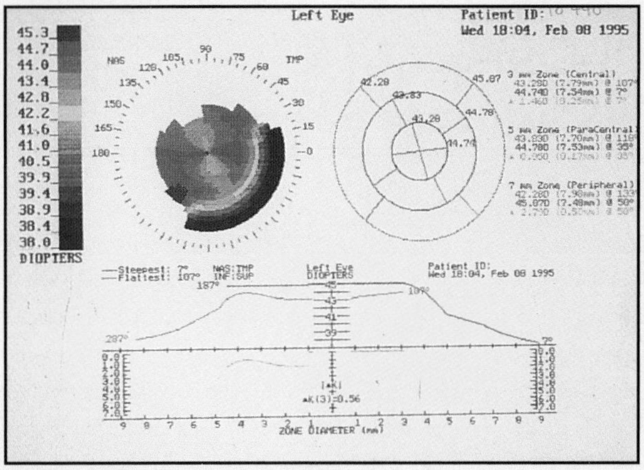

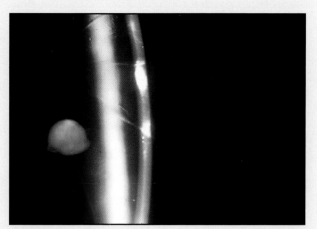

Figure C-2d.
Serial corneal videokeratography of C-2a demonstrating excellent stability of effect at 1 year post-LTK.

Figure C-3.
Postoperative view of Sunrise holmium LTK for consecutive hyperopia post-RK. The LTK procedure was performed 1 year post-RK. There was no radial incision gaping noted.

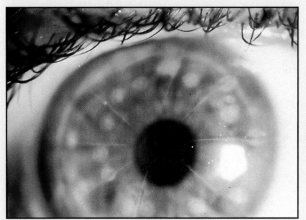

Figure C-4.
Postoperative view at 1 year of Sunrise holmium LTK for consecutive hyperopia post-RK. LTK spots were placed both between and on the radial incisions. Of clinical significance is the absence of corneal incision gaping.

cases (16.27%). Sixty-three cases (73.2%), reached their best corrected visual acuity without correction or with less than +1.5 D in spectacles despite showing some degree of regression. Mean postoperative refraction was +1.82 ± 0.63 D ($p<0.005$). A significant increase in the central K readings and videokeratoscopic evidence of corneal multifocality was obtained in many of these cases (Figures C-3 and C-4). In the whole series, spontaneous vision at 1 year was significantly better than preoperatively. Age of the patients and central pachymetric values showed a significant influence on the regression. Central K values are also another but less important factor. We have created a formula for anticipating preoperatively the percentage of potential postoperative regression:

$$\text{Percent of Regression} = \frac{\text{Average K}}{28} \times \frac{\text{Pachymetry}}{\text{Age}}$$

Overcorrection following myopic PRK was also treated by non-contact LTK. In these cases, a huge effect was obtained with less regression (Figures C-5a and C-5b). This is due to the lower central pachymetric values (ie, thin corneas). Also, the absence of Bowman's membrane in these cases helps the cornea yielding to the LTK spots. The application of the laser spots in these cases should be outside the previously ablated zone in order to avoid confluence of opacities.

Non-contact LTK offers a limited alternative for the correction of hyperopia >+3 D. Algorithms to improve the final results should include the induction of an initial calculated hypercorrection adjusted to variables that influence the regression, such as age and corneal thickness.

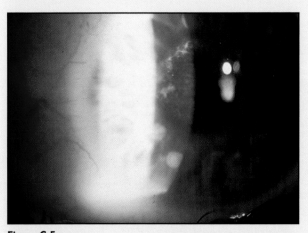

Figure C-5a.
Sunrise holmium LTK following PRK for consecutive hyperopia.

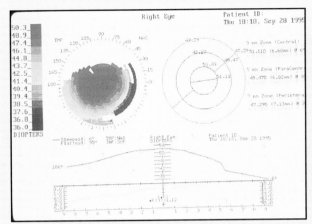

Figure C-5b.
Corneal videokeratography 15 months postoperatively demonstrating stability of effect with steep keratometry values.

References

1. Seiler T, Matallana M, Bende T. Laser thermokeratoplasty by means of a pulsed holmium:YAG laser for hyperopic correction. *Refract Corneal Surg.* 1990;6:99-102.

2. Moreira H, Campus M, Sawusch MR, McDonnell JM, Sand B, McDonnell PJ. Holmium laser keratoplasty. *Ophthalmology.* 1992;5:752-761.

3. Ismail MM, Alió JL. Correction of hyperopia by holmium laser. ESCRS Congress; October 2-5, 1994; Lisbon, Portugal.

4. Ismail MM. Non-Contact LTK for the correction of Hyperopia. 15 months follow-up. ISRS Congress; July 28-30, 1995; Minneapolis, Minn.

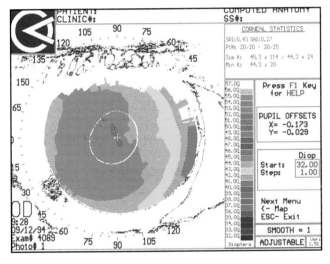

Figure 4-36a.
Spherical hyperopia correction with Sunrise LTK. Preoperative +1.50 +0.25 x 150.

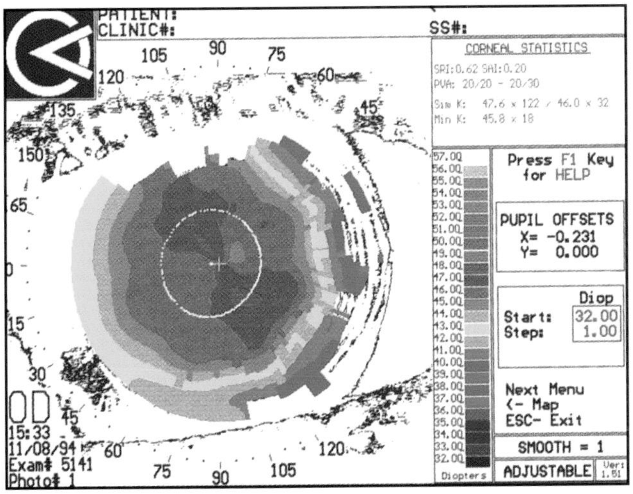

Figure 4-36b.
Post-LTK at 6 months plano +0.50 x 150 with single LTK ring at 7 mm. Uncorrected visual acuity 20/20.

Treatment of RK Overcorrection

Mahmoud M. Ismail, MD, and Jorge L. Alió, MD, PhD

The overcorrection following AK and RK is a significant complication of these techniques. This is due to the sudden demand of accommodation that a myope did not previously intend. In the PERK study, 10% of cases were shifted to hyperopia.[1] We treated these cases by corneal Merseline sutures in a published series[2-5] in an experience of 13 cases of RK overcorrections and 15 cases of AK overcorrections. In cases of RK overcorrections, a combination of a 10.0 Merseline purse-string suture at 5.5 mm of the optical zone and 11-0 Merseline

suturing of the radial incision of 7.5 mm of the visual axis induced a wide range of central corneal steepness and eliminated previous wound gaping respectively. The adjustment of the suture was done using a Placido ring under the operating microscope (Figures D-1a through D-1c). Only the combination of purse-string suture and radial incision suturing provided a stable result. Preoperative best corrected visual acuity was maintained in all cases. Suture removal at 6 months postoperatively did not seem to influence the refractive result. All cases were maintained within 1 D of emmetropia following 6 months after surgery.

Astigmatic overcorrection was reversed by suturing the astigmatic incision. One year after surgery, all 15 patients had gained two or more lines in the Snellen's chart, while two cases failed to improve. Refraction was stable in all cases following 12 months after surgery. The refractive result was less predictable than in RK overcorrections protocol. No significant complications were observed in any of those patients. The knot of the suture, especially in the purse-string suture, needs to be deeply buried into the corneal stroma as it can erode into the epithelium, leading to corneal thinning and neovascularization.

The results of our studies suggest that corneal sutures may be used safely and effectively to manage overcorrections after

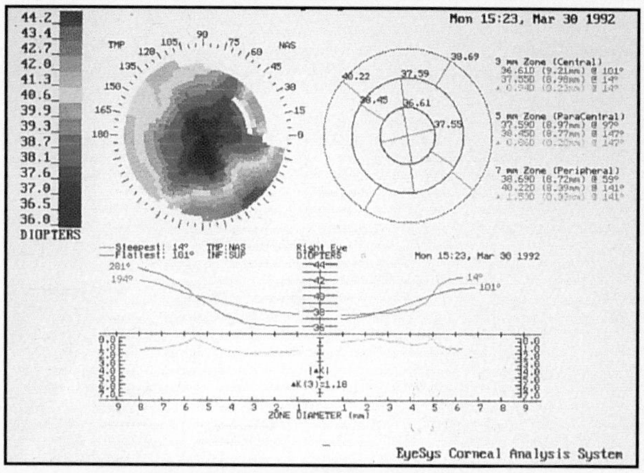

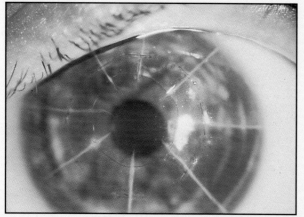

Figure D-1a.
Corneal videokeratography following RK with postoperative consecutive hyperopia and irregular astigmatism.

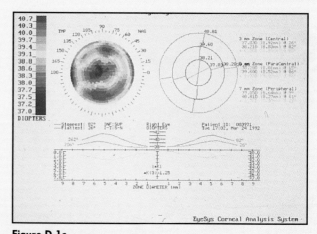

Figure D-1b.
Combined purse-string and radial suture technique for treatment of overcorrection and stabilizing of cornea.

Figure D-1c.
One year postoperative videokeratography of following corneal suturing technique with significantly improved refractive outcome and corneal regularity.

AK or combined RK/AK with satisfactory results. At this point, we have shifted to the treatment of both conditions with the non-contact LTK technique hoping for more predictable results (38 eyes operated). No complications were observed in treating such cases. The corrections obtained have been more or less stable than in virgin hyperopic cases. Superficial opening of an old RK incision (three cases) was only managed by 24-hour eyepatching. To avoid wound gape after LTK, we recommend the application of the laser spots on the previous RK incision. The laser spot retracts the incision to the interior of the cornea, thus preventing a separation wound.

References

1. Waring GO, Lynn MJ, Gelender H, et al. Results of the prospective evaluation of radial keratotomy (PERK) study one year after surgery. *Ophthalmology*. 1985;92:177-198.

2. Alió JL, Ismail MM. Management of radial keratotomy overcorrections by corneal sutures. *J Cataract Refract Surg*. 1993;19:195-199.

3. Alió JL, Ismail MM. Management of astigmatic keratotomy overcorrections by corneal suturing. *J Cataract Refract Surg*. 1994;20:13-17.

4. Alió JL, Ismail MM, Artola A. Cirugía de la hipermetropía post-queratotom a radial mediante suturas corneales. *Archivos Sociedad Española de Oftalmología*. 1994;66:211-218.

5. Ismail MM, Alió JL, Artola A. Tratamiento de las hipercorreciones post-queratotomía astigmatica. *Archivos Sociedad Española de Oftalmología*. 1994;67:167-172.

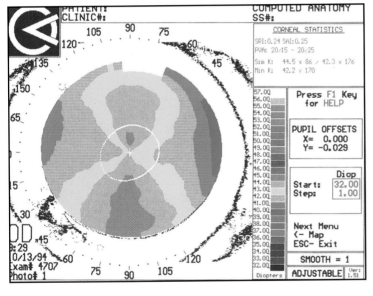

Figure 4-37a.
Sunrise LTK for cylinder correction. Preoperative +2.25 +2.25 x 85.

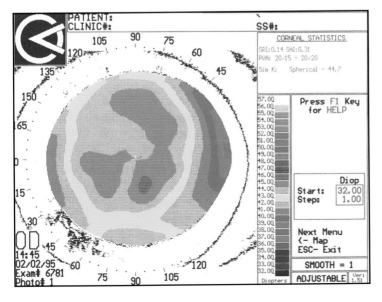

Figure 4-37b.
Postoperative +2 D sphere. Second procedure for spherical hyperopia correction.

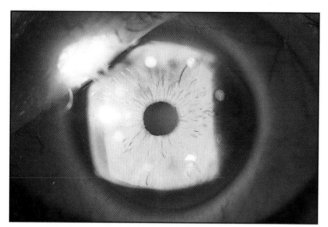

Figure 4-38a.
Well-centered Sunrise holmium LTK, single treatment for +1.50 D.

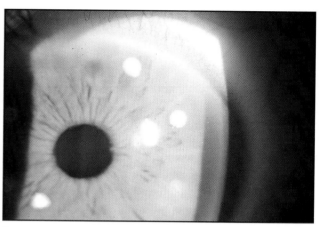

Figure 4-38b.
Higher magnification view of LTK treatment spots demonstrating epithelial crenation in the early postoperative phase.

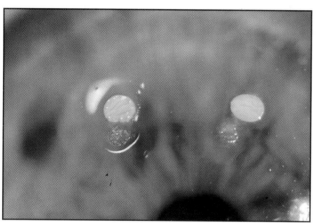

Figure 4-39.
High magnification view of Sunrise holmium LTK radial, double-ring technique.

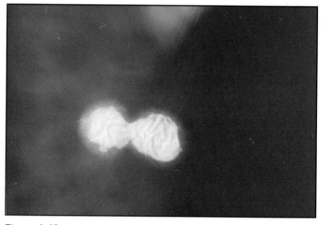

Figure 4-40.
Contiguous Sunrise holmium LTK spots clinically appear white, with crenated appearance on the first postoperative day.

over the burns of contact LTK, producing increased discomfort and increased need for pressure patching overnight.

Clinically, the procedure and the recovery are usually painless, although some patients requiring multiple rings complain of increased photophobia, tearing, and ocular discomfort. In the immediate postoperative period the vision can be clear or more commonly a little blurry because of epithelial irregularity produced by drying and induced irregular astigmatism. Rapid visual recovery is typical, with most patients improving significantly within days. Most patients, however, are myopic when measured the following day and often express improvement with respect to their near vision rather than their distance vision. Surprisingly, many patients report both excellent near and distance vision

as a result of creating a multifocal cornea. Regression of effect in the magnitude of 0.50 to 1.00 D is common, but greater degrees of regression are apparent with higher corrections. Regression of effect is the most significant associated problem observed with LTK. Clinically, patients over 40 years of age respond better to LTK, with patients over 50 years achieving superior stability of effect. LTK achieves good predictability up to +3.00 D with optimal results in patients less than +1.50 D. Poor results are observed for attempted corrections above 3 D of hyperopia, especially with younger patients. Holmium hyperopia correction is not recommended for candidates under 30 years of age or above 3 D of hyperopia. Cylinder predictability is even more variable, with 50% to 150% of cylinder correction obtained. In addition to age and degree of correction

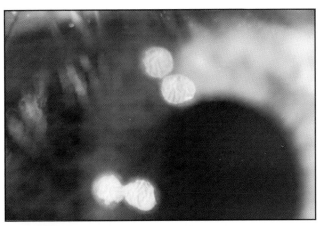

Figure 4-41.
Double Sunrise holmium LTK ring treatment for +2.50 D. Increased efficacy with radial alignment of LTK burns compared to skewed alignment.

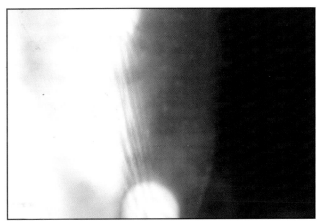

Figure 4-42.
Clinical appearance of induced corneal striae under high magnification between Sunrise holmium LTK treatment spots within days of primary treatment.

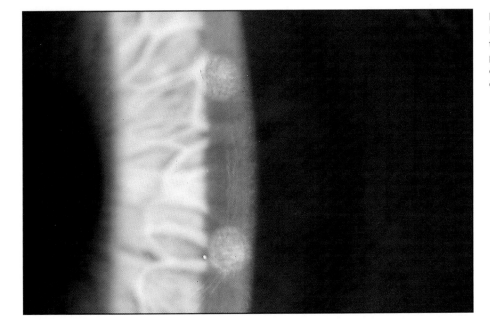

Figure 4-43.
Faded Sunrise holmium LTK treatment spots 1 month postoperatively. Corneal striae still evident. Good clinical effect still observed.

attempted, other factors which affect holmium efficacy include corneal diameter size, corneal curvature, corneal thickness, and treatment variables such as optical zone size. It appears that larger corneal diameters and larger optical zones increase the effectiveness of each laser ring placed.

Results

Following PRK, the effectiveness of holmium is dramatically improved. Excellent results can be achieved for both cylinder and spherical hyperopia correction even in younger patients. It appears that two mechanisms may be involved in increasing holmium LTK effectiveness post-PRK: corneal thinning and absence of Bowman's layer. Methods which may be used to increase the effectiveness of the holmium laser are to combine excimer phototherapeutic keratectomy (PTK) or LASIK with LTK. In treating overcorrected PRK patients, care should be taken not to overtreat these patients in light of the increased efficacy of LTK and only one 6- to 7-mm ring performed in each session. Depending upon corneal thickness, up to 5 D of hyperopia can be corrected with one single ring of holmium LTK. If the PRK was performed for high myopia expect a greater effect, if for low myopia expect good but reduced efficacy (Figures 4-38a through 4-48).

Figure 4-44.
Sunrise holmium LTK double-ring treatment of congenital hyperopia 1 month postoperatively for +2.25 D correction. Manifest refraction measured at -0.25 D.

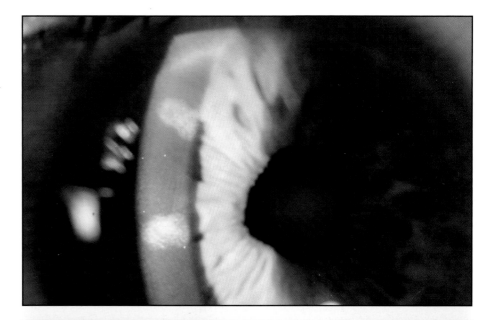

Figure 4-45.
Single holmium LTK ring at 1 month postoperatively for correction of PRK overcorrection. Prior to holmium LTK, patient was +2.25 D, with postoperative refraction of +0.25 D.

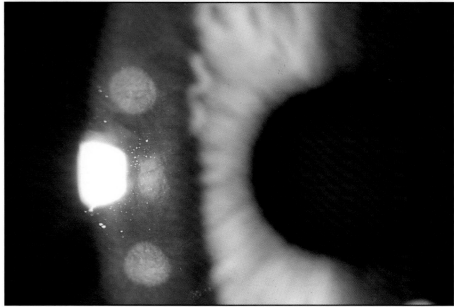

Corneal Findings Following PRK
Punctate Keratopathy

A punctate keratitis can be detected in 3% of patients related to medication toxicity, ultraviolet photokeratitis, or an underlying stromal inflammation. Symptoms include blurred vision, photosensitivity, and increased night glare. A myopic refraction may accompany the keratitis related to ciliary spasm. Patients who develop a non-specific mild superficial keratitis during the first month should be treated conservatively and reassured. Continue steroids and add lubrication (Figures 4-49 and 4-50).

Diffuse Iron Spot

It is not unusual for patients postoperatively to develop iron deposits in the basal epithelium in the region of the ablation. It often appears as a diffuse iron spot. This is related to the alteration in corneal curvature and stagnation of the tear film. Patients are asymptomatic.

Corneal Opacification

Corneal haze or subepithelial scatter is related to a multitude of causes, including, but far from limited to, depth of ablation. Haze is clearly related to steep contours,

Figure 4-46.
Postoperative examination 3 months following Sunrise holmium LTK for +1.50 D. Initial postoperative refraction at 1 week was -0.75 D, with 3-month refraction regressing to +0.25 D.

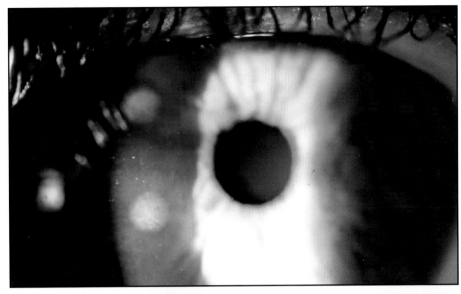

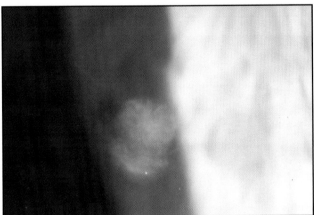

Figure 4-47.
Holmium LTK spot 6 months postoperatively with iron deposition with basal epithelium observed secondary to localized disturbance in tear flow.

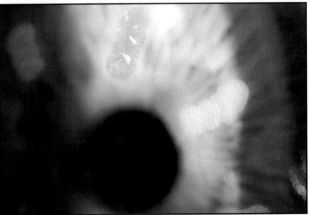

Figure 4-48.
Sunrise holmium LTK triple ring for treatment of +3.25 D of congenital hyperopia. Treatment spots were aligned radially. Excellent clinical effect achieved initially, with 3.00 D of myopic shift, however, significant regression occurred over 6 months, resulting in only 1.75 D of achieved effect.

intraoperative stromal hydration, and patient variability. Most corneas develop trace or mild reticular haze. Natural history of subepithelial haze includes onset, usually at 1 to 2 weeks, peaking at 3 months, and clearing over several months. Reticulated corneal haze is a normal part of the healing process. The only important distinction to be made when grading corneal haze is to discern clinically significant haze. As stated, the hallmark of clinically significant haze is confluence. Haze is further discussed in Chapters 5 and 6.

Confluent haze is associated with a higher risk of:

- Myopic regression both immediate and long-term
- Loss of best corrected visual acuity related to absolute degradation of vision, irregular astigmatism, and abnormal topography

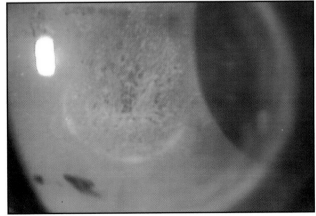

Figure 4-49.
Severe superficial punctate keratitis secondary to medication toxicity. Aminoglycoside antibiotics and NSAIDs most commonly responsible.

Figure 4-50.
Moderate superficial punctate keratitis following PRK. Typical onset at 1 to 2 weeks. Etiology includes topical medications, underlying stromal inflammation, and UV induced.

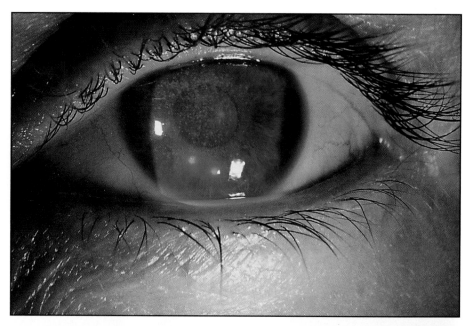

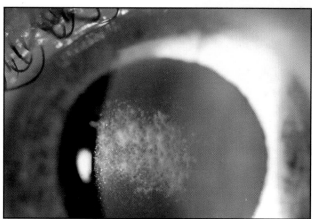

Figure 4-51a.
Dense confluent healing haze following PRK.

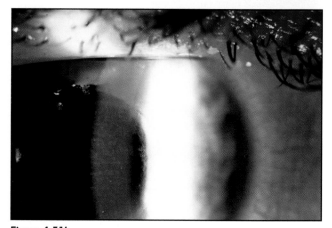

Figure 4-51b.
Medium magnification view of stromal surface following retreatment for the removal of haze and reversal of myopic regression. Clinical endpoint for retreatment is trace haze.

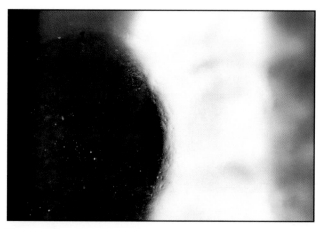

Figure 4-51c.
High magnification view of stromal surface following retreatment for the removal of haze and reversal of myopic regression. Clinical endpoint for retreatment is trace haze.

It is remarkable how much haze can be present without any loss of best corrected acuity. If a patient develops confluent haze, do not increase steroids, just retreat if regression and reduced visual acuity are noted. With good technique, retreatment is 80% effective and can be repeated safely.

As discussed, corneal haze and regression can be controlled but not eliminated with topical steroid administration. The natural history of dense corneal haze is gradual resolution over months to years. Retreatment is indicated for the removal of collagen plaques, utilizing a phototherapeutic modality to try to re-establish the originally sculpted corneal contour (Figures 4-51a through 4-51c). Trace haze, and not a clear cornea, is the goal in these cases; that is, to convert clinically significant haze to clinically insignificant haze. Clinically significant haze, even in severe myopes, is infrequent with proper techniques to improve wound contour (see Figures 4-52a through 4-54 in Chart 4-1). The main element of any haze grading scale is the presence of confluence.

LATE POSTOPERATIVE CARE

Most patients require very little care following the first 6 months other than to ensure stability. Table 4-3 illustrates the first 6-month clinical findings in a typical PRK patient. A cycloplegic refraction is performed to document stability at 6 and 12 months. Corneal clarity is reassessed and patients questioned with regards to their subjective visual quality and dissipation of night glare. Corneal videokeratography is very useful in evaluating postoperative outcome but

Indications for PRK Enhancement
- Cycloplegic refraction equal or greater than -1.00 D
- Uncorrected visual acuity of 20/40 or worse
- Moderate or severe confluent corneal haze affecting vision
- Corneal topographical abnormality affecting vision after 6 months

patient subjective visual quality must remain the focus (Figures 4-56a and 4-56b). Patients with residual refractive errors are considered for enhancement surgery once pharmacological management has failed. Disposable contact lenses can be fitted pending enhancement.

Mixed astigmatism is better treated with AK. The presence of subepithelial haze, even confluent haze, does not indicate the need for retreatment unless vision is affected.

TABLE 4-3
VISUAL ACUITY

Exam	Uncorrected Visual Acuity	Best Corrected Visual Acuity	Refraction (Spherical Equivalent)	Corneal Clarity
Day 10	Expect 20/50 Range 20/20 to 20/100	20/25	+1.00 D (± cyl)	Clear to trace
Month 1	Expect 20/30 Range 20/20 to 20/50	20/20	+0.50 D (± cyl)	Trace haze
Month 2	Expect 20/25 Range 20/20 to 20/40	20/20	+0.25 D (± cyl)	Mild haze
Month 3	Expect 20/20 Range 20/20 to 20/40	20/20	Plano (± cyl)	Mild haze
Month 6	Expect 20/20 Range 20/20 to 20/40	20/20	-0.25 D (±- cyl)	Trace haze

CHART 4-1
CORNEAL CLARITY GRADING: HAZE GRADES AND PATTERNS

Clinically Insignificant Haze

Clear 0.0, clear cornea, no discernible haze

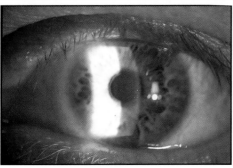

Figure 4-52a.
Clear cornea following right PRK treatment with Summit ExciMed UV 200 laser in early 1992. Diffuse iron spot observed. Preoperative refraction -3.50 D OD reduced to +0.25 D OD.

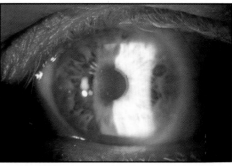

Figure 4-52b.
Clear cornea following left PRK treatment with Summit ExciMed UV 200 laser in early 1992. Diffuse iron spot observed. Preoperative refraction -3.50 D OS reduced to plano OS.

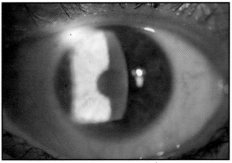

Figure 4-53a.
Clear cornea following right PRK treatment with VisX 20/20 excimer laser system for -5.50 D OD in early 1992. Current refraction -0.50 D OD.

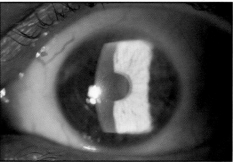

Figure 4-53b.
Clear cornea following left PRK treatment with VisX 20/20 excimer laser system for -6.00 D OS in early 1992. Current refraction -0.50 D OS.

Trace +0.5, barely perceptible, fine reticular haze

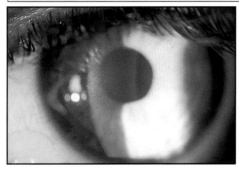

Figure 4-54.
Trace reticular haze following PRK treatment with Chiron Technolas Keracor 116 excimer laser system. Patient was treated late 1993 for -6.00 -2.00 x 180 achieving 20/25 uncorrected visual acuity with stable refraction after 6 months of +0.50 -0.50 x 180.

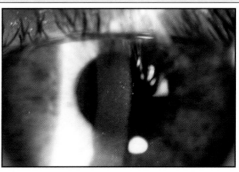

Figure 4-55a.
Trace reticular haze, normal PRK healing pattern.

CHART 4-1 (CONTINUED)
CORNEAL CLARITY GRADING: HAZE GRADES AND PATTERNS

Mild +1.0, easily visible, reticular haze

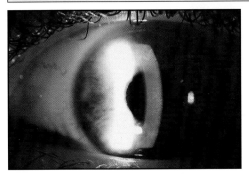

Figure 4-55b.
Mild reticular haze.

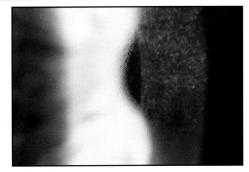

Figure 4-55c.
Mild reticular haze. High magnification view demonstrates non-confluent pattern of haze which will clear gradually over 6 months without further treatment.

Clinically Significant Haze

Moderate, +2.0, an area of confluence, focal pattern

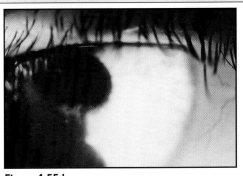

Figure 4-55d.
Focal confluent haze.

Moderate +3.0, diffuse areas of confluence, diffuse pattern

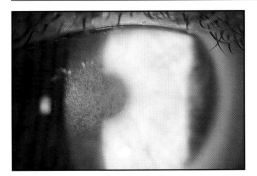

Figure 4-55e.
Moderate confluent haze, diffuse pattern.

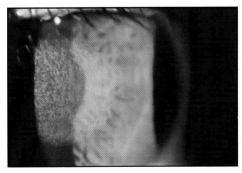

Figure 4-55f.
Diffuse clinically significant haze.

CHART 4-1 (CONTINUED)
CORNEAL CLARITY GRADING: HAZE GRADES AND PATTERNS

Severe +4.0, extensive confluent haze, iris visible, central pattern

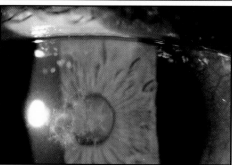

Figure 4-55g.
Severe confluent haze following PRK for extreme myopia. Dense collagen plaque produces myopic regression and reduced qualitative vision typically requiring retreatment.

Severe +4.0, extensive confluent haze, iris visible, arcuate pattern

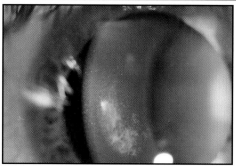

Figure 4-55h.
Arcuate confluent haze typically associated with steep wound margins.

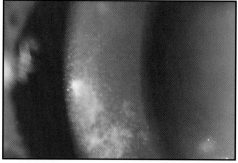

Figure 4-55i.
High magnification view of confluent arcuate haze.

Severe +5.0, opaque cornea, no iris details visible

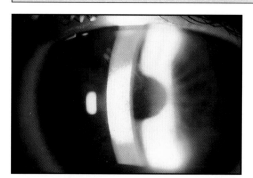

Figure 4-55j.
Dense plaque of confluent haze with no iris details visible. Grade +5.0.

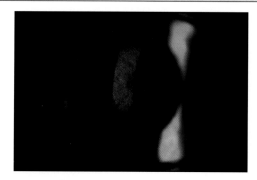

Figure 4-55k.
Dense collagen plaque following VisX 20/20 surface ablation for -10.00 D.

CHART 4-1 (CONTINUED)
CORNEAL CLARITY GRADING: HAZE GRADES AND PATTERNS

Severe +5.0, opaque cornea, diffuse pattern

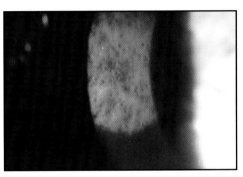

Figure 4-55l.
Diffuse collagen plaque.

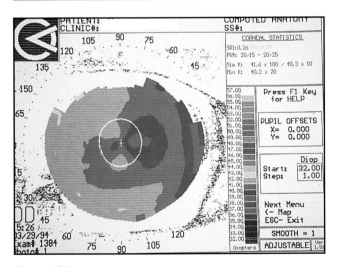

Figure 4-56a.
In properly evaluating postoperative videokeratography, one must also examine the preoperative map or perform a differential subtraction map to determine the quality of the ablation. The preoperative videokeratography of this patient must be used as a baseline to properly evaluate the postoperative change.

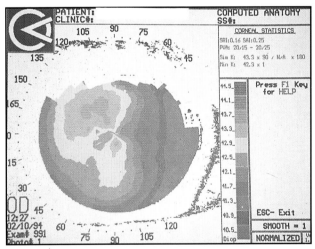

Figure 4-56b.
In this patient, the clinical appearance of the postoperative videokeratography gives the impression that the surgical outcome would be poor, since the classic smooth circular blue area of flattening is not observed. In fact, the patient was 20/15 uncorrected with excellent qualitative vision. It is only after one examines the preoperative videokeratography and compares the steeper and flatter areas on both maps that the impression of a symmetrical and even ablation is apparent. The principle to be drawn here is that the postoperative videokeratography alone does not always give the entire postoperative clinical picture.

CHAPTER 5

PRK Complications and Their Management

The safety of excimer photorefractive keratectomy (PRK) is currently being evaluated at multiple sites across North America. Preliminary reports indicate that PRK appears to be both safe and predictable in correcting low to moderate degrees of myopia. However, there has been a general trend toward minimizing the risks associated with PRK. The adverse side effects and known complications have received only limited exposure. Many of the problems encountered in PRK patients, such as under- and overcorrections, are similar to those experienced by radial keratotomy (RK) patients and do not come as any surprise. Other complications, such as central islands and corneal haze, however, are specific to the excimer laser. In order to prevent and determine how to best manage them, it is essential to understand these complications.

COMPLICATIONS RELATED TO UNPLANNED DEVIATIONS FROM INTENDED CORRECTION

OVERCORRECTION

Clinical: The risk of overcorrection is greatest in patients over 40 years of age with high myopia corrections, excessive steroid use, and with the Summit ExciMed gaussian beam profile. The Summit OmniMed series has a reduced risk of overcorrection as it possesses a somewhat

Overcorrection associated with:

- Age > 40 years
- Gaussian energy beam profile excimer laser
- Small optical zone
- Excessive topical steroid use
- Excessive stromal drying intraoperatively secondary to slow mechanical debridement, alcohol debridement, gas blow
- Excessive pretreatment or "anti-island" software program
- Non-cycloplegic preoperative refraction

flatter beam than its predecessors. Patients complain of poor reading vision, a decline in vision as the day progresses (diurnal fluctuation), and night glare.

Management: Overcorrections are probably one of the most difficult complications to manage. Initial management consists of tapering and/or withdrawal of topical steroids. If significant hyperopia is evident, greater than +2.00 D (unless Summit ExciMed), discontinue steroids. If between +1.25 and +2.00 D, decrease steroid frequency weekly. Rapid withdrawal of steroids promotes haze and regression. Restart steroids once regresses to +1.00 D. If a patient has been off topical steroids for some time, fit with extended wear contact lens to produce an anoxic irritative drive to promote further wound healing and regression. Failing the

Holmium LTK for the Correction of Both Primary and Post-PRK Hyperopia and Astigmatism

Louis E. Probst V, MD

Thermal keratoplasty alters the anterior corneal curvature by heating the stromal tissue to 60° to 65°C,[1] causing collagen to shrink to 30% to 50% of its original length[2] for up to 90% of the stromal thickness.[3,4] At higher temperatures, substantial additional shrinkage does not occur, however, thermal injury and necrosis can result.[4] This thermal processing of collagen produces dissociation of hydrogen bonds, partial unwinding and coiling of the triple helix, crosslinking between amino acid moieties, and changes in stromal hydration.[5] While the collagen of normal corneas has a half-life of approximately 20 years, the effect of collagen turnover on the long-term stability of thermal keratoplasty is unknown.[5]

Thermal keratoplasty has been performed in the past using a variety of techniques including heated objects, microwaves, and most recently lasers. Lans[6] was the first to study cautery in rabbit corneas in 1898. Rowsey and Doss[7] attempted thermal keratoplasty with radio frequency probe, however, this work was abandoned due to poor predictability. Fyodorov[8] devised the technique of inserting a heated needle into the stroma to produce temperatures of 600°C. Unfortunately, this method also suffered from regression and poor predictability and is no longer performed. The holmium:YAG laser offers the latest method of thermal keratoplasty. Advantages of laser thermal keratoplasty (LTK) include the excellent penetration of the laser wavelength into the cornea, relatively low cost, and the ease of use.[9]

Histopathological studies of the treated cornea after LTK have identified increased epithelial eosinophilia and hyperplasia with elongated nuclei,[4] increased hematoxylin uptake with a loss of distinct stromal lamellae,[4] and no stromal necrosis.[2] No morphological effects have been found on the endothelial cell structures of human corneas at the common energy densities used.[2] No morphological effects have been found on the endothelial cell structures of human corneas at the common energy densities used.[2] The maximal endothelial loss caused by LTK on the rabbit cornea, which is only 65% the thickness of the human cornea, was found to be 1.2% with an irradiance pattern of 32 spots at maximal laser fluence levels ≥20 mJ/cm²).[4]

The basic pattern for the treatment spots of the holmium:YAG laser involves eight radial sites spread over 360° in an octagonal pattern with the spots 45° apart (Figure A-1). Seiler

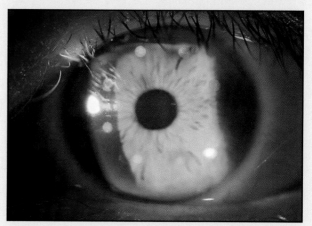

Figure A-1.
Sunrise holmium LTK, single treatment for +1.50 D.

and coworkers have identified a linear relationship between the clear zone diameter and the refractive change with approximately 5 D of myopic change at 5 mm and only 1 D of change at 9 mm.[9] Koch and coworkers have found that treatment pattern diameters 3.5 mm or less flatten the cornea centrally while diameters 6.0 to 7.0 mm steepen the central cornea and between 3.5 to 6.0 mm there is a null zone that produces little persistent change in cornea curvature.[10,11] Multiple rings of treatment can be applied at different diameters for higher degrees of hyperopia.[12] A radial pattern of multiple LTK rings of different diameters has been found to achieve a significantly better refractive outcome and faster visual rehabilitation than a skew pattern.[13] Astigmatic LTK steepens the flat corneal meridian by positioning the four to eight variable diameter treatment spots separated by 45° so that they straddle the flat corneal axis. With astigmatic LTK there is an associated steepening of the central cornea with a resultant hyperopic correction of 0.50 D for every 1.0 D of astigmatism correction.[9]

Currently, holmium:YAG LTK is mainly performed clinically with lasers from Summit Technology Inc. and Sunrise Technologies Inc. The Summit system is a contact laser that emits the 2.06-micron wavelength with 300 microsecond pulses at a 15 Hz repetition frequency and a pulse energy of approximately 19 mJ. Each treatment location receives 25 pulses. The laser is delivered through a fiber-optic handpiece focused with

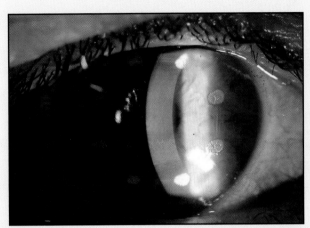

Figure A-2.
Single ring treatment of eight LTK spots at a 7.0 mm acheiving 2.00 D of myopic shift post-PRK.

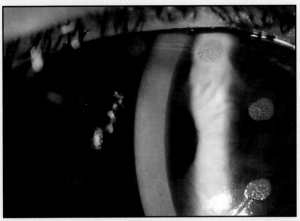

Figure A-3.
Sunrise holmium LTK for overcorrected PRK. Day 1 biomicroscopic slit lamp photo demonstrating corneal striae.

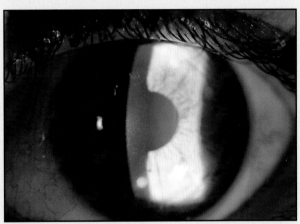

Figure A-4.
Postoperative clinical appearance of Sunrise holmium LTK for PRK overcorrection at 1 month demonstrating more faded appearance of LTK spots and reduced corneal striae. Regression of effect noted with efficacy of myopic shift reduced from 2.00 to 1.5 D over first 4 weeks.

a sapphire tip which is applied to the corneal surface, producing 700-micron diameter treatment spot to a depth of approximately 450 microns.[9] The Sunrise system is a compact solid-state non-contact laser which emits the 2.13-micron wavelength with 250 microsecond pulses at a 5 Hz repetition frequency with pulse energies from 8 to 11 J/cm[2].[11] One to eight pulse exposures of 220 to 240 mJ can be applied to each treatment location, and this produces a 500- to 600-micron spot[11] which extends to approximately 75% of the corneal thickness.[2]

Durrie and coworkers[12] have reported follow-up data on eyes treated with the Summit holmium:YAG laser. A total of 79% of eyes with preoperative hyperopia between +2.0 to +6.62 D were within 1 D of the intended correction, and 75% achieved J2 or better near vision at 6 months follow-up. Two lines of best corrected visual acuity were lost by 7% of patients due to irregular astigmatism. Regression patterns stabilized at the 6-month follow-up; however, regression was identified in some patients at 1 year.[14] Small studies of the treatment of astigmatism have demonstrated continued regression each year after treatment, which in some cases resulted in keratometry values returning to their pretreatment values.[15,16] Regression was particularly noted in hyperopic astigmatism, younger patients, and with larger amounts of myopic astigmatism.[16]

The studies of the Sunrise LTK have found an initial hyperopic reduction of 1.4 D at 3 months.[17] Ismail found that 21% of eyes had virtually total regression of refractive correction at 15 months after surgery.[18] Pop and Arus found significant regression in the hyperopic correction up to 6 months postoperatively, leaving an average of 1.2 D of correction with similar regression of astigmatic correction. However, 80% of

eyes had a correction of at least 1 D at 1 year.[19] A strong correlation was found between the age of the patient and the degree of correction attained.[19] Koch and coworkers have reported 2-year post-treatment results after spherical hyperopic LTK with the Sunrise laser on 21 eyes.[5,20] The four eyes with clear zone diameters less than 6.0 mm had no long-term correction. The remaining eyes (n=7) were treated with a 6.0-mm clear zone diameter, 10 pulses, eight spots, and pulse radiant energies of 7.5 to 9.0 J/cm[2]. The mean change in the refraction in this group was 0.79 ± 0.74 D with a mean change in astigmatism of 0.1 D at 18-month follow-up[16] and a mean regression of only 0.1 D between 3 months and 2 years postoperatively. Mean uncorrected visual acuity improved from 20/150 to 20/50. No patient lost two or more lines of Snellen visual acuity and the only complication was an increase of refractive astigmatism of 0.5 to 1.0 D in four patients.

LTK with the Sunrise laser for post-PRK hyperopia has been found to produce an average change of 3.6 D at 12 months post-treatment with 21% to 63% regression from the initial postoperative correction.[21] The absence of Bowman's membrane and the thinner central cornea following PRK may increase the efficacy and stability of LTK.[21]

The results of non-contact Sunrise holmium LTK for the correction of primary hyperopia, post-PRK hyperopia, and post-LASIK hyperopia at TLC The Laser Center, Windsor, Canada, were retrospectively reviewed—a total of 32 eyes of 17 patients with primary hyperopia. Twenty eyes of 20 patients with post-PRK hyperopia and four eyes of four patients with post-LASIK hyperopia were treated. The eyes were divided into either group A with <+3.0 D spherical equivalent and <1.0 D astigmatism or group B with ≥+3.00 D spherical equivalent and ≥1.0 astigmatism. In the primary hyperopia group with average follow-up of 5.9 months (range: 1 to 11 months), 100% of eyes (15/15) achieved at least 20/40 visual acuity. Eighty-seven percent of eyes (13/15) were within 1 D of emmetropia, and 13% of eyes (2/15) required retreatment in group A (Figures A-2 and A-3). In group B, 47% of eyes (8/17) achieved at least 20/40 visual acuity. Fifty-three percent of eyes (9/17) were within 1 D of emmetropia, and 41% of eyes (7/17) required retreatment. The results for post-PRK hyperopia with average follow-up of 3.5 months (range: 1 to 9 months) were 85.7% of eyes (12/14) achieved at least 20/40 visual acuity, 64.3% of eyes (9/14) were within 1 D of emmetropia, with none of the eyes requiring retreatment in group A. In group B, 33% of eyes (2/6) achieved at least 20/40 visual acuity, 33% of eyes (2/6) were within 1 D of emmetropia, and 33% of eyes (2/6) required retreatment. For post-LASIK hyperopia with all eyes, +3.0 D SE and only one patient with ≥1.0 D astigmatism with average follow-up of 1.5 months (range: 1 to 3 months), 100% of eyes (4/4) achieved at least 20/40 visual acuity, 75% of eyes (3/4) were within 1 D of emmetropia, and none of the eyes required retreatment. Significant hyperopic regression was noted in the eyes with longer follow-up and greater amounts of correction (Figure A-4). Undercorrection was the only complication observed. These results indicate that non-contact holmium LTK is effective in correcting primary hyperopia, post-PRK hyperopia, and post-LASIK hyperopia with <-3.0 D SE and <1.0 D astigmatism, but far less successful with higher degrees of hyperopia and astigmatism.

FDA Phase IIa studies with 1-year follow-up using modified protocols of two treatment rings at 6 and 7 mm with 10 pulses achieved a mean correction of 1.7 D.[5] Further modification of the treatment variables using three rings with only five pulse treatments gave 3.5 D of correction at 6 months follow-up.[5]

Most investigators agree that LTK is effective for less than 2 to 3 D of hyperopia with minimal astigmatism, and treatment should be limited to patients 40 years or older.[3,19,22] Although persistent regression has been noted, the treatment is relatively easy to perform, post-treatment recovery is fast, and patient acceptance is high.[3] No vision-threatening complications have been reported to date.[5] Further modifications of the treatment parameters that minimize keratocyte injury and maximize collagen shrinkage should improve the long-term regression, efficacy, and predictability of this procedure.[5]

References

1. Shaw EL, Gasset AR. Thermokeratoplasty (TKP) temperature profile. *Invest Ophthalmol Vis Sci.* 1974;13:181-186.

2. Ariyasu RG, Sand B, Menefee R, et al. Holmium laser thermal keratoplasty of 10 poorly sighted eyes. *J Refract Surg.* 1995;11:358-365.

3. Yanoff M. Holmium laser hyperopia thermokeratoplasty update. *Eur J Implant Ref Surg.* 1995;7:89-91.

4. Moreira H, Campos M, Sawusch MR, et al. Holmium laser thermokeratoplasty. *Ophthalmology.* 1993;100:752-761.

5. Koch DD. Holmium laser thermal keratoplasty with slit-lamp delivery system. American Academy of Ophthalmology Meeting; October 30-November 3, 1995; Atlanta, Ga.

6. Lans LJ. Experimentelle Untersuchungen uber die Entstehung von Astigmatismus durch nicht-perforierende Corneawunden. *Graefes Arch Clin Ophthalmol.* 1988;45:117-152.

7. Rowsey JJ, Doss. Electrosurgical keratoplasty: update and retraction. *Invest Ophthalmol Vis Sci.* 1987;28:224.

8. Fyodorov SN. A new technique for the treatment of hyperopia. In: Schachar RA, Levy NS, Schachar L, eds. *Keratorefractive Surgery.* Denison, Texas: LAL Publishing; 1989.

9. Thompson VM, Seiler T, Durrie DS, Cavanaugh TB. Holmium:YAG laser thermokeratoplasty for hyperopia and astigmatism: an overview. *Refract Corneal Surg.* 1993;9(Suppl):S134-S137.

10. Koch DD, Abarca A, Menefee RF, et al. Holmium:YAG laser thermal keratoplasty (LTK) for corrections of spherical refractive errors. Current Research: Refractive and Cataract Surgery Symposium; November 1993; Minneapolis, Minn.

11. Koch DD, Berry MJ, Vassiliadis A, et al. Noncontact holmium:YAG laser thermal keratoplasty. In: Salz JJ, McDonnell PJ, McDonald MB, eds. *Corneal Laser Surgery.* St. Louis, Mo: Mosby; 1995.

12. Durrie DS, Schumer J, Cavanaugh TB. Holmium:YAG laser thermokeratoplasty for hyperopia. *J Refract Corneal Surg.* 1994;10(Suppl):S227-S280.

13. Azzolini M, Vinciguerra P, Epstein D, et al. Laser thermokeratoplasty for the correction of hyperopia, a comparison of two different application patterns. *Invest Ophthalmol Vis Sci.* 1995;36(4):S716.

14. Yanoff M. Holmium laser hyperopia thermokeratoplasty update. *Eur J Implant Ref Surg.* 1995;7:89-91.

15. Hennekes R. Holmium:YAG laser thermokeratoplasty for correction of astigmatism. *J Refract Surg.* 1995;11(Suppl):S358-S360.

16. Cherry PMH. Holmium:YAG laser to treat astigmatism associated with myopia or hyperopia. *J Refract Surg.* 1995;11(Suppl):S349-S357.

17. Fucigna RJ, Gelber E, Belmont S. Laser thermal keratoplasty for the correction of hyperopia: a retrospective study of 35 patients. 1995 ISRS Pre-Academy Conference and Exhibition; October 26, 1995; Atlanta, Ga.

18. Ismail MM. Non-contact LTK by holmium laser for hyperopia: 15 month follow-up. 1995 ISRS Mid-Summer Symposium and Exhibition; July 28-30, 1995; Minneapolis, Minn.

19. Pop M, Aras M. Regression after hyperopic correction with the holmium laser: one year follow-up. 1995 ISRS Mid-Summer Symposium and Exhibition; July 28-30, 1995; Minneapolis, Minn.

20. Koch DD, Villarreal R, Abarca A, et al. Two-year follow-up of holmium:YAG thermal keratoplasty for the treatment of hyperopia. *Invest Ophthalmol Vis Sci.* 1995;36(4):S2.

21. Alió JL, Ismail M. Management of post-PRK hyperopia by holmium laser. 1995 ISRS Pre-Academy Conference and Exhibition; October 26, 1995; Atlanta, Ga.

22. Mathys B, Van Horenbeeck R. Contact holmium laser thermokeratoplasty (LTK) for hyperopia surgery: follow-up of our first clinical cases. 1995 ISRS Pre-Academy Conference and Exhibition; October 26, 1995; Atlanta, Ga.

extended wear contact lenses there have been anecdotal reports of mechanical debridement retriggering wound healing and promoting myopic regression. Refractory cases of overcorrection can be managed surgically with holmium laser thermokeratoplasty (LTK) (see Chapter 4).

UNDERCORRECTION

Clinical: Patients complain of poor distance acuity and increased night glare. Undercorrection is due to inadequate initial treatment often related to a young patient, high myopia, or a moist cornea intraoperatively.

Management: If mild undercorrection is attained (<-1.00 D), maintain steroids qid for up to 12 weeks, then taper over 4 to 6 weeks. If significant undercorrection (>-1.00 D), complete steroid regimen, then retreat when stable. If the patient is in the presbyopic age group, consider monovision.

INDUCED ASTIGMATISM

Regular Astigmatism

Clinical: Patients complain of a doubling of images and blurred vision.

Management: Induced or residual cylinder can be treated with repeat PRK if still myopic or astigmatic keratotomy (AK) when mixed astigmatism is detected.

Irregular Astigmatism

Clinical: Patients often have some degree of irregular astigmatism early in their healing response. This was most common with the VisX 20/20 Model B early software programs and nitrogen blow techniques. It is related primarily to intraoperative corneal hydration or irregular epithelium. It results in reduced spectacle best corrected visual acuity during the first weeks following PRK. Coexisting irregular astigmatism is the reason patients seem unable to accom-

modate minimal hyperopic refractions early on.

Management: No specific treatment is recommended or proven efficacious; this usually clears spontaneously. Artificial tears may help if epithelium irregularities are a contributing factor.

REGRESSION

Severe Regression With/Without Haze

Clinical: A certain degree of regression is planned for in the computer algorithm, however, excessive regression may

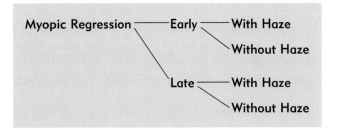

Myopic regression associated with:

- Young age
- High dioptric corrections
- Flat corneas
- High cylindrical treatments
- Steep wound margins
- Gaussian beam profile lasers
- Rapid steroid withdrawals
- Fellow eye healing response
- Hormonal imbalance/pregnancy
- Possibly female gender
- Possibly ultraviolet light exposure
- Haze formation

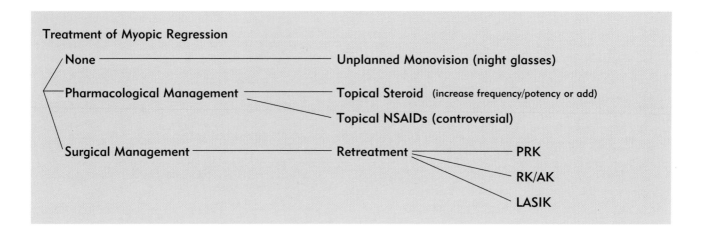

Treatment of Myopic Regression

None ——————————————— Unplanned Monovision (night glasses)

Pharmacological Management ——————— Topical Steroid (increase frequency/potency or add)

Topical NSAIDs (controversial)

Surgical Management ——————— Retreatment ———— PRK

RK/AK

LASIK

occur. Related factors include small optical zones, steep wound edges, high myopia, young patient age, and single zone treatment. Regression may occur immediately following steroid withdrawal or later, 6 to 18 months postoperatively. A "second wave of haze," a focal area of confluent haze which expands, is associated with most of these cases of late regression.

Management: There are two methods of therapy.
1. Restart topical steroids, typically fluorometholone 0.1% qid, then taper more slowly over 6 to 8 weeks
2. Retreatment once stability is reached

In general, topical medication should be attempted first unless more than -2.00 D of myopia is noted. Never restart topical steroids if regression reoccurs a second time once topical steroids have been withdrawn, since steroid dependency will only result in long-term steroid use and unacceptable steroid-induced complications. If significant haze is present, retreatment is almost always required and a steroid trial can be avoided. Stability of refraction means two refractions 1 month apart, off steroids within 0.25 to 0.50 D with unchanged videokeratography (see Chapter 4). Long-term use of NSAIDs for the prevention or reversal of

---

Surgical Retreatment Approach
 Mechanical Debridement
   Regression without haze
   Central island
 Transepithelial Approach
   Regression with haze
   Complex/asymmetric topographical abnormalities

---

myopic regression is controversial and I do not recommend it. The instillation of NSAIDs for modulation of refractive error early in the healing course may actually increase haze formation.

Ultraviolet-Induced Regression

Clinical: There have been a number of anecdotal reports of regression following intense ultraviolet light exposure during the initial 6 months following PRK in seemingly stable patients. Skiing has been most commonly associated. Altitude may also be a factor.

Management: Sunglasses with ultraviolet protection are recommended for all patients following PRK, especially during the first 6 months. Treatment is identical for other causes of regression, with a topical steroid trial followed by retreatment if significant confluent haze is not present.

Pregnancy-Induced Regression

Clinical: Patients should be screened for pregnancy, as this not only alters refraction, but alters wound healing (Figure 5-1). Six patients who became pregnant either immediately before or shortly after PRK surgery evidenced the definite hormonal effect upon wound healing. The more morning sickness and hormone imbalance each patient experienced, the more haze and regression were evident. Two of the six women had severe haze coinciding with significant hormone fluxes. The least affected patient, at -0.50 D and a clear cornea, had no topical steroids instituted and was associated with an "easy pregnancy," working until her delivery date (see Clinical Note in Chapter 2).

Management: Treatment consists of retreatment following delivery. If patient is breast-feeding, treatment should be further postponed.

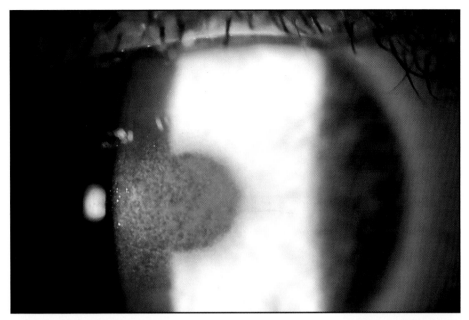

Figure 5-1.
Severe corneal haze, diffuse pattern with onset related to pregnancy during critical first 3 months of PRK wound healing.

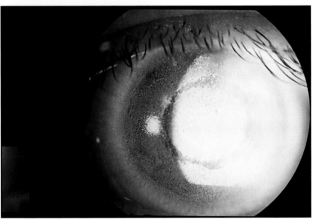

Figure 5-2a.
Diffuse Ciloxan precipitates adherent to bandage contact lens observed on second postoperative day following PRK.

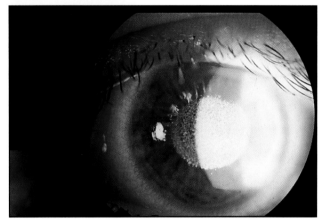

Figure 5-2b.
Following removal of bandage contact lens Ciloxan precipitates were found to be strongly adherent to denuded stroma.

COMPLICATIONS RELATED TO POSTOPERATIVE MEDICATIONS

ORAL NARCOTIC-RELATED
Vasovagal Reactions

Clinical: Patients may become vasovagal secondary to narcotic use for pain control. Nausea, vomiting, facial pallor, perspiration, and light-headedness are associated. Patients may also feel faint immediately following the PRK procedure.

Management: Patients should be warned not to overmedicate themselves. If a patient becomes faint, immediately place the patient in a supine position with legs elevated. Do not walk the patient to a chair. A cool compress to the forehead is helpful. Instruct your staff accordingly.

ANTIBIOTIC-RELATED
Allergic

Clinical: Neomycin and sulfa reactions are most common. Conjunctival and lid edema, as well as injection, are evident.

Management: Avoid these agents or exchange for alternate antibiotic. Combination steroid-antibiotic, TobraDex (Alcon), is commonly used following PRK, but a fluoroquinolone such as Ocuflox (Allergan) provides better

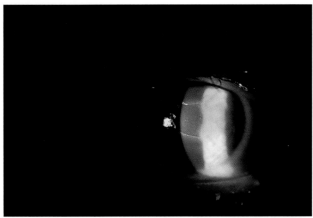

Figure 5-2c.
Following careful debridement with blunt spatula, delayed epithelial healing was observed. Minute Ciloxan crystals were noted along advancing edge of epithelium. Complete epithelial healing required 21 days and resulted in confluent haze formation.

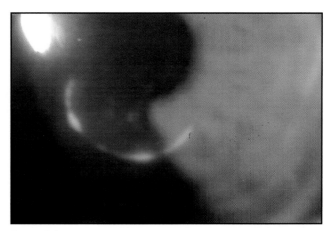

Figure 5-3.
Immune ring secondary to NSAID use.

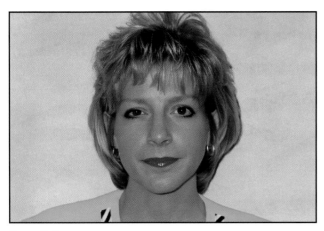

Figure 5-4.
Ptosis secondary to topical steroid use.

broad spectrum coverage with a low incidence of allergic sensitivity.

Toxicity

Clinical: Aminoglycoside toxicity is most common, producing keratitis and delayed epithelial healing.

Management: Gentamicin and neomycin are more epitheliotoxic than tobramycin. Polytrim (tromethoprim sulfate and polymyxin B sulfate) or fluoroquinolones are less toxic to the epithelium. Ciloxan (Figures 5-2a through 5-2c) produces debris and precipitates beneath the therapeutic contact lens, but does not appear to significantly affect wound healing except in unusual cases. Ofloxacin 0.3%, another fluoroquinolone, has not been associated with precipitates and is recommended. Lubrication is help-

ful. Tobramycin works well, but does not cover streptococcal bacterial well, and gram-positive bacteria are most likely culprits of microbial corneal ulceration (see Clinical Note on Fluoroquinolones in Chapter 4).

Preservative-Related Toxicity

Clinical: Keratitis and delayed epithelial healing appear clinically.

Management: Discontinue offending agent and add nonpreserved lubrication.

NSAID-RELATED
Immune Reactions

Clinical: Paracentral infiltrate or immune ring (Figure 5-3) may be associated with short-term use of topical nonsteroidals such as Voltaren (diclofenac sodium 0.1%, CIBA) and Acular (ketorolac tromethamine 0.5%, Allergan). Stromal melt has also been reported with excessive topical NSAID use.

Management: Discontinue NSAID and start topical steroids. Monitor closely for stromal melting. A full-strength topical steroid such as dexamethasone phosphate 0.1% or prednisolone acetate 1% is recommended every 1 to 2 hours initially. An infectious agent must be excluded (see Clinical Note in Chapter 4).

Toxicity

Clinical: Diffuse/inferior punctate keratitis and delayed epithelial healing. Frequent use of topical NSAIDs can have a dramatic impact on epithelial healing rates and must be closely monitored.

Complications of Corticosteroids After PRK: Literature Review

Louis E. Probst V, MD

Topical corticosteroids are commonly used following PRK to reduce the risk of haze and myopic regression. Some investigators, however, have elected not to use postoperative corticosteroids following PRK for low to moderate myopia because of their well-known ocular complications, which include elevated IOP and posterior subcapsular cataracts.

CORTICOSTEROID-INDUCED OCULAR HYPERTENSION

While Kim and coworkers have reported an incidence of steroid-induced ocular hypertension after PRK in only 0.14% of 2920 eyes treated with 0.25% prednisolone acetate postoperatively,[2] most investigators have reported a considerably higher rate of this condition even when lower concentrations of less potent corticosteroids were used. Epstein and coworkers found a 13% rise in IOP greater than 24 mmHg when topical dexamethasone was used postoperatively.[3] The Italian Study Group on Excimer Laser Keratectomy reviewed 1236 PRK procedures treated with either fluorometholone 0.25% or dexamethasone 0.1% and found that 25.3% of eyes had an IOP greater than 26 mmHg postoperatively.[4] Gartry and coworkers have reported and IOP rise greater than 21 in 21% of their patients treated with tapering dexamethasone 0.1% postoperatively, which included 7.5% with IOPs between 30 to 40 mmHg and 1.7% with IOPs greater than 45 mmHg.[5,6] In these studies, the increased IOP was easily controlled by cessation of the topical corticosteroid and/or the use of topical beta-blockers.[3,5] Seiler has correlated the incidence of corticosteroid-induced ocular hypertension with the degree of myopia by demonstrating an IOP rise of 6 mmHg at more than 1 month postoperatively to be 26% to 32% with less than 9 D of correction and 50% with greater than 9 D of correction when dexamethasone 0.1% was used on a tapering schedule postoperatively.[7]

More recent studies have used topical fluorometholone 0.1% following PRK to reduce the incidence of steroid-induced complications. Maguen and coworkers found that the postoperative IOP rise greater than 21 mmHg in 10.8% of cases and greater than 25 mmHg in 1.7% of cases, with their highest pressure measuring 32 mmHg while using fluorometholone 0.1%

on a tapering schedule.[8] Salz and coworkers also used tapering fluorometholone 0.1% and reported an incidence of IOP rise of greater than 24 mmHg in 3% of 160 eyes.[9] Talley and coworkers[10] reported IOPs greater than 24 mmHg in only 2.2% of 91 PRK eyes, and Tong and coworkers[11] found less than 1% of 108 eyes developed steroid-induced ocular hypertension when treated with fluorometholone 0.1% postoperatively.

Interestingly, Piebenga and coworkers[12] reported one patient with elevated IOP after PRK who had not been treated with any steroids postoperatively. A detailed past ocular history revealed that this patient had had periodic IOP elevations preoperatively.

Schipper, Senn, and colleagues have provided an additional consideration to the postoperative IOP by demonstrating that the central cornea IOP measurements after PRK give a 2 to 3 mmHg lower value than the measurements outside the ablation zone, suggesting that incidence of postoperative corticosteroid-induced ocular hypertension may be in fact underestimated.[13]

POSTERIOR SUBCAPSULAR CATARACTS

Despite the 4-month tapering course of topical steroids generally used after PRK, very few cases of posterior subcapsular cataracts have been reported from the thousands of cases studied. Three cases of posterior subcapsular cataracts have been reported following PRK with postoperative dexamethasone for which the steroid frequency and duration varied from four times a day for 3 months to every 2 hours for 8 months to control regression.[14]

OTHER COMPLICATIONS

Herpes simplex keratitis reactivation has been demonstrated in animal studies[15] and clinically following PTK[16] and PRK[17] treated postoperatively with topical steroids. In view of these reports, it is recommended that corneal sensation be tested in all patients prior to photokeratectomy.[17] Seiler and coworkers reported postoperative ptosis of more than 1 mm in 1% of 193 eyes which lasted for 3 months, but resolved between 3 and 6 months.[7] One case of permanent ptosis following PRK occurred in the Cedars-Sinai series which was corrected with a Muller muscle-conjunctival resection.[14] Another complication occasionally attributed to topical steroids is toxic superficial keratopathy.[14]

References

1. McDonald MB, Talamo JH. Myopic photorefractive keratectomy: the experience in the United States with the VisX excimer laser. In: Salz JJ, McDonnell PJ, McDonald MB, eds. *Corneal Laser Surgery.* St. Louis, Mo: Mosby; 1995.

2. Kim JH, Sah WJ, Hahn TW, et al. Some problems after photorefractive keratectomy. *J Refract Corneal Surg.* 1994;10(Suppl): S226-S230.

3. Epstein D, Fargerholm P, Hamberg-Nystrom H, Tengroth B. Twenty-four-month follow-up of excimer laser photorefractive keratectomy for myopia. Refractive and visual results. *Ophthalmology.* 1994;101:1558-1564.

4. Brancato R, Tavola A, Carones F, et al. Excimer laser photorefractive keratectomy for myopia: results in 1165 eyes. *Refract Corneal Surg.* 1993;9:95-104.

5. Gartry DS, Kerr Muir MG, Marshall J. Photorefractive keratectomy with an argon fluoride excimer laser: a clinical study. *Refract Corneal Surg.* 1991;7:420-435.

6. Gartry DS, Kerr Muir MG, Marshall J. Photorefractive laser keratectomy. 18 month follow-up. *Ophthalmology.* 1992;99:1209-1219.

7. Seiler T, Holschbach A, Derse M, et al. Complications of myopic photorefractive keratectomy with the excimer laser. *Ophthalmology.* 1994;101:153-160.

8. Maguen E, Salz JJ, Nesburn AB, et al. Results of excimer laser photorefractive keratectomy for the correction of myopia. *Ophthalmology.* 1994;101:1548-1557.

9. Salz JJ, Maguen E, Nesburn AB, et al. A two-year experience with excimer laser photorefractive keratectomy for myopia. *Ophthalmology.* 1993;100:873-882.

10. Talley AR, Hardten DR, Sher NA, et al. Results one year after using the 193 nm excimer laser for photorefractive keratectomy in mild to moderate myopia. *Am J Ophthalmol.* 1994;118:304-311.

11. Tong PPC, Kam JTK, Lam RHS, et al. Excimer laser photorefractive keratectomy for myopia: six-month follow-up. *J Cataract Refract Surg.* 1995;21:150-155.

12. Piebenga LW, Matta CS, Deitz MR, et al. Excimer photorefractive keratectomy for myopia. *Ophthalmology.* 1993;100:1335-1345.

13. Schipper I, Senn P, Thomann U, Suppiger M. Intraocular pressure after excimer laser photorefractive keratectomy for myopia. *J Refract Surg.* 1995;11(5):366-370.

14. Maguen E, Machat JJ. Complications of photorefractive keratectomy, primarily with the VisX excimer laser. In: Salz JJ, McDonnell PJ, McDonald MB, eds. *Corneal Laser Surgery.* St. Louis, Mo: Mosby; 1995.

15. Pepose JS, Laycock KA, Miller JK, et al. Reactivation of latent herpes virus by excimer laser photorefractectomy. *Am J Ophthalmol.* 1992;116:101-102.

16. Vrabec MP, Durrie DS, Chase DS. Recurrence of herpes simplex after excimer laser keratectomy. *Am J Ophthalmol.* 1992;116:101-102.

17. Seiler T, Schmidt-Petersen H, Wollensak J. Complications after myopic photorefractive keratectomy, primarily with the Summit excimer laser. In: Salz JJ, McDonnell PJ, McDonald MB, eds. *Corneal Laser Surgery.* St. Louis, Mo: Mosby; 1995.

Management: Reduce frequency or discontinue use. Lubrication and topical steroids indicated. In general, topical non-steroidal agents should not be used more than 3 days and limited to 2 days in cases of retarded re-epithelialization. The frequency should not exceed qid, and bid may be adequate in most cases. Concomitant topical steroid use is always indicated to avoid sterile infiltrates.

STEROID-INDUCED COMPLICATIONS
Ptosis

Clinical: Ptosis is most common in young females (Figure 5-4). It is primarily related to frequency and potency of topical steroid use. Ptosis usually measures 1 to 2 mm. There can be tremendous diurnal variation related to dosing. It may also be related to postoperative lid edema and the eyelid speculum utilized.

Management: Ptosis always improves and usually, but not always, resolves with discontinuation of topical steroids. The frequency, potency, and duration should be reduced whenever possible once ptosis becomes evident.

Glaucoma

Clinical: Raised intraocular pressure (IOP) related to topical steroid use occurs more frequently with high potency steroids such as FML Forte 0.25% and dexamethasone phosphate 0.1%. The reported incidence of elevated IOP over 30 varies from 1.5% to 8%, depending upon the frequency and potency of the topical steroid. Some patients describe blurred vision, especially upon waking, or a pressure or pulling sensation. Most are asymptomatic.

Management: In general, use the minimum drops required. Avoid high potency topical steroids, fluorometholone 0.1% preferable. Monitor IOP every month at a minimum. If IOP is elevated above 22 mmHg or raised by more than 8 mmHg, reduce topical steroids and/or add a topical beta-blocker when no contraindications are present. Follow IOP more closely, as field loss has been reported.

Posterior Subcapsular Cataracts

Clinical: Posterior subcapsular cataracts (Figure 5-5) have been reported following use of dexamethasone phosphate 0.1%, but not with fluorometholone 0.1% or 0.25%. In

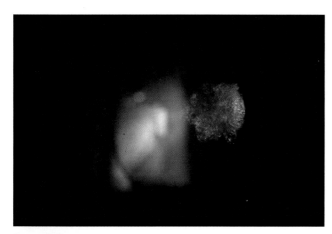

Figure 5-5.
Posterior subcapsular cataract secondary to dexamethasone phosphate 0.1%. Despite the fact that the patient was only -3.50 D preoperatively, she experienced considerable regression immediately following steroid withdrawal. The referring doctor maintained patient on steroids for 9 months to sustain 20/20 uncorrected vision. Postoperative PRK regimens consisting of potent topical steroids and/or prolonged courses exceeding 6 months significantly increase the risk of cataract formation.

general, avoid dexamethasone phosphate following PRK.

Management: Same as for cataracts of other etiologies. Prevention is the key, in that the low potency steroids should be the agent of choice in the management of the post-PRK patient, even fluorometholone 0.25% should be routinely avoided.

HSV Keratitis Reactivation

Clinical: Reactivation of HSV has been reported; however, a remote history of HSV is not an absolute contraindication, only a relative one. Patients with a history of HSV have been treated with no reactivation; prophylactic coverage with oral acyclovir 400 mg five times per day starting 2 days preoperatively for 1 week may be helpful. If the patient has had a recurrence within the past year and/or a history of stromal or uveitic involvement, treatment is contraindicated. Topical steroids, ultraviolet radiation, and surgical trauma are all possible mechanisms that may reactivate the virus.

Management: Treatment of HSV keratitis following PRK consists of discontinuation of topical steroids, institution of viroptic topically every 2 hours, and oral acyclovir systemically.

Keratoconjunctivitis Sicca

Clinical: Dry eye is one of the most common problems encountered postoperatively, related to both the PRK procedure and topical steroid use. It may affect vision, but usual-ly produces only ocular irritation. Patients with a history of dry eye preoperatively should be warned that the procedure and drops may exacerbate their symptoms. Dry eye in general is not a contraindication. Most candidates with contact lens intolerance in fact have dry eye. Patients with severe dry eye and epithelial breakdown should be avoided. Symptoms are exacerbated in winter with forced heat, summer with air conditioning, and in offices and airplanes.

Management: Lubrication with tears and ointment. Humidification at home (bedroom) or office helpful. Punctal plugs recommended.

COMPLICATIONS RELATED TO THERAPEUTIC CONTACT LENS USE

TIGHT CONTACT LENS SYNDROME

Clinical: Patients should be fitted with the steepest base curve which prevents excessive movement, usually base curve 8.4. Excessive movement will increase pain and delay epithelial healing. A tight lens will actually feel more comfortable. Tight contact lens syndrome may produce stromal edema, ciliary flush, or an injected and chemotic eye. Pain is variable. Epithelial healing will become stagnant (see Chapter 4). A contact lens that fits snugly but does not induce corneal hypoxia and allows for rapid re-epithelialization is optimal.

Etiology of Postoperative Pain
- Corneal nerve plexus damage
- Thermal energy inflammation
- Ultraviolet keratitis

Management: Remove the bandage contact lens and fit with a flatter base curve (base curve 8.8) if no significant corneal edema, ciliary flush, or chemosis is evident. One may increase the potency and/or frequency of the topical steroid in the postoperative regimen as needed. If significant edema, remove bandage contact lens and patch with antibiotic-steroid ointment such as TobraDex (Alcon). In general, do not use a therapeutic contact lens beyond 3 to 4 days as the risk of infection and other problems increases rapidly. Instead patch daily until healed. Therapeutic collagen shields have not been found to be effective and may actually increase pain and inhibit rapid re-epithelialization.

Figure 5-6.
Severe corneal ulcer secondary to gram positive bacteria following PRK. Culture demonstrated pneumococcal bacteria following intensive fortified antibiotic therapy. Patient eventually regained 20/40 uncorrected vision, although best corrected vision was reduced to 20/30.

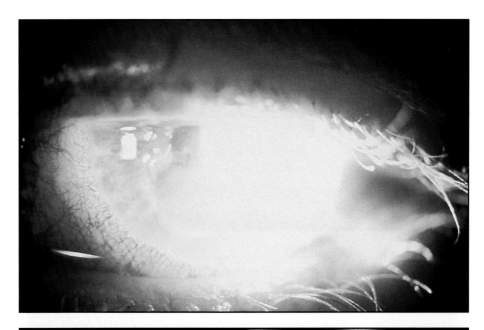

Figure 5-7.
Postoperative PRK infection in a physician who put in his own contact lens and questionably his own solution. The infection resolved with some subepithelial haze. He subsequently underwent PTK and his vision is 20/25 best corrected. Courtesy of Dr. Neal Sher.

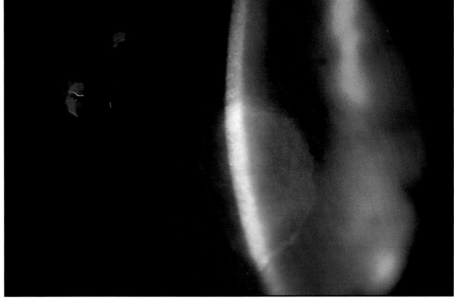

STERILE CORNEAL INFILTRATES

Clinical: Peripheral superficial infiltrates, usually small and along the limbus, can sometimes be observed and are likely related to hypoxia. Although not always sterile, they typically are if associated with an intact epithelium. More central and larger infiltrates must be considered suspicious for infection.

Management: In all cases where a true infiltrate is discovered, the contact lens must be removed and an antibiotic alone or in combination with steroid therapy initiated. Peripheral infiltrates with intact epithelium should be treated with combination antibiotic-steroid therapy. A fluoroquinolone such as ciprofloxacin or ofloxacin is the recommended antibiotic, although TobraDex (tobramycin 0.3%–dexamethasone 0.1%, Alcon) is commonly prescribed. Central and pericentral infiltrates are more likely to be infectious or sterile and NSAID related, but must be considered infectious if the epithelium is denuded. All suspicious infiltrates must be cultured and treated as infectious with an hourly fluoroquinolone or a fortified antibiotic drop regimen. Clinical judgment develops with clinical experience, and all infiltrates should be monitored very closely, even twice daily, when the diagnosis is unclear.

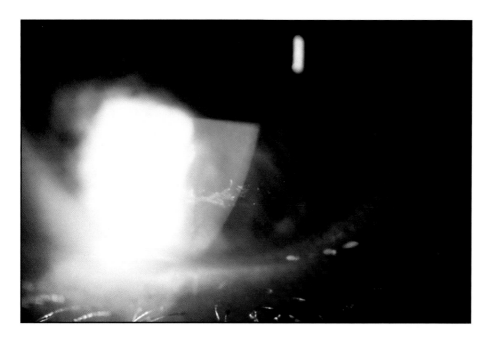

Figure 5-8.
Basement membrane changes at site of recurrent corneal erosion following 5-mm Summit ExciMed UV 200 ablation for -4.00 D. Patient achieved 20/15 uncorrected vision but experienced classic recurrent corneal erosion symptoms. Area of breakdown was outside ablative zone but within area of epithelial debridement. Patient failed to respond to conservative hyperosmotic therapy and was treated successfully with 5 micron PTK locally.

COMPLICATIONS RELATED TO EPITHELIAL HEALING

PAIN

Clinical: Pain usually peaks early and is often most severe within the first 6 to 12 hours postoperatively. Increased irritation occurs during the final 6 to 12 hours of epithelial healing as well, and is likely related to contact lens use. Patients often describe two types of pain: a superficial, irritative type of pain and a deep, dull pain. The pain can be quite severe and I have found that it is not well tolerated by some male patients. It is unrelated to the severity of the myopia corrected.

Management: Only the deeper pain is responsive to oral narcotic medication. The most common systemic analgesic combination used in the United States is Demerol (meperidine 50 mg) and Phenergan (promethazine 25 mg) in the form of Mepergan Fortis. I have had the clinical experience of attempting post-PRK pain management without the benefit of bandage contact lenses and topical NSAIDs, which had required Percocet (oxycodone), morphine sulfate, codeine, and Toradol (oral/injectable ketorolac tromethamine). Unbelievable as it may sound, a small number of patients continued to experience severe pain despite these strong systemic analgesic agents. Some surgeons continue to pressure patch patients to virtually eliminate their risk of microbial infection associated with contact lens use, a common practice in Australia. If it were my eye, however, I would accept the 1/1000 risk of infection and use a steeply

fit contact lens and Voltaren (diclofenac sodium 0.1%) to alleviate or at least dramatically reduce the anticipated postoperative pain. The bandage contact lens in combination with topical non-steroidals is truly effective in 90% of patients in relieving both types of pain. One in 10 patients still complains of severe pain. Cycloplegics are generally ineffective and only exacerbate photophobic symptoms. A cool compress to the eyes and a dark room or dark sunglasses are helpful adjuncts. Increased activity tends to increase pain. A loose contact lens is also very painful and slows re-epithelialization, therefore, the contact lens should fit snugly.

DELAYED EPITHELIAL HEALING

Clinical: Most patients (99%) are healed in 72 hours. Range is 2 to 7 days. Transepithelial approach produces faster healing related to distinct epithelial wound margins. Age is a factor. Patching speeds healing but reduces comfort. A very loose or tight bandage contact lens and severe dry eye slow epithelial healing. Collagen vascular disease may seriously affect healing (see below). Haze increases.

Management: Delayed epithelial healing is usually noted on the second or third day when inadequate progress in re-epithelialization is observed. The bandage contact lens fit should first be reassessed and an excessively tight or loose lens refitted. If by the third postoperative day less than two thirds of the epithelial defect has closed, the bandage contact lens should be removed and the eye pressure patched. Delayed epithelial healing is most commonly observed in

Haze Following PRK: Literature Review

Louis E. Probst V, MD

Animal studies have indicated that superficial stromal haze after PRK is associated with increased basal epithelial cells, vascularization at the epithelial-stromal junction, fragmentation of the reformed basement membrane, increased fibroblast in the anterior stroma, and the deposition of type III collagen.[1,2] Visually significant postoperative corneal haze has been reported to be maximal at 3 months, after which there is a steady reduction in severity for at least 18 months.[3] The amount of postoperative haze has been found to be associated with greater amounts of treatment, a younger patient age, the male sex, ablation zones less than 4.5 mm, nitrogen flow, premature cessation of postoperative steroid drops, and slow postoperative re-epithelialization.[3-5] Untreated allergic conjunctivitis has been recently identified as another risk factor for regression and haze following PRK.[6]

Haze can be graded on a scale from 0 to 3:

- Grade 0 for a totally clear cornea
- Grade trace for faint corneal haze seen by indirect broad tangential illumination
- Grade 1 for mild haze easily visible with direct focal slit illumination
- Grade 2 for moderate haze with dense opacity that partially obscures iris detail
- Grade 3 for severe haze with a dense opacity that obscures the detail of intraocular structures.[7]

The FDA Phase III clinical trial with the VisX 20/20 excimer laser found that 6.9% of all PRK cases demonstrated significant haze at 1 month, and this decreased to approximately 1% at 12 months.[4] The Summit arm of this trial found that 12 months after surgery, 89.3% of patients were free of clinically significant haze and no patients suffered marked haze.[8] Epstein and coworkers found that 24 months after PRK, 3% of eyes had a haze grading of 2+, and 1% had a haze grading of 3+.[9] Similar results were reported by Salz and coworkers, who found a 3% incidence of haze greater than grade 1 and a less than 1% incidence of haze of grade 2.5 over 2 years of follow-up.[10] The Italian Study Group on Excimer Laser Keratectomy found that haze was related to regression and a significant reduction of haze occurred over the 12 postoperative months; however, they were unable to find a significant correlation between haze and decreased best corrected visual acuity.[11] Seiler and coworkers have differentiated normal heal-ing haze from postoperative manifest scars occurring within 12 months postoperatively, for which they have reported an incidence of 0% for up to -3.0 D correction, 1.1% for -3.1 to -6.0 D correction, 17.5% for -6.1 to -9.0 D correction, and 16.7% for greater than -9.1 D correction.[12]

Haze generally resolves without treatment by 6 months postoperatively.[13] Persistent haze can be treated with topical steroids or retreatment with PRK if there is associated myopic regression. Seiler and coworkers reported no recurrence of haze after retreatment with up to 21 months of follow-up.[12] Scraping the hyperplastic epithelium has been found to reduce the myopic regression associated with haze by greater than 1 D.[14] Recently, topical diclofenac has also been shown to decrease corneal haze in rabbits in the early postoperative period, suggesting possible therapeutic applications.[15] Marshall and coworkers have suggested that the plasmin/plasminogen system activation following PRK may be responsible for myopic regression and haze and they are investigating methods of controlling this effect.[16] Finally, the control of dry eyes in the immediate postoperative period has been suggested as a method of reducing haze in some patients.[17]

References

1. Fantes FE, Hanna KD, Waring GO III, et al. Wound healing after laser keratomileusis in monkeys. *Arch Ophthalmol.* 1990;108:665-675.

2. Hanna KD, Pouliquen Y, Waring GO III, et al. Corneal stromal wound healing in rabbits after 193 nm excimer laser surface ablation. *Arch Ophthalmol.* 1989;107:895-901.

3. Caubet E. Cause of subepithelial corneal haze over 18 months after photorefractive keratectomy for myopia. *Refract Corneal Surg.* 1993;9(Suppl):S65-S69.

4. Maguen E, Machat JJ. Complications of photorefractive keratectomy, primarily with the VisX excimer laser. In: Salz JJ, McDonnell PJ, McDonald MB, eds. *Corneal Laser Surgery.* St. Louis, Mo: Mosby; 1995.

5. Ditzen K, Anschutz Schroder E. Photorefractive keratectomy to treat low, medium, and high myopia: a multicenter study. *J Cataract Refract Surg.* 1994;20(Suppl):234-238.

6. Yang H, Toda I, Bissen-Miyajima H, et al. Allergic conjunctivitis is a risk factor for regression and haze after PRK. 1995 ISRS Pre-AAO Conference & Exhibition; October 26, 1994; Atlanta, Ga.

7. Kim JH, Hahn TW, Young CL. Photorefractive keratectomy in 202 myopic eyes: one year results. *Refract Corneal Surg.* 1993;9(Suppl):S11-S16.

8. Thompson KP, Steinert RF, Daniel J, Stulting D. Photorefractive keratectomy with the Summit excimer laser: The phase III US

results. In: Salz JJ, McDonnell PJ, McDonald MB, eds. *Corneal Laser Surgery.* St. Louis, Mo: Mosby; 1995.

9. Epstein D, Fagerholm P, Hamberg-Nystrom H, et al. Twenty-four-month follow-up of excimer laser photorefractive keratectomy for myopia. *Ophthalmology.* 1994;101:1558-1564.

10. Salz JJ, Maguen E, Nesburn AB, et al. A two-year experience with excimer laser photorefractive keratectomy for myopia. *Ophthalmology.* 1993;100:873-882.

11. Brancato R, Tavola A, Carones F, et al. Excimer laser photorefractive keratectomy for myopia: results in 1165 eyes. *Refract Corneal Surg.* 1993;9:95-104.

12. Seiler T, Holschbach A, Derse M, et al. Complications of myopic photorefractive keratectomy with the excimer laser. *Ophthalmology.* 1994;101:153-160.

13. Talley AR, Hardten DR, Sher NA, et al. Results one year after

using the 193-nm excimer laser for photorefractive keratectomy in mild to moderate myopia. *Am J Ophthalmol.* 1994;118:304-311.

14. Loewenstein A, Lipshitz I, Lazar M. Scraping the epithelium for treatment of undercorrection and haze after photorefractive keratectomy. *J Cataract Refract Surg.* 1994;10(Suppl 2):S274-S276.

15. Nassaralla BA, Szerenyi K, Wang XW, et al. Effect of diclofenac on corneal haze after photorefractive keratectomy in rabbits. *Ophthalmology.* 1995;102(3):469-474.

16. Lohmann CP, Marshall J. Plasmin- and plasminogen-activator inhibitors after excimer laser photorefractive keratectomy: new concepts in the prevention of myopic regression and haze. *Refract Corneal Surg.* 1993;9(Suppl):300-302.

17. Tervo T, Mustonen R, Tarkkanen A. Management of dry eye may reduce haze after excimer laser photorefractive keratectomy. *Refract Corneal Surg.* 1993; 9(Suppl):306. Letter.

patients who exhibited loose epithelial adherence upon mechanical debridement of their epithelium intraoperatively. If the eye appears dry, lubrication should be added. If a toxic medication effect is considered, suspicious agents such as NSAIDs and aminoglycosides should be discontinued. In fact, NSAIDs should routinely be discontinued or tapered the second day if re-epithelialization is even somewhat retarded. These patients must be monitored closely, not only for infection, but for stromal melts. Vitamin C 1500 mg daily may promote epithelial healing (D. Schneider, MD).

MICROBIAL CORNEAL ULCER

Clinical: Painful red eye with central or paracentral infiltrate within denuded area of epithelium (Figures 5-6 and 5-7). Infectious infiltrates likely occur with an incidence of 0.2% but respond rapidly to removal of the bandage contact lens and topical antibiotics. Severe corneal ulcers occur in about 0.1% of treated eyes. Aggressive lid hygiene preoperatively reduces risk of severe corneal ulcers to 0.05% or less.

Management: Culture and start hourly fortified antibiotics immediately. Await results and manage accordingly. Newer studies indicate that hourly (around the clock) fluoroquinolones may be equally effective in corneal ulcer management pending cultures.

RECURRENT CORNEAL EROSIONS

Clinical: Patients sometimes complain of brief, sharp pains, usually in the morning hours upon waking, associated with tearing, photosensitivity, and possibly blurred vision. These episodes usually resolve within an hour and may or may not recur. These most likely represent episodes of recurrent corneal erosions (RCE). The erosions are evident in the area outside the ablative zone, but within the area

of epithelial debridement. Microcysts, non-random tear film staining, or basement membrane excrescences are sometimes visible at the slit lamp (Figure 5-8).

Management: The treatment for RCE syndrome following PRK is identical to that of other traumatic etiologies with lubrication and hypertonic ointments forming the mainstay of therapy. Excimer PTK of 5 to 7 microns can be performed, if conservative therapy fails, over a persistent area of epithelial breakdown with exceptionally good results. Use a surgical spear to debride the loose epithelium prior to treatment.

CORNEAL ULCERATION RELATED TO AUTOIMMUNE DISEASE

Clinical: One case of stromal melt leading to perforation has been described by Theo Seiler, MD. The patient failed to heal postoperatively and required a corneal transplant to restore ocular integrity. She was subsequently diagnosed with systemic lupus erythematosus.

Management: All patients with collagen vascular disorders or other autoimmune diseases which can affect wound healing are contraindicated and should be specifically screened for preoperatively. Each patient must be followed closely until his or her epithelium is intact. Intrastromal techniques reduce the risk of stromal melt in these patients; however, refractive surgery should be avoided in any patient with active collagen vascular disease.

Clinical Note

Autoimmune and Collagen Vascular Disorders

Theo Seiler, MD, submitted a case report of a middle-aged woman with undiagnosed systemic lupus erythematosus who was treated with PRK and who developed a

Figure 5-9.
Corneal melt with uveal prolapse following PRK in a patient with undiagnosed systemic lupus erythematosus. Courtesy of Dr. Theo Seiler.

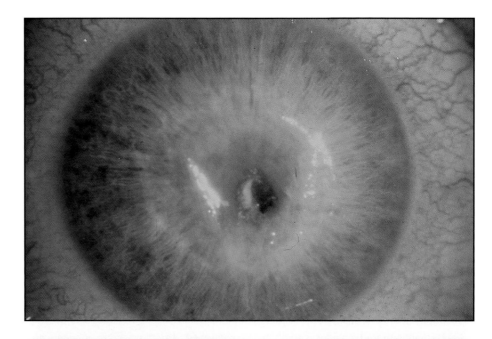

Figure 5-10.
Central corneal haze with evidence of early confluence. Grade +2.0.

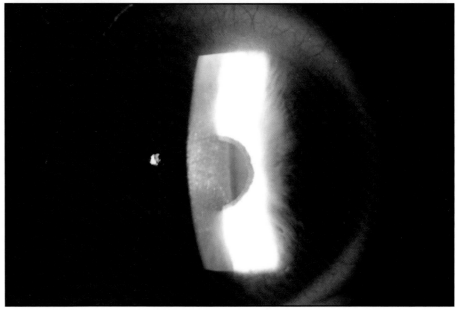

corneal melt and perforated centrally, requiring corneal transplantation. The patient was on no medications and the only prior history was one of polyarthritis 10 years preoperatively. Autoimmune and collagen vascular disorders (Figure 5-9) have been contraindicated for PRK for fear of developing a stromal melt; however, by ablating intrastromally and leaving the epithelium intact, LASIK is not contraindicated. I have treated four patients with rheumatoid arthritis antibodies and two patients with lupus antibodies (after considerable preoperative discussion with each patient) with no complications or adverse healing patterns observed. In general, patients with active autoimmune disease or vasculitides, not simply seropositive, are contraindicated.

NON-TOXIC KERATITIS

Clinical: A small percentage of patients develop a diffuse non-specific central keratitis, reducing visual acuity, and producing glare, with mild irritation. The fine punctate keratitis usually starts 1 week following PRK and resolves

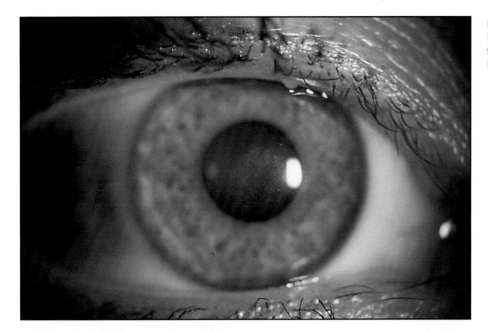

Figure 5-11.
Dense corneal haze observed centrally following Summit ExciMed UV 200 PRK treatment. Grade +3.0.

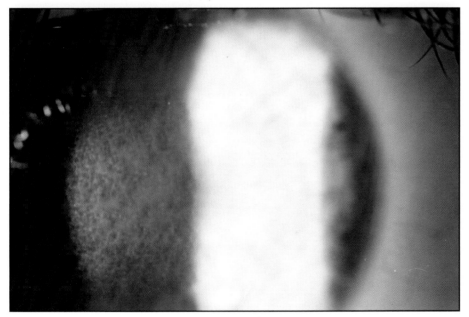

Figure 5-12.
Diffuse confluent haze.

by the fourth week.

Management: Lubrication, especially with non-preserved formulations of ointments at bedtime, is helpful. Humidification at bedtime also aids recovery.

IRITIS

Clinical: The incidence is probably less than 0.1%, usually in patients with a past history of iritis or who are determined to be HLA-B27 positive. The iritis usually flares up immediately following surgery and resolves rapidly within the first week with topical steroids.

Management: A history of idiopathic iritis does not appear to be a contraindication. Cycloplegics and topical steroids are indicated.

COMPLICATIONS RELATED TO STROMAL WOUND HEALING

SUPERFICIAL STROMAL OPACIFICATION (HAZE)

Clinical: Corneal haze or subepithelial scatter is related to a multitude of causes including, but far from limited to,

Figure 5-13a.
Confluent central haze under medium magnification demonstrating pronounced reticular haze with developing areas of confluence. Grade +3.0.

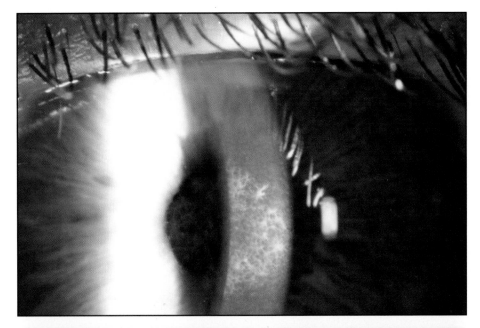

Figure 5-13b.
Confluent central haze under high magnification demonstrating pronounced reticular haze with developing areas of confluence. Grade +3.0.

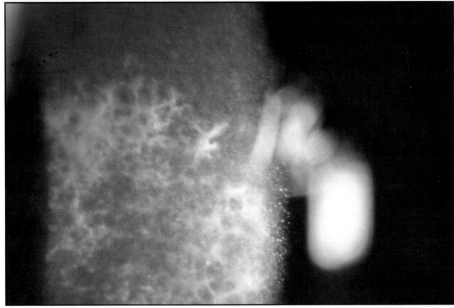

depth of ablation. Haze is clearly related to steep contours, intraoperative stromal hydration, and patient variability. Reticulated corneal haze is a normal part of the PRK healing process.

The only important distinction to be made when grading corneal haze is to discern clinically significant haze from clinically insignificant haze.

Any confluent area of haze, the hallmark for clinically significant haze, is associated with:

- Regression, both immediate and long-term
- Loss of best corrected visual acuity related to absolute

degradation of vision, irregular astigmatism, and/or abnormal topography (Figures 5-10 through 5-12)

It is remarkable how much haze can be present without any loss of best corrected acuity (Figure 5-13a and 5-13b).

Management: Corneal haze and regression can be controlled, but not eliminated, with topical steroid administration. Clinically significant haze, even in severe myopes, is infrequent with proper techniques to improve wound contour (larger optical zones and multi-multizone techniques) and with proper attention to adequate intraoperative stromal hydration.

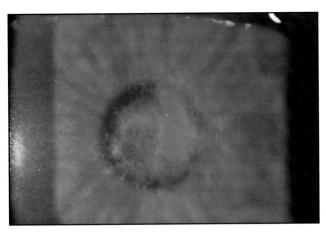

Figure 5-14.
Confluent central haze. Grade +4.0.

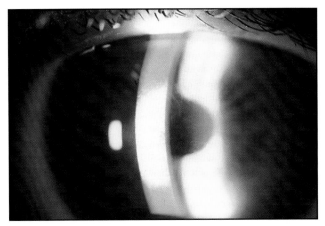

Figure 5-15.
Dense plaque of confluent haze with no iris details visible. Grade +5.0.

COLLAGEN PLAQUE FORMATION

Clinical: Patients with dense collagen plaques complain of poor qualitative and quantitative vision. Their uncorrected vision is reduced because of the associated myopia, and the best corrected vision is reduced because of the opacification (Figures 5-14 and 5-15). Dense plaques can be diffuse, central, arcuate, semi-circular, or focal. It is difficult to visualize iris details through the plaques.

Utilizing proper techniques, the risk is:
- 0.5% low myopes <-3.00 D
- 1.0% moderate myopes -4.00 to -6.00 D
- 2% to 3% severe myopes -7.00 to -9.00 D
- 4% to 5% extreme myopes -10.00 to -15.00 D

Loss of Best Corrected Visual Acuity
- Related to collagen plaque
- Related to abnormal topography
- Related to irregular astigmatism

Management: The natural history of dense corneal haze is gradual resolution over months to years. Retreatment is indicated for the removal of collagen plaques, utilizing a combined PRK/PTK modality, to try to re-establish the originally sculpted corneal contour. Trace haze, and not a clear cornea, should be the goal. The premise behind this is that "You did the right surgery, the patient just healed wrong." (The retreatment technique is described in Chapter 6.)

COMPLICATIONS RELATED TO ERRORS IN ABLATION

DECENTRATION OF ABLATION ZONE

Clinical: Greater than 1 mm of decentration is usually clinically significant and more than 2 mm creates significant monocular diplopia, asymmetric night glare, and blurred visual acuity symptoms (Figures 5-16 and 5-17). Within 0.5 mm is ideal, and 0.5 to 1 mm of decentration is often asymptomatic. Unlike RK, the cornea is not multifocal but ideally unifocal, so that small decentrations are forgiven, especially with larger ablative zones. Small optical zones 5 mm or under must always be well centered to avoid symptoms (see Chapter 3). Newer excimer laser systems such as CIBA—Autonomous Technologies Corporation, which has the LADAR eyetracking system described in Chapter 1, may eliminate problems of decentration in the future.

Management: There is no easy answer. Patients will often adjust to small decentrations, but significant decentrations are problematic. If the patient is undercorrected, the best answer in some cases may simply be to enlarge the optical zone maximally and still center the retreatment

---

Decentration Symptoms
- Asymmetric night glare or halos
- Monocular diplopia
- Induced regular cylinder
- Induced irregular astigmatism
- Reduced image quality
- Loss of best corrected vision

Optical Aberrations Following PRK: Starburst, Halos, and Decentration

Louis E. Probst V, MD

Disturbances in night vision occur preoperatively in approximately 21% of refractive surgery patients, while postoperatively 45% of patients complain of some disturbance of night vision and 15% find it a significant problem.[1] Night vision problems include the starburst effect and halos.[1] Recently, it has been suggested that increased postoperative corneal asphericity alone may also contribute to some of the bothersome glare symptoms experienced during night driving.[2,3]

Corneal haze results in the starburst phenomenon, which is the scattering of light around bright light sources at night. The scattered component of light can degrade visual function and reduce contrast sensitivity. Haze is generally first apparent about 4 weeks postoperatively and is maximal at 2 to 4 months. In over 90% of patients, the starburst effect is reduced to an insignificant level after the first 3 postoperative months, as the corneal haze gradually diminishes.[4]

Halos have been described as a shimmering circular zone extending from a point source of light and are generated by differential light refraction along the treated and untreated zones of the circular ablation edge.[1,5] Halos tend to be a problem at night in young patients when the pupil dilates larger than the edge of the ablation zone.[6] The halos after PRK are similar in their severity to those associated with soft contact lenses and spectacle correction, and less significant than the halos associated with hard contact lenses.[4] Gartry and coworkers found that 78% of their patients reported halos in the early postoperative period after a 4-mm ablation.[7] The magnitude of the halo effect as measured by the amount of negative lens required to eliminate the halo was found to be directly correlated to the pupil size and the amount of induced refractive change. At 1-year follow-up, the incidence of halos had decreased to 10% of patients but was severe enough to discourage the affected patients from having their other eye treated. Gimbel and coworkers[6] found 50% of patients with 4.5- to 5-mm ablation zones complained of halos 8 months postoperatively. Kim and coworkers[8] used a 5-mm ablation zone and found the incidence of severe halos changed from 30.4% at 3 months to 8.7% at 2 years. A loss of visual acuity under glare conditions has also been associated with smaller ablation zones.[3]

The mean pupil size between the ages of 20 to 30 years has been found to be 7.5 mm, and between 33 to 45 years, 6.5 mm.[9] Theoretical calculations indicate that the ablation zone used for PRK should be at least as large as the entrance pupil to avoid foveal and parafoveal glare.[10] Patients with bilateral PRK correction have identified significantly less halos with the 5-mm as opposed to the 4-mm ablation zone.[11] In another study, less than 1% of patients with a 6-mm ablation zone complained of significant halos.[12] A study of 5.0-, 5.5-, 6.0-, and 7.0-mm ablation zones found the lowest incidence of halos in the 7.0-mm ablation zone group.[9]

Multipass/multizone PRK allows larger diameter ablations while decreasing the depth of the overall ablation. A recent study using this protocol with the VisX 20/20 excimer laser reported persistent halos in less than 1% of patients at 6 month follow-up.[3] Machat reported night glare in 75% to 80% of cases with a 4-mm ablation zone, 35% to 40% of cases with a 4.5-mm ablation zone, 20% of cases with a 5-mm ablation zone, 5% with a 6-mm ablation zone, and less than 0.5% of cases when 7-mm multizone ablation was used.[12]

PRK ablations should be centered on the pupillary center.[13] Asymmetric halos and astigmatism can result if the ablation is eccentric to the pupil, particularly with smaller ablation zones. Maloney calculated that a 1-mm decentration of a 4-mm ablation zone would result in a ghost image and monocular diplopia.[14] The Italian Study Group on Excimer Laser Keratectomy reported an incidence of decentered ablations in 10.6% of their patients.[15] Cantera reported decentration of 0.5 mm in 30.3% of patients and more than 1 mm in only 5.1%.[16] Similarly, Lin and coworkers found that 2% of ablations were more than 1 mm outside the pupillary center with the greatest amount of decentration being 1.5 mm.[17] Decentered ablations have been reported to reduce acuity[18] and result in an asymmetrical halo effect.[5] Schwartz-Goldstein and coworkers found that decentration was associated with decreased patient satisfaction but not associated with best corrected vision, predictability, astigmatism, and their glare/halo ranking, although half of their patients with greater than 1-mm decentration demonstrated a high glare/halo grade.[19] While they are best avoided, decentered ablations can still be associated with excellent visual acuity.[20]

Haze causing a starburst effect generally resolves with time and requires no further treatment unless it is also associated with myopic regression.[4] Persistent significant halos can be treated with negative lens overcorrection or miotic therapy[11] but these treatments are not well tolerated.[12] When a clear disparity exists between the pupillary and ablation zone diameters in a patient with residual myopia, retreatment with enlargement of the optical zone may be beneficial.[12] Eccentric ablations can be similarly retreated by a second PRK eccentrically opposite to the original ablation if patients complain about asymmetric halos or are experiencing decreased visual acuity.[3]

References

1. O'Brart DP, Lohmann CP, Fitzke FW, et al. Disturbances of night vision after excimer laser photorefractive keratectomy. *Eye.* 1994;8(Pt 1):46-51.

2. Assil KK. Halos, starburst and comets: significance of optical aberrations associated with keratorefractive procedures I & II. 1995 ISRS Pre-AAO Conference & Exhibition; October 27, 1995; Atlanta, Ga.

3. Seiler T, Schmidt-Petersen H, Wollensak J. Complications after myopic photorefractive keratectomy, primarily with the Summit excimer laser. In: Salz JJ, McDonnell PJ, McDonald MB, eds. *Corneal Laser Surgery.* St. Louis, Mo: Mosby; 1995.

4. Lohmann CP, Fitzke FW, O'Brart DP, et al. Halos—a problem for all myopes? A comparison between spectacles, contact lenses, and photorefractive keratectomy. *J Refract Corneal Surg.* 1993;9 (Suppl):S72-S75.

5. Gartry DS, Kerr Muir MG, Marshall J. Photorefractive keratectomy with an argon fluoride excimer laser: a clinical study. *Refract Corneal Surg.* 1991;7:420-435.

6. Gimbel HV, van Westenbrugge JA, Johnson WH, et al. Visual, refractive, and patient satisfaction results following bilateral photorefractive keratectomy for myopia. *J Refract Corneal Surg.* 1993;9(Suppl):S5-S10.

7. Gartry DS, Kerr Muir MG, Marshall J. Excimer laser photorefractive keratectomy. 18 month follow-up. *Ophthalmology.* 1992; 99:1209-1219.

8. Kim JH, Hahn TY, Lee YC, Sah WJ. Excimer photorefractive keratectomy for myopia: two year follow-up. *J Cataract Refract Surg.* 1994;20(Suppl):229.

9. Anschutz T. Pupil size, ablation diameter, halo incidence of dependence after PRK. 1995 ISRS Pre-AAO Conference & Exhibition; October 26, 1995; Atlanta, Ga.

10. Roberts CW, Koester CJ. Optical zone diameters for photorefractive corneal laser surgery. *Invest Ophthalmol Vis Sci.* 1993;34:2275-2281.

11. O'Brart DP, Lohmann CP, Fitzke FW, et al. Night vision disturbances after excimer laser photorefractive keratectomy: haze and halos. *Eur J Ophthalmol.* 1994;4(1):43-51.

12. Maguen E, Machat JJ. Complications of photorefractive keratectomy, primarily with the VisX excimer laser. In: Salz JJ, McDonnell PJ, McDonald MB, eds. *Corneal Laser Surgery.* St. Louis, Mo: Mosby; 1995.

13. Uozato H, Guyton DL. Cantering corneal surgical procedures. *Am J Ophthalmol.* 1987;103:264-275.

14. Maloney RK. Corneal topography and optical zone location in photorefractive keratectomy. *Refract Corneal Surg.* 1990;6:363-371.

15. Brancato R, Tavola A, Carones F, et al. Excimer laser photorefractive keratectomy for myopia: results in 1165 eyes. *Refract Corneal Surg.* 1993;9:95-104.

16. Cantera E, Cantera I, Olivieri L. Corneal topographic analysis of photorefractive keratectomy in 175 myopic eyes. *Refract Corneal Surg.* 1993;9:S19-S22.

17. Lin DTC, Sutton HF, Berman M. Corneal topography following excimer photorefractive keratectomy for myopia. *J Cataract Refract Surg.* 1993;19:149-154.

18. Salz JJ, Maguen E, Nesburn AB, et al. A two-year experience with excimer laser photorefractive keratectomy for myopia. *Ophthalmology.* 1993;100:873-882.

19. Schwartz-Goldstein BH, Hesh PS, The Summit Photorefractive Keratectomy Topography Study Group. Corneal topography of phase III excimer laser photorefractive keratectomy. Optical zone centration analysis. *Ophthalmology.* 1995;10(2):951-962.

20. Maguire LJ, Zabel RW, Parker P, Lindstrom RL. Topography and raytracing analysis of patients with excellent visual acuity 3 months after excimer laser photorefractive keratectomy for myopia. *Refract Corneal Surg.* 1991;7:122-128.

on the previous ablation. If the patient is not undercorrected, tailoring the treatment so as to treat only the untouched central cornea becomes a risky and artistic procedure if attempted. Properly centering the new ablation may induce cylinder, hyperopia, and monocular diplopia as it overlaps with the previously decentered ablation. It may be best to utilize a transepithelial approach to blend in the new well-centered treatment using the epithelium as a mask, creating a more refined transition between the old and new treatment zones. Future scanning lasers which incorporate topography may solve these problems (see Chapter 6).

Inadequate Ablation Zone Size (Halos)

Clinical: Disturbances in vision under conditions of reduced illumination were the most significant adverse effect associated with early excimer lasers. Halos and even starbursts were commonly reported by patients with excellent visual acuities. Some 20/15 patients actually felt unsafe to drive at night. Halos are directly related to pupil size in dim light exceeding the effective optical zone size, a pronounced form of spherical aberration (Figures 5-18a and 5-18b).

Halos are unrelated to corneal haze, although certain patterns of haze may alter topography, reducing the size of the effective optical zone as well as inducing myopic regres-

Figure 5-16.
Corneal videokeratography
demonstrating eccentric PRK ablation.

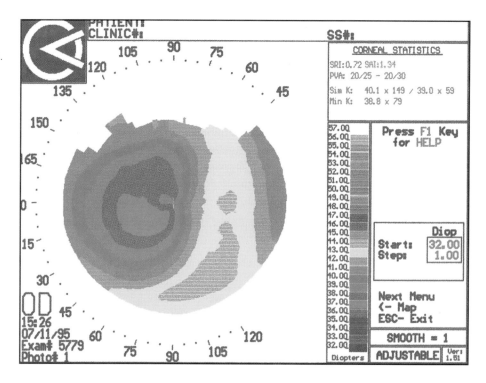

Figure 5-17.
Patient with eccentric ablation evident
on corneal videokeratography.
Uncorrected visual acuity 20/30 with
best corrected vision unchanged at
20/25.

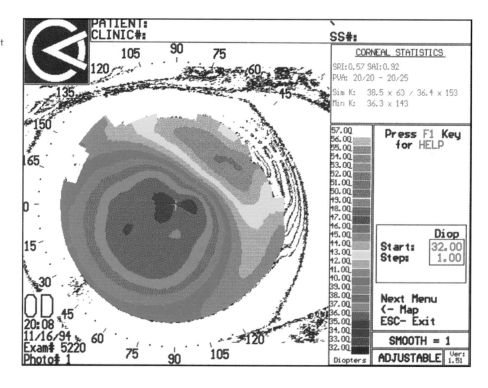

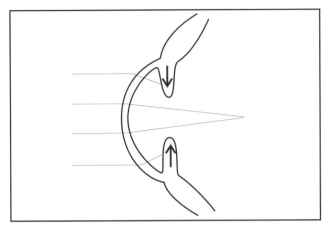

Figure 5-18a.
Light ray path when the pupil is small preventing night glare.

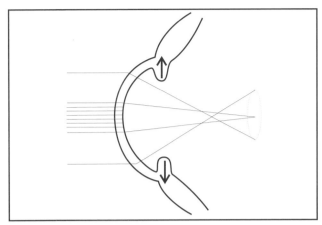

Figure 5-18b.
Light ray path creating glare when the pupil is large.

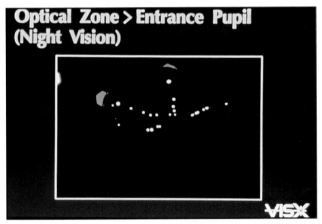

Figure 5-19a.
Demonstration of the amount of night glare perceived when PRK treatment zone exceeds size of entrance pupil. Note the minimal degree of night visual disturbances.

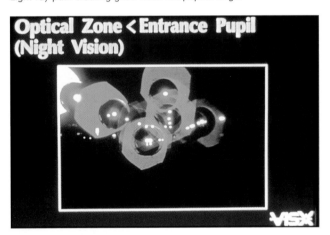

Figure 5-19b.
Demonstration of the amount of night glare when the entrance pupil size exceeds the PRK treatment area. Clinically significant night visual disturbances are produced with halo formation.

sion. These are the only mechanisms by which haze produces halos. There have been patients with absolutely clear corneas who have severe glare and patients with dense haze who have no glare (Figures 5-19a and 5-19b). The incidence of halos varies directly with optical zone size utilized.

Management: A 6-mm optical zone capability is manda-

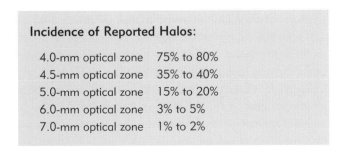

Incidence of Reported Halos:

4.0-mm optical zone	75% to 80%
4.5-mm optical zone	35% to 40%
5.0-mm optical zone	15% to 20%
6.0-mm optical zone	3% to 5%
7.0-mm optical zone	1% to 2%

tory. A multizone or aspheric technique should always be utilized to minimize depth of ablation and improve wound contour.

It is extremely disappointing to have a 20/20 patient dissatisfied because of severe night glare. Fortunately, most patients improve with time and with their fellow eye treatment. Retreatment for glare with a larger optical zone must be performed in patients who are also undercorrected to achieve a good result. A transepithelial approach to blend the old wound edge into the new surface contour is recommended. Treatment of any residual myopia is very helpful in itself and slightly overcorrected spectacles with anti-reflective coating can be prescribed. Night driving glasses should be discussed preoperatively, especially with high myopes and those considering monovision.

Figure 5-20.
Central island formation following VisX 20/20 Model B PRK treatment for -6.00 D with single zone technique. Best corrected visual acuity was reduced to 20/30 with monocular dyplopia and ghosting of images.

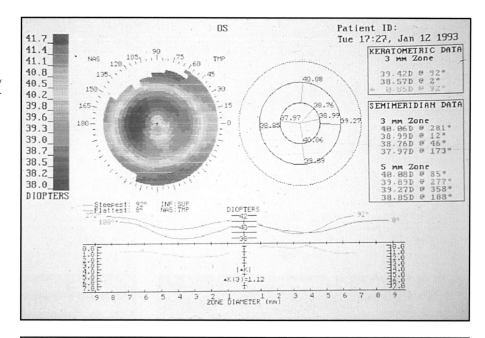

Figure 5-21.
Abnormal topography with peninsula formation following PRK retreatment.

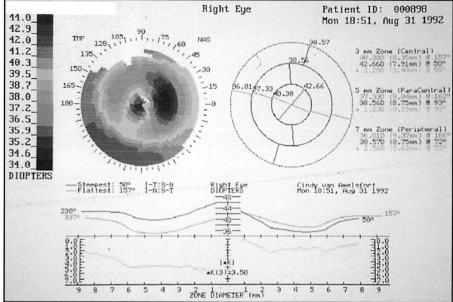

The definition of a central island is a central or pericentral steepening of:

- At least 1 to 3 D in height
- A diameter of at least 1 to 3 mm
- Measured at least 1 month postoperatively
- Associated with clinical symptoms of monocular diplopia, ghosting of images, or qualitative visual changes

ABNORMAL ABLATION PATTERNS
Central Islands

Clinical: Central islands are the most significant topographical abnormality observed both in incidence of diagnosis and clinical symptoms experienced by the patient. The problem of central islands was most notable with broad beam excimer lasers such as the VisX 20/20 Model B and VisX 20/15 (Taunton) lasers. Many theories have been advanced about central islands, including that they are a transient anomaly. The simple fact is that central islands are real, may persist indefinitely, and can create clinically sig-

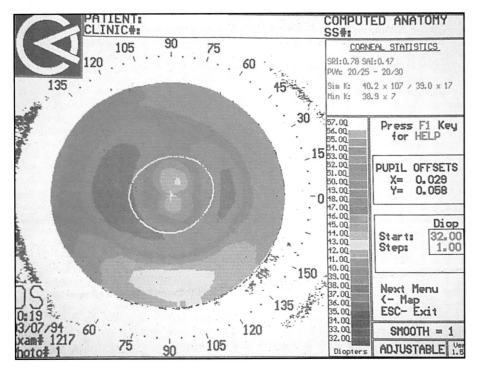

Figure 5-22.
Central island formation following PRK with Chiron Technolas Keracor 116 multizone ablation with inadequate pretreatment. Preoperative cylinder is evident within area of central undercorrection. Larger central island size corresponds to larger 7-mm treatment area.

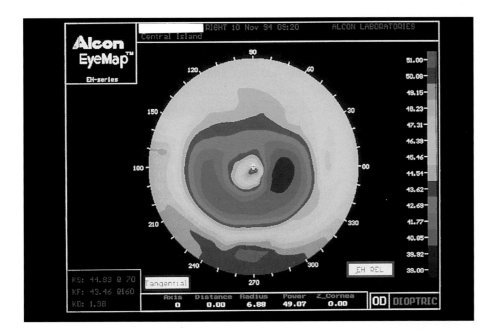

Figure 5-23.
Central island formation following PRK.

nificant visual disturbances (Figures 5-20 through 5-23). The incidence of central islands is as high as 80% at 1 week with broad beam laser delivery systems, but reduces to 15% by 3 months and less than 5% by 6 months. Newer software programs have further reduced the incidence and improved the rate of resolution of most central islands.

"Focal epithelial hyperplasia" was proposed as the cause

Factors increasing central islands include:
- Lasers with homogeneous or flat energy beam profiles
- Single zone techniques
- Large optical zones
- Moderate or severe degrees of myopia
- Moist corneas intraoperatively

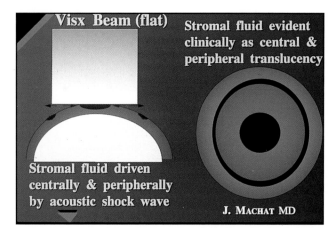

Figure 5-24.
Schematic diagram illustrating proposed mechanism for central island formation. Diagram demonstrates how energy beam profile producing characteristic acoustic shockwaves determines intraoperative hydration pattern creating central fluid accumulation. Increased central hydration corresponds with central undercorrection of topographical islands.

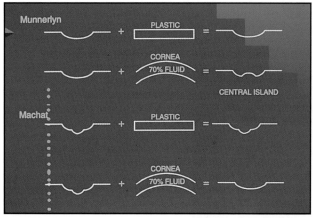

Figure 5-26.
Schematic diagram illustrating clinical importance of adjusting theoretical lenticular ablation patterns for hydrated corneal stroma in order to prevent central island formation. Classic Munnerlyn formula provides refractive correction on PMMA plastic but may create central islands under specific situations in patients. Machat modification increases central treatment beyond theoretical lenticular curve in order to compensate for hydrated corneal stroma.

There are four main theories as to the cause of central islands:

1. Focal central epithelial hyperplasia
2. Vortex plume theory
3. Degradation of laser optics
4. Acoustic Shockwave theory/Differential Hydration

Central island formation is likely multifactorial.

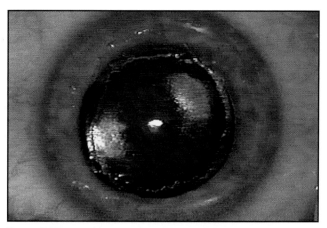

Figure 5-25.
Central translucency indicating increased hydration of central stroma during PRK photoablation. Central island formation related to differential hydration status of stroma intraoperatively.

of central islands based upon both suppositions and fact. The primary evidence in favor of the epithelium producing central islands were reports that epithelial debridement alone had improved patients with central islands and, even more importantly, focal epithelial hyperplasia was demonstrated in cases of central islands with confocal microscopy. The most significant difficulties with this theory are that it failed to explain why the epithelium would heal differently with different laser systems and larger ablation zones and why laser in situ keratomileusis (LASIK) would have an even higher incidence for central islands when the epithelium is undistorted.

The Vortex Plume Theory proposed that the emitted plume of ablative debris forms a random vortex, centrally blocking successive pulses. This theory was advanced by Stephen Klyce, PhD, based upon the observation that central islands were detected once nitrogen blow was discontinued in February 1992. However, central islands, although observed with the VisX, Taunton, and Technolas lasers, were essentially nonexistent with the Summit ExciMed UV 200 unit. The Summit ExciMed had no vacuum aspiration system and a pulse repetition rate twice that of the VisX, leaving half the time for plume dissipation which should have resulted in a higher incidence of central islands based upon the vortex plume theory.

Other investigators have proposed that degradation of the beam optics centrally would result in less ablative effect centrally. Central islands, however, have been observed with normal calibration test plastics and following replacement of optics, as well as on new laser systems. Central island effects can be demonstrated on calibration test plastics occasionally, especially with degraded optics. The central por-

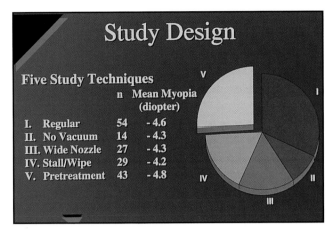

Figure 5-27.
Pie chart demonstrating the five study groups evaluating the mechanisms and possible treatments for central islands. Group I served as the control group with 54 eyes treated with a standard PRK no-blow technique and mechanical debridement. Group II consisted of 14 eyes treated without vacuum aspiration. Group III consisted of 27 eyes treated with a standard no-blow technique and a vacuum aspiration with a wider, less turbulent nozzle. Group IV consisted of 29 eyes treated with a stall and wipe technique by which multiple interruptions of the treatment were made and the accumulated central fluid wiped away with a blunt spatula. Group V evaluated 43 eyes that were pretreated in the central 2.5 mm with 1 micron/D. Mean preoperative myopia ranged from -4.20 to -4.80 D in the five study groups.

tion of the optic absorbs the greatest energy flow and therefore degrades centrally first.

My theory which seems to have gained acceptance is that based upon the Acoustic Shockwave model. Each pulse produces an acoustic shockwave, the pattern of which is related to the energy beam profile of the laser. Intraoperative stromal hydration patterns are determined by the acoustic shockwave pattern. The presence of physical shockwaves secondary to the recoil forces following plume ejection has been documented by Bor et al utilizing laser-based high-speed photography. Flat or homogeneous energy beam profiles produce central fluid accumulation intraoperatively, which result in reduced ablation centrally (Figures 5-24 and 5-25). Blowing nitrogen would reduce islands by drying this central fluid pocket. A more recent theory advanced by David Lin, and consistent with the Acoustic Shockwave theory, is the Differential Hydration model which relates central island formation to the naturally increased stromal hydration in the central anterior one third of the cornea. Scanning excimer lasers which produce minimal acoustic shockwaves do not develop central islands as predicted by the Differential Hydration model but not by the Acoustic Shockwave model. However, it appears clear that these two theories are centered around hydration as the key element in central island formation, and both likely play a role.

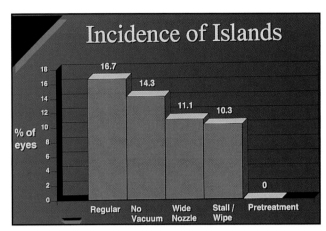

Figure 5-28.
Bar graph demonstrating the incidence of central islands at 3 months in the five study groups. The highest incidence was recorded in the control group with 16.7% manifesting central islands, and lowest incidence in the pretreatment group with a 0% incidence.

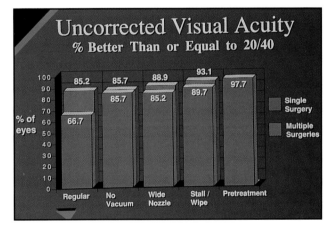

Figure 5-29.
Bar graph illustrating visual results before and after retreatment in the various study groups. Group I, serving as the control group, achieved 20/40 or better uncorrected vision in only 66.7% of eyes after one treatment, increasing to 85.2% with retreatment. This is sharply contrasted with the stall and wipe technique, where over 90% of eyes achieved 20/40 or better uncorrected visual acuity. The pretreated group was able to achieve even better results with about 98% achieving 20/40 or better after a single procedure. Group V patients also commented on the improved qualitative vision they achieved compared to fellow eyes when treated with other techniques.

Julian Stevens, MD, one of the most noted authorities on corneal-laser interaction, questioned whether the central fluid accumulation could be related to cell lysis, which occurs to a greater extent centrally with myopic PRK. The most significant difficulty with this model is that phototherapeutic keratectomy (PTK) at 6 mm will result in central island formation, despite the fact that the entire ablative area receives the same amount of laser exposure.

All lasers with a flat, hat-top type of energy beam profile produce central islands, but improved stability with little regression of effect. The Summit Eximed UV 200 laser has a gaussian energy beam profile with a higher energy density centrally, preventing central islands but resulting in a greater regression of effect. Therefore, the Summit ExciMed algorithm is set higher so that immediate postoperative hyperopia is greater than +2.00 D, more than double that of the other lasers (see Chapter 1). Although central islands were virtually unheard of with the Summit ExciMed series with 5-mm optical zone capability, users of the Summit OmniMed series with a more homogeneous beam profile and 6.5-mm capability have reported a number of cases, particularly with LASIK.

Management: First, it must be recognized that most central islands resolve spontaneously with time and do not require intervention, only patient reassurance and encouragement. Second, it is important to understand excimer ablation dynamics based upon the corneal stroma as a fluid model rather than a test plastic. Intraoperative stromal hydration, although it increases the incidence of central islands, improves patient fixation and reduces both corneal haze and irregular astigmatism. Therefore, techniques which leave the cornea moist are advocated; however, software modification must be made to apply additional pulses centrally to compensate for the accumulated moisture (Figure 5-26).

Central islands can be prevented by pretreating the stroma with additional pulses preoperatively after epithelial removal. A pretreatment of 1 micron per diopter in the central 2.5 mm has been calculated to be adequate to prevent islands with the VisX 20/20 in patients under -6.00 D. New VisX software 4.01 incorporates additional pulses centrally to counteract central island formation and improve qualitative vision.

Multizone treatment decreases the amount of pretreatment required for higher myopes—about 0.6 microns per diopter is adequate. The pretreatment required for the Technolas is greater than that for the VisX because of the beam profile and larger optical blend zone. The pretreatment is blended into the ablation with the full treatment. Patients are not overtreated because the pretreatment only removes tissue that should have been removed, that is, it removes tissue before the fluid builds.

In general, eyes tolerate a facet visually much better than a bump. Epithelium is incredibly forgiving. Excessive pretreatment of 2 microns per diopter with the VisX will result in a refractive effect, inducing hyperopia and possibly increasing haze.

Pretreatment is programmed in the VisX 20/20 Model B by inputting half the spherical correction at 2 to 2.5 mm—one can read the depth off the screen. That is, for a 6-mm -5.00 D correction, input a pretreatment of -3.00 D at 2.3 mm, which equals about 5 microns. With the elliptical program, an elliptical pretreatment: -3.00 -1.50 x 180 correction at 6 mm is pretreated with -1.50 -1.50 x 180 at 2.5 mm. VisX has introduced the central island factor (CIF) software to automatically introduce additional pulses beyond the theoretical lenticular curvature calculation in the 4.01 software.

Clinical Note

Central Islands and the Evolution of the Pretreatment Technique

When first developing the pretreatment technique in 1992, my theory developed from the observation that during VisX PRK treatment, increased translucency was observed centrally. This translucency represented an increased area of central hydration, which could be dried by wiping with a blunt spatula, sponged with a surgical spear, or allowed to evaporate naturally or with vacuum aspiration. The more rapid I became with mechanical epithelial debridement, the more moisture I observed. My first patient to develop a central island was a 29-year-old female patient from my general practice who was contact lens intolerant in her left eye. She was the first patient I had treated on a VisX 20/20 after performing about 100 Summit surface ablations myself and examining over 600 Summit-treated eyes. I had asked her to wait for a larger optical zone in light of her pupil size of 6.0 mm, as we were limited to 4.5- and 5.0-mm ablations with the Summit ExciMed UV 200. I was very surprised by the clinical appearance of the cornea during the VisX ablation as the stromal surface became quite gray and opaque, which was radically different from the diffusely translucent Summit stromal surface during ablation. I observed two other very different clinical features: first, that the patient had more difficulty fixating intraoperatively, and second, that the excellent acuity patients often exclaimed immediately upon completion of the Summit ExciMed ablation was absent. The patient, however, achieved a crisp 20/15 uncorrected visual acuity which has remained stable for over 3 years.

Her right eye was treated a few months later, as I became more proficient with the VisX 20/20 Model B laser and epithelial debridement. Intraoperatively, an area of central translucency was observed, which helped improve intraoperative fixation, but immediate postoperative vision was still quite blurry. Postoperatively, the patient complained of monocular diplopia, ghosting, and experienced a loss of best corrected vision of three lines from 20/15 to 20/30. Uncorrected vision was 20/40, with a refraction of -2.75 +1.50 x 80 which added only one additional line of Snellen vision. I observed my first central island on EyeSys videokeratography. After no clinical improvement in 6 months, I mechanically debrided the epithelium and attempted to retreat the patient with the cycloplegic refraction over 6.0 mm. The clinical outcome was +1.50 -1.00 x 170 with a peninsular island and no improvement in qualitative or quantitative vision. The patient has remained unchanged on videokeratography for 3 years with no resolution of the topographical abnormality or return of best corrected vision. The patient functions quite well because of the excellent acuity in her left eye (see Figures 5-20 and 5-21).

In retrospect, the central island retreatment should have ignored the refraction and performed a 3.0-mm ablation centrally for 6 microns as calculated from the videokeratography and Munnerlyn formula (see Chapter 6). The VisX 20/20 Model B would be programmed with approximately 50% of the original refraction at 2.5 to 3.0 mm. The thinking behind this approach was developed from the assumption that each pulse produces increased central hydration on the stromal surface and every other pulse removes fluid instead of stromal tissue. Therefore, 50% of the original refractive error should be targeted at an optical zone equivalent to that of the fluid accumulation, which is typically equal to that of the central island on videokeratography.

The excimer laser, when first introduced, utilized a small optical zone of 4.0 mm or less in an attempt to limit the depth of ablation. From L'Esperance's original patents it can be seen that he discussed removing only Bowman's layer within the procedure, 12 to 15 microns, which entails an optical zone of 3.0 mm in order to correct 4.00 or 5.00 D of myopia. Depth increases exponentially with the square of the diameter of the optical zone used; therefore, small optical zones were selected so as to maintain an extremely shallow ablation to hopefully prevent scar tissue or stromal haze formation within the visual axis. Unfortunately, spherical aberration produced severe night glare as the mid-peripheral and peripheral cornea were still myopic and refracted light rays myopically when the pupil was naturally dilated at night. Also, small optical zone treatments produced steep wound contours and incited haze formation rather than preventing it, especially when higher corrections were attempted. With a 4.0-mm optical zone, 75% of patients over -6.00 D developed severe night

glare and 15% to 20% developed severe stromal haze, reducing best corrected visual acuity.

As both Summit and VisX excimer laser systems moved toward larger optical zones, both night glare and corneal haze incidence were reduced substantially and treatments of higher degrees of myopia became more effective. There was also a movement toward a more physiologically hydrated cornea intraoperatively as Don Johnson, MD, and other Canadian investigators demonstrated improved VisX results without nitrogen blow. VisX altered their FDA protocol and technique to a no-blow technique. Nitrogen blow was a technique whereby gas was blown across the corneal surface to push the plume or ablative debris from the preceding pulse away and out of the pathway of the succeeding pulse. The early nitrogen blow technique studies demonstrated increased stromal haze, irregular astigmatism, early loss of best corrected visual acuity, and regression with slower visual rehabilitation. By 3 years postoperatively, Phase IIIa patients treated with nitrogen blow technique recovered their best corrected vision within one line, with 62% achieving a refraction within 0.50 D of emmetropia. The no-blow technique employed by Summit and other excimer laser systems was incorporated by VisX with more consistent results, however, central islands were observed with this change in technique.

In my first 100 VisX 20/20 Model B 6.0-mm single zone procedures, I observed 17 central islands, compared to none in the first 1000 Summit ExciMed 5.0-mm procedures I examined, treated by Joe Weinstock, MD, Fouad Tayfour, MD, and myself. The clinical difference in the intraoperative hydration pattern was the most dramatic to me. I began a clinical study to evaluate the parameters that differed between the Summit ExciMed and VisX 20/20 Model B laser, which could affect stromal hydration and central island formation.

The prevailing theory at the time was the Vortex Plume Theory proposed by Stephen Klyce, PhD, which stated that the photoablative plume created by each pulse created a random vortex which could block the central beam and result in central islands. The theory is supported by high speed photography which demonstrated the plume, and the fact that central islands were only observed following the discontinuation of nitrogen blow. My problem with the Vortex Plume Theory in 1992 was that the Summit ExciMed did not have a vacuum aspiration device and had double the pulse repetition rate of the VisX 20/20 Model B, which cut the time for plume dissipation between pulses in half. One would have expected an increased incidence of central islands, rather than a 0% incidence in 1000 Summit ExciMed cases using similar techniques. The intraoperative clinical differences in the hydration pattern produced by the two lasers struck me as the most likely etiology, as the size of central islands on videokeratography corresponded to the size of the intraoperative fluid accumulation. Following the control group, I began to experiment first with the vacuum aspiration device of the VisX system, both in respect to placement of the nozzle and intensity setting of the vacuum suction, which could alter the stromal hydration pattern.

The next parameter technique evaluated involved wiping the stromal surface with a blunt paton spatula, which was an attempt to keep the central fluid from accumulating and resulting in an undertreatment centrally. It was impossible to keep the central stroma dry with an even hydration status within the ablative field, as fluid accumulated too rapidly. That is, every pulse produced fluid and there were five pulses applied per second of treatment. The only solution was to program the application of additional pulses to the central 2.5-mm area, prior to or following the treatment. It was decided, based upon fundamental PRK principles, that additional central treatment should be applied prior to the full treatment, as the treatment would then blend in the central pretreatment. A handful of patients were first pretreated with 100% of the original refraction at 2.5 mm, followed by their full refraction at 6.0 mm, but this resulted in an overcorrection of +1.00 to +2.00 D in all these study eyes, although no central islands were observed. It was then surmised that 50% was a more realistic pretreatment amount since the accumulated central fluid does not block the entire central treatment, but approximately every other pulse. With a 50% pretreatment for patients up to -6.00 D single zone technique, no central islands were observed in 120 consecutive eyes (Figures 5-27 through 5-33).

The patient who most dramatically emphasizes the real importance of the pretreatment technique was treated one eye at a time for -6.00 D, 1 month apart. A standard 6.0-mm single zone technique was used for both eyes, but immediately following epithelial debridement of the second eye, I applied -3.00 D at 2.5 mm, 50% of the correction at the diameter I observed the fluid accumulation. This only amounted to an additional 6 microns beyond the 72-micron single zone VisX ablation profile. The patient spontaneously commented 1 week postoperatively that the "vision" in the recently pretreated eye was better than the first eye despite the fact that the patient was 20/20 uncorrected with +0.50 D in the first eye and only 20/30 uncor-

rected in the pretreated eye at the time. No central islands were apparent clinically in either eye on videokeratography. Although the patient was reading the Snellen chart better with his first eye, his qualitative vision was better in his pretreated eye, despite the absence of a central island in the first eye. Even 1 year postoperatively, when both eyes were measured at 20/20 and +0.25 D, the qualitative vision remained better subjectively in the pretreated eye, which continues to this day to surprise me. Typically, the non-pretreated eye "catches up" after 6 months or so. What this told me is that there is often a central undercorrection which may not reduce quantitative vision, but reduces the optical performance of the cornea.

Pretreatment improves qualitative vision in addition to reducing the incidence of central island formation. The issue of qualitative vision with respect to refractive surgery is often poorly examined. Daytime qualitative vision as discussed earlier in the book is reliant upon the quality of ablation in the central 3 mm, and night qualitative vision is derived from the outer 5 to 7 mm of treatment. Summit ExciMed patients treated with 4.5- and 5.0-mm optical zones often appeared clinically to have better qualitative vision than early VisX 20/20 Model B patients in well-illuminated environments, such as a sunny day outdoors. Under low levels of illumination, the small optical zone size of the ExciMed resulted in unacceptable night visual disturbances for many patients. Not only was the small optical zone responsible for preventing central islands, but so was the gaussian beam profile of the original Summit ExciMed laser. The higher energy density centrally of the ExciMed beam inhibited central island formation, in much the same way that the pretreatment technique did. The advantage of the pretreatment technique was that unlike the ExciMed beam, it was not associated with significant myopic regression requiring an initial hyperopic overshoot of 2.00 D or more; therefore, visual recovery was more rapid.

The analogy I developed for understanding intraoperative central fluid accumulation was that of the cornea acting more like a pool of water than a piece of polymethylmethacrylate plastic, which was reasonable in light of the fact that the cornea consists of 70% water. Based on clinical observation, the cornea appeared to become more hydrated centrally and peripherally, much like a what occurs when one drops a hoop or ring into a pool of water. The ripple effect pushes fluid both centrally and peripherally. The peripheral fluid would not interfere with ablation and is of no clinical concern, but the central fluid accumulation would result in central island formation. The cause of the ring pattern is based on the pattern of energy distribution of each pulse or energy beam profile which creates an acoustic shockwave. The larger the optical zone, the larger the ring dropped into the water, and the greater the central fluid accumulation and central island incidence. The acoustic shockwave is both audible with all broad beam lasers and visible with specialized photography demonstrating the ripple and recoil effects of the acoustic shockwave. The gaussian energy beam profile of the Summit ExciMed, greater energy centrally, acts more like a rock being tossed into the pool of water with all ripples going outward. No central islands are seen. However, if the beam becomes larger and flatter as it did with the Summit OmniMed series, one would predict the occurrence of central islands, which were reported. Similarly, applying that beam with LASIK at an optical zone of 6.0 mm or greater to the deeper stroma, which is more hydrated, results in a high incidence of central islands. Similarly, VisX users who utilized 10% to 20% ethyl alcohol to debride the epithelium did not encounter central islands, as the stroma became relatively dehydrated, altering the intraoperative hydration status of the cornea. Therefore, the pattern of energy distribution or energy beam profile of the laser system and optical zone best predict the formation of central islands. It is not the absolute energy difference in fluence between the Summit (180 mJ/cm^2) and VisX (160 mJ/cm^2) laser systems as my work was interpreted by Dr. Aron-Rosa, one of the well-known experts in the field of excimer laser surgery, but the difference in energy beam profiles (macrohomogeneity) which resulted in a higher incidence of central islands for the VisX compared to the Summit ExciMed.

The primary concern of VisX was that only 15% of patients develop central islands, and most resolve spontaneously over 6 months, reducing the incidence to 3% to 5% without treatment. Therefore, pretreatment would overtreat or unnecessarily treat 85% to 97% of patients. My view was that not only does the eye tolerate a facet better than a bump, but that pretreatment improves qualitative vision in all patients even in the absence of a central island, as demonstrated by the patient described earlier. Central islands may permanently reduce qualitative and quantitative visual function, and if nothing else, may delay full visual recovery for 6 to 12 months. Pretreatment compensates for the hydration status of the stroma and helps preserve best corrected vision and speed visual recovery.

The concept of pretreatment is independent of the timing of the additional pulses. The concept of pretreatment is the application of additional pulses to the central cornea, in addition to the pulses required to create a theoretical lenticular curve for any given dioptric correction as defined by Munnerlyn et al. That is, pretreatment is a modification of the Munnerlyn formula or a theoretical lenticular curve to compensate for the hydration status of the cornea.

Following my work on pretreatment, VisX then developed the CIF software which increased the amount of central treatment for all patients. Early versions of the software created hyperopic overcorrection and increased haze and did not eliminate central islands as evaluated by Lin and Machat in separate studies. Lin compared pretreatment, early VisX anti-island software and controls, and determined that pretreatment was most effective in reducing central islands without resulting in overcorrections. Improvements by VisX over the past 2 years have resulted in the anti-island 4.01 software, which has managed to produce a significant reduction in central islands without the hyperopic overcorrections of earlier versions.

The Chiron Technolas Keracor 116 laser incorporated my pretreatment technique to counteract central island formation. When first developed and used in Europe, no central islands were identified in the first 1000 procedures because of the use of 20% to 25% alcohol to debride the epithelium. Upon discontinuation of alcohol and a shift toward manual debridement, central islands were encountered. I had anticipated the development of central islands because of the homogeneous (flat) energy beam profile of the laser system. The larger 7.0-mm optical zone and specific beam profile required a larger pretreatment of over 1 micron per diopter at a 3.0-mm optical zone. The incidence of central island formation varies from 0% to 35%, depending upon the technique and excimer laser system utilized. The use of small optical zones less than or equal to 5.0 mm, multizone techniques, alcohol epithelial debridement, gas blow techniques, gaussian beam profile lasers, and scanning laser systems all reduce central island formation.

The move toward scanning delivery systems, which are associated with minimal acoustic shockwave effect, as evidenced by the quietness of the scanning procedures, has resulted in virtually no central islands. David Lin's Differential Hydration model which states that central islands are a result of the natural distribution of water in the cornea, being greater both centrally and within the deeper layers, explains many of the facts known about central islands and their occurrence. However, the model as I understand it does not predict that scanning lasers should be exempt from central islands, as the increased central

Figure 5-30a.
A 48-year-old female patient treated with PRK for -13.50 D. Developed 5.00 D central island postoperatively. Videokeratographies Figure 5-30a through Figure 5-30d demonstrate gradual resolution over 9 months. No treatment as patient continued to improve.

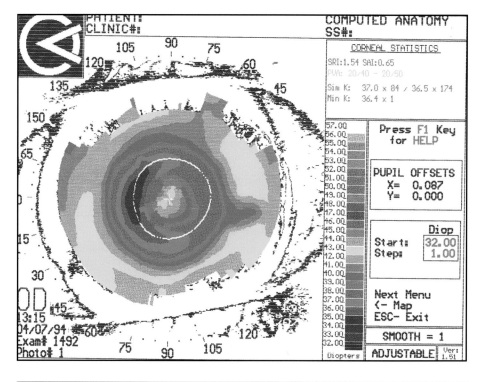

Figure 5-30b.
Demonstration of gradual resolution over 9 months. No treatment as patient continued to improve.

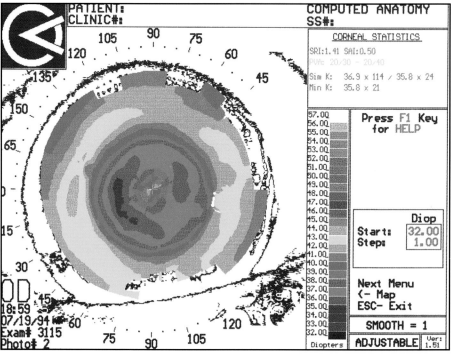

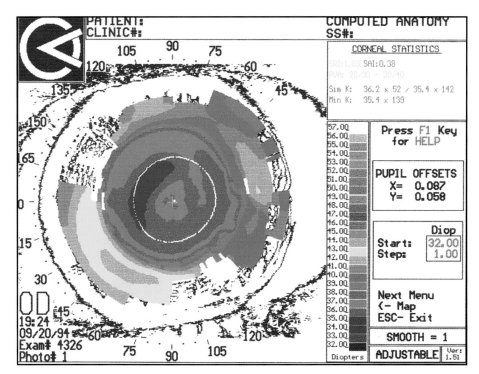

Figure 5-30c.
Demonstration of gradual resolution over 9 months. No treatment as patient continued to improve.

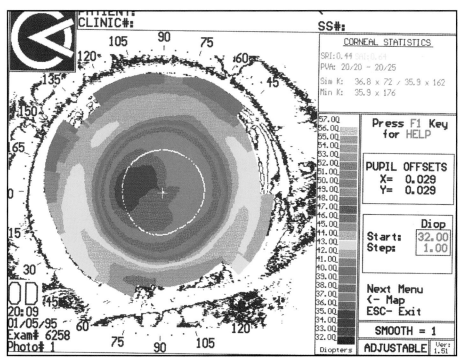

Figure 5-30d.
Demonstration of gradual resolution over 9 months. No treatment as patient continued to improve.

Figure 5-31.
Videokeratography demonstrating small 1 to 2 D central island. Clinically asymptomatic with 20/20-2 uncorrected visual acuity. No treatment as clinically insignificant.

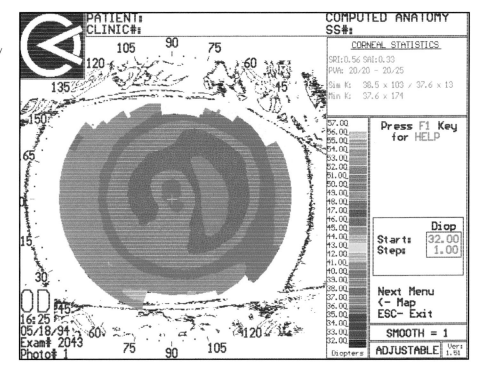

Figure 5-32a.
Central Island with toric ablation. Preoperatively: -15.75 +6.00 x 90. Postoperatively: -1.25 +0.50 x 175. Gradual resolution over 3 months. No treatment.

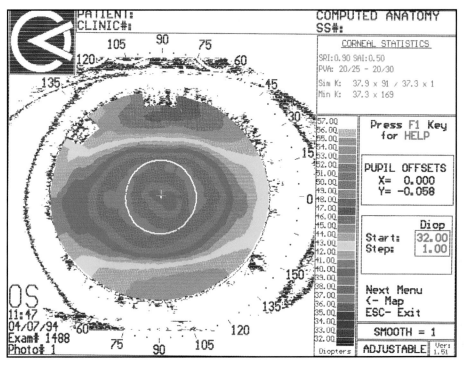

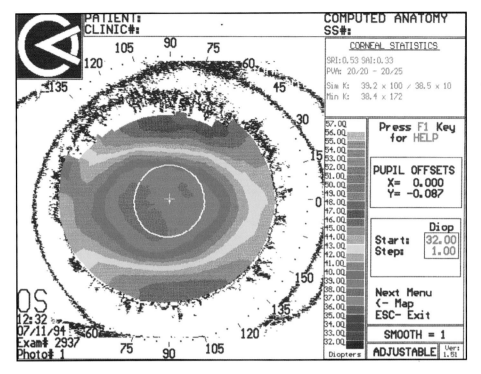

Figure 5-32b.
Central island with toric ablation. Preoperatively: -15.75 +6.00 x 90. Postoperatively: -1.25 +0.50 x 175. Gradual resolution over 3 months. No treatment.

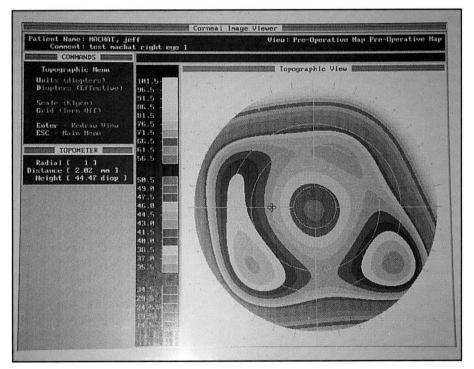

Figure 5-33.
PAR topographical or true elevation map with clinical appearance of central island. This map is actually that of the author's right eye which has never been treated with refractive surgery. Not all central islands represent topographical abnormalities, are clinically significant, or require treatment.

Figure 5-34.
Difference map illustrating ablation pattern achieved. Postoperative semi-circular topographic pattern (A). Preoperative with-the-rule cylinder (B). Difference map explains that semi-circular videokeratography pattern related to large central island formation. Ideal difference map would be solid blue circular pattern.

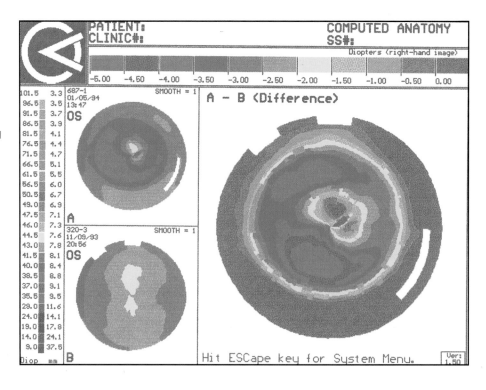

Figure 5-35.
Semi-circular ablation pattern with peninsula/central island continuum evident.

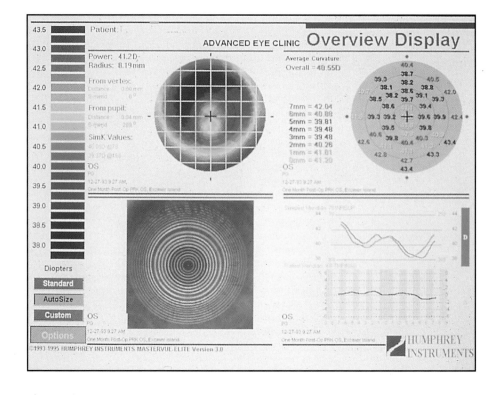

hydration should still block full treatment and result in a central undercorrection. The Acoustic Shockwave model, however, correctly predicts that scanning delivery systems which do not produce appreciable acoustic shockwaves should not produce central islands. It remains that multiple factors play a role in central island formation, but that stromal hydration is central to their etiology and that both the Acoustic Shockwave model and Differential Hydration model best explain the importance of hydration.

Although central islands only occur in 15% of VisX 20/20 Model B cases at 3 months, all eyes can be safely pretreated. Qualitative visual improvement is seen in fellow eyes of patients who achieved 20/20 OU that were only pretreated in their second eye.

Transepithelial approach with the VisX 20/20 laser requires pretreatment as well, since PTK induces islands. A pretreatment of 5 to 6 microns for epithelium (55 microns), 1 micron for every 10 microns of PTK, is necessary. Transepithelial ablation with the Technolas requires about 10 microns of pretreatment at 3 mm. The pretreatment can be performed on the surface of the epithelium prior to PTK or just prior to the PRK on the epithelial plug. The VisX transepithelial program incorporates the CIF software and, if installed, will not require additional pretreatment.

In order to treat an island, a study of the preoperative attempted correction and the topographical map must be made. One can calculate the height and diameter of the island from the map using the Munnerlyn formula.

An island is usually treated with 50% of the preoperative refraction over a 2- to 3-mm area. Typically a -5.00 D 6-mm treatment will result in a 5-micron 2.5-mm island. A transepithelial PTK approach or mechanical debridement are both recommended to remove epithelium, followed by a PRK treatment of the island. The same nomogram is used as for pretreatment (see Chapter 6). An additional 2 microns can be input. Therefore, this patient can be treated with -3.00 D correction at 2.5 or 2.6 mm in diameter, with an ablation depth of 6 to 7 microns (see below).

Semicircular Patterns

Clinical: Various topographical abnormalities (Figures 5-34 and 5-35) have been described following excimer ablation. Lin et al identified four topographical patterns:
1. A uniform circular ablation 44% to 45%
2. A central island of steepened cornea within the ablative

$$\text{Ablation depth} = \frac{\text{optical zone}^2 \times \text{refractive change}}{3}$$

$$\text{Ablation depth} = \frac{(2.5 \text{ mm})^2 \times 3.00 \text{ D}}{3}$$

$$\text{Ablation depth} = 6.25 \text{ microns}$$

zone 10% to 26%
3. A keyhole ablative pattern 12%
4. A semi-circular ablative pattern 18% to 33%

Management: No treatment unless symptomatic. Treatment is tailored to patient based upon refraction and topography once stable.

Clinical Note
Semi-Circular Ablation Pattern

A 38-year-old female patient (Figures 5-36a through 5-36c) who had a 25-year history of gas permeable lens wear underwent PRK after a 6-week discontinuation of contact lens use and apparent stabilization of videokeratography and refraction at -6.00 +1.75 x 85. Postoperatively, the patient developed an asymmetric superior semi-circular ablation pattern with residual myopic astigmatism. Cycloplegic refraction was -2.75 +1.25 x 85 with a better than anticipated uncorrected vision of 20/70- but a reduced best corrected vision of 20/30. The better than expected uncorrected visual acuity had been suggestive of a central island component. The patient was retreated after 6 months for the full refractive error measured over 6.0 mm with manual epithelial debridement, without any specific attempt to restore topography, resulting in mixed astigmatism with a semi-circular ablation pattern. In retrospect, a transepithelial approach should have been performed (see Chapter 6). A third procedure was performed to help correct the residual mixed astigmatism and help restore topography. The procedure performed was incisional, with an inferior AK arc placed to reduce cylinder and flatten the cornea locally. This was successful with 20/25 uncorrected visual acuity and improved videokeratography. The fellow eye -7.75 +1.25 x 90 was treated 2 years later with LASIK achieving +0.25 D sphere, 20/30 uncorrected vision, equivalent to preoperative best corrected vision.

Figure 5-36a.
Semi-circular ablation pattern observed following PRK.

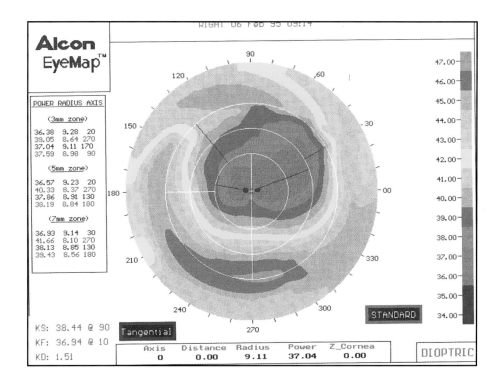

Figure 5-36b.
Semi-circular ablation pattern following PRK retreatment for myopia and astigmatism without addressing topographical abnormality with transepithelial approach.

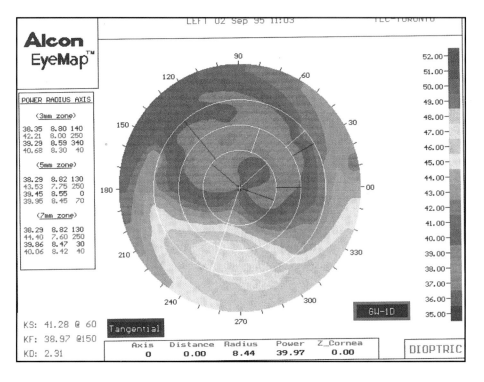

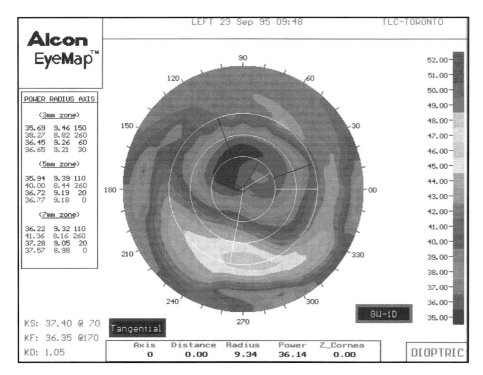

Figure 5-36c.
Semi-circular ablation pattern treated with inferior AK to flatten cornea locally.

Keyhole Patterns

Clinical: Both the keyhole patterns and the semi-circular patterns demonstrate inadequate inferior ablations predominantly. Visual acuity was still excellent with best corrected visual acuity often maintained (Lin). The most significant topographical abnormality observed with respect to patient symptoms was the central island (Figures 5-37 and 5-38).

Management: No treatment unless symptomatic. Treatment is tailored to patient based upon refraction and topography once stable. If an "island" component is evident, treatment is the same as for central islands.

MISCELLANEOUS COMPLICATIONS

DECOMPENSATED PHORIA (DIPLOPIA)

Clinical: As has been reported following RK, the dissociation of the two eyes and loss of fusion which occurs following unilateral treatment can result in manifestation of a previously compensated for phoria with binocular diplopia.

Management: Ocular motility testing is prudent preoperatively to uncover such tendencies.

ANISOCORIA

Clinical: Occasionally, a patient develops a dilated but reactive pupil postoperatively. No IOP rise or trauma associated. Etiology unknown. Mild glare symptoms.

Management: No specific therapy.

CORNEAL GRAFT REJECTION FOLLOWING PTK

Clinical: There have been reports of PTK inducing corneal transplant rejection. In general, the excimer laser does not produce predictable results with grafts, and regression of effect appears to be the rule.

Management: Same as for PKP rejection of other etiology.

PERSISTENT OCULAR TENDERNESS

Clinical: A small percentage of patients complain about ocular tenderness and sensitivity upon rubbing their eyes. Ocular tenderness appeared postoperatively and was more common in patients who were patched, but also did occur after therapeutic contact lens use. It was unrelated to degree of correction or postoperative pain level. It persists for months, if not indefinitely. It can occur in one eye in patients treated bilaterally. It is likely related to aberrant corneal nerve regeneration.

Management: Reassurance and lubrication with artificial tears.

Figure 5-37.
Videokeratography demonstrating large central island extending to periphery, forming classic peninsula pattern. Myopic refraction and loss of two lines of best corrected vision acuity.

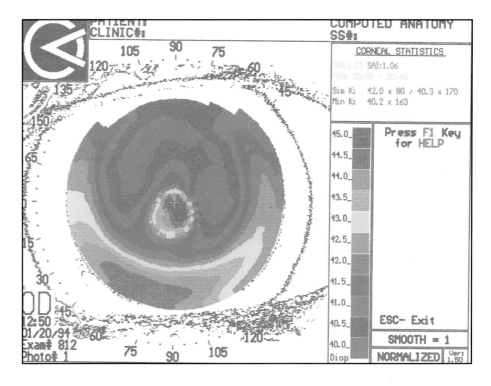

Figure 5-38.
Keyhole or peninsula pattern observed on videokeratography. Over 2.00 D of oblique cylinder evident on topography and clinically. Best corrected vision reduced three lines acuity to 20/40.

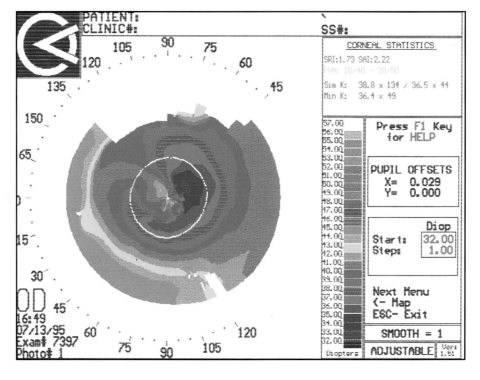

CHAPTER 6

PRK Retreatment Techniques and Results

INDICATIONS FOR PRK RETREATMENT

There are four indications for retreatment:
1. Undercorrections/regression
2. Haze/collagen plaque
3. Corneal topographical abnormalities
4. Decentered treatment zone

PRINCIPLES AND TECHNIQUE

The technique varies with the indication for retreatment and differs both in regard to the principles maintained and the purpose for each. Once a patient has had surgery, PRK or RK, the cornea behaves differently. The epithelial adherence is altered and the epithelium may be thicker than normal (60 to 80 microns vs. 50 to 55 microns). The surface also appears to be more sensitized to additional procedures, and so caution must be taken to avoid inducing increased haze. Lastly, corneal topography has been altered and must be accounted for whenever a retreatment is considered.

In general, uncorrected visual acuity should always be reduced to less than or equal to 20/40 prior to considering a retreatment. Exceptions to this basic rule are certain topographical abnormalities, in which qualitative visual reduction is the chief complaint. If the principles are maintained,

there appears to be no defined upper limit to the number of surgeries which can be performed within reason and without imposing undue risk to the patient.

Basic Principles of Retreatment
- Be conservative. Avoid hyperopia (you can always go back).
- Always leave trace haze, not a clear cornea, when retreating for haze.
- Mixed astigmatism is better treated with astigmatic keratotomy, not PARK.
- Account for central island formation induced by PTK with transepithelial approach.
- Topography plays a much more vital role.
- Maintain contour. Leave no sharp edges. Blend, blend, blend.

Clinical Note

One patient underwent five treatments over 2 years, the primary procedure with the Summit followed by four retreatments for regression and haze. The fifth treatment was performed with the Technolas. The patient remains at 20/20/+0.50 D/trace haze/no glare 2 years following the fifth procedure. Some of these principles have been learned the hard way.

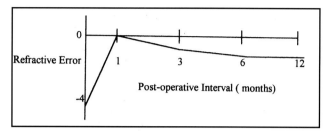

Figure 6-1.
Graphic of undercorrection, demonstrating inadequate initial surgery.

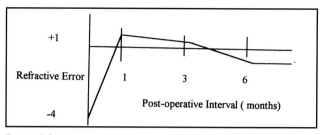

Figure 6-2.
Graphic of regression, demonstrating adequate initial surgery with greater than anticipated myopic shift usually following withdrawal of topical steroids.

WHEN TO RETREAT?

Investigators state that retreatment must be performed after 6 months. In actual fact, stability of refraction and topography can vary from 3 months to at least 18 months. My definition of stability is based upon two refractions performed 1 month apart that are within 0.25 D with no significant alteration in the accompanying topographical map.

Retreatment Results

- Usually safe
- Usually effective
- Usually no increased risk of haze with proper technique
- Restores topography
- Improves uncorrected and best corrected vision
- Reduces glare
- Reduces distortion
- Allows for near perfect results

RETREATMENT OF MYOPIC OR ASTIGMATIC REGRESSION AND UNDERCORRECTIONS

The difference between an undercorrection and regression is subtle. In an undercorrection, the amount of surgery performed was inadequate, and very early in the postoperative course—usually even by 1 month—the undercorrection becomes apparent (Figure 6-1). The cornea has clinically insignificant haze. This response is more common in young patients. Often, the cornea was very moist intraoperatively.

In myopic regression, the patient usually appears stable

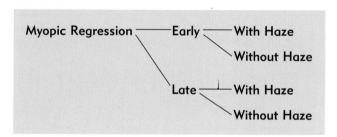

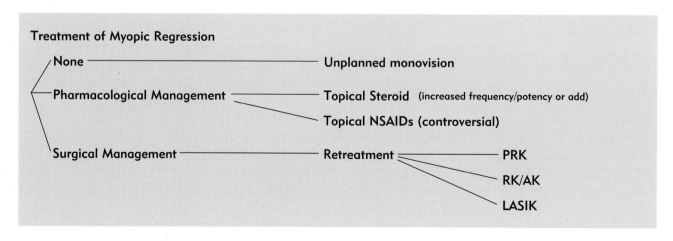

but then becomes myopic at a later point in time, often following the withdrawal of steroids (Figure 6-2). The cornea may or may not have clinically significant haze; however, severe haze is always associated with myopic regression. The normal regression pattern is followed initially, but then continues with a steeper curve and fails to plateau. Regression is more common with single zone techniques, smaller optical zones, and gaussian energy beam profile lasers. A dry cornea, such as that produced by blowing nitrogen in the preliminary VisX Phase IIIa FDA trials, is likely not only to induce more haze and irregular astigmatism, but may also induce regression.

What constitutes an undercorrection varies with the

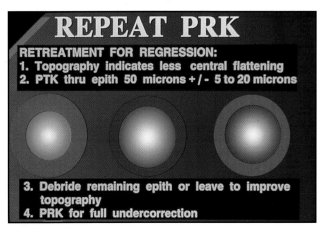

Figure 6-3.
Schematic diagram of PRK retreatment for myopic regression. Diagram on left illustrates preoperative topographical map with inadequate central flattening and small effective optical zone. Central diagram illustrates green pseudofluorescence observed intraoperatively with transepithelial approach. In standard PRK retreatment without haze, epithelium can also be mechanically debrided. Diagram on right illustrates postoperative topographical map with improved central flattening and larger effective optical zone.

Etiology of Undercorrections
- Wound healing/patient variability
- Intraoperative stromal hydration
- Laser calibration/programming

Advantages of Transepithelial Approach
- Reduces haze
- Eliminates epithelial adherence problems
- Helps correct topographical abnormalities

---

patient and surgeon. Most patients feel that -1.00 D is unacceptable, unless their fellow eye compensates, or if they are over 40 and enjoy reading. Some patients find -0.50 D difficult to cope with, especially for night driving. Education, reassurance, and explanation of the pros and cons of being minimally undercorrected becomes crucial.

RETREATMENT TECHNIQUE FOR UNDERCORRECTIONS/REGRESSION (WITHOUT HAZE)

The transepithelial approach in general is recommended for retreatments if haze is evident, if there is abnormal topography, or by surgeon preference. If the cornea is clear, mechanical debridement can be utilized safely and effectively. For the transepithelial approach, turn room lights down. Reduce intensity of microscope illumination once the patient is positioned and aligned. A moistened surgical spear to gently smooth the tear film can be used if the tear film is patchy. A central island pretreatment should always be performed with the VisX (if no CIF software) and Technolas PTK or transepithelial programs. An additional 1 to 2

microns of pretreatment is recommended for every 10 microns of PTK. The pretreatment can be performed on the surface of the epithelium prior to epithelial removal or following epithelial removal.

The laser should be set to a maximal optical zone and the patient warned of the startling noise. Perform one to two pulses to train the patient and observe the green pseudofluorescence pattern for abnormalities, as these will be transmitted through to the stroma.

Once the patient is comfortable with the snapping sound, 50 microns or 200 pulses are usually required to ablate through the epithelium. The endpoint is best observed with the microscope light completely off. The stroma will appear black in contrast to the fluorescence of the epithelium. The preoperative appearance of the topography is important in defining the endpoint and improving postoperative topography.

If the topography demonstrates a circular homogeneous flat (blue) ablation pattern (Figures 6-3 and 6-4), the fluorescence usually clears peripherally first. The remaining epithelium may clear roughly simultaneously, or more commonly with a thicker epithelial plug, often 60 to 80 microns centrally. It is best to do an extra 10 microns, but do not try to eliminate the central plug completely. Stopping after a 1-mm ring of black stroma develops along the edge of the ablation is the desired endpoint. Some investigators have tried to remove the plug with a blunt spatula. Lastly, a PRK protocol of 10 to 15 microns can be set for thicker plugs.

Figure 6-4.
Well-centered postoperative videokeratography of myopic regression without haze following PRK. Diameter of optical zone decreases and mean keratometry increases. Preoperative refraction -8.00 D. At 4 months, patient was plano with 20/20 uncorrected visual acuity. At 8 months, patient regressed to -1.50 D with 20/80 uncorrected vision requiring enhancement. Stromal blackness usually appears peripherally first. After additional ablation, the endpoint is reached where epithelium remains over the flattest topographical areas. At this point the residual refractive error is treated with the PRK mode. Epithelium is used as a natural blocking agent, protecting the flattest areas on topography, thereby helping to improve the ablation pattern.

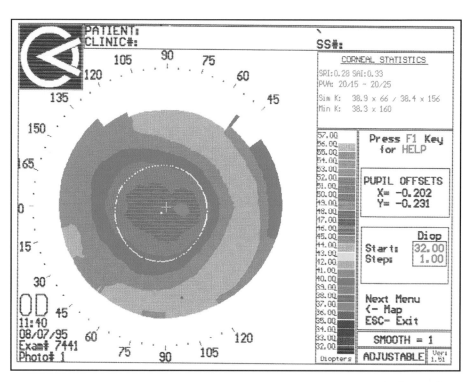

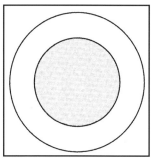

Figure 6-5.
Schematic illustration of transepithelial technique. During initial ablation of epithelium, the entire 6-mm treatment zone will exhibit a green pseudofluorescence when the microscope and room lights are dimmed.

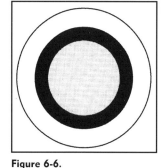

Figure 6-6.
Schematic illustration of endpoint for transepithelial technique in eyes without prior refractive surgery or with normal postoperative ablation patterns. With homogeneous energy beam profile lasers, the peripheral epithelium will be ablated first and the stroma will appear black when encountered. PTK of the epithelium should be stopped when a 1-mm ring of stromal blackness is observed.

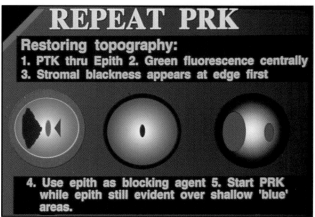

Figure 6-7.
Schematic illustration of PRK technique for improving corneal topography following PRK or other refractive surgery. Diagram on left is a clinical example of an abnormal topography with a small central island and two asymmetrical areas of pronounced flattening. The central and right diagrams illustrate the expected pseudofluorescence pattern when the epithelium is ablated. In the central diagram, stromal blackness appears centrally first, as the epithelium is thinnest over the steepest topographical area.

The risk, of course, is hyperopic overcorrection; thus, it is best to be conservative. The cause of these undercorrections is clearly epithelial hyperplasia, which can improve spontaneously over 6 to 12 months with epithelial thinning. Therefore, the endpoint should be a small epithelial plug 4 to 5 mm in diameter (1 to 2 mm smaller than the transep-ithelial optical zone) (Figures 6-5 and 6-6).

If the topographical map demonstrates shallow (deep blue) and elevated (red) areas within the ablative zone (Figure 6-7), it should be understood that the epithelium is often thicker over the shallow areas and thinner over the elevated areas. As one ablates through the epithelium and

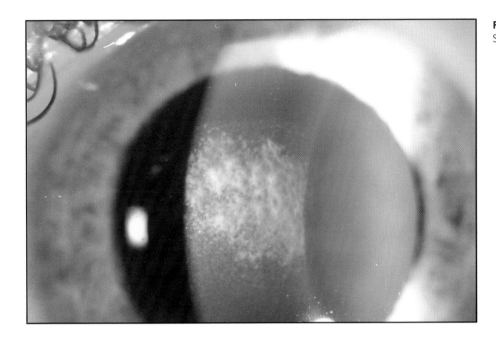

Figure 6-8.
Subepithelial collagen plaque.

nears the endpoint, the epithelium often clears first, both peripherally and over the elevated regions. The shallow areas often retain fluorescence later. The endpoint is once the stroma is black in all regions except where the topography appears to have shallow, darker blue areas. The epithelium will act as a blocking agent and help smooth the postoperative topography, flattening the steeper areas and steepening the shallower areas.

Start the PRK procedure once the endpoint is reached. If the epithelium is mechanically debrided, the retreatment procedure is similar to the primary PRK procedure. The epithelial adherence is usually loose with VisX, Technolas, and other lasers that produce a smooth ablative surface. The original Summit ExciMed often had a very adherent epithelium observed upon mechanical debridement for retreatment. In general, the amount of undercorrection targeted should be less than that measured and in keeping with the uncorrected vision. That is, it is not uncommon to measure a -2.00 D and have a patient read 20/60 uncorrected. The target in this example should be only -1.25 D in keeping with the uncorrected vision.

Undercorrected cylinder should only be corrected if associated with myopia. Hyperopic astigmatism may result when attempting residual astigmatism correction with the VisX sequential program. The VisX elliptical program is preferred, but an equal amount of myopia and cylinder must be present. The Technolas and scanning lasers, such as the Nidek EC-5000 and the Aesculap-Meditec MEL 60, are able to treat a plano-cylindrical correction. In general, astigmatic

keratotomy is preferable if mixed astigmatism alone is present (eg, +0.50 -2.00 x 180).

RETREATMENT OF HAZE AND COLLAGEN PLAQUE FORMATION

A transepithelial approach is almost mandatory in cases of clinically significant haze and regression. If dense haze is evident, a retreatment is invariably necessary. Although the natural history of haze is gradual resolution, this process can take years. With proper technique, significant haze will not return in 80% of cases and a good visual result can still be achieved. That is, collagen plaques are treatable.

Collagen plaques, if diffuse, induce corneal steepening and myopia. Collagen plaques are subepithelial (Figure 6-8); asymmetric plaques can induce abnormal topography. Night glare can also be induced from a reduced effective optical zone and the induced myopia.

There are a few critical differences in treating regression with haze compared with regression without haze described above. The primary objective is different in that the surgery is performed with the understanding that "the surgeon did the correct amount of surgery, the patient just healed wrong." Therefore, if one could clear the haze, or transform it from clinically significant to clinically insignificant haze, the patient would be 20/20 with a plano refraction theoretically (Figures 6-9a through 6-10b). In other words, there is really no necessity to treat the associated myopia.

Figure 6-9a.
Dense central collagen plaque prior to retreatment.

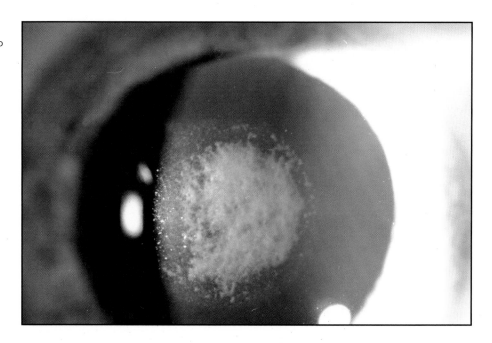

Figure 6-9b.
Immediate postoperative view demonstrating excellent corneal clarity following retreatment for haze.

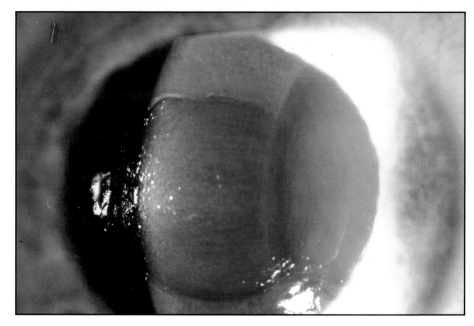

RETREATMENT TECHNIQUE FOR HAZE AND COLLAGEN PLAQUE FORMATION

The epithelium is ablated with a PTK approach with all laser systems (Figure 6-11). The endpoint is a mottled "stromal" or "haze" surface, as this represents bits of epithelium within the surface of the plaque. The optical zone should be maximal (Figures 6-12a through 6-12c), at least as large as the primary procedure. The epithelium should ablate in 200 pulses or 50 microns. Collagen plaques are typically 20 to 40 microns in thickness (mean: 30 microns). PTK is recom-

mended for gaussian beam profile and PRK for homogeneous (flat) beam profile systems once the mottled surface is reached. An additional 60 to 80 pulses, or 15 to 20 microns, of PTK can be performed. It is the number of microns depth, not the dioptric correction, that is important in clearing the haze (Figures 6-13a and 6-13b).

The patient should then be taken to the slit lamp and examined. A trace amount of residual haze is ideal (Figures 6-14a through 6-14c). A clear cornea might make the surgeon happy, but it may leave the patient hyperopic (Figures

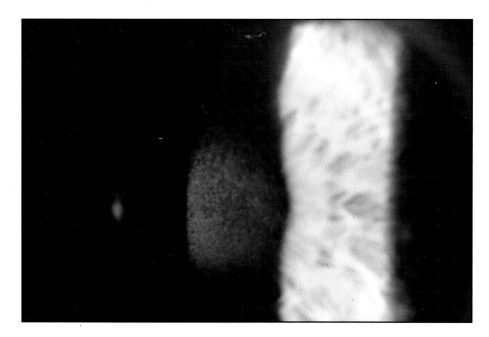

Figure 6-10a.
Clinically significant (3+) confluent haze following PRK.

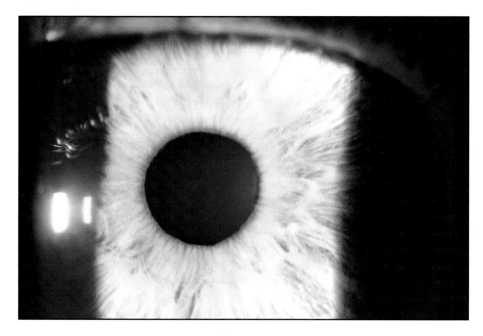

Figure 6-10b.
Postoperative view of Figure 6-10a 6 months following retreatment, demonstrating restoration and preservation of corneal clarity.

6-15a through 6-15c), which would necessitate topical steroid withdrawal and increased haze postoperatively. If excessive haze is still evident, the patient should be taken back to the laser and an additional 5 to 15 microns ablated. The patient should be re-examined after each treatment to avoid overtreatment. This titration method of haze removal with blending is vital to achieve optimal results.

A PRK approach can be performed following the ablation of the epithelium. The only important distinction is that the associated myopia should not be fully treated (about 50% to 60%) and the depth of ablation carefully monitored. This approach is often more suitable for lasers with flat energy beam profiles (Figure 6-16) because PTK induces central islands and a PRK approach treats the central area of the collagen plaque more. A central island pretreatment should always be performed with the VisX and Technolas PTK programs (Figures 6-17a through 6-19b). Once again, the principle is to titrate the treatment to avoid overcorrections, with an emphasis placed on number of microns ablated rather than diopters corrected. That is, treat the patient,

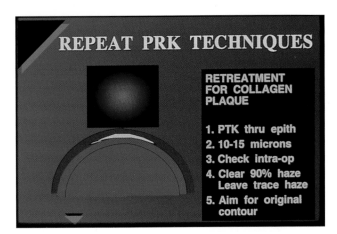

Figure 6-11.
Schematic diagram illustrating subepithelial position of collagen plaque and removal technique. Concept of retreatment is based upon re-establishing original contour following initial PRK treatment. Ablation of plaque should convert haze from clinically significant to clinically insignificant grade with trace haze being optimal. Until clinical experience is gained patient should be taken frequently to slit lamp for titration of treatment recognizing that confluent haze typically varies from 20 to 40 microns in thickness.

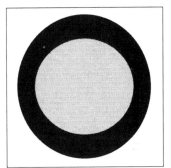

Figure 6-12a. Schematic illustration of PRK retreatment for confluent haze. Transepithelial approach recommended with green pseudofluorescence evident during laser ablation of epithelium. Room and microscope lights must be dim or off.

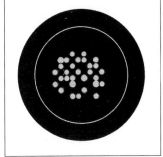

Figure 6-12b. Mottled green and black clinical endpoint representing epithelial nests within honeycomb surface of collagen plaque. Once clinical endpoint is achieved PRK or PTK mode may be used to remove collagen plaque. Typically, 60% of refractive error can be programmed with PRK mode carefully noting micron depth.

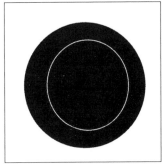

Figure 6-12c. Once collagen plaque is removed, diffuse stromal blackness should be observed. Endpoint of procedure is trace clinical haze which is only discernible at slit lamp examination.

not the numbers. Another manual approach recommended by some investigators: following manual epithelial debridement, the edge of the collagen plaque can occasionally be pulled back as a single sheet, leaving a relatively smooth ablative surface. A few pulses of PTK to polish the surface is then recommended. This method has been effective in select cases, but the majority cannot be treated in this manner. Also, manipulation of the plaque and ablative surface often results in recurrent haze postoperatively.

Asymmetric Haze

Asymmetric haze must be treated on a case-by-case basis. Semi-circular, arcuate, and symmetrically crescentic areas of haze are well-recognized patterns observed. The semi-circular and arcuate patterns are related to sharp wound edges, whereas the symmetric crescents are most commonly related to the VisX sequential cylindrical troughs formed. No procedure should be undertaken if uncorrected vision is not affected, despite clinical appearance. That is, what often bothers the surgeon does not bother the patient (Figures 6-20a and 6-20b). A transepithelial approach is still recommended with asymmetric haze; however, a manual debridement approach has been advocated by some investigators. When asymmetric haze is present, laser ablation of the epithelium becomes as much a challenge of restoring topography as haze reduction. The epithelium is often thinner over the area of haze, therefore, the epithelium acts as a partial blocking agent. Once the mottled surface of the asymmetric haze becomes apparent, care should be taken to protect the remaining stroma with methylcellulose, Healon, or artificial tears. A blocking agent should always be smoothed over the surface, as for any PRK procedure, to allow for selective ablation of the collagen plaque. Once the haze is reduced adequately, the entire surface should be blended with a fraction of the associated correction using a PRK approach. The objective once again is not to obtain a clear cornea, but to debulk the collagen plaque, eliminate the associated refractive error, and restore topography. A topographical mapping system is critical for surgical planning in these cases.

A manual approach to asymmetric haze involves removing epithelium only over the area of haze, followed by wide area therapeutic (PTK) or refractive (PRK) ablation using the remaining epithelium as a 50-micron thick blocking agent. For the PRK approach, either the current refraction or a portion of the preoperative refraction is advocated.

Induced astigmatism does not need to be treated often in these complex cases, since it is the abnormal topography

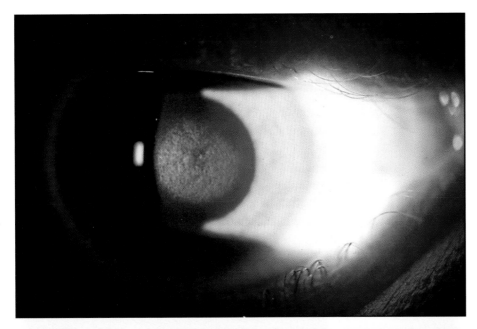

Figure 6-13a.
Central dense confluent haze following Summit ExciMed UV 200 PRK for -7.00 D. Patient was treated with 5.0-mm ablation zone for identical corrections in both eyes. Fellow eye achieved 20/20 uncorrected vision following 4-month topical steroid tapering regimen. Clinically significant haze developed following cessation of steroids at 6 weeks by patient.

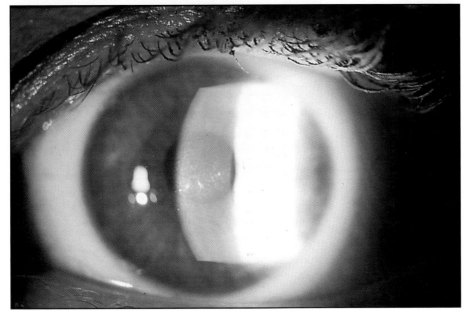

Figure 6-13b.
Mild reticular haze, clinically insignificant, at 3-month examination following retreatment for haze. Examination 2 years following retreatment demonstrated 20/20 uncorrected vision OU with +0.50 D refractive error in the retreated eye and barely perceptible trace corneal haze.

which induces the cylinder. Therefore, by eliminating the topographical abnormality with spherical PRK or a PTK approach, the cylinder is often simultaneously eliminated.

Post RK Retreatment

PRK following RK reduces residual myopia and astigmatism, reduces night glare through improved topography (Figures 6-21a through 6-22b), and may reduce diurnal fluctuation in some patients through epithelial hyperplasia. However, the treatment of residual refractive errors following RK is associated with an increased incidence of corneal opacification and need for retreatment (Figures 6-23 through 6-24e). The incidence of clinically significant corneal haze is approximately 5%, despite the fact that most corrections are performed for small amounts of residual myopia less than 3.00 D (Figure 6-25). The incidence of clinically significant haze in virgin corneas is less than 1% for mild myopia, so this represents a five- to ten-fold increase in the incidence of postoperative haze formation. Similarly, the incidence of retreatment is approximately 30% post-RK, at least a seven- to ten-fold increase compared to congenital myopia with similar refractive errors.

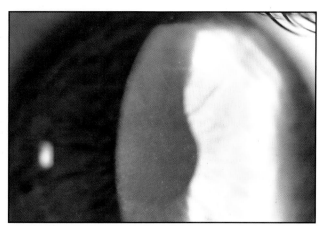

Figure 6-14a.
Clinical photo demonstrating ideal endpoint following PRK retreatment for haze. Low magnification view of trace haze following collagen plaque ablation.

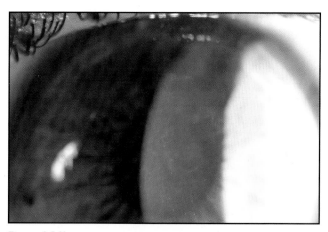

Figure 6-14b.
Clinical photo demonstrating ideal endpoint following PRK retreatment for haze. Medium magnification view of trace haze following collagen plaque ablation.

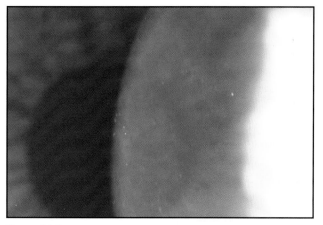

Figure 6-14c.
Clinical photo demonstrating ideal endpoint following PRK retreatment for haze. High magnification view of trace haze following collagen plaque ablation.

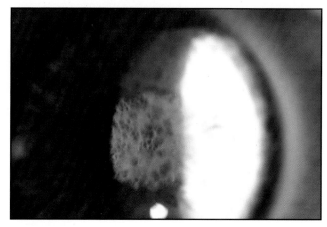

Figure 6-15a.
Preoperative medium magnification view of dense confluent haze prior to retreatment. Reticular and confluent areas coalescing preoperatively.

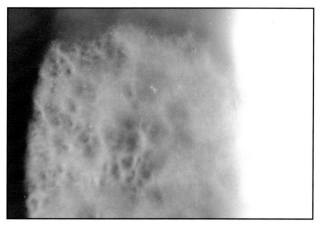

Figure 6-15b.
Preoperative high magnification view of dense confluent haze prior to retreatment. Reticular and confluent areas coalescing preoperatively.

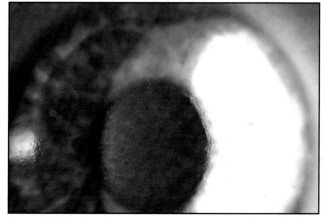

Figure 6-15c.
Trace reticular haze observed following retreatment. Absolutely clear corneas following retreatment may be associated with significant hyperopic overcorrections.

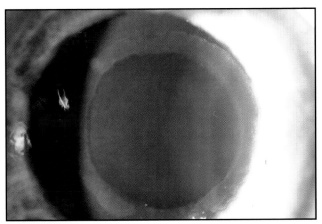

Figure 6-16.
Postoperative view of very trace reticular haze following collagen plaque removal. PTK ablation of epithelium and PRK ablation of collagen plaque. Final PRK zone programmed to exceed PTK ablation by 1 mm to blend peripheral margin. Ring of ablated epithelium evident.

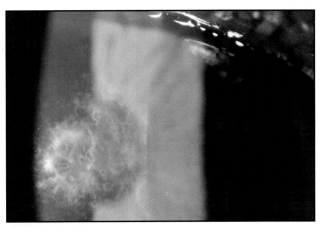

Figure 6-17a.
Preoperative photo of dense central confluent haze 3 to 4 mm in diameter following -19.00 D surface ablation.

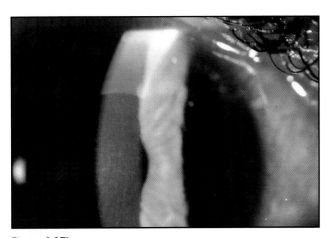

Figure 6-17b.
Postoperative examination reveals trace haze following collagen plaque retreatment.

Clinical Note

The treatment of residual myopia and cylinder following maximal RK is more complex than retreatment following PRK. Predictability is reduced, with undercorrections and overcorrections more common. At least a 20% reduction in expected predictability with a five- to ten-fold increase in the incidence of confluent haze formation. A conservative approach is therefore warranted with undercorrections of 0.50 to 1.00 D of myopia targeted to avoid overcorrections. A higher retreatment rate is understood, with 20% to 25% requiring an additional procedure. Despite the limitations, excellent surgical outcomes can be achieved with reductions in spherical myopia and cylinder and improvements in both night glare and fluctuating vision. The epithelium often becomes hyperplastic, dampening fluctuations and the effective optical zone enlarged, as illustrated in Figure 6-22b. A morning cycloplegic refraction is required to establish the least myopia experienced by the patient, and that measure becomes the maximum target input. Topical steroids are mandatory and must be tapered slowly, as late haze is not uncommon. Additionally, gentle debridement or a transepithelial approach with a moist stromal bed technique help reduce the haze formation incidence. Large optical zones not only reduce night glare but reduce epithelial hyperplasia. Preoperative counseling is mandatory.

Treatment of Collagen Plaque
- Goal is to remove 85% to 90% of collagen plaque, not 100%. Debulked collagen will clear naturally.
- Aim to re-establish original contour from primary procedure.
- Do not treat associated myopia.
- Do not overtreat. Clear cornea usually means overtreatment and significant hyperopia. Lower hyperopia allows topical steroid use postoperatively. Overtreatment means sharp wound edge margins.

Figure 6-18a.
Central 2-mm area of mixed confluent and reticular haze following PRK for moderate myopia.

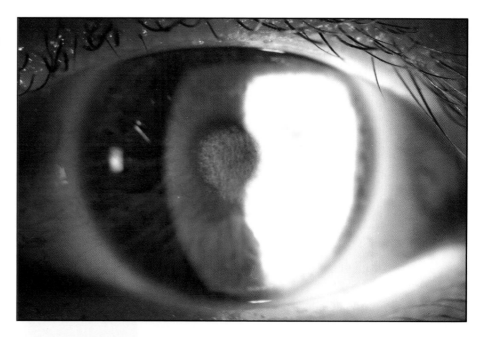

Figure 6-18b.
Immediate postoperative view of clear cornea following retreatment.

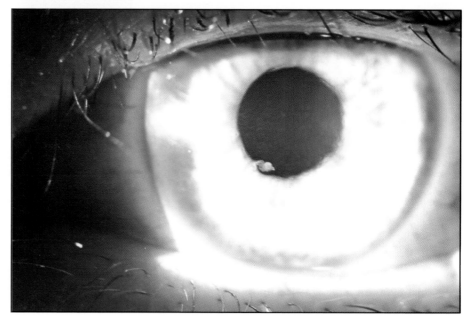

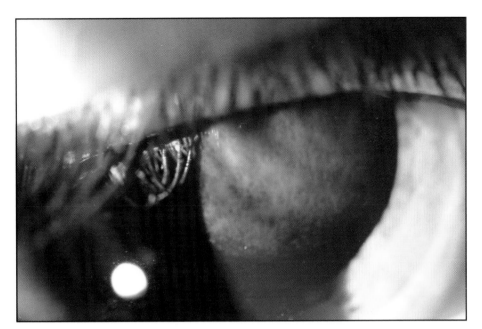

Figure 6-19a.
Diffuse confluent haze over 6-mm ablation zone.

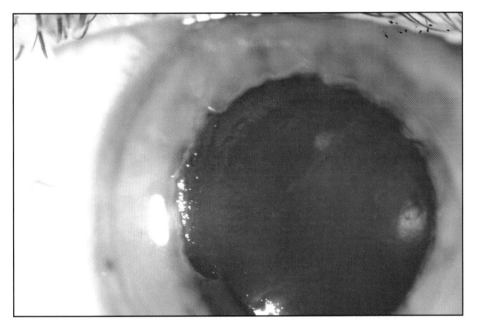

Figure 6-19b.
Trace reticular haze evident postoperatively following retreatment.

Figure 6-20a.
Asymmetric confluent haze with superior arcuate plaque.

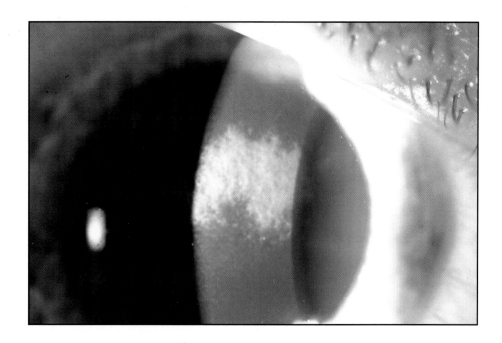

Figure 6-20b.
Treatment with transepithelial approach over entire 6-mm area performed utilizing epithelium as natural blocking agent. Mottled epithelial-haze endpoint observed superiorly, while inferior stroma protected by epithelium. Homogeneous trace haze evident, symmetry restored.

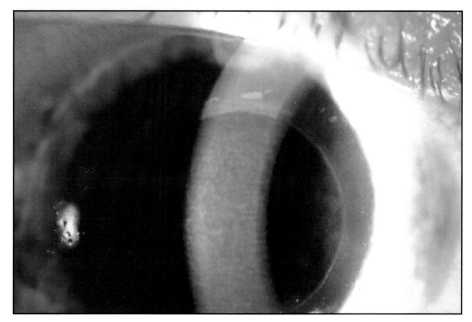

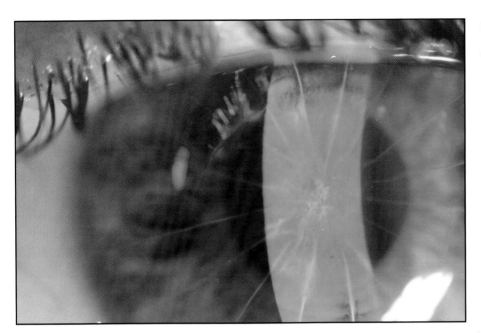

Figure 6-21a.
Epithelial healing day 3 following RK enhancement with excimer PRK.

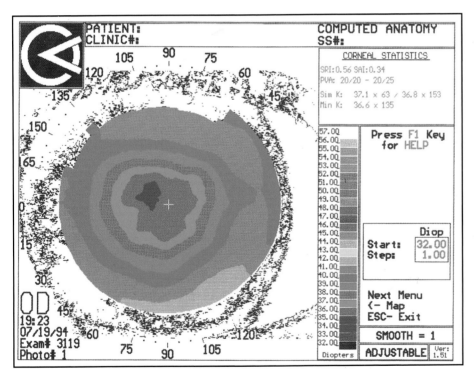

Figure 6-21b.
Corneal videokeratography demonstrates multizone appearance to central corneal flattening post-RK.

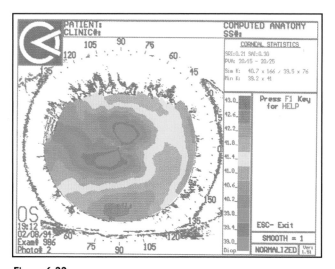

Figure 6-22a.
RK enhancement with PRK. Preoperative: -4.50 -1.25 x 140. Note that the difference in scales makes a comparison of preoperative and postoperative maps more difficult.

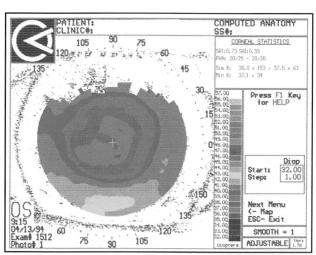

Figure 6-22b.
Postoperative -1.00 D refraction. Improved corneal topography and reduction of residual myopia. Uncorrected vision improved to 20/40 with no haze.

Figure 6-23.
Postoperative view of trace to mild reticular haze following PRK treatment of undercorrected RK. Haze grade was clinically insignificant, but patient was monitored more closely and topical steroids tapered more slowly.

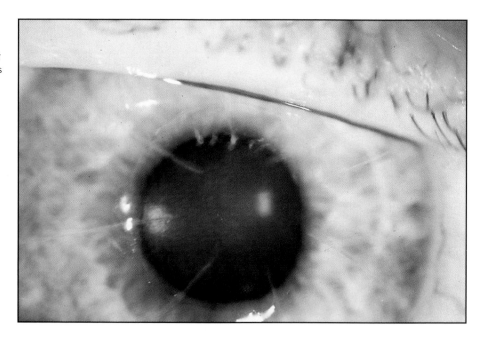

The important issues in treating residual myopia are first the recognition that an increased incidence of haze is encountered for proper preoperative counseling and patient selection, and second for developing techniques to minimize complications. Reduced predictability is also observed when retreating RK patients, with an increased standard deviation, producing both significant undercorrections and overcorrections. Although all RK patients appear to be sensitized, a subset of RK patients who are at increased risk for haze formation possess three clinical findings:

1. Greater than eight incisions
2. Smaller than 3.0-mm optical zone
3. Increased corneal scarring and splay of radial incisions (Figures 6-26 and 6-27).

When treating RK patients, special care must be taken when debriding the epithelium to avoid opening the radial and transverse incisions (Figures 6-28a and 6-28b). Gentle mechanical debridement is also recommended in an attempt to avoid stimulating the stromal surface to produce stromal collagen formation. Intraoperatively, the stroma should be

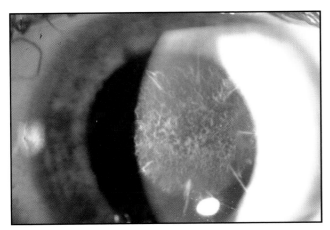

Figure 6-24a.
Postoperative view of confluent haze following PRK treatment of undercorrected RK.

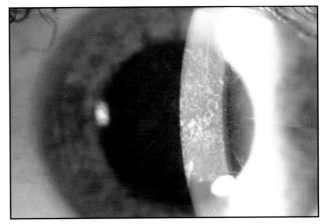

Figure 6-24b.
Reticular haze pattern progressing to confluent areas with associated myopic regression and reduced qualitative vision.

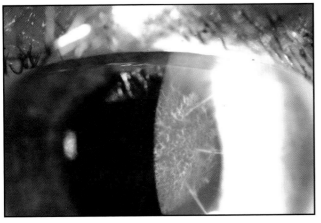

Figure 6-24c.
Postoperative view of confluent haze following PRK treatment of undercorrected RK. Iron deposits observed secondary to disturbed tear flow.

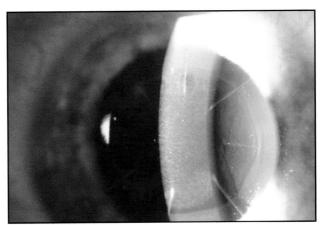

Figure 6-24d.
Following confluent haze retreatment, only trace haze evident.

left somewhat moist, which helps preserve corneal transparency. An early morning cycloplegic refraction should be used to calculate the target refractive error and an undercorrection should be routinely targeted.

Retreatment for haze formation post-RK is similar to that for haze formation post-PRK, utilizing the same blending principles and transepithelial approach (Figures 6-29a through 6-30b). A transepithelial approach can also be used for the primary PRK procedure following RK, as the risk of disturbing the corneal incisions is eliminated, corneal topographical abnormalities may be smoothed, and the stroma remains moist. The difficulty with this approach is simply that the beam homogeneity must be excellent, an increased incidence of central islands may be observed, and the variability of epithelial thickness post-RK may complicate predictability.

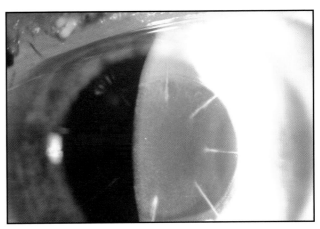

Figure 6-24e.
Following confluent haze retreatment, only trace haze evident.

Figure 6-25.
Dense, clinically significant haze following PRK for residual myopia post-RK.

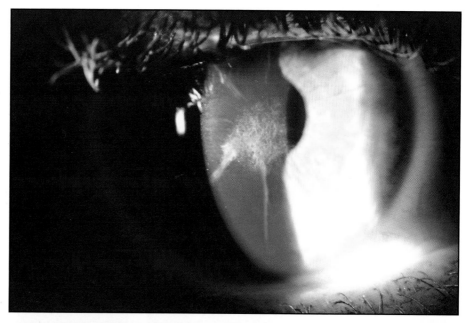

Figure 6-26.
Preoperative photo of 18-incision RK with overlying hexagonal keratotomy and corneal scarring. Patient presented with -2.00 -4.25 x 78, 3 years following last refractive procedure. Patient was informed of high incidence of haze, overcorrection, and further loss of best corrected vision. Transepithelial approach with PRK performed, achieving -1.25 -0.50 x 92 with an uncorrected visual acuity of 20/70 and a single line improvement in best corrected vision to 20/25.

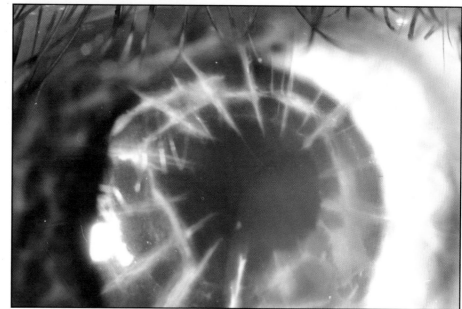

RETREATMENT OF CORNEAL TOPOGRAPHICAL ABNORMALITIES

Central islands are treated with the same philosophy as other topographical abnormalities with an understanding of their cause. The central or pericentral topographical steepening is related to a preferential undercorrection of the central stroma due to fluid accumulation intraoperatively. Acoustic shockwaves generated by each pulse drive fluid centrally and peripherally. The central fluid accumu-

lation blocks the central portion of successive pulses, reducing their effectiveness. Depending upon the preoperative hydration status, method of epithelial removal, size of the optical zone utilized, number of zones programmed, and degree of preoperative myopia, the incidence of clinically significant central islands varies (see Chapter 5).

Understanding the method of formation, roughly half the pulses have their central portion blocked. Theoretically and simply stated, one pulse removes central stroma tissue but produces central fluid, so that the next pulse is "busy" removing fluid instead of its share of

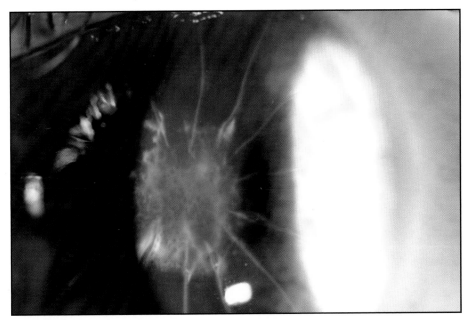

Figure 6-27.
Dense confluent haze developing in patient with 16-incision RK following PRK treatment of residual myopia. Note the healing of the RK incisions and small optical zone, both risk factors for confluent haze development.

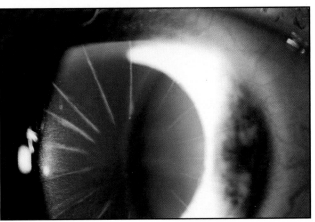

Figure 6-28a.
Sixteen-incision RK with 2.75-mm optical zone. PRK performed for residual myopia with undercorrection targeted in light of higher risk of overcorrection and haze with incisional RK.

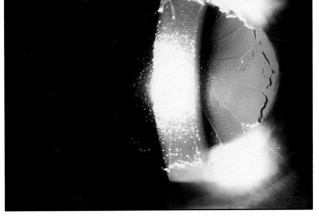

Figure 6-28b.
Repeat PRK performed with mechanical debridement in the absence of haze. Smooth ablative surface observed postoperatively. Refraction following RK was reduced from -11.00 D to -4.00 -1.00 x 160, following initial PRK, refraction reduced to -1.75 D, and following repeat PRK -0.75 D.

tissue. A central island therefore represents about half the dioptric power of the attempted correction in the 2- to 3-mm diameter equal to the area of fluid accumulation. Larger central islands are produced when larger optical zones are utilized.

TECHNIQUE FOR CENTRAL ISLAND TREATMENT

A transepithelial or manual debridement approach is recommended (3- to 4-mm optical zone). Utilizing videokeratography, one can calculate both the height and diameter of the central island. The height or depth of the central

Treatment of Topographical Abnormalities

- Treatment is based upon establishing proper topography

- Use epithelium and other blocking agents

- Do not treat associated cylinder with islands (unless preoperative cylinder)

- Avoid overtreatment

Figure 6-29a.
High magnification view of confluence.

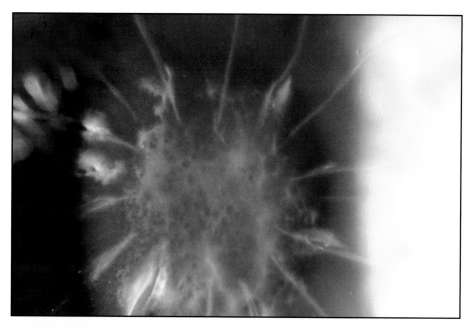

Figure 6-29b.
Following retreatment, clear cornea is evident.

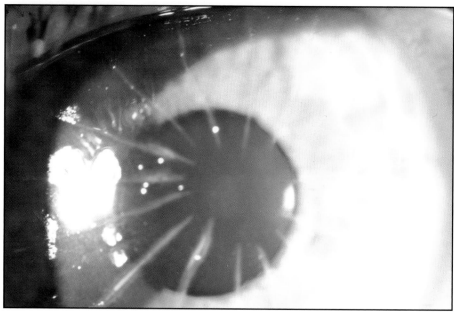

island is calculated using the Munnerlyn formula: the depth is equal to the diameter (optical zone) of the island squared, then multiplied by the dioptric height divided by three. For example, a central island that is 2.00 D in height (color differences) and 3 mm in diameter would be 6 microns high.

A preoperative refraction of a -6.00 D patient, treated with a single 6-mm zone, may create the central island example in Figures 6-31a and 6-31b. Treat this central island with a PRK treatment of 50% of the preoperative refraction at 2.5 mm; that is, -3.00 D at 2.5-mm optical zone = 6.25 microns. This correlates well with the depth calculation. If the island is larger, increase the optical zone up to 3 mm

(Figures 6-32a and 6-32b). In general, a correction of 1 micron per diopter of preoperative myopia is needed with islands in patients under -6.00 D with the VisX 20/20 Model B system. The Technolas requires a slightly greater correction than 1 micron per diopter at 3-mm optical zone.

Another approach is to treat the central island with 100% of the preoperative refraction at 2.5 to 3 mm, which is advocated by Don Johnson, MD. Since the eye tolerates a facet much better than a bump, the epithelium smooths any depression, and this technique works well. A concern with utilizing 100% of the preoperative refraction is overtreatment and haze. If too deep a facet is produced, circular haze

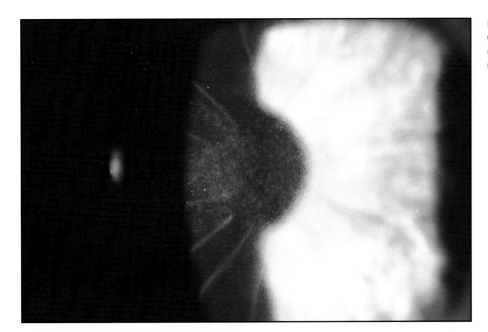

Figure 6-30a.
Corneal haze (Grade 1.5) and regression following PRK for residual myopia post-RK.

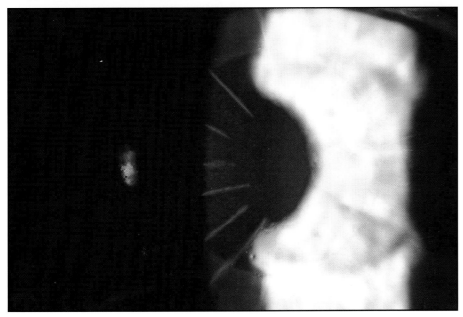

Figure 6-30b.
Transepithelial retreatment for haze and myopia.

may develop related to the steep edges with symptomatic glare, or more commonly hyperopic overcorrection. These problems are usually related to the combination of too deep a transepithelial PTK ablation and the 100% treatment.

KEYHOLE/PENINSULA AND SEMI-CIRCULAR ABLATION PATTERNS

The approach to these patterns is similar to that for central islands and asymmetric haze. They usually result from asymmetric stromal hydration intraoperatively related to the acoustic shockwave and vacuum aspiration system of

the VisX. They also may be related to abnormalities in the optical pathway and preoperative corneal topography. In general, treating central topographical abnormalities are foremost. Beware that the induced cylinder is likely only related to the topography. Don Johnson, MD, uses the epithelium as a blocking agent over the well-treated flat areas and manually debrides over the steep portions only; he has found this effective. Again, treatment is on a case-by-case basis. The principles remain the same. I personally treat asymmetric topographical abnormalities in the same manner as asymmetric haze.

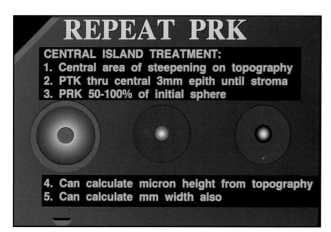

Figure 6-31a.
Schematic diagram of central island retreatment. Surgeon view utilizing transepithelial approach. Mechanical debridement equally acceptable and even preferable with some laser systems. Left-hand diagram illustrate central area of steepening on corneal topography. Central diagram illustrates PTK ablation of epithelium at 3-mm diameter. Right-hand diagram illustrates stromal blackness once epithelium is ablated. Fifty percent of initial sphere is programmed for PRK correction of central island. Micron depth of central island should be calculated from topography utilizing Munnerlyn formula and correlated with planned treatment.

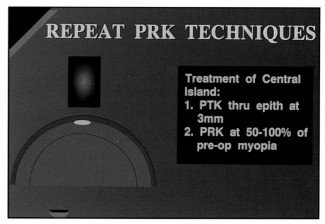

Figure 6-31b.
Profile view of central island representing central stromal bump of several microns beneath epithelium. Treatment concept revolves about establishing original planned curvature over treatment of central island may result in hyperopia and possibly increased haze, therefore, conservative approach is warranted and correlation with height on topographical map necessary. Maximal 50% of preoperative sphere recommended.

MANAGEMENT OF PRK DECENTRATION

The management of decentration is as much an art as a science, but is based upon the same fundamental principles utilized in all retreatment techniques. There are a number of retreatment techniques ranging from performing a PRK equally decentered in the opposite direction (O'Brart) to performing multiple small PRK treatments along the edge of the ablation in an effort to enlarge the treatment zone (Jackson). My concerns with these techniques are the induction of irregular astigmatism and haze by introducing a step or unevenness between the treatment zones. An unclear endpoint is estimated, which invites error into the amount of treatment performed.

My retreatment technique for decentration is similar to that I described for treating asymmetric haze or asymmetric topographical abnormalities. I advocate a transepithelial approach with a large optical zone of at least 6 mm. The technique is based on the principle that surface epithelium is thicker or hyperplastic over treated stroma than untreated stroma. Therefore, by using the epithelium as a natural masking agent, the thicker epithelium protects the treated stroma while allowing ablation of the untreated area.

The laser is placed in PTK mode for the transepithelial

ablation, which is centered appropriately. As the ablation proceeds through the epithelium, the entire 6-mm area appears clinically as green pseudofluorescence in a darkened room. An arc of stromal blackness will appear over the untreated stroma, while the previously treated stroma with a thicker surface epithelial layer continues to pseudofluorescence indicating that it is being protected. This provides the surgeon with a surgical cue as to the starting point. At this point, a PRK mode is used to treat the residual refractive error, modified for uncorrected visual acuity and induced cylinder. That is, if the uncorrected day vision is 20/40, a -3.00 D correction is excessive and should be reduced to -1.00 or -1.25 D. Furthermore, if there is 3.00 D of induced cylinder, this is likely related to the decentration and should not be treated.

Some surgeons debride the epithelium manually over the untreated stroma prior to treating the residual refractive error (Johnson). My concern with this approach is that a 50-micron step is introduced which may incite haze formation secondary to overtreatment.

The PTK mode can also be utilized if no significant refractive error exists. PTK ablation is performed until the epithelium over the decentered zone just clears, which provides the surgeon with a clear endpoint. Since the epithelial masking agent is just clearing, we know that the decentered area has been protected and not further ablated. The number

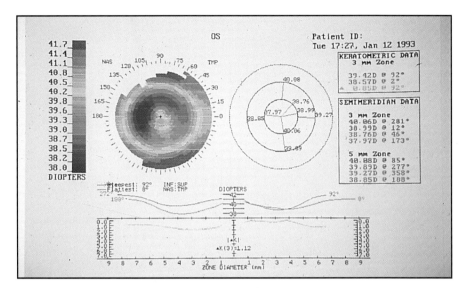

Figure 6-32a.
EyeSys corneal videokeratography demonstrating central island formation following 6-mm single zone PRK for moderate myopia with VisX 20/20 Model B excimer laser system.

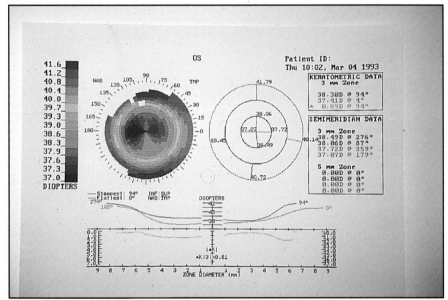

Figure 6-32b.
EyeSys corneal videokeratography following retreatment of central island. Profile graph demonstrates flattening of central elevation.

of pulses required between the starting point when the arc of stromal blackness appeared over the untreated stroma and the endpoint when the decentered area stopped fluorescing, indicates the amount of treatment required to correct the topographical decentration. With this technique we also know that no step exists between the retreatment and decentered treatment zones. This clear endpoint thereby provides the surgeon with two pieces of clinical information: first, that no excessive treatment has been performed and second, that a smooth transition zone has been created.

In this manner, the untreated area becomes part of the original contour and becomes centered. As well, the smooth transition reduces the incidence of haze formation and irregular astigmatism.

Surgical Retreatment Approach

Mechanical Debridement
    Regression without haze
    Central island

Transepithelial Approach
    Regression with haze
    Complex/asymmetric topographical abnormalities

CHAPTER 7

PRK Clinical Issues and Results

LOW MYOPIA

As with radial keratotomy (RK), the predictability of excimer photorefractive keratectomy (PRK) is greatest for patients with low myopia of less than 3 D. It is always best to treat a low myope as your first patient, rather than a high myope, since the procedure is simplified and the results are almost uniformly excellent. Despite the natural assumption that a surgeon can do no wrong by performing PRK on a high myope since there will be at least some improvement, the fact remains that not only do higher myopes have equally high expectations, but their risk of complications is greater.

> It must be recognized that there are no sharp edges on the human body nor should there be on the eye. As the body will reject sharp contours by inciting a wound healing response.

> It is always best to treat a low myope as your first patient.

Conversely, despite candidates with milder degrees of myopia having the greatest statistical probability of achieving emmetropia and the lowest statistical probability of developing a postoperative complication, an excellent outcome can never be assured and should never be guaranteed.

At least 95% of low myopes achieve 20/40 or better vision, with the majority (70% to 80%) achieving 20/25 or better vision in most series with all laser systems. Associated cylinder of 1.00 D or greater in these candidates decreases the predictability considerably, by as much as 10%. Visual recovery is typically more rapid, especially in younger patients. The incidence of complications such as infection and pain are equal to that of more severe candidates, however, the risk of subepithelial haze and loss of best corrected visual acuity is significantly reduced to 0.5% or less. Central islands are encountered much less frequently. Monovision should always be considered for patients unilaterally treated and a trial of monovision attempted whenever possible in pre-presbyopic and presbyopic candidates.

Retreatment for residual myopia is required in less than 5% of patients in light of the excellent predictability. It should be noted, however, that most candidates will desire retreatment unless 20/30 or better, and a number demand 20/25 or better. It should never be assumed that 20/40 is adequate to please most myopes, despite the fact that this level of visual acuity is quoted to patients preoperatively.

MODERATE MYOPIA

Moderate myopes between -3.10 and -6.00 D are the most common candidates for PRK, with a mean of -3.50 to -3.75 D. Once again, these candidates do well, with approx-

One to Two Year Results of PRK for Low to Moderate Myopia

Louis E. Probst V, MD

The results of PRK in the low to moderate myopia groups are summarized in Table A-1. The studies originate from nine different countries and date back to 1991. There is some overlap of the data, as some groups have published more than once on the same group of patients.[6,8,13,15] Most of the PRK was done with the Summit ExciMed, with less done using the VisX 20/20. The ablation zone size has increased from 3.5 mm in 1991[1] to 7.0 mm in 1994.[2]

The attempted correction generally ranged from -1.0 to -7.0 D. In the low to moderate myopia groups, 40% to 100% of eyes were within 1 D of the intended correction.[2,20] Between 25% to 100% of eyes achieved at least 20/40 uncorrected visual acu-

ity,[2,14] and the percentage of eyes reaching this level of vision almost always exceeded those within 1 D of intended correction. The studies reported in 1994 tend to report better results, with 80% of patients within 1 D of emmetropia and over 90% achieving better than 20/40 visual acuity.[12-19]

The loss of two or more Snellen lines of visual acuity ranged from 0% to 5%.[9,13] IOP elevations following PRK were found in 2% to 28% of eyes.[4,14] Halos and night glare were reported to occur in 10% to 70% of eyes.[6,15] Decentrations of greater than 1 mm have been reported to occur in 5% to 20% of eyes.[12,14]

TABLE A-1
RESULTS OF PRK FOR LOW TO MODERATE MYOPIA

Author/Year	Country	Laser Type	Ablation Zone (mm)	Number of Eyes	Follow-Up	Attempted Correction	± 1 D (%)	20/40+ Uncorrected (%)	Loss of Two Snellen Lines (%)	↑ IOP (%)	Other 12 Month Complication
Seiler et al, 1991[1]	Germany	Summit ExciMed	3.5	26	12	-1.4 to -9.25	92	96	0	3.1	2.8% corneal scars
Gartry et al, 1991[2]	UK	Summit ExciMed	4.0	120	12	-1.5 to -7.0	40-90	25-90	2.5	12	10% significant halos
McDonald et al, 1991[3]	USA	VisX 20/20	4.25-5.0	7	12	-2.00 to -5.0	57	86	0	NR	18% astigmatism in high myopia group
				10	12	-5.00 to -8.0	18	18	18		
Seiler et al, 1993[4]	Germany	Summit ExciMed	4.0-5.0	42	12	-1.25 to -3.0	98	100	1	28	15.4% stromal scarring with ≥ 6 D myopia
				85	12	-3.1 to -6.0	92	97			
Lavery et al, 1993[5]	Ireland	Summit ExciMed	3.0-4.3	99	12	-1.25 to -9.6	93	84	1	NR	1% glare+ decentration
Kim et al, 1993[6]	Korea	Summit ExciMed	5.0	135	12	-2.0 to -7.0	91	99	8.1	14	10% glare/halos 21% blurred vision
				67	12	-7.25 to -13.5	52	63	17.9	24	
Brancato et al, 1993[7]	Italy	Summit ExciMed	3.5 -5.0	146	12	-0.8 to -6.0	71	NR	1.4	25	9% anisocoria 10% >1mm decentration
				145	12	-6.1 to -9.9	35	NR	2.1		
				39	12	-10.0 to -25.0	28	NR	7.7		
Salz et al, 1993[8]	USA	VisX 20/20	5.0-5.5	71	12	-1.25 to -7.5	84	91	1.4	3	1% significant haze
				12	24		92	100	0		

TABLE A-1 (CONTINUED)
RESULTS OF PRK FOR LOW TO MODERATE MYOPIA

Author/Year	Country	Laser Type	Ablation Zone (mm)	Number of Eyes	Follow-Up	Attempted Correction	± 1 D (%)	20/40+ Uncorrected (%)	Loss of Two Snellen Lines (%)	↑ IOP (%)	Other 12 Month Complication
Piebenga et al, 1993[9]	USA	VisX 20/20	4.0-5.0	70	12	-1.0 to -6.0	71	75	0	3	2% stromal reaction
			(+nitrogen)	25	24	-1.0 to -5.0	58	67			
				20	36	-2.0 to -8.0	60	70			
Gimbel et al, 1993[10]	Canada	Summit ExciMed	4.5-5.0	52	15.5	-5.6 ± 1.6	43	96	NR	NR	50% halos
				52	9	-5.9 ± 1.5	45	92			
Tengroth et al, 1993[11]	Sweden	Summit ExciMed	4.3-4.5	420	12	-1.5 to -7.5	86	91	NR	13	26% halos
				194	15		87	87			
Shimizu et al, 1994[12]	Japan	Summit ExciMed	4.5	11	12	-2.0 to -3.0	100	NR	NR	9	5% >1 mm, decentration
				45	12	-3.1 to -6.0	76	NR			
				41	12	> -6.1	44	NR			
Maguen et al, 1994[13]	USA	VisX 20/20	5.0 -5.5	122	12	-1.00 to -7.75	79	89	4	11	2% recurrent erosions
				48	24		86	92	5		
				9	36		90	90	0		
Talley et al, 1994[14]	USA	VisX 20/20	6.0-7.0	23	12	-1.0 to -3.12	100	100	1	2	20% decentration ≥1 mm
				21	12	-3.25 to -4.37	100	100			2% central island
				41	12	-4.5 to -7.50	85	95			
Kim et al, 1994[15]	Korea	Summit ExciMed	5.0	45	24	-2.0 to -6.0	91	98	4	16	70% halos/glare
Epstein et al, 1994[16]	Sweden	Summit ExciMed	4.3-4.5	495	24	-1.25 to -7.5	86	91	0.4	13	3% ≥2+ haze
Dutt et al, 1994[17]	USA	Summit ExciMed	5.0	47	12	-1.5 to -6.0	80	94	0	11	42% halos
FDA Study- VisX, 1994[18]	USA	VisX 20/20	NR	521	12	-1.0 to -6.0	79	86	1	5	10% retreatment
FDA Study- Summit, 1994[19]	USA	Summit ExciMed	5.0-58%	585	12	-1.0 to -6.0	78	91	3	NR	no endothelial cell loss
			4.5-42%								
Amano et al, 1995[20]	Japan	Summit ExciMed	5.0	11	24	-2.0 to -3.0	100	NR	NR	NR	3% ≥2+ haze
				28	24	-3.1 to -6.0		75	NR		
				21	24	-6.1 to -14.0		52	NR		

References

1. Seiler T, Wollensak J. Myopic photorefractive keratectomy with the excimer laser. One year follow-up. *Ophthalmology.* 1991;98:1156-1163.

2. Gartry DS, Kerr Muir MG, Marshall J. Photorefractive keratectomy with an argon fluoride excimer laser: a clinical study. *Refract Corneal Surg.* 1991;7:420-435.

3. McDonald MB, Liu JC, Byrd RJ, et al. Central photorefractive keratectomy for myopia: partially sighted and normally sighted eyes. *Ophthalmology.* 1991;98:1327-1337.

4. Seiler T, Wollensak J. Results of a prospective evaluation of photorefractive keratectomy at 1 year after surgery. *Ger J Ophthalmol.* 1993;2(3):135-142.

5. Lavery FL. Photorefractive keratectomy in 472 eyes. *Refract Corneal Surg.* 1993;9(2 Suppl):S98-S100.

6. Kim JH, Hahn TW, Lee YC, et al. Photorefractive keratectomy in 202 myopic eyes: one year results. *Refract Corneal Surg.* 1993;9(2 Suppl):S11-S16.

7. Brancato R, Tavola A, Carones F, et al. Excimer laser photorefractive keratectomy for myopia: results in 1165 eyes. *Refract Corneal Surg.* 1993;9:95-104.

8. Salz JJ, Maguen E, Nesburn AB, et al. A two-year experience with excimer laser photorefractive keratectomy for myopia. *Ophthalmology.* 1993;100:873-882.

9. Piebenga LW, Matta CS, Deitz MR, et al. Excimer photorefractive keratectomy for myopia. *Ophthalmology.* 1993;100:1335-1345.

10. Gimbel HV, Van Westenbrugge JA, Johnson WH, et al. Visual, refractive, and patient satisfaction results following bilateral photorefractive keratectomy for myopia. *Refract Corneal Surg.* 1993;9(2 Suppl):S5-S10.

11. Tengroth B, Epstein D, Fagerholm P, et al. Excimer laser photorefractive keratectomy for myopia. Clinical results in sighted eyes. *Ophthalmology.* 1993;100:739-745.

12. Shimizu K, Amano S, Tanaka S. Photorefractive keratectomy for myopia: one-year follow-up in 97 eyes. *J Refract Corneal Surg.* 1994;10(Suppl):S178-S187.

13. Maguen E, Salz JJ, Nesburn AB, et al. Results of excimer laser photorefractive keratectomy for the correction of myopia. *Ophthalmology.* 1994;101:1548-1557.

14. Talley AR, Hardten DR, Sher NA, et al. Results one year after using the 193-nm excimer laser for photorefractive keratectomy in mild to moderate myopia. *Am J Ophthalmol.* 1994;118:304-311.

15. Kim JH, Hahn TW, Lee YC, Sah WJ. Excimer laser photorefractive keratectomy for myopia: two-year follow-up. *J Cataract Refract Surg.* 1994;20(Suppl):229.

16. Epstein D, Fagerholm P, Hamberg-Nystrom H, Tengroth B. Twenty-four month follow-up of excimer laser photorefractive keratectomy for myopia. Refractive and visual acuity results. *Ophthalmology.* 1994;101:1558-1564.

17. Dutt S, Steinert RF, Raizman MB, Puliafito CA. One-year results of excimer laser photorefractive keratectomy for low to moderate myopia. *Arch Ophthalmol.* 1994;112:1427-1436.

18. McDonald MB, Talamo JH. Myopic photorefractive keratectomy: the experience in the United States with the VisX excimer laser. In: Salz JJ, McDonnell PJ, McDonald MB, eds. *Corneal Laser Surgery.* St. Louis, Mo: Mosby; 1995.

19. Thompson KP, Steinert RF, Daniel J, Stulting D. Photorefractive keratectomy with the Summit excimer laser: the phase III US results. In: Salz JJ, McDonnell PJ, McDonald MB, eds. *Corneal Laser Surgery.* St. Louis, Mo: Mosby; 1995.

20. Amano S, Shimizu K. Excimer laser photorefractive keratectomy for myopia: two year follow-up. *J Refract Surg.* 1995;11(Suppl):S253-S260.

imately 90% achieving 20/40 or better and 50% achieving 20/25 or better uncorrected visual acuity in most series with various laser systems. About 85% of the myopic population has less than 6 D of myopia. In general, the mean predictability of a single PRK procedure for 20/40 or better uncorrected vision exceeds 90% for the majority of the myopic population. Once again, there are qualifications to be made, in that most patients are unsatisfied with 20/40 uncorrected visual acuity and require retreatment for an acceptable 20/25 level of vision. Furthermore, most reported series have an abundance of young lower spherical myopes which skew data toward better uncorrected visual acuities. Young patients with better accommodative amplitudes accept greater degrees of hyperopia and therefore have a more rapid apparent visual recovery as well.

The fact that little or no cylinder was evident in most of these candidates improves expected predictability in these series. Parallel to RK results, predictability falls off somewhat between -5.00 and -6.00 D. Although the retreatment incidence may begin to increase at this level of myopia, the ability of PRK to treat higher degrees of myopia relative to RK remains without question. Depending upon the age and gender of the patient, PRK has a decided advantage over RK for myopes above -4.00 or -5.00 D. It becomes both a philosophical and financial question as to when RK ceases to be a viable alternative to PRK. For lower myopes, the risks and benefits of RK and PRK appear to be equivalent, but in more moderate myopes treated with more advanced PRK techniques, PRK is able to achieve greater predictability with

lower complication rates. Increasing the number of incisions and decreasing the size of the surgical optical zone in RK only serves to destabilize the cornea and invite fluctuating vision, night glare, and possibly progressive hyperopia.

It must be appreciated that moderate myopia in the -4.00 to -6.00 D range still represents the middle of the refractive envelope for PRK. Retreatment rates of about 10% to 15% are reported in most series, but can be reduced to as little as 3% with aggressive steroid regimens. The risk of night glare begins to increase, as it is directly related to the degree of preoperative myopia, especially in those with larger pupils. Moderate myopes treated both with single zone techniques and with homogeneous broad beam excimer laser systems (ie, VisX 20/20 Model B or Chiron Technolas Keracor 116) are at greater risk for central islands. The incidence of clinically significant confluent haze requiring retreatment is highly dependent upon the PRK technique and laser system utilized, but ranges from 1% to 5%, with a mean of 1% to 2%. Reticular haze is a normal part of the healing pattern post-PRK and resolves over several months. Most corneas develop trace to mild reticular haze with moderate myopia and clear to trace haze with mild myopia correction. The incidence of loss of best corrected visual acuity of at least two lines is approximately 1% with advanced PRK techniques and laser systems, reduced from 3% to 5% with previous PRK applications. Since confluent haze following PRK is treatable in almost all cases, PRK may very well be the procedure of choice for candidates with moderately severe myopia.

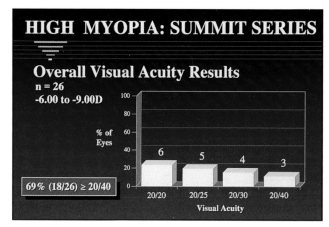

Figure 7-1.
Graphic illustration of uncorrected visual acuity results following Summit ExciMed UV 200 excimer laser PRK for high myopia. Preoperative myopia was between -6.00 to -9.00 D in the 26 eyes treated. Eighteen of the 26 eyes (69%) achieved 20/40 or better uncorrected visual acuity after one procedure with 6 to12 months follow-up. All eyes treated by the author and Fouad Tayfour, MD.

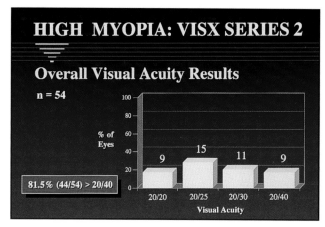

Figure 7-2.
Graphic illustration of VisX 20/20 excimer laser visual acuity results for high myopia following surface PRK. VisX Series 2 represents visual outcomes in 54 eyes treated with a four zone technique commencing with a 2.5-mm pretreatment. Over 80% (44/54) of eyes treated achieved 20/40 or better unaided vision results. All eyes treated by the author.

SEVERE MYOPIA

Early reports found a dramatic fall-off in refractive predictability and stability for PRK above -6.00 D, which resulted in the FDA limiting the early US trials to low and moderate myopia. The technique utilized for these early cases of high myopia was a single zone technique with a small optical zone of 4.00 to 4.25 mm in order to limit the depth of ablation. It was at the Phillips Eye Institute where larger optical zones were demonstrated to be more effective in the treatment of high myopia. Additionally, multizone techniques have managed to reduce depth of ablation while maximizing optical zone size and improving wound contour. Larger optical zones not only reduce night glare, but also improve wound contour, which reduces regression and improves long-term stability.

The Summit ExciMed UV 200 excimer laser system, which had a maximum optical zone of 5 mm and a gaussian energy beam profile, seems to be the least effective in correcting higher degrees of myopia and producing a stable result. In general, about 70% of higher myopes in my series (Figure 7-1) between -6.00 to -9.00 D were corrected 20/40 or better unaided. A small degree of myopic regression was often noted in these Summit ExciMed patients long-term, especially in these more severe cases, further reducing the predictability. Visual recovery was quite prolonged in some cases and haze more evident. Intrastromal techniques have been used internationally by Summit ExciMed users to achieve high myopia corrections. The Summit OmniMed series, with larger optical zone capabilities and a more homogeneous energy beam profile, has demonstrated improved high myopia results. The Summit multizone program, which produces a continuous aspheric ablation pattern, has been reported to achieve superior and more stable high myopia results relative to the original ExciMed series.

The high myopia results I achieved with the VisX 20/20 unit equipped with a 6.0-mm optical zone and a homogeneous energy beam profile utilizing a multizone approach for high myopia were better, with about 80% achieving 20/40 or better from -6.10 to -9.00 D with a single surgical procedure (Figure 7-2). The VisX multizone approach I utilized corrected 50% of preoperative correction at 4 mm, 30% at 5.0 mm, and 20% at 6.0 mm. An alternative VisX multizone algorithm uses 5.0, 5.5, and 6.0 mm; however, this increases depth ablation without any reported improved clinical

> **The smaller optical zone is always performed initially to blend with larger zones and create a smoother surface.**

results. The smaller optical zone is always performed initially to blend with larger zones and create a smoother surface. The same principle applies to the change by VisX of the movement of the iris diaphragm from out to in when first introduced, to the current industry standard of in to out.

The Chiron Technolas Keracor 116 system high myopia results vary considerably with the technique utilized. With a

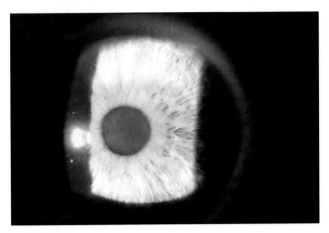

Figure 7-3a.
Low magnification view of clinically significant confluent haze following PRK for high myopia.

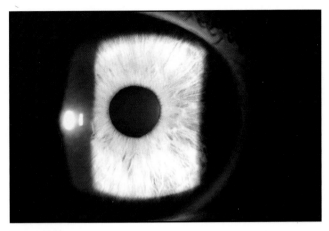

Figure 7-3b.
Low magnification view of clinical appearance of same cornea (Figure 7-3a) following collagen plaque removal.

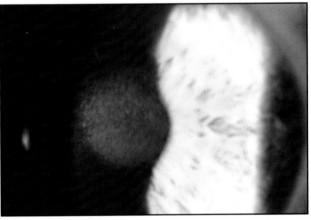

Figure 7-3c.
High magnification view of the same eye (Figure 7-3a) demonstrating density of the confluent haze, which was associated with reduced best corrected vision of two lines.

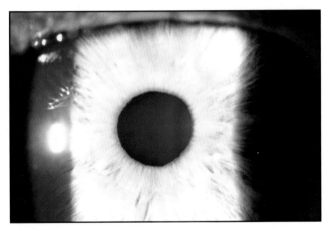

Figure 7-3d.
High magnification view of the same eye (Figure 7-3a) demonstrating restored corneal clarity following haze retreatment with return of best corrected vision.

single zone technique and 5.0-mm optical zone, 20% to 30% regression of effect was observed by a number of international investigators over 6 to 12 months, whereas the 7-mm multi-multizone technique for high myopia has reduced the degree of regression observed to less than half. In patients between -6.10 and -9.00 D, 86% achieved visual acuity within three lines of their best corrected vision, most within 2 to 3 weeks in our series.

Retreatment rates for high myopia are definitely higher, as the incidence of undercorrection and myopic regression increases with increasing degrees of preoperative myopia. In general, retreatment rates of between 10% to 25% are expected between -6.10 and -9.00 D with PRK depending on technique, laser system, optical zone size, and topical steroid regimen utilized. The risk of haze is related to depth

> The risk of haze is related to depth of ablation; however, it is not simply because of the greater induction of wound healing with depth, but also due to the dramatic alterations in wound contour.

> Multizone techniques, transition zones, and aspheric ablation patterns will all improve the PRK wound profile, and are most important when treating high myopia.

of ablation; however, it is not simply because of the greater induction of wound healing with depth, but also due to the dramatic alterations in wound contour. That is, a single zone technique with small diameter to limit depth of ablation will

Long-Term Results of VisX PRK for Very High Myopia

D. Keith Williams, FRCSC, FACS, FRCOphth

All patients had a minimum 1-year follow-up, with 44 patients in each of the severe and extreme myopia groups reaching 2-year follow-up.

- 281 patients
- Range: -6.00 to -20.75 D
- 208 patients -6 to -10 D
- 73 patients >-10 D
- Astigmatism up to 6.00 D

Corneal topography pre- and postoperatively on all patients:

- Ages 23 to 57 years (mean: 40 years)
  (>-10 D, 43.5 years)
  (<-10 D, 36.5 years)
- 175 males, 106 females
- 126 right eyes, 155 left eyes

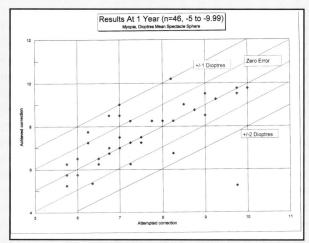

Figure B-1.
One-year results (n=46, -5 to -9.99 D).

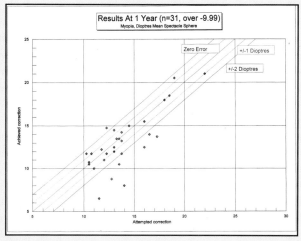

Figure B-2.
One-year results (n=31, over -9.99 D).

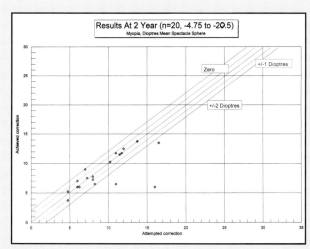

Figure B-3.
Two-year results (n=20, -4.75 to -20.5 D).

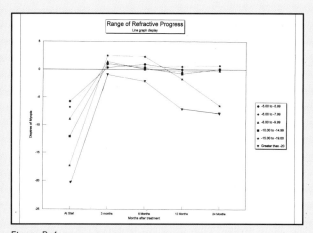

Figure B-4.
Range of refractive progress.

	TABLE B-1	
	REGRESSION	
<-10 D	-10 to -15 D	>-15 D
8%	25%	47.5%

Four patients (all greater than -10 D preoperatively) regressed between 1 to 2 years and were not reversed with steroid drops.

Twenty patients regressed between 3 months and 1 year. All were reversed with prompt use of steroid drops irrespective of preoperative myopia.

TABLE B-2		
PERCENTAGE OF LOST LINES OF BEST CORRECTED VISUAL ACUITY		
	1 Year	2 Years
Loss of one line best corrected visual acuity <-10 D	8.5%	2.5%
Loss of two lines best <-10 D	0%	0%
corrected visual acuity >-10 D	10%	10%

TABLE B-4		
REFRACTIVE PREDICTABILITY		
	1 Year	
	-6 to -10 D	>-10.00 D
±2 D	95%	70%

TABLE B-3				
UNCORRECTED VISUAL ACUITY RESULTS				
Uncorrected Visual Acuity	-6.00 to -10.00 D		>-10.00 D	
	1 Year	2 Years	1 Year	2 Years
20/20	40%	39%	10%	8%
20/40	86%	80%	54%	48%

VisX 20/20 excimer laser:

- 193 nm
- Rep. rate: 5 Hz
- Fluence: 160 mJ/cm^2
- Ablation rate: 0.20 to 0.25 m
- Manual removal of epithelium (20 seconds average)
- Multizone (3)
    - 5.0 mm   50% correction
    - 5.5 mm   30% correction
    - 6.0 mm   20% correction and cylinder
        - (elliptical or sequential)
- Lowest: -4.00 -4.00 x 180, 305 pulses, 65 microns
- Highest: -19.50 -2.50 x 160, 869 pulses, 174 microns

Postoperative regimen:

1. Voltaren one drop every 2 hours for 12 hours postoperatively. Patch.

2. Tobramycin or Ciloxan first day postoperatively until epithelium healed (average: 3 days).
3. No steroid drops below -4 preoperatively, or if high hyperopic shift at 1 week to 1 month postoperatively.
4. FML qid 1 week, tid 1 week, bid 1 week, once daily between -4 to -6 if small hyperopic shift to all patients.
5. FML or FML Forte to all patients for longer, -6 to -10 and above depending on hyperopic shift.

- Retreatments: Three patients
- IOP: Three patients
- Central islands: Four patients (series 3), one persisted >1 year, zero patients (series 4)
- Glare: Five patients
- Halos: Five patients
- Overcorrection: Six patients (+0.25 to +1.00 D)
- Retinal detachment: Two patients
- Haze: All patients. Related to degree of myopia (ie, greater the myopia, the more severe the haze). Overall, the haze is less using the series 4 software.

create sharp wound edges at the margins as well as steep walls. Investigators have reported 10% to 20% significant haze and regression with 4-mm optical zones treating high myopia. The wound healing response may produce arcuate haze along the steep edges or diffuse haze across the entire ablative surface. Multizone techniques, transition zones, and aspheric ablation patterns will all improve the PRK wound profile and are most important when treating high myopia. In general, despite the best techniques, about 2% to 3%, with a range of up to 5%, will develop clinically significant confluent haze and regression utilizing multizone and various scanning and blending techniques for myopia correction between -6.10 and -9.00 D. Most patients develop reticular haze, which clears over several months and is not clinically significant.

Although multizone techniques and larger optical zones reduce night glare, higher myopes are still more likely to experience night visual disturbances. Most highly myopic patients have some degree of night glare preoperatively and should not expect this to go away, as they often do. In fact, night glare in higher myopes is clearly exacerbated by all forms of refractive surgery and requires several months for improvement through cortical integration. Treatment of the fellow eye (even with inadequate optical zone) is nececessary for night glare to improve, as cortical integration of the images between the two eyes requires them to be balanced. The risk of losing two lines or more of best corrected visual acuity is definitely higher for severe myopes. Various investigators have reported the risk to be between 1% to 10%. The causes for loss of best corrected visual acuity in severe myopes include:

- Irregular astigmatism
- Confluent haze
- Abnormal topography including central islands and decentration

The mean incidence for loss of best corrected visual acuity of two or more lines in severe myopes is likely in the order of 2% to 3%. Most investigators still consider PRK a viable and preferred refractive surgery treatment method for severe myopia correction, but many, especially those with less advanced laser systems and techniques, have shifted toward laser in situ keratomileusis (LASIK).

EXTREME MYOPIA

The treatment of extreme myopia with PRK, defined as myopia greater than -9.00 D, is somewhat controversial, with many laser refractive surgeons performing LASIK exclusively for these patients. Despite the fact that many anecdotal reports exist (including those of my own) of extremely myopic patients of -15.00 and -20.00 D that have been treated successfully with PRK, the high degree of regression and increased risk of complications indicate LASIK as the procedure of choice. Even with LASIK, patients with greater than -15.00 D experience greater clinical regression, slower visual recovery, and a higher associated incidence of loss of best corrected visual acuity of two or

more lines. Up to -12.00 D, good results can be achieved with more advanced PRK techniques and laser systems.

The refractive envelope of PRK is expanding with further refinements in both the procedure and technology, but the primary limitation remains patient variability in wound healing. Dr. Marguerite McDonald has cited the development of new wound healing modulators as an important evolutionary step in expanding the refractive envelope of PRK and improving clinical results within the realm of current PRK guidelines. What appears to be more surprising is any ability to achieve stable, near emmetropic refractive errors in cases of extreme myopia, while preserving corneal clarity. Clearly, it is not the amount of tissue removed but the technique by which it is removed. Retreatment rates of 25% to 100% are reported with the final outcome in many cases simply being a dramatic reduction in the degree of myopia, typically to within 1.00 to 2.00 D of emmetropia. The complications associated with PRK for extreme myopia chiefly center upon haze and irregular astigmatism. Confluent haze occurs in 4% to 15% of these cases, with optimal techniques developing opacification in only 4% to 5% of patients. The development of confluent haze typically requires retreatment and prolongs visual recovery (Figures 7-3a through 7-3d). Irregular astigmatism similarly improves with time and delays visual rehabilitation, but is not amenable to medical or surgical intervention. Although not the norm, it should be recognized that visual recovery in certain PRK-treated cases of extreme myopia may require several months or longer. The incidence of irregular astigmatism approaches 100% immediately postoperatively but drops to about 10% after 1 month and 2% to 3% by 6 months. Only 1% to 2% of these extremely myopic candidates will experience a permanent loss of best corrected visual acuity of two or more lines with advanced PRK techniques for high myopia correction. The most common visual complaint, however, is related to the tremendous disturbances in night vision that these patients perceive. Additionally, extremely myopic patients with large pupils will complain of poor qualitative vision in any condition with low illumination as spherical aberration is induced.

SUMMARY OF MYOPIA TREATMENT

In summary, approximately 95% of mild myopes achieve 20/40 uncorrected visual acuity, with 75% measuring 20/25 or better. At least 90% of moderate myopes below -6.00 D achieve 20/40 or better vision uncorrected visual acuity, with about half exceeding 20/25. Severe myopes

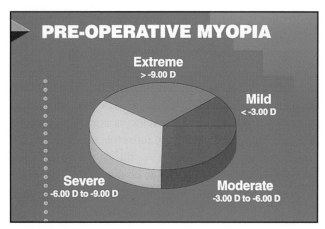

Figure 7-4.
Pie chart of 392 eyes entered into Chiron Technolas multi-multizone PRK treatment study. The patients were divided into study groups based upon their level of preoperative myopia, with the largest group having a spherical equivalent between -6.00 and -9.00 D. All eyes treated by the author.

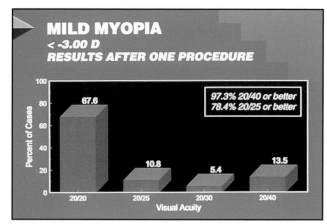

Figure 7-5.
Mild myopia (-1.00 to -3.00 D) PRK treatment group uncorrected visual acuity results. All eyes had 6 to 12 months follow-up. After one procedure, 97.3% of eyes attained 20/40 uncorrected visual acuity with 78.4% 20/25 or better.

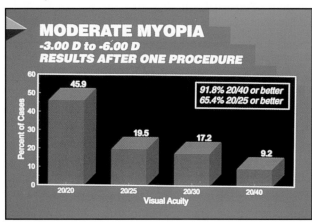

Figure 7-6.
Moderate myopia (-3.10 to -6.00 D) PRK treatment group uncorrected visual acuity results. All eyes had 6 to 12 months follow-up. After one procedure, 91.8% of eyes attained 20/40 uncorrected visual acuity with 65.4% 20/25 or better.

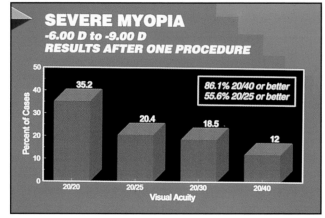

Figure 7-7.
Severe myopia (-6.10 to -9.00 D) PRK treatment group uncorrected visual acuity results. All eyes had 6 to 12 months follow-up. After one procedure, 86.1% of eyes attained 20/40 uncorrected visual acuity with 55.6% 20/25 or better.

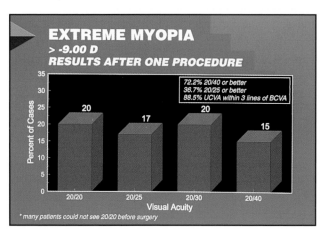

Figure 7-8.
Extreme myopia (>-9.10 D) PRK treatment group uncorrected visual acuity results. All eyes had 6 to 12 months follow-up. After one procedure, 72.2% of eyes attained 20/40 uncorrected visual acuity with 36.7% 20/25 or better. More impressive clinical results were achieved when reduced best corrected vision was taken into account, but a subset of patients demonstrated clinically significant side effects, most commonly night glare and complications. Dense confluent haze reducing best corrected visual acuity by two or more lines was observed in just under 5%. Retreatment for continued myopic regression over 12 months was performed in approximately one in four patients.

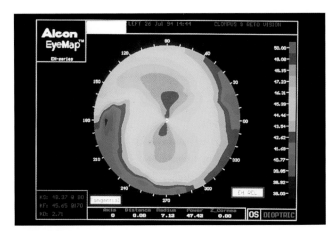

Figure 7-9a.
EyeMap corneal videokeratography demonstrating preoperative with-the-rule cylinder.

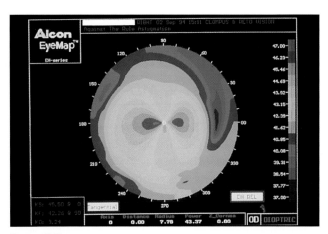

Figure 7-9b.
EyeMap corneal videokeratography demonstrating preoperative against-the-rule cylinder.

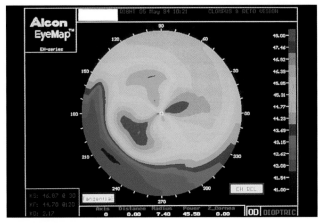

Figure 7-9c.
EyeMap corneal videokeratography demonstrating preoperative oblique symmetrical cylinder.

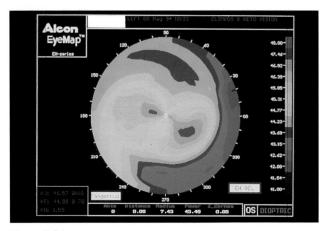

Figure 7-9d.
EyeMap corneal videokeratography demonstrating preoperative oblique symmetrical cylinder.

between -6.00 and -9.00 D achieve 20/40 uncorrected vision in about 75% of patients with about one third reading 20/25 or better. The results above -9.00 D for cases of extreme myopia less than -15.00 D are highly variable and much less predictable as myopic regression occurs in a high percentage over the first year. In general, about 50% are able to achieve an uncorrected visual acuity within three lines of their best corrected vision, which is often reduced, after one procedure, with only 10% to 15% reaching within one line of their best corrected vision. Above -15.00 D, multiple procedures are required and the final outcome is variable.

Although newer software algorithms and laser systems demonstrate improved predictability below and above -9.00 D, PRK above -9.00 D is clearly associated with more complications. Some series with newer scanning and multizone algorithms demonstrate an almost equivalent predictability

between moderate and severe myopes with about 90% of these candidates achieving 20/40 uncorrected visual acuity. Significantly improved extreme myopia results up to -15.00 D are observed with these newer PRK applications with 70% to 80% of patients capable of reading within three lines of their best corrected visual acuity after a single procedure. The results in the severely myopic population remain a challenge and have been quite variable as well as technique and laser dependent (Figures 7-4 through 7-8).

ASTIGMATISM

In general, astigmatism correction is not as predictable as myopia correction. Two issues of concern with respect to cylinder predictability are magnitude of correction and axis

Results of PRK for High Myopia

Louis E. Probst V, MD

The results for PRK for varying degrees of high myopia are summarized in Table C-1. The studies originate from nine different countries and date back to 1993. While the Summit ExciMed is the most common excimer laser, the VisX 20/20 and 20/15, the Aesculap-Meditec MEL 60, and the Chiron Technolas Keracor 116 were also used. Some surgeons used multizone ablations in order to decrease the ablation depth,

myopic regression, and haze.[3,4,6,8,10,13-15]

Attempted ablations ranged from -6.0 to -27.0 D. Between 28% to 85% of eyes were within 1 D of emmetropia, with better results for the less than -10.0 D corrections.[1,13-15] Uncorrected visual acuity of 20/40 or better was achieved by 26% to 100% of patients, again with better results with less than -10.0 D corrections.[10,13] Up to 33% of patients lost two or more

TABLE C-1
RESULTS OF PRK FOR HIGH MYOPIA

Author/Year	Country	Laser Type	Ablation Zone (mm)	Number of Eyes	Follow-Up	Attempted Correction	± 1 D (%)	20/40+ Uncorrected (%)	Loss of Two Snellen Lines (%)	↑ IOP (%)	Other 12 Month Complication
Brancato et al, 1993[1]	Italy	Summit ExciMed	3.5 -5.0	39	12	-10.0 to -25.0	28	NR	8	25	9% anisocoria 10% >1 mm decentration
Kim et al, 1993[2]	Korea	Summit ExciMed	5.0	67	12	-7.25 to -13.5	52	63	18	24	10% glare/halos 21% blurred vision
Heitzmann et al,1993[3]	USA	VisX 20/20	4.0+5.0 +6.0	23	12	-8.0 to -19.5	39	57	0	NR	30% regression ≥1.75 74% halos/starburst
Rogers et al, 1994[4]	Australia	Summit ExciMed	3.6-4.5 +5.0	14	12	-10.25 to -20.5	71	NR	0	NR	50% retreatment for regression and haze
Sher et al, 1994[5]	USA	VisX 20/20 or 20/15	5.5-6.2	47 / 40	6 / 12	-8.0 to -15.25	40 (47) / 58 (81)	49 / 60	NR / 15	0	23% retreatments () at 6 to 16 months
Krueger et al, 1995[6]	USA	VisX 20/20	4.0+5.0+6.0 5.0+5.5+6.0 (+nitrogen)	14	6	-10.37 to -24.5	29	NR	21	NR	29% retreatment 14% severe haze
Amano et al, 1995[7]	Japan	Summit ExciMed	5.0	21	24	-6.1. to -14.0	52	NR	NR	NR	3% ≥2+ haze
Rajendran et al, 1995[8]	India	Summit OmniMed	4.5+5.0+6.0	124	6	-8.0 to -22.5	NR	48	33	NR	25% retreatment
Chan et al, 1995[9]	Singapore	Summit ExciMed	5.0	66	12	-6.2 to -11.9	34	75	0	8	3% moderate haze
Menezo et al, 1995[10]	Spain	Aesculap-Meditec MEL 60	7.0 (tapered)	88 / 45	12 / 12	-6.0 to -12.0 / -12.5 to -22.0	78 / 37	NR / 26	0 / 7	10	1% haze in high myopia
Hardten et al, 1995[11]	USA	VisX 20/15	5.0 -6.2	65	6	-8.0 to -15.0	47	76	12	NR	10% haze ≥ 2
VisX 20/15 Study, 1995[11]	USA	VisX 20/15	5.0-6.2	45	12	-10.4 ± 1.6	42 (53)	NR	22	NR	29% retreatment ()
Durrie et al, 1995[12]	USA	Summit ExciMed	NR	10	12	-6.0 to -9.0	60	100	0	NR	
Pop et al, 1995[13]	Canada	VisX 20/20	2.5 +3.5-6.0 (multizone)	92 / 37	6 / 6	-6.0 to -10.0 / -10.1 to -27.0	85 / 60	92 / 60	2 / 19	NR	minimal haze no central islands

lines of best corrected Snellen acuity, with many studies demonstrating this level of loss in about 20% of eyes.[2,6,8,11,13] Ocular hypertension was noted following the PRK in 0% to 25% of eyes.[1,5] Retreatment rates were very high in many of the studies at 23% to 50%.[4-6,8,11]

Recent studies utilizing multizone ablation patterns have reported the most successful results, with 81% to 85% of eyes within 1 D of emmetropia and 74% to 92% of eyes with at least 20/40 uncorrected visual acuity for corrections from 6.0 to -10.0 D of myopia.[13,14] The results for greater than -10.0 D corrections are less impressive, with 70% to 80% of eyes within 1 D of emmetropia and 60% to 69% of eyes with at least 20/40 uncorrected visual acuity.[13,14] The loss of two or more Snellen lines of best corrected visual acuity for 6% to 33% of eyes in the greater than -10.0 D multizone corrections is concerning.[6,8,13,15]

The PRK results for high myopia are far less impressive than those for the mild to moderate myopia groups.[1,2,7] The efficacy, predictability, and safety of PRK for myopia appears to diminish as the level of attempted correction is increased. While multizone ablation protocols have improved the results of surface PRK for less than -10.0 D corrections, preliminary studies indicate that LASIK may be more successful for high myopia.[13,16]

References

1. Brancato R, Tavola A, Carones F, et al. Excimer laser photorefractive keratectomy for myopia: results in 1165 eyes. *Refract Corneal Surg.* 1993;9:95-104.

2. Kim JH, Hahn TW, Lee YC, et al. Photorefractive keratectomy in 202 myopic eyes: one year results. *Refract Corneal Surg.* 1993;9(Suppl 2):S11-S16.

3. Heitzman J, Binder PS, Kassar BS, et al. The correction of high myopia using the excimer laser. *Arch Ophthalmol.* 1993;111:1627-1634.

4. Rogers CM, Lawless MA, Cohen PR. Photorefractive keratectomy for myopia of more than -10 diopters. *J Refract Corneal Surg.* 1994;10(Suppl):S171-S173.

5. Sher NA, Hardten DR, Fundingsland B, et al. 193-nm excimer photorefractive keratectomy in high myopia. *Ophthalmology.* 1994;101:1575-1582.

6. Krueger RR, Talamo JH, McDonald MB, et al. Clinical analysis of excimer laser photorefractive keratectomy using a multiple zone technique for severe myopia. *Am J Ophthalmol.* 1995;119:263-274.

7. Amano S, Shimizu K. Excimer laser photorefractive keratectomy for myopia: two year follow-up. *J Refract Surg.* 1995;11(Suppl):S253-S260.

8. Rajendran B, Janakiraman P. Multizone photorefractive keratectomy for myopia of 8 to 23 diopters. *J Refract Surg.* 1995;11(Suppl):S298-S301.

9. Chan W-K, Heng WJ, Tseng P, et al. Photorefractive keratectomy for myopia of 6 to 12 diopters. *J Refract Surg.* 1995;11(Suppl):S286-S292.

10. Menezo JL, Martinez-Costa R, Navea A, et al. Excimer laser photorefractive keratectomy for high myopia. *J Cataract Refract Surg.* 1995;21:393-397.

11. Hardten DR, Sher NA, Lindstrom RL. Correction of high myopia with the excimer laser: VisX 20/15, VisX 20/20, and the Summit experience. The VisX 20/15 excimer laser. In: Salz JJ, McDonnell PJ, McDonald MB, eds. *Corneal Laser Surgery.* St. Louis, Mo: Mosby; 1995.

12. Durrie DS, Schumer J, Cavanaugh TB, Gubman DT. Correction of high myopia with the excimer laser: VisX 20/15, VisX 20/20, and the Summit experience. The Summit experience. In: Salz JJ, McDonnell PJ, McDonald MB, eds. *Corneal Laser Surgery.* St. Louis, Mo: Mosby; 1995.

13. Pop M, Aras M. Multizone/multipass photorefractive keratectomy: six month results. *J Cataract Refract Surg.* 1995;21:633-643.

14. LaFond G, Balazsi G, Kadambi D, et al. Photorefractive keratectomy for low and medium myopia and astigmatism with the Chiron Technolas Keracor 116 excimer laser system: the Canadian experience. ISRS Mid-Summer Symposium and Exhibition; July 28, 1995; Minneapolis, Minn.

15. McGhee CNJ, Weed KH, Bryce IG, Anastas CN. Results of three zone, single pass PRK and PARK in eyes with greater than -8.00 D of myopia. ISRS Mid-Summer Symposium and Exhibition; July 28, 1995; Minneapolis, Minn.

16. Machat JJ. Multizone PRK versus multizone LASIK for high myopia: principles and results. ISRS Mid-Summer Symposium and Exhibition; July 29, 1995; Minneapolis, Minn.

of correction. A poorly understood relationship exists between the axis and magnitude of cylinder identified topographically and that identified on cycloplegic refraction (Figures 7-9a through 7-9d). Also, the cylinder axis and magnitude often differ on cycloplegic refraction compared to manifest refraction, and topographically, the degree and axis of the cylinder may differ once the epithelium has been debrided. The refractive astigmatism represents the net astigmatism, which is the sum product of the lenticular and corneal astigmatism, both anterior corneal and posterior corneal. Cylinder may be symmetric or asymmetric (Figures

> **Axis misalignment of 15° reduces efficacy by 50%.**

> **Cylinder correction least effective for very low (<1.00 D) and very high (>3.00 D) degrees.**

7-10a and 7-10b), despite the fact that spectacle correction is the same for both of these varieties. It may be orthogonal or nonorthogonal (Figure 7-11).

Noel Alpins, MD, has attempted to analyze astigmatism

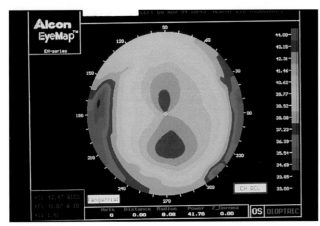

Figure 7-10a.
EyeMap corneal videokeratography demonstrating preoperative mild with-the-rule asymmetrical cylinder.

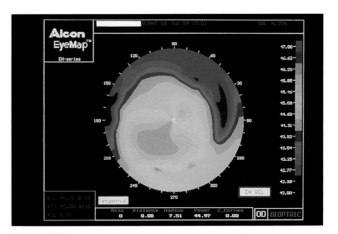

Figure 7-10b.
EyeMap corneal videokeratography demonstrating preoperative severe with-the-rule asymmetrical cylinder.

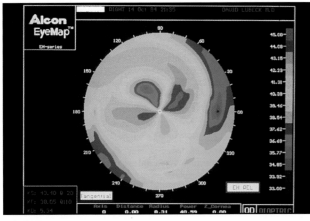

Figure 7-11.
EyeMap corneal videokeratography demonstrating preoperative non-orthogonal cylinder.

results utilizing a vector model. His analogy of a golfer putting is particularly appropriate, in that the putt may miss the cup related to either a stroke that is too strong, too weak, misdirected, or as a result of a combination of these factors. An error in cylinder axis will result in a significant loss of corrective effect in cylinder magnitude. Furthermore, the supine position may result in incyclotorsion of unknown significance. Point fixation of the eye, such as with forceps, often results in significant torsion of the eye with further induced cylinder errors.

TORIC ABLATION
Techniques

There are a variety of PRK approaches used to perform toric ablations with broad beam and scanning excimer laser

systems. Photoastigmatic refractive keratectomy (PARK) is an important element in achieving optimal clinical results, as 50% of candidates possess some degree of astigmatism. PARK approaches range from the Emphasis erodible mask developed by Summit Technologies to the scanning modality of the Chiron Technolas.

Clinical Note
Astigmatism Correction Delivery Systems

Broad Beam Astigmatic Delivery Systems

VisX 20/20 and STAR: Computer-controlled rotatable slit which expands along minus cylinder axis either alone (sequential program) or in combination with contraction of iris diaphragm (elliptical program). Large beam diameter passed through blades with rate of blade expansion controlling degree of cylinder correction.

Coherent-Schwind Keratom I/II: A broad beam is passed through a series of enlarging slit and oval apertures to create an elliptical ablation pattern.

Summit Apex Plus Erodible Mask: The Apogee system incorporates the Emphasis erodible mask to perform toric ablation patterns. The erodible mask corrects cylinder through a shape transfer process. Once again, a broad beam is used, but this time it is passed through a polymethylmethacrylate toric mask. Once the beam ablates through the thinnest portions of the mask, the ablation of the stromal surface begins at that site, reproducing the pattern of the mask onto the cornea. Any ablation pattern can be created and custom ablation patterns effected. The surface is also exquisitely smooth in the absence of diaphragmatic ridges. The erodible mask is inserted within a car-

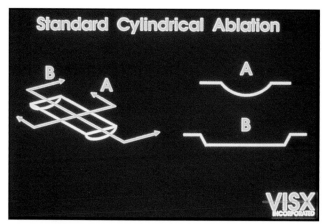

Figure 7-12a.
Graphic illustration of VisX sequential astigmatic ablation program. Note the steep contours created at the ends of the cylindrical trough which may be associated with arcuate haze formation.

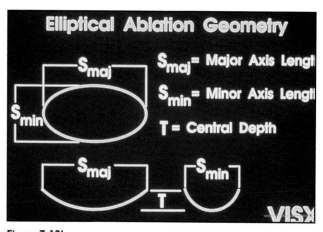

Figure 7-12b.
Graphic illustration of VisX elliptical astigmatic ablation program. Note the smoother contours of the astigmatic wound margin.

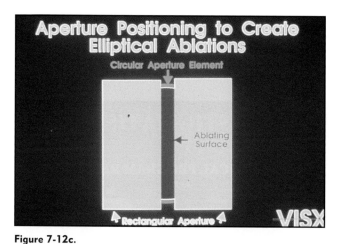

Figure 7-12c.
Schematic depiction of delivery system elements for VisX astigmatic programs. Rotatable and expandable linear slit is oriented along minus cylinder axis during sequential and elliptical astigmatic ablation programs. Circular iris diaphragm which contracts in concert with elliptical program.

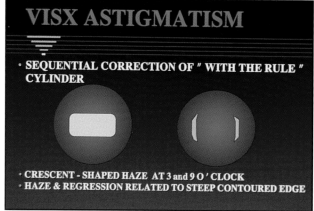

Figure 7-13.
Schematic representation correlating VisX sequential astigmatism program and arcuate haze formation along steep wound margins of cylindrical trough.

tridge and introduced into the optical rail. Previous attempts with the OmniMed series to place the mask, supported on a quartz window (ultraviolet light transmissible), in an eyecup on the surface of the eye presented difficulties with respect to both alignment and refractive predictability. The introduction of the mask in the rail SVS Apex Plus system has improved both predictability and the ease of performance of the procedure.

Scanning Astigmatic Delivery Systems

Aesculap-Meditec MEL 60: The scanning slit delivery system of the MEL 60 uses a rotating hand-held mask that is placed over the eye. The laser scans a 2.0 by 7.0 mm vertical slit beam across the mask which is specifically designed for creating cylindrical ablation patterns. The mask rotations create an asymmetric ablation pattern, rather than the symmetrical patterns created with spherical myopic and hyperopic treatments.

Chiron Technolas Keracor 116/117: The hybrid delivery system of the Technolas Keracor 116 treats myopia with an expanding iris diaphragm, and astigmatism with a scanning program. The Technolas Keracor 117 uses all scanning technology to treat both myopia and astigmatism. The scanning program creates toric ablations by

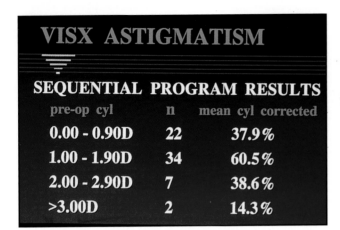

Figure 7-14a.
Refractive results following VisX sequential astigmatic treatment of 65 eyes with preoperative cylinder ranging from 0.50 to 4.75 D. Mean percentage of cylinder corrected was analyzed based upon degree of preoperative astigmatism. The sequential astigmatic program appeared to be most effective for moderate levels of preoperative astigmatism, and least effective for very low and very high degrees of cylinder.

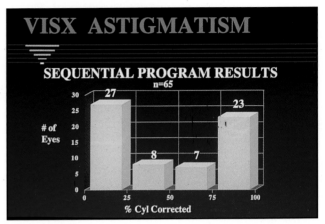

Figure 7-14b.
Bar graph demonstrating number of eyes treated with the VisX sequential astigmatic program that achieved 0% to 25%, 25% to 50%, 50% to 75%, and 75% to 100% of their preoperative cylinder corrected. The overall pattern of the graph illustrates that of the 65 treated eyes, roughly 40% did poorly, achieving less than 25% cylinder correction with approximately the same number demonstrating impressive clinical results, achieving greater than 75% cylinder correction. That is, the program either appeared to work very well or not at all, with little middle ground. Poor results were associated with arcuate haze and regression.

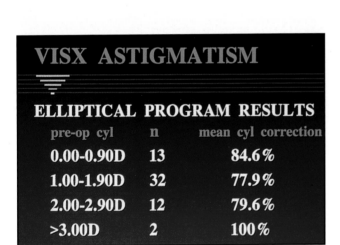

Figure 7-15a.
Refractive results following VisX elliptical astigmatic treatment of 59 eyes with preoperative cylinder ranging from 0.50 to 3.75 D. Mean percentage of cylinder corrected was analyzed based upon degree of preoperative astigmatism. The elliptical astigmatic program appeared to be almost equally effective for all degrees of preoperative astigmatism.

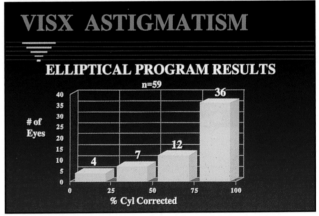

Figure 7-15b.
Bar graph demonstrating number of eyes treated with the VisX elliptical astigmatic program that achieved 0% to 25%, 25% to 50%, 50% to 75%, and 75% to 100% of their preoperative cylinder corrected. The overall pattern of the elliptical software graph illustrates that the majority of the 59 treated eyes, roughly two thirds, achieved greater than 75% cylinder correction. This pattern of cylinder outcomes is in direct contrast to the clinical results noted in Figure 7-14b with the sequential program. Less than a handful of eyes attained less than 25% cylinder correction. No cases of arcuate haze were observed, although diffuse reticular haze was evident in a number of patients.

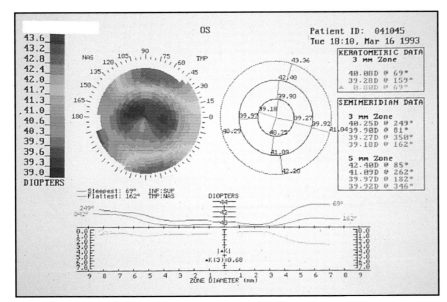

Figure 7-16.
Postoperative corneal videokeratography following VisX elliptical astigmatic ablation of -3.00 -3.00 x 180. Patient achieved 20/40 uncorrected visual acuity with residual spherical refractive error of -1.00 D.

ablating along the minus cylinder axis with an enlarging circular beam, increasing from about 1 to 4 mm in diameter. A trough, about 4 by 12 mm, is created with blended edges, helping prevent regression and haze formation.

Nidek EC-5000: The Nidek system uses a scanning slit which rotates 120° with each pass to improve blending. The astigmatic program scans a toric ablation pattern by preferentially scanning the minus cylinder axis to create an elliptical ablation pattern as horizontal blades expand.

LaserSight Compak-200 Mini-Excimer, CIBA— Autonomous Technologies Corporation Tracker-PRK laser system, Novatec LightBlade (non-excimer) laser system: These scanning systems all utilize flying spot delivery systems to create a toric ablation pattern. The correction of myopia with the LaserSight Compak-200 involves scanning layers of the cornea in a contiguous linear path, with each layer scanned in a semi-random angle to improve blending. The CIBA—Autonomous Technologies Corporation Tracker-PRK and Novatec LightBlade systems use a spiral program to treat myopia. The Novatec LightBlade is a solid-state titanium sapphire unit which utilizes approximately 213-nm (range: 200- to 215-nm) ultraviolet light to perform spherical and toric PRK.

VisX 20/20 Excimer Laser System
Elliptical and Sequential Programs

The VisX 20/20 Model B is equipped with two toric ablation programs: the sequential program and the elliptical program (Figures 7-12a and 7-12b). The elliptical program can only perform cylinder corrections if the accompanying

> **Percentage of cylinder corrected with VisX:**
> - Mean elliptical cylinder correction: 81%
> - Mean sequential cylinder correction: 49%

myopic sphere is equal or greater than the cylinder. It creates an elliptical ablation pattern by first correcting the cylinder with an expanding rotatable slit, followed by the contraction of the iris diaphragm for the spherical correction (Figure 7-12c). The sequential program creates a cylindrical trough through the expansion of the iris slit alone. It is utilized to correct cylinder in cases where it exceeds the degree of accompanying sphere. The elliptical program creates a smooth ablation pattern, whereas the cylindrical trough formed by the sequential program leaves steep edges which may result in greater regression of effect and crescentic haze (Figure 7-13). The sequential cylinder must be blended in with myopic sphere to smooth the trough edges; it should be programmed with an optical zone of 3.5 to 4.5 mm maximum. The smaller the optical zone, the greater the blending, but the smaller the visual window. It is the sphere correction, however, that will provide contour and reduce night glare with the sequential program. Plano-cylindrical corrections with the sequential program achieve variable clinical results.

In my clinical series, comparing the VisX elliptical and sequential astigmatic programs (Figures 7-14a through 7-15b), the elliptical program was able to achieve superior clinical results with less regression of effect (Figure 7-16). The toric ablation pattern produced by the sequential program appeared clinically either to produce excellent results

Figure 7-17a.
Preoperative corneal videokeratography of moderate oblique cylinder, with slightly non-orthogonal appearance.

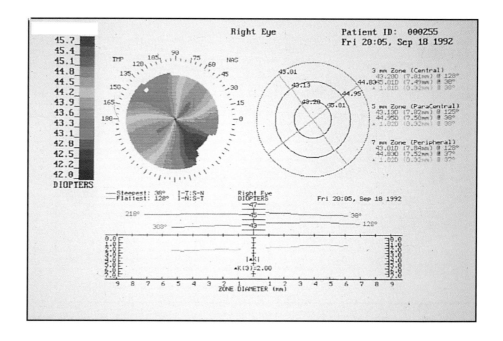

Figure 7-17b.
Postoperative corneal videokeratography demonstrating flattening along minus cylinder axis following VisX 20/20 Model B orthogonal toric ablation with elliptical program. Excellent clinical result achieved with 20/25 uncorrected vision 1 year postoperatively with 0.75 D of mixed astigmatism remaining.

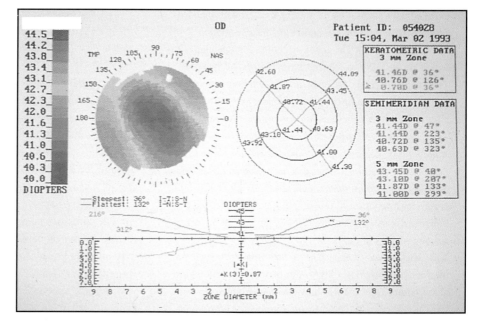

with preserved corneal clarity or arcuate haze and regression of effect with negligible benefit. While most VisX investigators prefer the elliptical program for cylinder correction whenever possible, surprisingly some investigators have reported superior clinical results with their sequential programs. The pattern of the cylindrical ablation with the sequential program compared to the elliptical program, however, violates fundamental principles by leaving a steep edge, which may invite haze and regression, as was observed clinically. That is, based upon the ablation profile, the clinical outcome was predictable. While approximately

40% of patients obtained greater than 75% correction with clear corneas and no regression, an additional 40% of patients obtained less than a 25% cylinder correction with crescentric haze and regression. Clinically, the steep edges left by the sequential program may result in haze and secondary regression if not adequately blended, which is dependent upon the attempted correction.

The VisX elliptical program created elliptical central islands and therefore requires an elliptical pretreatment, the amount of which was half the sphere with the same cylinder and axis at a 2.5-mm optical zone. As discussed in Chapter 5, central islands are created because of increased central hydration, resulting in reduced ablative efficacy centrally. A dry cornea increases effect of cylinder correction, and hydration plays an essential role in the magnitude of correction obtained. The elliptical software undercorrects sphere because of significant moisture produced during the cylindrical correction (Figures 7-17a and 7-17b). Drying the cornea with a blunt spatula helps to increase the spherical and cylinder effect while decreasing the formation of central islands.

Clinical Examples of VisX
Astigmatic Approaches
1. -1.00 -2.00 x 180

    Option 1: Sequential for 2.00 D at 4 mm followed by sphere for 1.00 D at 6 mm.

    Option 2: Sequential for 1.00 D at 4 mm followed by elliptical for -1.00 -1.00 x 180 at 6 mm.

    Option 2 is preferable because of improved wound healing, but both are commonly employed by VisX users.

2. -2.00 -2.00 x 180

    Option 1: Elliptical correction.

    Option 2: Sequential for 2.00 D at 4 mm followed by sphere at 6 mm.

    Option 1 is clearly preferable.

3. Plano -2.00 x 180

    Option 1: Sequential correction at 5 or 6 mm since no sphere to blend with. No other option, but results are variable. RK or a scanning excimer system is recommended.

4. +0.50 -2.00 x 180

    Option 1: Radial keratotomy or holmium.

    Not an excimer candidate at this time since sphere in minus cylinder form is hyperopic, even though the spherical equivalent is myopic. Could only be considered in a young patient where hyperopic outcome is acceptable.

Most investigators will correct as little as 0.50 D of cylinder for mild to moderate myopia and 0.75 D of cylinder for more severe cases. If topographical cylinder is in the same axis as that measured on refraction, and especially if of greater magnitude, then small amounts of cylinder correction are indicated.

Examples
1. Refraction: -4.00 -0.50 x 180

    Videokeratography:

a. -1.00 D at 180	Treat cylinder	
b. -1.00 D at 90	Do not treat cylinder	
c. Spherical	Surgeon discretion (usually no)	

2. Refraction: -4.00 D sphere

    Videokeratography:

a. Spherical	Treat sphere only	
b. -1.00 D at 180	Treat sphere only	
	(usually ok to leave WTR cyl)	
c. -1.00 D at 90	Surgeon discretion	
d. -1.50 D at 180	Surgeon discretion	
	(usually do partial correction if significant, eg, 0.50 to 0.75 D)	

Unfortunately, there are no absolute solutions and only clinical experience will help dictate personal guidelines. If there is a discrepancy between the videokeratography and refraction of a significant nature, the refraction should always be repeated. The treatment of the manifest refraction primarily, with influence of the videokeratography, is the guiding principle.

Treatment of spherical refractive errors with spherical PRK while ignoring with-the-rule cylinder of greater than 1.00 D may result in both spherical refractive outcomes and with-the-rule astigmatic outcomes. That is, I have treated patients with spherical refractive errors with astigmatic videokeratography based upon refraction alone, only to have their full cylinder manifest in their refraction postoperatively. On other occasions, I have treated identical patients similarly based upon their spherical refractive error only, and achieved emmetropia with no manifest cylinder, despite the residual cylinder on postoperative videokeratography. Therefore, preoperatively I attempt to push cylinder into the refraction at the videokeratographic axis in an attempt to discern individuals who may manifest postoperative cylinder. Intraoperatively, I will attempt partial correction of their cylinder if more than 1.00 D of cylinder is evident on videokeratography. The rationale behind Example 2d is that spherical treatment may result in plano -1.50 x 180, therefore intermediate treatment may be indicated.

More subtle problems arise where the axis on videokeratography and that of refraction measure differently. If 170° on manifest and cycloplegic refraction and 180° on videokeratography, 175° is a reasonable compromise. However, even a 5° shift will reduce the efficacy of the magnitude correction and may induce off-axis cylinder.

Toric ablation results are more predictable when cylinder magnitude and axis on videokeratography corresponds with that measured on refraction. The videokeratography should be used as a guide when performing the refraction to seek correspondence. The main determinant for attempted cylinder refraction should always be the manifest refraction and not the videokeratography values. That is, if manifest and cycloplegic refractions indicate 1.00 D or more cylinder

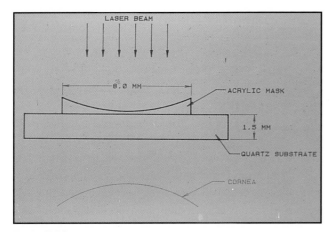

Figure 7-18.
Summit erodible mask performs toric ablations based upon shape transfer process rather than mechanical iris diaphragms. Masks act as a template during the ablation process, correcting cylinder by varying the thickness of mask along different meridians.

Figure 7-20.
Summit SVS Apex Plus with Emphasis erodible mask cartridge inserted into the optical rail.

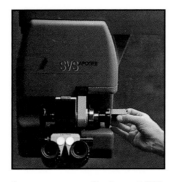

at 90° and videokeratography demonstrates cylinder at 180°, treat at 90°. If less than 1.00 D of cylinder, I will often ignore the cylinder and treat the spherical equivalent. When in doubt, treat the manifest/cycloplegic refraction.

SUMMIT OMNIMED EXCIMER LASER SERIES
Erodible Mask

The theory behind the erodible mask is unparalleled in that any toric ablation can be produced, whether symmetrical or asymmetrical, orthogonal or non-orthogonal (Figure 7-18). In addition, a smooth surface without steep edges or circular diaphragmatic ridges can be created. In clinical practice, however, the results of toric ablations have been variable, with approximately 50% predictability. Initially, the erodible mask was placed within an eyecup and balanced on the corneal surface. The mask was aligned with six red helium-neon beams which ensured the mask was perpendicular to the eye. The eyecup was further developed to maintain hydration, remove ablative debris, and better illuminate the mask intraoperatively. The combination of astigmatic keratotomy and PRK, which many international users opted for,

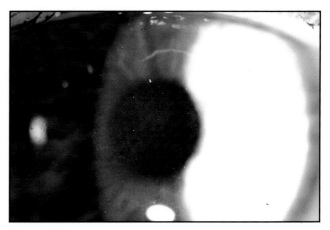

Figure 7-19.
Clinical photo of combined astigmatic keratotomy and PRK for compound myopic astigmatism correction.

was more predictable (Figure 7-19). Summit has currently developed a system to introduce the erodible mask into the optical rail system, which has improved predictability considerably to levels comparable to those achieved with diaphragmatic and scanning systems (Figure 7-20).

Clinical Note
Summit Vision Systems Apex Plus: Cylinder Correction

The SVS Apex Plus incorporates the mask in rail system for the correction of astigmatism and other refractive errors. The advantages of the erodible mask are unparalleled smoothness and unlimited potential for complex ablation profiles. In the original designs, the erodible mask-quartz substrate was supported within an eyecup manually held over the eye. Alignment and centration difficulties precluded reproducible clinical results. The clinical results of the prototype masks were disappointing. The incorporation of the Emphasis erodible mask into the optical pathway has not only simplified the procedure, but improved clinical results. The appropriate toric erodible mask is selected and inserted into the cartridge. The cylinder axis can then be dialed to the appropriate meridian. Performance of the actual PRK procedure is identical to that without the mask once inserted.

Variable correction of cylinder was previously observed, with a mean cylinder correction of approximately 50% recorded. Preliminary Italian results with myopic astigmatism correction observed slight overcorrection of sphere and slight undercorrection of cylinder (Brancato). Six-month results of 67 eyes treated for myopic astigmatism demonstrated 89% 20/25 or better uncorrected visual

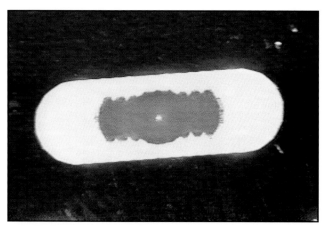

Figure 7-21a.
Chiron Technolas Keracor 116 excimer laser system ablation pattern of planocylindrical toric ablation pattern.

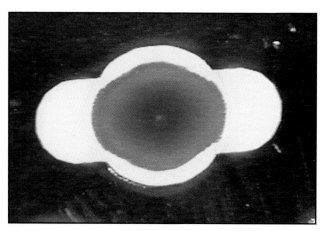

Figure 7-21b.
High myopia toric ablation pattern.

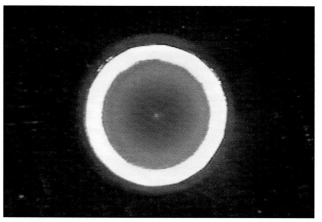

Figure 7-21c.
Spherical multi-multizone ablation pattern. White blend zone evident with all ablation patterns to reduce regression and haze formation.

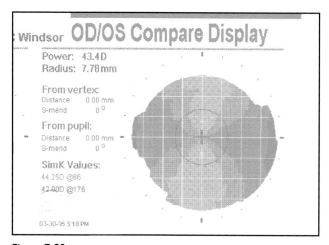

Figure 7-22a.
Preoperative Humphrey MasterVue Ultra corneal videokeratography demonstrating 2.25 D with-the-rule astigmatism.

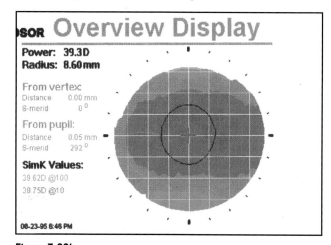

Figure 7-22b.
Postoperative Humphrey MasterVue Ultra corneal videokeratography demonstrating toric ablation pattern with 0.87 D of residual topographical cylinder, but spherical cycloplegic refraction.

acuity (Carones). Preliminary Australian astigmatic results with the Summit Apex Plus system have been very favorable, with approximately 70% cylinder correction, which is quite comparable to other excimer laser delivery systems (Rogers). The formation of central islands was noted, the pathology of which was likely the combination of a large optical zone (6.0 to 6.5 mm) and the more homogeneous (flatter) beam profile of the Apex Plus.

Preliminary hyperopic PRK results have been impressive, with more than 4.00 D of stable hyperopic correction reported (Rogers). In fact, overcorrection of hyperopia was observed, indicating that nomogram development may enable low and moderate degrees of mask hyperopic correction. Refinements will likely yield further clinical improvements with this technology.

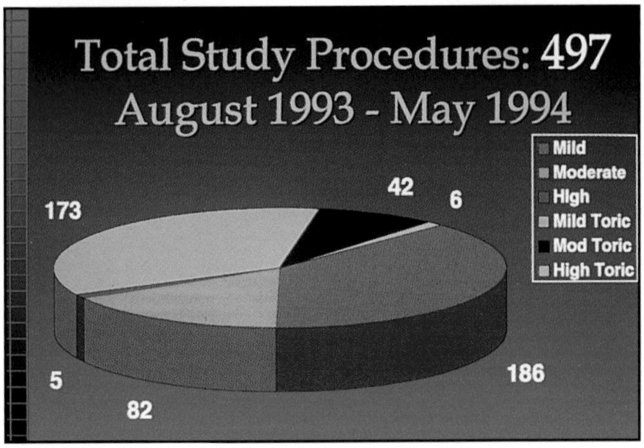

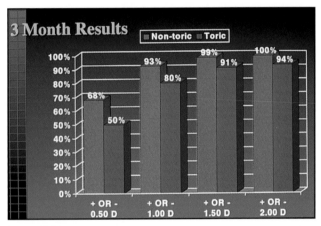

Figure 7-23a.
Canadian multicenter PRK trials of Chiron Technolas Keracor 116 excimer laser system. Pie chart illustration outlines preoperative degree of myopia and treatment protocols for 497 eyes enrolled for spherical and toric ablations during first 6-month phase of Canadian trials.

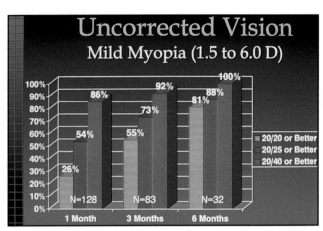

Figure 7-23b.
Efficacy of the Chiron Technolas Keracor 116 is reviewed with respect to quantitative vision. Uncorrected visual acuity results for spherical correction of mild to moderate myopia subset (<-6.00 D) PRK ablation results yielded 20/40 or better in all eyes in this group with 88% achieving 20/25 or better, and 81% attaining 20/20 or better unaided visual acuity at 6 months.

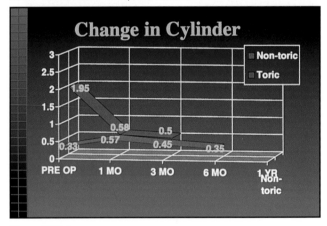

Figure 7-23c.
Refractive predictability results for toric and non-toric PRK ablations with at least 3 months follow-up. Toric ablations were not as effective as non-toric PRK ablations, with 80% of eyes within 1.00 D of emmetropia compared to 93% for spherical corrections.

Figure 7-23d.
Graph indicating improvement in cylinder from preoperative mean of 1.95 D to a postoperative mean of 0.50 D. Of equal clinical significance was that overall, spherical ablations were essentially astigmatism neutral.

CHIRON TECHNOLAS KERACOR 116
Scanning Toric Ablation

The Technolas Keracor 116 corrects astigmatism using the scanning mode of the laser with multiple PRKs performed along the minus cylinder axis 50 microns apart (Figures 7-21a through 7-22b). With each pass along the axis, the diameter of the ablation enlarges. The edges are blended leaving no sharp edges, and the cylindrical correction is not dependent upon the myopic correction, so that plano -6.00 x 180 can be treated and corrected. Although the cylindrical correction is performed sequentially, the scanning mode enables smooth contours to be created. Arcuate haze related to steep cylindrical edges is not observed with this PARK program. In general, combined myopic astigmatism is always better treated. Chiron Technolas mean cylinder correction is equivalent to that of the VisX elliptical program, with 80% efficacy. The limitations of axis and magnitude correction discussed throughout this chapter prevent the clinical results of cylinder correction from matching those achieved with spherical correction.

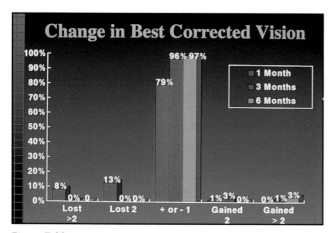

Figure 7-23e.
Safety of myopic PRK with the Chiron Technolas Keracor 116 was investigated, with no eyes reporting a loss of best corrected visual acuity in the specific study group at 6 months.

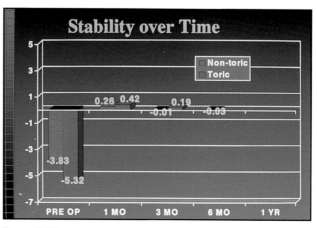

Figure 7-23f.
Stability of the Canadian Chiron Technolas Keracor 116 excimer laser clinical results was almost uniformly excellent by 6 months.

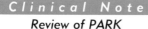

Review of PARK

Clinical results with myopic astigmatism correction have not been as impressive as those achieved in the treatment of spherical myopia. Clinical results have improved, however, with the evolution of excimer laser systems, nomograms, and increased insight into the variables limiting cylinder correction. Accurate axis alignment is one of the major limiting factors. Noel Alpins, MD, has performed a great deal of analysis in this complex area in an effort to better define the variables and provide methods by which we can analyze them. In one series, Taylor, Kelly, and Alpins compared 20 patients treated for myopic astigmatism with 32 patients treated for myopia alone. At 6 months, 85% (17/20) of the toric ablation group were within 1.00 D of emmetropia with 95% (19/20) reading 20/40 uncorrected, while 88% (28/32) of the spherical ablation group achieved the same refractive and visual result. In a later study with the VisX 20/20 laser, the same investigators

reported a larger series involving 139 consecutive PARK treatments compared with 107 spherical PRK procedures. The 12-month clinical results of the largest PARK series by the same Australian investigators are summarized in Table 7-1. In the PARK group, 68% of eyes were within 1.00 D of emmetropia with 72% achieving 20/40 uncorrected visual acuity. The spherical PRK group was observed to have a better outcome, with 87% of the 107 eyes at 6 months stabilizing to within 1.00 D of plano and 90% achieving 20/40 or better unaided visual acuity.

In another series reported by Spigelman, Albert et al, 70 patients treated with VisX 20/20 toric ablations were followed for 6 to 12 months with a mean postoperative sphere -0.14 D and mean postoperative cylinder of -0.54 D. Seventy-one percent at 6 months achieved 20/40 or better uncorrected visual acuity. The clinical results remained stable or improved slightly between 6 and 12 months.

Kim et al reported a series of 168 elliptical ablations. Mean preoperative astigmatism was reduced from 1.51 ±

TABLE 7-1
12-MONTH RESULTS FOR 333 PARK EYES

Degree of Myopia	Uncorrected Vision Better Than 20/20	Refraction Better Than 20/40	±1 D	±2 D
Low (<5 D)	47%	87%	89%	99%
High (5 to 10 D)	25%	71%	62%	88%
Extreme (>15 D)	2%	27%	28%	50%

0.81 D to 0.67 ± 0.60 D at 6 months. Overall reduction of cylinder was 55.6%, with the least improvement noted in patients with less than 1.00 D of preoperative cylinder. The axis of astigmatism also varied postoperatively, with less than half remaining within 10° of their preoperative axis.

The VisX 20/20 uses a mechanical iris diaphragm and rotating slit to create toric ablations. Utilizing the Aesculap-Meditec MEL 60 scanning excimer laser system and hand-held hourglass mask design, Dausch and coworkers found similar results. The metal mask rotates regularly over 360° and performs cylindrical ablations by varying the angular distances, increasing the depth of ablation in the desired meridian. With the ExciMed UV 200 laser, and even during erodible mask prototype development with the OmniMed series, Summit investigators combined AK and PRK to effectively manage compound myopic astigmatism. Ring, Hadden, and Morris compared a series of 40 eyes of spherical PRK combined with AK to a second series of 179 eyes treated with PRK alone. Preoperative myopia ranged from -1.50 to -13.50 D with a mean preoperative cylinder of -1.73 D, ranging from -0.75 to -4.00 D. The mean postoperative spherical equivalent in the 40 eyes was emmetropia, with mean residual cylinder of 0.32 D. This compared very favorably to the 179 eyes who received PRK alone. Uncorrected visual acuity was 20/40 or better in 75% of the PRK/AK treated eyes, with almost half achieving 20/20 unaided. Over 90% of the spherical myopia group achieved 20/40 or better uncorrected.

Hersh and Patel reported preliminary Summit erodible mask results from 25 eyes of 25 patients enrolled in the Phase IIb FDA clinical trial. In this trial, the hand-held ablatable mask system was utilized. Fifteen eyes received spherical ablations and 10 eyes toric ablations for up to 2.75 D of cylinder. All eyes measured less than 6.00 D of myopia. In the 10 eyes treated for compound myopic astigmatism, mean astigmatism decreased by less than half, from 1.48 to 0.86 D. Eighty-six percent of spherical myopes and 63% of astigmatic myopes achieved 20/40 or better uncorrected vision. Despite the theoretical advantages of the erodible mask shape transfer process, eliminating the need for a mechanical iris diaphragm and creating a smoother ablative surface, the preliminary spherical myopia results are worse than those reported by Summit without the hand-held mask. One third of eyes had a decentered ablation zone greater than 1.0 mm. As the erodible mask design evolved and was introduced into the optical rail in the SVS Apex Plus series, the clinical results also improved (see Clinical Note on Summit mask).

Overall, PARK is an effective modality in the treatment of myopic astigmatism. Alpins has developed a statistical regression formula based upon vector analysis and has reported a 90% success rate in cylinder reduction, but for the most part, 75% to 80% success rates remain the standard.

Clinical Results of the Technolas Keracor 116

Preliminary clinical results have demonstrated exceptional safety and efficacy. The preliminary 6-month data representing the overall Canadian Chiron Technolas Keracor 116 experience treated at five investigational sites are reviewed below (Figures 7-23a through 7-23f).

Spherical and Toric Corrections

Myopia <6.00 D: In the Canadian experience, for myopia less than -6.00 D, 104 eyes with less than 1.00 D of cylinder were treated, with 97 eyes (93%) achieving 20/40 or better and 75% achieving 20/25 uncorrected visual acuity. Mean preoperative myopia in this group was -3.79 D. Only one eye (1%) lost two lines of best corrected visual acuity. Ninety-two eyes (88%) were within 1 D of the intended correction. Toric ablations were performed on an additional 112 eyes with a mean sphere of -3.41 D in this range of myopia with up to 5.00 D of preexisting cylinder, with 86% achieving 20/40 or better uncorrected visual acuity and 69% achieving 20/25 or better vision. Preoperative mean cylinder was reduced from 1.58 to 0.65 D at 6 months. Eighty percent of eyes were within 1.00 D of the planned refraction at 6 months.

Myopia -6.00 to -10.00 D: Forty-two eyes with spherical myopia in the range of -6.00 to -10.00 D and a mean sphere of -7.70 D received non-toric ablations; 35 eyes (83%) achieved 20/40 or better uncorrected vision and 49% achieved 20/25 or better. No eyes lost two lines or greater of best corrected visual acuity. Thirty-three eyes (79%) were within 1 D of the target correction. Toric ablations were performed on an additional 36 eyes with 6 months data and a mean sphere of -8.03 D. Preoperative cylinder ranged from 1.00 to 12.00 D of myopia with a mean preoperative cylinder of 1.74 D, and was reduced to 0.53 D at 6 months. Uncorrected visual acuity was 81% for 20/40 or better and 55% for 20/25 or better for the toric treatment group. Seventy-nine percent were within 1.00 D of the attempted correction. One eye (3%) treated with a toric ablation and 6.00 to 10.00 D of myopia lost two or more lines of best corrected vision at 6 months.

Myopia >-10.00 D: Only eight eyes with more than

Clinical Results of PRK Following RK

Louis E. Probst V, MD

RK has been found to leave residual myopia in about 30% of eyes 1 year after surgery.[1] Undercorrected cases of RK tend to occur because of inadequate surgery with shallow incisions, inappropriate surgery with too few incisions and too large an optical zone, or unresponsiveness of the eyes to RK.[2] Further incisional surgery may not be possible because of maximal treatment and can produce an unpredictable result, with increased glare and increased diurnal variation.[3] Since PRK has been shown to be extremely effective for the treatment of simple or compound myopia, it is not surprising that a number of investigators have reported the use of PRK for the treatment of residual myopia after RK.

Many series have reported good results of PRK following RK with relatively few complications. McDonnell and coworkers were the first to report early results with a successful refractive effect in two eyes 3 months following surgery.[4] Seiler and Jean next presented the results of five eyes treated with PRK following RK and achieved results similar to those of PRK alone.[5] Hahn and coworkers[6] performed PRK on 10 undercorrected RK eyes, and found that 9 months following PRK, the visual acuity ranged from 20/25 to 20/50 in all cases and the mean manifest refraction decreased from -5.06 D preoperatively to -0.66 D postoperatively. Persistent haze in one eye at 9 months postoperatively was the only complication noted. Meza and coauthors[7] also performed PRK on 10 undercorrected eyes after RK, and achieved an uncorrected visual acuity of at least 20/40 in 80% (8/10) of eyes at 3 months and 100% (3/3) of eyes at 12 months follow-up. A hyperopic deviation of the refraction was noted over the 12 months of follow-up, and one eye developed increased haze with a transient loss of two lines of best corrected Snellen acuity. Durrie and coworkers[8] reported the results of 91 eyes of 71 patients who had previous RK, RK and AK, and AK alone. At 1 year, uncorrected visual acuity of at least 20/40 was achieved in 89.7% of eyes, and 75.9% of eyes were within 1 D of their intended correction. Subepithelial haze caused a loss of greater than two lines of Snellen acuity in 6.5% (2/29) of eyes at 12 months follow-up. Nordan and colleagues[9] achieved at least 20/40 visual acuity in 92% (11/12) of eyes previously treated with RK. One eye was overcorrected to +3.12 D SE and one eye developed mild haze which resolved at 6 months follow-up. Kwitko and coworkers[10] achieved at least

20/40 in 90% (9/10) eyes at 6 months follow-up; the incidence of haze was not reported. Finally, Lee and coworkers[11] reported the results of eyes with at least 24 months follow-up after PRK following RK. Eyes were divided into group 1 for residual myopia of -6.00 D or less, and group 2 for residual myopia of greater than -6.00 D. Uncorrected visual acuity of 20/40 or better was achieved in 86% (12/14) of group 1 and 50% (2/4) of group 2. Predictability within 1 D was achieved in 71.4% (10/14) of group 1 and 75% (3/4) of group 2. Complications included a persistent myopic shift through the 24-month follow-up in group 2 and significant corneal haze in one eye (6%).

Maloney and coworkers[12] have recently reported the results of the Summit Therapeutic Clinical Trial of PRK for the correction of residual myopia following RK. Interestingly, the results of this report were significantly less impressive than those of the previous studies, with a much higher incidence of complications. One hundred seven eyes underwent PRK for residual myopia after RK (90/107), AK (7/107), RK and AK (7/107), hexagonal keratotomy (1/107), and cataract surgery (2/107), and had 1-year follow-up. Only 74% achieved at least 20/40 or better visual acuity and 63% were within 1 D of intended correction. An alarming 29% of eyes lost two or more lines and 11% lost four or more lines of best corrected visual acuity. Moderate to severe central corneal haze in 8% of eyes and irregular astigmatism were felt to be responsible for the visual loss. The remarkable contrast of the results of this study with those of previous reports suggests that post-RK patients may be a very heterogeneous popoulation with a variable response to surgery.[2]

The recent results for TLC The Laser Center for the correction of residual myopia with PRK were reviewed. A Chiron Technolas Keracor 116 excimer laser was set to correct 60% to 70% of the residual myopia, recognizing that these eyes can have a variable refractive response. A sample of 39 recent cases with 6-month follow-up were reviewed. The mean preoperative SE residual myopia was -2.68 ± 2.31 D (range: -0.62 to -8.75 D) and the mean postoperative SE refractive error was -0.32 ± 0.75 D (range: +0.75 to -1.87 D). Ninety-two percent (36/39) of eyes achieved at least 20/40 visual acuity, and 79% of eyes were within 1 D of emmetropia. Retreatments were performed in 35.9% (14/39) of eyes. Four eyes (10%) lost two or more lines of best corrected Snellen acuity due to haze associated with regression; these eyes were retreated and all recovered to a loss of less than two lines of Snellen acuity.

These studies suggest that PRK offers an effective treatment for residual myopia following RK with an increased risk of postoperative haze. Conservative PRK with retreatments can still lead to excellent results despite the variable refractive response to PRK after RK. The postoperative haze and loss of best corrected visual acuity that can occur may be treated by enhancement procedures in most cases.

References

1. Waring GO III, Lynn MJ, Gelender H, et al. Results of the Prospective Evaluation of Radial Keratotomy (PERK) study one year after surgery. *Ophthalmology.* 1985;92:177-198.

2. Binder PS. A multicenter trial of photorefractive keratectomy for residual myopia after previous ocular surgery. *Ophthalmology.* 1995;102:1042-1053. Discussion.

3. Rashid ER, Waring GO III. Complications of radial and transverse keratotomy. *Surv Ophthalmol.* 1989;34:73-106.

4. McDonnell PJ, Garbus JJ, Salz JJ. Excimer laser myopic photoradial keratectomy after undercorrected radial keratotomy. *Refract Corneal Surg.* 1991;7:146-150.

5. Seiler T, Jean B. Photorefractive keratectomy as a second attempt to correct myopia after RK. *Refract Corneal Surg.* 1992;8:211-214.

6. Hahn TW, Kim JH, Lee YC. Excimer laser photorefractive keratectomy to correct residual myopia after radial keratotomy. *Refract Corneal Surg.* 1993;9(Suppl):S25-S29.

7. Meza J, Perez-Santonja JJ, Moreno E, et al. Photorefractive keratectomy after radial keratotomy. *J Cataract Refract Surg.* 1994;20:485-489.

8. Durrie DS, Schumer J, Cavanaugh TB. Photorefractive keratectomy for residual myopia after previous refractive keratotomy. *Refract Corneal Surg.* 1994;10(Suppl):S235-S238.

9. Nordan LT, Binder PS, Kassar BS, Heitzman J. Photorefractive keratectomy to treat myopia and astigmatism after radial keratotomy and penetrating keratoplasty. *J Cataract Refract Surg.* 1995;21:268-273.

10. Kwitko ML, Gow JA, Bellavance F. Excimer photorefractive keratectomy after undercorrected radial keratotomy. *J Refract Surg.* 1995;11(Suppl):S280-S283.

11. Lee YC, Park CK, Sah WJ, et al. Photorefractive keratectomy for undercorrected myopia after radial keratotomy: two year follow-up. *J Refract Surg.* 1995;11(Suppl):S274-S279.

12. Maloney RK, Chan W-K, Steinert R, et al. A multicenter trial of photorefractive keratectomy for residual myopia after previous ocular surgery. *Ophthalmology.* 1995;102:1042-1053.

-10.00 D of myopia and less than 1.00 D of cylinder had 6-month data available within this series, with a mean preoperative sphere of -11.49 D. Uncorrected visual acuity of 20/40 or better was achieved in 83% (five of the six) of eyes with data available, and none of the eyes lost more than two lines of best corrected visual acuity. Only four of the eight eyes (50%) were within 1.00 D of the attempted correction. There were an additional 11 eyes with 6-month data that were treated for myopia greater than 10.00 D and cylinder ranging from 1.00 to 5.0 D. The preoperative mean cylinder was reduced from 2.43 to 0.61 D. Half of all eyes reached 20/40 or better uncorrected visual acuity with only 13% obtaining 20/25 or better uncorrected vision at 6 months. Three of the 11 eyes within this severity of myopia and astigmatism lost two or more lines of best corrected vision after 6 months.

OVERVIEW

The more highly myopic a patient, the greater the degree of cylinder encountered. Over half of our patients over -9.00 D have 1.25 D or more of associated cylinder with a mean of 2.00 D and a range up to 6.00 D. Therefore, not only are higher myopes more likely to have combined myopic-astigmatic treatments, but the cylinder treated is usually more substantial. This will invariably reduce the predictability of clinical results with high myopia.

In addition, the nomogram for cylinder correction is 10% to 20% less predictable than that for spherical correction, typically undercorrecting. An adjustment is often introduced by the surgeon to compensate, which varies with the degree of cylinder attempted. In general, undercorrected cylinder is tolerated better than overcorrected cylinder. Also, a small amount of residual with-the-rule cylinder is stated to be better tolerated, although some series have expressed the reverse observation.

Most patients will tolerate 0.75 D of cylinder, especially if in the same axis as that to which they are accustomed. Most patients with 1.00 D or greater usually require further treatment. If associated with myopia, spherocylindrical, or even plano-cylindrical treatment can be performed once stable, typically at 6 months. Two refractions 1 month apart within 0.25 D, with no alteration in videokeratography, defines stability. AK is very effective in cases of residual mixed astigmatism.

Comparison of PRK and RK

It is difficult to compare the clinical efficacy of RK and PRK (Table 7-2) without addressing the limitations and risks of both procedures and placing them within the context of the marketplace, which always provides the final verdict. Both procedures alter the anterior corneal curvature, but through different well established mechanisms. Each procedure can be utilized to enhance the surgical outcome of the other procedure. The laser has been utilized to improve the results of patients who have had maximal RK, but not without increased risk of clinically significant haze and overcorrection. Similarly, patients have had RK/AK after the PRK to eliminate residual astigmatism and myopia.

The clinical efficacy and safety of RK and PRK appear equal for mild myopia correction, and for the most part moderate myopia as well, but PRK has a greater refractive envelope and is the decisive victor for higher degrees of myopia correction, especially in young female candidates. It is important to compare these procedures utilizing the most current RK and PRK techniques. Proponents for each often compare newer PRK techniques with the PERK study or newer RK nomograms and techniques with antiquated PRK studies with first generation laser delivery systems.

The primary benefit for PRK is the ability of the procedure to treat higher degrees of myopia without corneal destabilization which may produce fluctuating vision or even progressive hyperopia. Most importantly, PRK allows the new refractive surgeon to achieve good clinical results immediately and safely because of a shallower learning curve relative to RK. Both refractive procedures are relatively quick and painless for the patient. PRK remains attractive to both patients and surgeons alike because of the aura which surrounds lasers with respect to both precision and marketability.

The primary issues for RK are speed of visual rehabilitation, lower cost to both the patient and surgeon, and reduced postoperative care and medications.

Reduced postoperative discomfort is often cited by RK proponents but the introduction of Voltaren and a bandage contact lens by Neal Sher, MD, has truly provided an effective means of pain control for the overwhelming majority of PRK patients. The most impressive clinical factor for myopic candidates still appears to be the rapid recovery of vision which often allows RK patients to see well the same or the following day. Most RK patients

TABLE 7-2
COMPARISON OF RK AND PRK

	PRK	RK
Surgeon Skill Dependence	+	+++
Patient Ease of Procedure	++++	+++
Efficacy		
Mild Myopia Correction	++++	++++
Moderate Myopia Correction	++++	+++
Severe Myopia Correction	++	+
Enhancements	+	+++
Side Effects		
Intraoperative Comfort	++++	++++
Postoperative Comfort	+	+++
Visible Scarring Early	++	+
Visible Scarring Late	-	+
Fluctuating Vision	-	++
Night Glare	+	++
Postoperative Care		
Postoperative Recovery	+	+++
Visual Rehabilitation	+	+++
Postoperative Medications	+++	+
Topical Steroid Requirements	+++	-
Safety	++++	++++
External Corneal Infection Risk	+++	+
Intraocular Infection Risk	-	+++
Visual Axis Involvement	++++	-
Corneal Integrity	++++	++
Invasiveness	+	++++
Long-Term Stability	+++	+++
Myopic Shift	++	+
Hyperopic Shift	-	+
Economic Cost	+++	+
Surgeon	+++	+
Patient	++++	++

return to work and daily routines within 48 hours. PRK takes several days for driving vision and a month for full visual recovery. Stabilization of vision with both procedures may take several months. Bilateral simultaneous surgery is easier to perform with RK, as the rapid visual rehabilitation does not incapacitate the patient for a considerable length of time as is sometimes the case with PRK. Fluctuating vision and night visual disturbances, although observed with both refractive procedures, are notably more problematic for RK patients. Incisional refractive surgery requires a higher enhancement rate to achieve equivalent refractive predictability compared to surface photoablation. RK enhancements, however, can be performed earlier and are associated with a much more rapid patient recovery.

PRK appears to have an edge in preserving ocular integrity, in light of the fact that RK incisions are almost full thickness, whereas PRK incisions only penetrate about 10% depth. Although the eye is more vulnerable to injury with RK, it is not a realistic argument for PRK proponents as the injury would have had to be so severe so as to have risked loss of the eye even if surgery had never been performed.

The incidence and variety of postoperative infections also differs in that the external infection risk is slightly higher following PRK than RK, but a perforating RK incision may produce infective endophthalmitis.

The clinical appearance of the eye following incisional refractive surgery differs considerably from that of surface photoablation. Visible signs of scarring are always identifiable with RK, but microscopic corneal changes associated with PRK become invisible over time. Most PRK patients develop trace degrees of haze during remodeling of the anterior corneal stroma, which clears completely after a year. Although RK has the distinct advantage of avoiding the visual axis, rare patients who develop severe stromal haze reducing vision can be retreated effectively with therapeutic modalities with few exceptions. In practice, central corneal scarring no longer appears to be a major concern with PRK for mild to moderate myopia correction.

Night glare is common with all refractive procedures, but newer PRK techniques and laser delivery systems which treat a larger effective optical zone have reduced the incidence of night visual disturbances considerably.

Starbursting of car headlights at night following RK is common but usually disappears or reduces in intensity after about 6 months. The degree of myopia treated and the size of the surgical optical zone remain the most important determinants of persistent night glare for both refractive procedures.

Diurnal variation in vision as stated is a complaint typically associated with incisional refractive procedures, not PRK, and is quite debilitating in some RK patients, necessitating multiple pairs of glasses. Many refractive surgery patients require night driving glasses independent of the refractive procedure performed. The multifocal nature of the RK cornea actually enables some RK patients to have excellent near and distance vision, avoiding reading glasses, a phenomenon which is rare following PRK.

Long-term stability and efficacy has yet to be fully determined for PRK and has been better evaluated with RK, which has been performed for over two decades. PRK has been performed for less than a decade and less than 5 years with any significant volume. The same can be said of RK, in that the RK of today differs considerably from that of the RK performed a decade ago. An active controversy remains concerning the true risk of hyperopic shift following RK, which has been reported in 10% to 30% of patients in some long term RK series. New instrumentation and more conservative RK techniques are anticipated to provide improved long-term stability. No hyperopic shift with PRK has been observed, and European data have not shown any long term safety issues with PRK. The removal of 50 to 100 microns of anterior stromal tissue does not appear to destabilize the cornea, a fact previously noted with lamellar procedures. The overwhelming majority of PRK patients remain stable after several months.

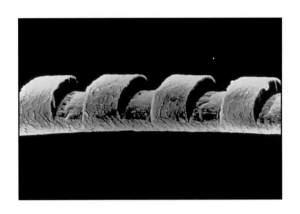

Section II
LASIK

CHAPTER 8

LASIK: Fundamental Concepts and Principles

Laser in situ keratomileusis, or LASIK, is a procedure that combines well-established lamellar surgical techniques practiced for three decades with the precision of photorefractive keratectomy (PRK). The primary limitation of PRK is wound healing. LASIK addresses this limitation by performing the ablation within the relatively inert stromal bed, which dramatically improves visual rehabilitation, and reduces both postoperative pain and susceptibility to infection, while virtually eliminating stromal haze formation. LASIK, however, is associated with a new set of limitations, primarily those associated with the creation of the corneal flap.

There is no procedure that is ideal for every patient; LASIK, however, is very likely the closest to an all-encompassing procedure at present. Requiring greater technical skill than PRK, LASIK represents a more complex procedure for altering the refractive properties of the cornea utilizing the excimer laser. LASIK is a procedure which is still rapidly developing, both in terms of technique and perioperative patient management. The long history of lamellar surgery provides us with an abundance of fundamental principles upon which the lamellar aspects of LASIK should evolve. The parameters of performing photoablation within the stromal bed must be re-evaluated, however, since factors such as altered mid-stromal wound healing, greater midstromal hydration, and proximity to the endothelium must all be considered. LASIK is still an evolving technique. The greatest areas of evolution for LASIK will be improvements

in microkeratome and laser software design. My clinical experience has been with the Chiron-Steinway microkeratome unit.

ROLE OF LASIK IN REFRACTIVE SURGERY

Refractive surgery can be subdivided into four areas:
1. Incisional techniques
2. Lamellar techniques, such as automated lamellar keratoplasty (ALK) and myopic keratomileusis
3. Laser techniques, such as PRK and laser thermokeratoplasty (LTK)
4. Intraocular and corneal lenses

Techniques such as LASIK combine both lamellar and laser techniques.

Incisional techniques include both AK and RK. In the 1890s, Leendert Jan Lans performed the first systematic study of incisional surgery for the management of astigmatism. In 1943, Tutomu Sato performed the first human keratotomy, utilizing an anteroposterior keratotomy approach, as the importance of the endothelium was not adequately appreciated at the time, resulting in corneal decompensation. In 1960, Fyodorov pioneered modern RK with an anterior keratotomy approach, which was introduced to the United States in 1978 by Leo Bores.

There have been a number of significant advances in

Development of LASIK

Ioannis Pallikaris, MD

As a modality, LASIK was introduced, designed, and developed at the University of Crete and the Vardinoyannion Eye Institute of Crete (VEIC) in 1988. Its introduction in the international literature is as follows. The first animal studies began in 1987, using a Lambda Physik excimer laser and a specially designed microkeratome (Figure A-1). The keratome was thus designed to produce a 150-micron flap instead of a cap. The whole idea came from the fact that an operation like PRK would destroy the Bowman's layer and affect corneal innervation and healing. The first studies were thus aimed in this direction.[1] Having the parameters and optics of the excimer laser determined, studies were performed on wound healing reaction on rabbit eyes, using the first specially designed microkeratome and the Lambda Physik excimer laser.

LASIK, the acronym for laser in situ keratomileusis, is a term that I suggested to describe a combination of excimer laser in situ keratomileusis under a hinged corneal flap (Figure A-2).[2] Many ophthalmologists refer to techniques similar to LASIK, creating confusion. For example, Buratto's technique,[3] although an in situ keratomileusis using the excimer laser, is performed under a cap. It does not use a flap; it is not LASIK. Laser intrastromal keratomileuses with other lasers does not involve flaps; they are not LASIK.

The breakthrough in my philosophy was the thought to create a corneal flap and to combine it with the excimer laser submicron accuracy of stromal tissue removal. My initial theory was that a flap would assure better fitting of tissues after removing the intrastromal tissue with laser and would not affect the anatomic relations of corneal layers mainly by two ways: preservation of Bowman's layer and better integrity of the nervous net at the superficial part of the cornea, as the latter follows at a great length its route through the base of the flap. Other important factors were the reduction of maneuvers and total time required for the operation. It is not coincidental that later on, during the 1993 American Academy of Ophthalmology meeting, LASIK was given the temporary name "Flap & Zap" by George Waring, MD. It reflects the alacrity of the operation. After all of these thoughts and studies, the next move was to design an appropriate keratome to perform the flap with and to study the healing factors.

On the other hand, the idea of a corneal flap is actually not

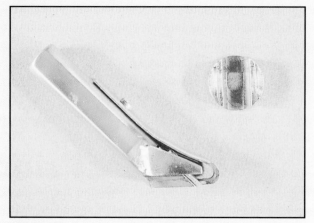

Figure A-1.
The first specially designed microkeratome for animal studies in LASIK.

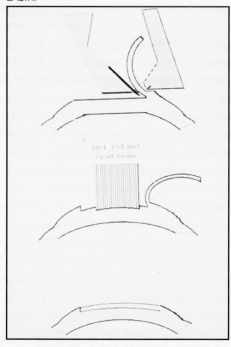

Figure A-2.
The first published diagram for LASIK.[2]

new. It was suggested much earlier by Pureskin, back in the late 1960s.[4] He attempted to do a flap manually and cut out the in situ part with a trephine; fairly crude by today's standards, but the idea was there. In the meantime, the first successful attempt of removal of corneal stromal tissue using the argon-fluoride excimer laser was published in 1983.[5] An earlier attempt to

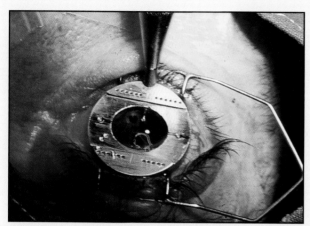

Figure A-3.
Application on the first blind eye of the specially modified microkeratome for LASIK. Note the oval opening and the side plugs along the path of blade excursion.

remove corneal tissue using a carbon dioxide laser had failed because of considerable tissue coagulation and scarring.[6] Other lasers, such as erbium-YAG, were reported as successful in modifying the corneal curvature by ablation of stromal tissue.[7]

The first papers on LASIK were presented during the Seventh European Congress of the ESCRS in Zurich in August 1989, and subsequently published in 1990.[1] The first LASIK on a blind human eye was performed in June 1989 (Figure A-3), part of an unofficial blind eye protocol. To date, we have published several articles concerning healing of partially sighted eyes,[8,9] results on partially sighted eyes,[10] a comparative study of PRK laser in situ keratomileusis in partially sighted eyes,[11] and a series of normal sighted eyes with 2-year follow-up.[12]

References

1. Pallikaris I, Papatzanaki M, Georgiadis A, Frenschock O. A comparative study of neural regeneration following corneal wounds induced by an argon fluoride excimer laser and mechanical methods. *Lasers Light Ophthalmol*. 1990;3:89-95.

2. Pallikaris I, Papatzanaki M, Stathi EZ, Frenschock O, Georgiadis A. Laser in situ keratomileusis. *Lasers Surg Med*. 1990;10:463-468.

3. Buratto L, Ferrari M, Rama P. Excimer laser intrastromal keratomileusis. *Am J Ophthalmol*. 1992;15(3):291-295.

4. Pureskin N. Weakening ocular refraction by means of partial stromectomy of the cornea under experimental conditions. *Vestn Oftalmol*. 1967;8:1-7.

5. Trokel SL, Srinivasan R, Braren R. Excimer laser surgery of the cornea. *Am J Ophthalmol*. 1983;96:710-715.

6. Peyman GA. Modification of rabbit corneal curvature with the use of carbon dioxide laser burns. *Ophthalmic Surg*. 1980;11:325-329.

7. *Ophthalmology*. 1989;96:1160-1170.

8. Pallikaris IG, Papatzanaki ME, Siganos DS, Tsilimbaris MK. A corneal flap technique for laser in situ keratomileusis. *Arch Ophthalmol*. 1991;109(12):1699-1702.

9. Pallikaris IG, Papatzanaki ME, Siganos DS, Tsilimbaris MK. Tecnica de colajo corneal para la queratomileusis in situ mediante laser. Estudios en Humanos. *Arch Opthalmol* (Ed Esp). 1992;3(3):127-130.

10. Siganos DS, Pallikaris IG. Laser in situ keratomileusis in partially sighted eyes. *Invest Ophthalmol Vis Sci*. 1993;34(4):800.

11. Pallikaris IG, Siganos DS. Excimer laser in situ keratomileusis and photorefractive keratectomy for correction of high myopia. *J Refract Corneal Surg*. 1994;10(15):498-510.

12. Pallikaris IG, Siganos DS. Corneal flap technique for excimer laser in situ keratomileusis to correct moderate and high myopia: two year follow-up. Best papers of Sessions. ASCRS symposium on Cataract, IOL, and Refractive Surgery. 1994;9-17. *J Cataract Refract Surg*. In press.

improving RK in both technology and technique. The introduction of diamond and biphasic blades, ultrasonic pachymetry, microscopes, nomogram developments, and technique alterations in both the number and length of incisions have enhanced RK with respect to both safety and efficacy. Charles Casebeer, MD, revolutionized RK in the early 1990s, creating a systematic approach to RK and RK enhancements, with the development of conservative age- and gender-based nomograms and instructional courses. Publication of the 10-year Prospective Evaluation of Radial Keratotomy (PERK) study conducted by George Waring, MD, demonstrated good safety and efficacy, but reduced predictability compared to current RK techniques. The PERK study remains one of the best prospective evaluations of any medical procedure to date. The ARC-T multicenter trials similarly helped define parameters for AK and was headed by Richard Lindstrom, MD. Current

nomograms and RK techniques with biphasic blades developed by both Charles Casebeer, MD, and Kerry Assil, MD, achieve 20/40 or better uncorrected visual acuity in 93% to 99% of candidates with low to moderate myopia. Recognition of corneal instability resulting in progressive hyperopia from RK techniques utilized during the PERK study have led to the Mini-RK concept and technique, pioneered by Richard Lindstrom, MD. The current direction of RK has become part of a comprehensive refractive surgery strategy limiting RK to lower degrees of myopia, with more conservative nomograms utilizing larger optical zones with fewer and shorter corneal incisions. With the introduction of the excimer laser, and in a concerted effort to minimize RK side effects, reduce corneal instability, and maximize predictability, the envelope of RK is limited to the correction of lower degrees of myopia, usually less than 4.00 to 5.00 D of myopia.

Overview of Lamellar Refractive Surgery

Stephen G. Slade, MD

The following text is intended to provide a general summary of the current status of lamellar refractive surgical techniques, primarily ALK and LASIK.

DEVELOPMENT

Automated lamellar keratoplasty (ALK) and LASIK are relatively new techniques in the family of lamellar refractive keratoplasty. Lamellar refractive keratoplasty has its roots in the work of Jose Barraquer, MD, beginning in 1949 in Bogota, Colombia (Figure B-1). Dr. Barraquer developed myopic keratomileusis, which used the cryolathe to shape the cornea for a

refractive change (Figures B-2 through B-4). The main difficulties with myopic keratomileusis were the learning curve of the keratectomy and the complexity of the cryolathe. A keratome driven across the eye by hand is very dependent upon the speed of the passage to determine the thickness of the cut (Figures B-5 through B-7). Any irregularity in this cut will be exposed as irregular astigmatism in the patient.[1] The cryolathe itself was also a difficult instrument to master and maintain. Complications with myopic keratomileusis and lamellar keratoplasty included all the normal complications and risks with eye surgery in general, along with specific problems, such as

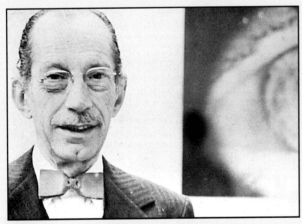

Figure B-1.
Jose Barraquer, MD, the father of modern lamellar refractive surgery.

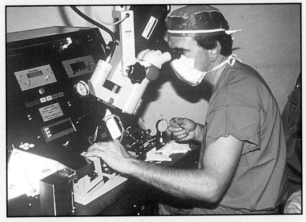

Figure B-2.
The cryolathe and master operator, Richard N. Baker, OD, FAAO.

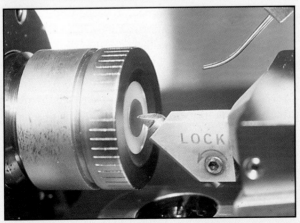

Figure B-3.
The corneal disc has been dyed and frozen to the lathe head and is ready for lathing.

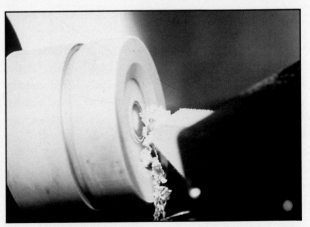

Figure B-4.
The lathe head spins and the cornea is lathed into a lens.

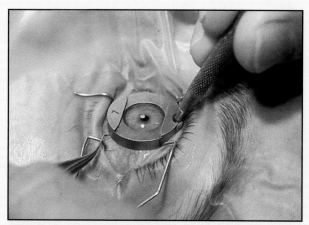

Figure B-5.
The single suction ring was set for one diameter. The ring fixates the globe, raises the pressure, and provides a track for the keratome.

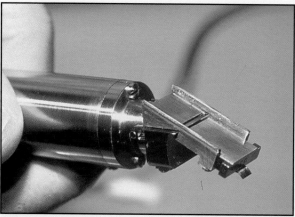

Figure B-6.
The Barraquer manual keratome had to be pushed across the eye by hand, requiring extensive training and skill.

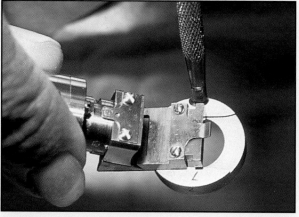

Figure B-7.
The keratome fit into the two dove-tail groves, but no mechanism was provided for forward movement.

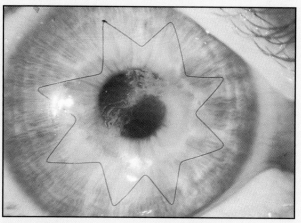

Figure B-8.
Epithelium in the interface in a MKM patient with the sutures still in, within 2 weeks postoperatively.

epithelial implantation of the stromal interface, and irregular astigmatism (Figure B-8). Good results were obtained initially by several investigators; however, the technique did not prove to be usable to a large number of surgeons in general (Figure B-9).[2,3] Several techniques were devised to improve results and simplify lamellar surgery, such as epikeratoplasty, where the surgeon was not required to perform the lathing and keratectomy (Figures B-10 and B-11).

The concept of raising a corneal flap and removing central tissue from the bed (keratomileusis in situ) was first described by Pureskin in 1966 (Figure B-12). Barraquer also worked with the keratome to remove tissue from the bed as a refractive cut, but preferred the cryolathe. Luis Ruiz, MD, working in Bogota, developed ALK to the current technique (Figure B-13). It was

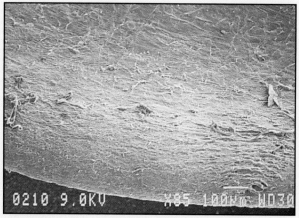

Figure B-9.
A scanning EM view of a cryolathed disc showing the fine surface.

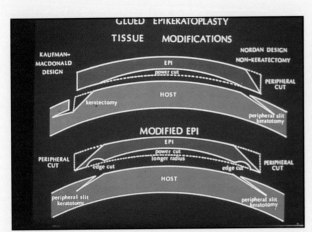

Figure B-10.
A schematic of epikeratoplasty of various techniques.

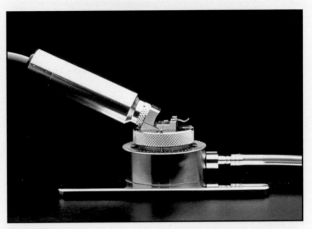

Figure B-11.
The Barraquer-Krumeich-Swinger keratome was an improvement over previous designs and introduced the concept of keratomileusis to many.

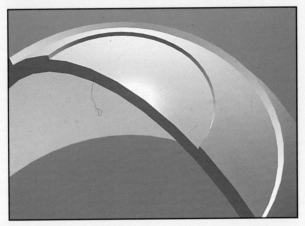

Figure B-12.
A schematic of keratomileusis in situ showing the two lamellar resections.

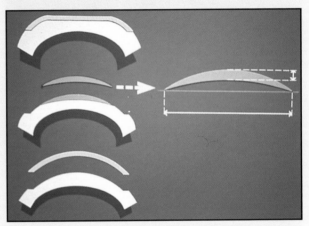

Figure B-13.
An early drawing of in situ keratomileusis showing the theoretical lenticle that was supposed to be removed.

the automated, or geared, keratome developed by Ruiz that made the technique available to a large number of surgeons (Figures B-14 and B-15).

THEORY

Barraquer developed several techniques that aimed to change the anterior curvature of the cornea by the addition or subtraction of tissue. This is in contrast to ectasia or bending procedures such as radial keratotomy and hyperopic ALK. In myopic keratomileusis (MKM), a subtraction technique used for myopia, a lamellar disc of anterior cornea is removed with the microkeratome and a cryolathe is used to remove tissue for the refractive change. In ALK, the keratome is used to make both the access and refractive cuts. In ALK, a lamellar, not lenticular, second disc of tissue is removed to reduce the myopia (Figure B-16). The effect depends on thinning the cornea and providing a knee effect at the edge of the keratectomy (Figures B-17 and B-18). An advantage of this knee is that the effective optical zone is larger than the resected cut (Figure B-19). LASIK, or excimer laser in situ keratomileusis, uses the keratome to make the access cut, and the excimer to remove the tissue for the refractive cut. The blended edge in typical LASIK produces a slightly smaller effective optical than the ablation (Figure B-20). Additional procedures such as keratophakia place a lens of tissue or synthetic material beneath a corneal flap.

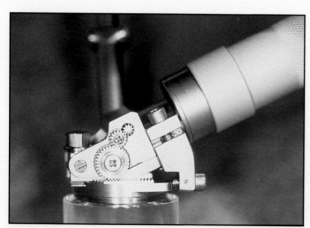

Figure B-14.
The geared keratome developed by Luis Ruiz and produced by Eric Weinberg, along with Hansa research and Chiron Vision.

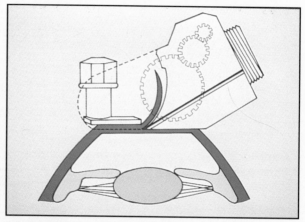

Figure B-15.
A schematic of the Ruiz keratome that demonstrates the gear mechanism that both propels the keratome across the eye and oscillates the blade.

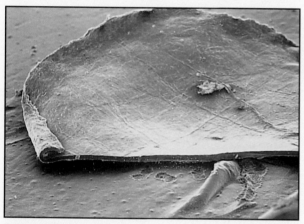

Figure B-16.
A SEM view of the actual lamellar disc that is produced in ALK-M by the keratome.

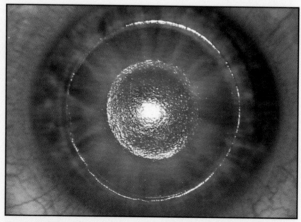

Figure B-17.
The actual bed of the cornea after the two resections.

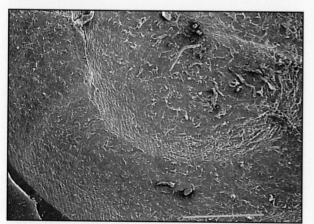

Figure B-18.
A SEM view comparable to Figure B-17.

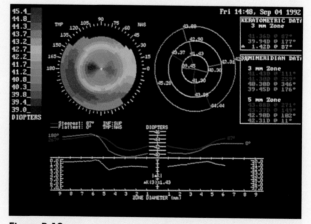

Figure B-19.
A topography view of ALK-M, which demonstrates that the cornea begins to bend at a larger diameter than the 4.2 resection.

Bending Procedures	Subtraction Procedures	Addition Procedures
RK	PRK	Keratophakia
ALK-H	ALK-M	Epikeratoplasty
LTK	LASIK	

Lamellar Procedure Resected	Access Cut	Refractive Cut	Lenticle
MKM	Microkeratome	Cryolathe	Lenticular
ALK	Microkeratome	Microkeratome	Lamellar
LASIK	Microkeratome	Excimer Laser	Lenticular

SURGICAL TECHNIQUE

Lamellar refractive surgery is done in an outpatient setting with topical anesthesia. As with all refractive surgery, extensive patient education and counseling is required. The patient must have an adequate knowledge of the procedure and realistic expectations. Oral sedation may be used but is not necessary. The patient is prepped and draped in the usual sterile fashion. It is important during the draping to create a clear path for the microkeratome. The patient is instructed to look at the microscope light and an inked marker is used to delineate the optical center, a pararadial line for orientation of the flap, and a 10-mm line close at the limbus to center the microkeratome (Figure B-21). A spacer device, or plate, is placed in the microkeratome to determine the thickness of the cut. This is typically 160 microns (Figure B-22). A suction ring is placed on the eye and engaged.

The suction ring fixates the globe, provides a geared path for the microkeratome, and raises the intraocular pressure so that a smooth keratectomy may be obtained (Figure B-23). A stopper device is often used to ensure the creation of a corneal flap (Figure B-24). After the first cut, which has a planned diameter of 7.5 to 8.0 mm, the suction ring is removed. The diameter ring is reset to 4.2 mm typically, and a second plate is placed which corresponds to the planned myopic correction. The suction ring is then replaced and a second cut is made after checking the diameter and the IOP of the eye (Figure B-25). The flap is then replaced and positioned, usually without sutures. The patient's eye is not patched and the patient is released from the clinic on antibiotic drops. The eye is examined the next day.

In LASIK, two different techniques are used (Figure B-26). The operation may proceed the same as ALK, but once the flap is made, the laser is used to ablate tissue from the bed in the planned correction, both sphere and cylinder. Alternatively, with the Buratto technique, a thick disc of tissue from 300 to 350 microns is removed completely from the eye. This is then placed beneath the laser stroma side up and ablated with the excimer laser (Figures B-27 and B-28). The disc of tissue, now a lens, is replaced on the eye. The treatment of hyperopia with ALK is an ectasia procedure. A thick flap cut is made, allowing the residual cornea to bow forward and steepen. Typically, this single cut must be at least 60 to 70% of the thickness of the cornea. The effect is graded by altering the diameter of the flap cut.

POSTOPERATIVE MANAGEMENT AND COMPLICATIONS

The patient is placed on topical antibiotics and steroids for the first 5 days. The first examination at day 1 is critical. The

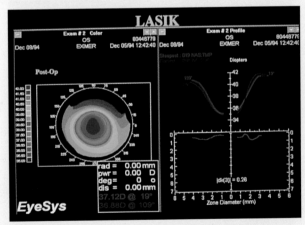

Figure B-20.
A LASIK topography that shows the smaller optical zone produced with a 7-mm multizone, broad beam LASIK algorithm.

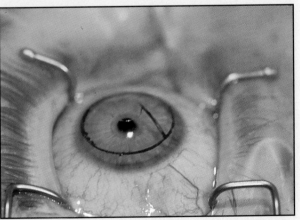

Figure B-21.
The cornea with good exposure, a clear mark, and ready for the keratectomy.

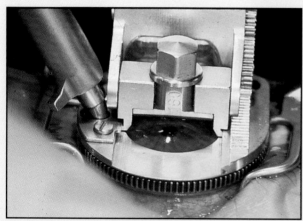

Figure B-22.
The keratome, 160 micron, in place being driven across the cornea.

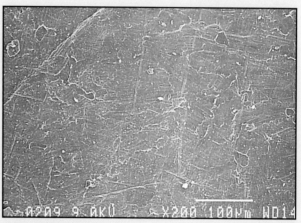

Figure B-23.
A SEM view at 200 power that demonstrates the fine smoothness that is produced with the geared Chiron keratome.

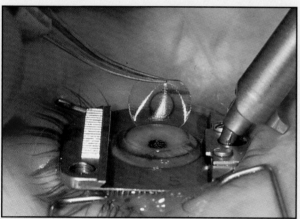

Figure B-24.
The 160-micron flap is lifted after the keratectomy.

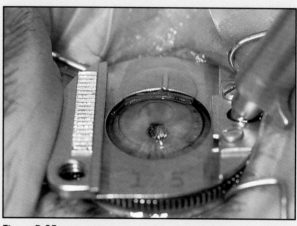

Figure B-25.
The second resection has been made, and the flap is now ready to be replaced.

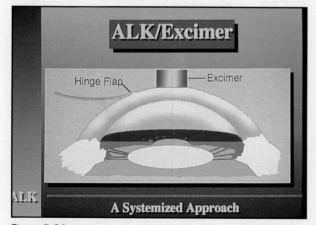

Figure B-26.
ALK combined with the laser in an in situ fashion was the beginning of LASIK.

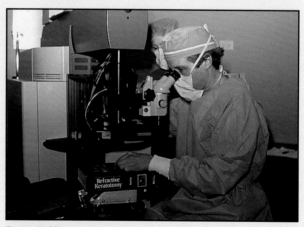

Figure B-27.
The author ablating the undersurface of a corneal disc during a Buratto technique LASIK.

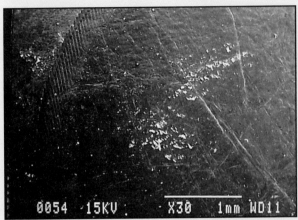

Figure B-28.
A SEM view of the edge of the keratectomy and the ablation. Note that the smoothness of the ablated area approaches that of Bowman's.

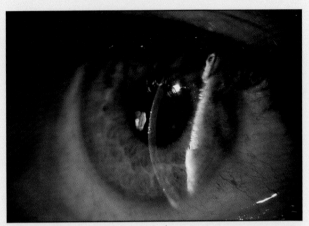

Figure B-29.
A LASIK patient demonstrating the clarity of the cornea 1-hour postoperatively.

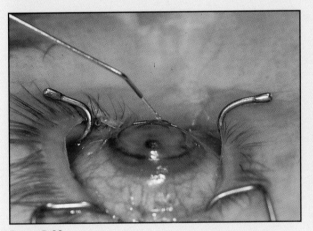

Figure B-30.
Irrigation of the interface in an attempt to avoid debris.

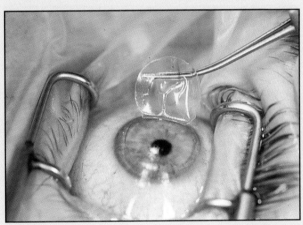

Figure B-31.
The LASIK flap may be lifted up months and even years after the original keratectomy.

vision should be in the range of 20/40 preoperative corrected vision. A determination must be made that the position of the cap is correct. There must be no edema (Figure B-29). No haze should be observed in the interface, although debris may be present (Figure B-30). The patient usually will not have pain but can experience a mild foreign body sensation. Assuming all the above are met, the patient may be seen again at 1 week to 1 month. The final visual result may take several weeks to obtain. If irregular astigmatism is present, this may take months or years to clear (Figure B-31).

While lamellar surgery lessens the problems associated with wound healing, other serious complications can occur. An extensive presurgical Preflight checklist should be reviewed before each case. This will help ensure that the keratome is in perfect working order, avoiding many potential complications. During surgery, decentration and malfunction of the keratome may occur. Centration depends on the first placement of the suction ring and must be as accurate as possible. If there is poor centration of the suction ring, the case should be aborted. The most serious complication in ALK is perforation of the globe by the microkeratome. This can occur when the plate is improperly placed or left out altogether. This and many other complications can be largely avoided by the strict usage of the Preflight checklist.

Postoperatively, complications can be both mechanical and refractive. The flap may be loose or in poor position. This must

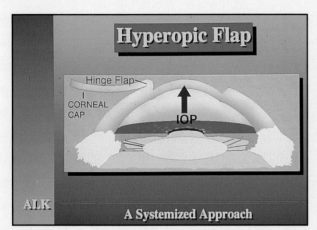

Figure B-32.
A schematic of ALK for hyperopia demonstrating the ectasia mechanism.

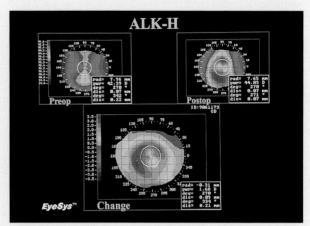

Figure B-33.
A change map topography of ALK-H which shows the corneal steepening postoperatively.

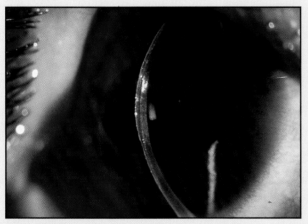

Figure B-34.
A 1-day postoperative view of a keratophakia cornea showing the flap and the clear tissue lens.

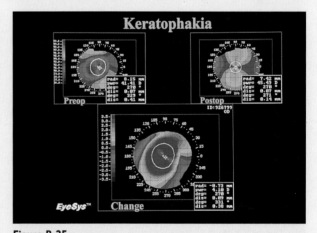

Figure B-35.
A change map topography of keratophakia demonstrating the dramatic amount of corneal steepening and astigmatically neutral character of the surgery.

be replaced with sutures if necessary. Poor flap placement may induce irregular astigmatism. Epithelium in the interface may occur by the actual ingrowth of epithelium from the keratectomy edge, implanted rests of cells from the surgery, or arise from preexisting epithelium, such as plugs in RK incisions. This epithelium should be removed if it is progressing, causing stromal melt, blocking the vision, or creating astigmatism.

Infections, while rare, may occur and should be treated aggressively; removing the flap may be necessary in intralamellar infections to obtain good antimicrobial drug access.

Refractive complications may include over- and undercorrections. While residual myopia may be treated with RK or repeat ALK, induced hyperopia is more problematic. ALK is usually astigmatism neutral, but temporary or rarely permanent cylinder may be induced. As with all corneal refractive surgery, the quality of vision may be altered with glare, halos, or decreased contrast sensitivity.

ENHANCEMENTS

ALK at this time is not as accurate as it is desirable. Since there is a wide scatter of achieved vs. intended refractive results, the surgeon should aim for undercorrections so that the result will fall in the myopic range. Radial keratotomy can be used with existing nomograms and instrumentation to refine the results. The eye may be assumed to be stable at 3 months for RK. The patient with preexisting astigmatism may be operated on sooner, when the cylinder is stable. LASIK patients may be retreated with the laser by lifting the flap or beneath a repeat keratectomy (see Figure B-31).

HYPEROPIC LAMELLAR SURGERY

Hyperopic ALK may be used for 1 to 5 D of correction (Figures B-32 and B-33). In contrast to myopic ALK, the entire cornea is bent to achieve the refractive effect. This is similar to RK. The same complications such as centration, epithelium, and displaced caps may occur. Hyperopic ALK has also been used in the treatment of consecutive hyperopia after RK. This should be approached with considerable caution. An ectasia operation is being performed over an existing ectasia operation, and a keratoconus-like condition can result.

The very first lamellar refractive work done by Barraquer was keratophakia for hyperopia (Figure B-34). This involved

changing the anterior surface of the cornea by placing an insert of corneal tissue or synthetic material between layers of cornea. In the original procedure of keratophakia, the microkeratome was used to remove a layer of tissue, and then a pre-cut lens calculated to correct hyperopia was inserted and covered by the first layer.

There are several major variables in the success of keratophakia. When not using human tissue, the biocompatability and physical properties of the implant materials are crucial. High permeability and a high refractive index are necessary with any synthetic implant to allow sufficient corneal nutrition to the overlying stroma. There are also potential differences in the two available surgical techniques: a freehand pocket incision vs. a lamellar keratectomy with a microkeratome. Barraquer's original keratophakia worked by releasing Bowman's entirely, allowing it to drape over the insert. Other surgeries, such as intracorneal rings and implants where Bowman's is not incised, must depend upon Bowman's layer stretching over the implant. There have been early promising results reported with keratophakia.[4-6] Lane and Lindstrom, reporting in Brightbill, described 40 cases of polysulfone implants in myopic and aphakic eyes.[7] Fifty-three percent of the 23 myopic patients were 20/40 or better best corrected, and 23% of the aphakic eyes were 20/40 or better best corrected. Complications included scarring, refractive debris, lens subluxation, sterile infiltrates, and vascularization. Many other materials have been used, such as plexiglass, silastic, and hydrogel. At this point, only further investigations will confirm the potential of these operations. With improved microkeratomes, interest in keratophakia as a way to correct higher degrees of hyperopia and aphakia, especially where secondary lens implantation is contraindicated, has grown. Keratophakia does hold the

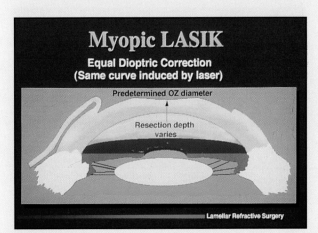

Figure B-36.
A schematic of myopic LASIK examining the relationship of depth and diameter in the ablation.

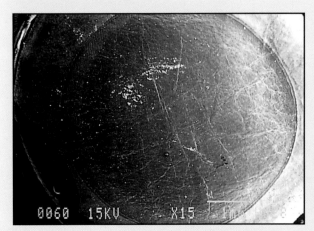

Figure B-37.
The view of the keratectomy, the lamellar characteristics.

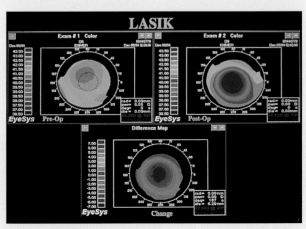

Figure B-38.
A change map topography of LASIK.

promise of producing large amounts of corneal steepening without the risk of an intraocular procedure (Figure B-35).

LASIK

In the future, LASIK may offer advantages over PRK (Figure B-36). ALK has proven very useful for high myopia, while still being limited by a lack of absolute accuracy. This had led researchers to explore ways other than the microkeratome to make the second critical refractive cut. Considering the fineness of cuts made with modern keratomes, this will be a difficult goal (Figure B-37). The excimer laser offers the potential accuracy to precisely remove corneal tissue, along with the ability to provide a lenticular rather than a lamellar cut (Figure B-38). Ioannis Pallikaris, MD, using an excimer ablation and a manual keratome, was an early researcher in situ photorefractive keratomileusis under a corneal flap on rabbit eyes.[8] Lucio Buratto, MD later reported good results in a large series of human eyes, placing an excimer ablation on the under surface of the 300-micron disc of tissue removed with the microkeratome or on the bed after a free cap had been removed.[9] Modern LASIK, using an automated keratome and the excimer, was first performed as part of the Summit Phase I ExciMed MKM study in 1992.

RESULTS

Despite a long history of lamellar surgery, little published data exist for ALK and LASIK. There are many studies in press and preparation that will add to our knowledge over the next few years. One can see the improvements that have occurred over the past few years by reviewing the available reports.

In 1991, Bas and Nano[10] reported on the first large series of MKM in situ and experienced the unpredictable nature of the technique as previously reported by Barraquer 20 years earlier. Early results have been reported by the ALK Study Group at the AAO in 1993 and 1994. The Study Group prospectively evaluated 100 consecutive cases from 10 surgeons, typically their first cases with the procedure. Eight of these surgeons had no previous MKM experience. Many of the patients were enhanced with RK. At 1 year follow-up, 75% of these eyes were within two Snellen lines of their preoperative best corrected acuity. At 1 year, two eyes were reported as losing more than two lines relative to their preoperative best corrected visual acuity. The predictability was good, generally within 1D of the planned correction. The refractive outcome was stable, with little change throughout the 1 year follow-up. ALK appears to be astigmatism neutral, affecting only the spherical component. The visual outcome was good, with 75% of the eyes achieving

20/40 or better uncorrected vision.[11]

The largest study of ALK is the US ALK Data Base. In this group of 10 surgeons, all cases are reported to Refractive Surgery Services in Kansas City. There were 1124 myopes and 370 hyperopes in the system as of February 1995. Uncorrected vision with the myopes was good, with 75% of the moderate myopes at 20/40 or better. This decreased to 66% of the -6 through -10 D and 51% of the -10 to -20 D. Sixty-six percent of the lower myopes were within 1.50 D of their intended correction. Hyperopes were somewhat better, with 71% of the +1.00 to +4.00 OD eyes at 20/40 uncorrected and 73% within 1.50 D of intended correction.

The use of an excimer laser in a large series was first reported by Lucio Buratto of Milan.[9] Buratto reported a prospective series of thirty consecutive eyes from -11.2 to 24.5 D, who underwent excimer laser MKM. A plano corneal disc was removed with the BKS microkeratome, followed by excimer ablation of either the resected disc (28 eyes) or on the stromal bed (two eyes). The excimer laser nomogram used was the standard PRK nomogram. The disc was then sutured into position. Recovery was rapid, with 83% of the corneas clear by 3 weeks. Fifty-seven percent of the eyes were within 1 D of the intended correction. Ten percent of the eyes were 20/40 or better uncorrected after surgery at 12 months, while 90% were 20/100 to 20/50.

The next large series of excimer MKM to be done was the Summit FDA protocol.[12] This was started in New Orleans by Stephen Brint and myself in Summer 1991. Uncorrected visual acuity at 1 day was excellent, with more than half of these patients seeing 20/40 or better. Visual acuity at 1 month continued to improve, with 13 out of the original 17 seeing 20/40 or better, and the only patients seeing 20/200 or worse were the patients who had poorly corrected best vision at the start of the case. With all lamellar cases, these patients tend to do better with time. Preoperative refraction ranges based on Stephen Brint's data with an initial range of -6.50 to -21.75 D have decreased to -.81 to +1.87 D at 24 months. Postoperatively the patients are in very little pain, usually far less than an RK or PRK patient. There does seem to be an initial correction to the plus side, which then levels out close to the intended correction.

The third large group series by Ruiz, Updegraff and myself in Bogota, Colombia, used the Chiron Technolas excimer laser to treat moderate to high myopia.[13] One hundred forty eyes on bilateral cases were enrolled and the early results were very promising. Long-term follow-up is needed to judge the stability and efficacy of these procedures, but early results indicate

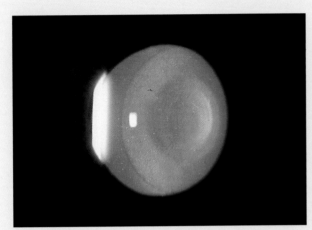

Figure B-39.
The ablation profile is "hidden" from wound healing in LASIK.

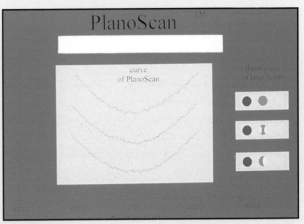

Figure B-40.
PlanoScan may offer smoother ablations with any beam, regardless of the purity or power. Graph shows sensitivity on beam homogeneity.

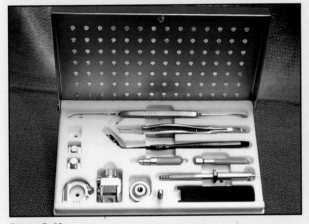

Figure B-41.
A LASIK keratome set.

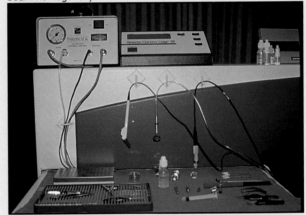

Figure B-42.
The additional equipment needed along with the laser for LASIK.

minimal effect on preexisting keratometric cylinder, as well as a similar refractive effect as PRK alone. Another large series with George Waring, MD, in Jeddah, Saudi Arabia, is currently underway. This is very much a procedure in current evaluation and evolution.

SUMMARY AND CONCLUSION

ALK for myopia and hyperopia and LASIK are members of the family of lamellar surgery pioneered by Jose Barraquer, MD. These techniques are powerful ways to alter the refractive state of the eye. Lamellar techniques offer reduced wound healing (Figure B-39). Often there are few other options for patients seeking correction. These techniques are also very much in development. Accuracy is not perfect and complications may occur. The surgeon who considers adding lamellar surgery to

his or her practice should invest in adequate training and have the capability of handling potential complications. Much work is being done on ALK to improve the accuracy. The keratome scope to inspect the blade and measure the gap, much like a RK knife, is one example. Improved ultrasonic pachymeters are also being employed to measure the thickness of cuts and depth of ablations. PRK algorithms must be altered and even new nomograms created for LASIK. We are just now learning about the excimer laser and what factors are important to consider.

New scanning techniques may prove better than the broad beam methods now in use (Figure B-40). More equipment is involved, and learning curves are steeper than that with PRK (Figures B-41 and B-42). While both ALK and LASIK take advantage of lamellar keratoplasty techniques, they do use a different method in making the second cut. Which will prove bet-

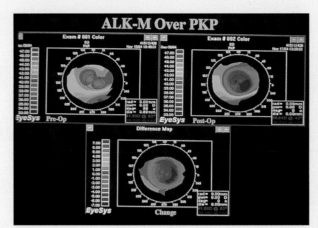

Figure B-43.
Lamellar surgery over a cornea with previous surgery, PKP.

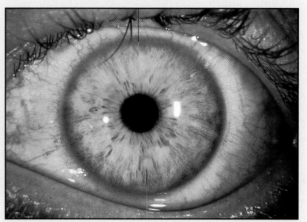

Figure B-44.
A typical 1-day postoperative LASIK cornea.

ter for the second cut: the microkeratome or the excimer? While ALK uses the same blade in a quick, relatively straightfoward fashion, the excimer laser is a complex, unwieldy, and expensive machine. Any significant improvements with the excimer over ALK will have to be weighed against the cost and availability of the excimer lasers. The excimer laser may have the edge in accuracy and offer other advantages, such as simultaneous treatment of astigmatism. Lamellar techniques may prove better for patients who have undergone previous corneal surgery, such as penetrating keratoplasty (Figure B-43). One may liken the acceptance of LASIK to that of phaco. More equipment, fewer but more serious complications, and a steeper learning curve, all to deliver results to the patient sooner in a more elegant fashion. Just as phaco replaced ECCE as the patient's choice, LASIK will largely replace PRK (Figure B-44).

References

1. Maguire LJ, Klyce SD, et al. Visual distortion after myopic keratomileusis: Computer analysis of keratoscopy photography. *Ophthalmic Surgery.* 1987;18:352-356.

2. Swinger CA, Barker BA. Prospective evaluation of myopic keratomileusis. *Ophthalmology.* 1984;91:785-792.

3. Nordan LT, Fallor MK. Myopic keratomileusis: 74 consecutive nonamblyopic cases with one year of follow-up. *J Refract Surg.* 1986;2:124-128.

4. Taylor D, Stern A, Romanchuk K. Keratophakia: clinical evaluation. *Ophthalmology.* 1981;88:1141-1150.

5. Friedlander MH, Werblin TP, Kaufman HE. Clinical results of keratophakia and keratomileusis. *Ophthalmology.* 1981;88:716-720.

6. Jester JV, Rodrigues MM, Villasenor RA, et al. Keratophakia and keratomileusis: histopathologic, ultrastructural and experimental studies. *Ophthalmology.* 1984;91:793-805.

7. Carey BE. In: Brightbill FS, ed. *Synthetic Keratophakia: Corneal Surgery.* St. Louis, Mo: CV Mosby; 1986.

8. Pallikaris IG, Papatzanaki ME, Stathi EZ, et al. Laser in situ keratomileusis. *Lasers Surg Med.* 1990;10:463-468.

9. Buratto L, Ferrari M, Rama P. Excimer laser intrastromal keratomileusis. *Am J Ophthalmol.* 1992;113:291-295.

10. Bas AM, Nano HD. In-situ myopic keratomileusis results in 30 eyes at 15 months. *Refract Corneal Surg.* 1991;7:223-231.

11. Slade SG, et al. Keratomileusis in-situ: a prospective evaluation. Poster presentation of American Academy of Ophthalmology; 1993.

12. Slade SG, Brint SJ, et al. Phase I myopic keratomileusis with the Summit Excimer Laser. In preparation.

13. Slade SG, Ruiz L, Updegraff SA. A prospective single-center clinical trial to evaluate ALK and ALK combined with PRK using the excimer laser versus PRK alone for the surgical correction of moderate to high myopia. Bogota, Colombia. In preparation.

Concurrent to the development of RK, the evolution of lamellar techniques to correct higher refractive errors was pioneered by Jose Barraquer, MD, the father of lamellar surgery. Over three decades, from the 1940s to the 1970s, keratomileusis evolved, but variable results reported by other surgeons, the complexity of the cryolathe, and the steep learning curve prevented widespread acceptance. In the 1980s, a number of modifications of Barraquer's tech-

niques to simplify the procedure were introduced, with the most important advance being the abandonment of the cryolathe. The Barraquer-Krumeich-Swinger (BKS) non-freeze technique and manual microkeratome were the first such efforts of non-freeze in situ keratomileusis.

The fundamental aspects of the procedure and the basic design of a suction ring and microkeratome introduced by Barraquer remain unchanged. Strengths of lamellar surgery

> The appeal of the excimer laser for refractive surgery was the potential for unparalleled predictability.

> The combination of laser and lamellar surgery addresses the most important challenge facing PRK, that of individual variation in patient wound healing.

continue to be rapid visual recovery, minimal discomfort, preserved corneal stability, and large potential range of treatable myopia. The primary weakness of lamellar surgery beyond the technical challenges was limited predictability.

The appeal of the excimer laser for refractive surgery was the potential for unparalleled predictability, due to the submicron precision and submicron collateral damage of far ultraviolet light energy because of minimal thermal damage associated. Excimer PRK was first conceived and described by Stephen Trokel, MD, in 1983. Theo Seiler, MD, performed the first human application of the excimer laser creating astigmatic corneal incisions in 1987. L'Esperance performed the first human wide-area keratectomy with an excimer laser later that same year. Marguerite B. McDonald, MD, performed many of the landmark animal and primate studies, and later performed the first PRK (within the FDA trial) on a sighted eye in 1988. In contrast to RK, the clinical results of PRK have been less dependent upon surgical skill, with greater dependence upon wound healing, the laser system, and specific technique utilized.

> Speed of passage of microkeratome is important. Faster rates produce thinner flaps regardless of depth plate utilized.

As described in the previous section on PRK, the improvement of PRK techniques to incorporate larger optical zones, pretreatment, and multizone blending techniques, while maintaining a more physiological state of corneal hydration, have led to considerable improvements in both PRK safety and efficacy. Advancements in delivery system design, incorporating more homogeneous energy beam profiles, and scanning capabilities, with an emphasis upon improvements in both calibration, centration, and eye-tracking systems, have also dramatically aided clinical outcome. Improvements in surgical technique and laser tech-

nology have reduced not only visual recovery time, but topical steroid requirements in lower and even moderate degrees of myopia. Postoperative pain management with the introduction of topical NSAIDs, such as diclofenac 0.1% in combination with bandage contact lenses, has also dramatically improved patient acceptance. The ease and reproducibility of laser refractive surgery has created high surgeon acceptance worldwide. The treatment of mild, moderate, and even severe degrees of myopia combined with astigmatism has resulted in an expanded refractive armamentarium for the RK surgeon. In addition to the expanded refractive envelope, corneal stability is also preserved with PRK. The persistent limitations of haze and regression with PRK for the treatment of severe and extreme degrees of myopia directed efforts by investigators such as Lucio Buratto, MD, toward the development of intrastromal techniques.

The combination of laser and lamellar surgery addresses the most important challenge facing PRK, that of individual variation in patient wound healing. It is very clear that there were many pioneers instrumental in the development of LASIK. In the late 1980s, Ioannis Pallikaris, MD, likely performed the first rabbit series with stromal bed ablation followed by human trials, while Buratto simultaneously developed intrastromal techniques with ablation applied to the stromal surface of the cap, after experiencing myopic regression and haze formation with PRK high myopia treatment. Stephen Brint, MD, was the first US surgeon to perform LASIK in North America using a Summit ExciMed laser after visiting with Buratto. The Summit FDA LASIK trial included both treatment of the stromal bed and on the stromal aspect of the 300 microns of the disc (Buratto technique).

The three most important developments for the widespread acceptance of lamellar techniques occurred in the 1990s, first with the invention of the automated microkeratome by Luis Ruiz, MD. The speed of passage of the microkeratome was important in standardizing the flap thickness, as faster rates produce thinner flaps regardless of the depth plate utilized. The automation allowed for repro-

Evolution of Myopic Keratomileusis
- MKM freeze techniques with cryolathe
- MKM non-freeze BKS technique
- MKM Buratto technique excimer laser on cap
- MKM excimer laser in situ technique on bed

Chiron Automatic Corneal Shaper Instrumentation

Richard N. Baker, OD, FAAO

The automatic corneal shaper is an elegant, precisely machined instrument. The equipment included with this system consist of a power "pack", which provides electrical current for a suction pump and microkeratome.

The suction pump is connected to the suction ring handle by disposable tubing, which comes packaged with a disposable blade. The adjustable suction ring consists of four parts:

1. Suction handle
2. Great ring
3. Vacuum ring
4. Track ring

The suction handles screws onto the assembled adjustable suction ring. This handle is hollow to allow the vacuum suction through the vacuum ring and handle. The assembly of the adjustable ring is performed with a ring assembly tool. The great ring holds the vacuum ring and the track ring together. The adjustment of the great ring changes the separation of track and vacuum rings. This, in turn, determines the diameter of cornea exposed throughout the ring, which will be resected. The diameter is measured by an applanation lens. The unit comes with a series of applanation lenses that are labeled to the corresponding reticule diameter on the lens. The cornea that touches the applanation lens when inserted into the suction ring will be resected by the microkeratome.

The microkeratome can be separated into the motor and shaper head. The assembled shaper head consists of six parts:

1. The head itself
2. A blade holder
3. A blade
4. The neural collar
5. A depth plate
6. A stopper

The parts of the shaper head are cleaned with Palmolive soap and a toothbrush. Once cleaned, the blade holder is inserted into the cavity inside the shaper head. A blade is inserted over the blade holder with a magnetic tool. This allows the shaper head to be closed over the blade. Once closed, the neural collar screws over the rear of the shaper head. A depth plate is selected and inserted into the front of the shaper head. The plates have detents which correspond to small bar bearings inside the shaper head which "snaps" when put into the proper position. The plate contains a locking hex nut which is tightened when the plate is in position. The stopper is placed over the neural collar into position by a locking screw. The newer models of the keratome contain a built-in stopper to the head and a one-size non-adjustable ring used for LASIK.

After cleaning and assembly, the microkeratome is always tested to ensure proper action with no resistance the verify that the stopper is functioning to stop the keratome in the desired position.

ducible smooth lamellar incisions. The origination of the hinged flap technique replacing the free lenticle cap by Pallikaris, who coined the term LASIK, was the second important element in improving the safety of the procedure, reducing the risk of lost caps and irregular astigmatism. The third major advance in LASIK was the development of a sutureless technique, having recognized that adequate corneal flap adhesion without sutures was possible. These elements allowed LASIK to be performed without the high incidence of irregular astigmatism typically associated with lamellar surgery, and helped create a more reproducible lamellar procedure which could be performed by most ophthalmic surgeons.

The challenges which are encountered with LASIK are nomogram development, regression, interface opacities,

The three most important LASIK developments are:
1. Automated microkeratome producing standard flaps
2. Development of hinged flap technique
3. Development of sutureless technique

Irregular astigmatism remains an ever-present challenge with lamellar surgery.

epithelial ingrowths, dislodged corneal flaps, or free caps. Irregular astigmatism remains an ever-present challenge with lamellar surgery. The steep surgical learning curve associated with lamellar procedures continues to complicate

Clear Corneal Molder

Ricardo Guimarães, MD, PhD

The concept of this new microkeratome presents some important advantages over the commercially available models, such as:

- The surgeon sees the whole resection of the corneal disk, being able to interrupt it to leave a peduncle at the moment he or she wishes.
- It is a one-piece system, which means the surgeon needs only one hand to operate the microkeratome, leaving the other hand free (Figure C-1).
- It is possible to resect disks of virtually any size, as the whole cornea is exposed and the blade has an appropriate length.
- There is no contact of the blade with any part of the microkeratome, what avoids metallic particles on the interface. The blade shaft does not need to be lubricated, avoiding the presence of grease at the interface.
- It is possible to use a diamond blade with this microkeratome, as the movement of the blade may be very gentle (Figure C-2).
- The movement of the blade across the cornea may be easily automated.

The principle of the Clear Corneal Molder is very simple. A suction ring fixates the eye, exposing the cornea to a glass plate. The contact area of the cornea with the glass plate determines the size of the disk, and the distance between the blade and the glass plate determines the thickness of the disk to be resected. Once the desired disk diameter and thickness are set, the resection movement is started by stepping on a foot pedal. The blade is then driven through the cornea by pushing a knob with the thumb. As the surgeon sees the cutting, he or she may stop the movement at the precise point where he or she wants to leave a peduncle.

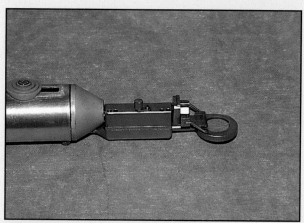

Figure C-1.
Clear corneal molder.

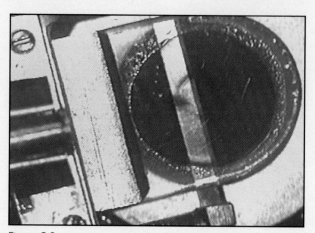

Figure C-2.
Intraoperative view of lamellar incision.

the rapid growth of intrastromal ablation in contrast with surface photoablation, despite the clinical benefits of improved comfort, rapid visual rehabilitation, and larger range of correction. Reduced postoperative steroid requirements, combined with the virtual elimination of stromal scarring even when treating severe myopia, clearly depicts LASIK as the procedure of choice for at least higher degrees of myopia correction.

THE ROLE OF THE EXCIMER LASER IN LASIK

It has been stated by Stephen Slade, MD, that "LASIK is 90% keratectomy and 10% laser." I believe this statement to be true. This does not, however, dismiss the 10% role of the excimer laser. Despite the incredible submicron precision of the excimer laser there is still great variabili-

The steep surgical learning curve associated with lamellar procedures continues to complicate the rapid growth of intrastromal ablation in contrast with surface photoablation, despite the clinical benefits.

ty in surface photoablation clinical results. Clearly, variability in wound healing is responsible for the distribution of refractive and visual results with PRK. The higher the degree of myopia treated, the greater the depth of ablation and the greater the healing response induced in any patient.

LASIK reduces but does not eliminate the following:
- The effects of wound healing, as the deeper stroma is less reactive. The corneal-laser interaction is less critical in the deeper stroma, as the epithelial-stromal interaction is fundamental to haze formation.
- The need for absolute beam homogeneity. The corneal flap helps smooth small ablation differences within the beam related to hot and cold spots.
- The need for smooth wound contours and blending. Sharp contours and steep wound margins are not associated with haze formation, as is evidenced by the refractive resection in ALK.

LASIK creates a spherical or toric lenticular pattern with tapered edges, whereas ALK creates a plano lamellar excision pattern with sharp margins.

The tapered wound edge profile of LASIK is masked by both the corneal flap and the increased stromal hydration of the deeper stroma.

The effective optical zone is larger than the treatment zone with ALK, and smaller than the treatment zone with LASIK.

LASIK reduces the influence of the excimer laser system utilized upon the refractive outcome. Improvements in ablation smoothness, blending, and beam homogeneity observed with newer laser delivery systems are of limited clinical significance with LASIK.

Inherent Limitations With ALK
- Limited optical zone size
- Double pass requires increased technical skill
- More complex instrumentation than for LASIK
- Plano excision of tissue, not lenticular
- Mechanical refractive cut accuracy ±10 microns
- Procedure predictability ±2.00 D
- High instrumentation care requirements
- Blade quality limitations

LASIK still requires multizone or aspheric ablation patterns to limit the depth of ablation, while maximizing the effective optical zone. It is important to minimize the depth of ablation to not only protect the endothelium, but to maintain long-term corneal stability. The residual corneal tissue pachymetry should ideally exceed 400 microns, to allow for a 160-micron flap and 240-micron stromal bed. Although smaller treatment areas of 4.2 to 5.0 mm were initially used to treat high myopia with LASIK in order to limit the amount of tissue ablated, the visual quality under low levels of illumination was often compromised. Ideally, a 6.0-mm area of ablation is utilized to provide adequate night vision quality; however, this limits the maximal treatment to less than -12.00 D unless multizone or aspheric programs are used. Depending upon the preoperative corneal pachymetry and ablation profile utilized, over 30 D of myopia can potentially be corrected. A patient with limited corneal thickness should be left undercorrected but with an adequate optical zone, rather than fully corrected with an inadequate optical zone.

LASIK creates a spherical or toric lenticular pattern

Central island formation is greater with LASIK because of the increased hydration status of the deeper stroma.

Original ablation nomograms for LASIK were based upon ALK concepts, later nomograms were tailored after PRK, but LASIK requires a combination approach.

Figure 8-1.
Chiron Corneal Shaper with adjustable three-piece suction ring for automated lamellar keratoplasty and LASIK. A smaller single piece suction ring is used for LASIK alone. Courtesy of Dr. Stephen G. Slade.

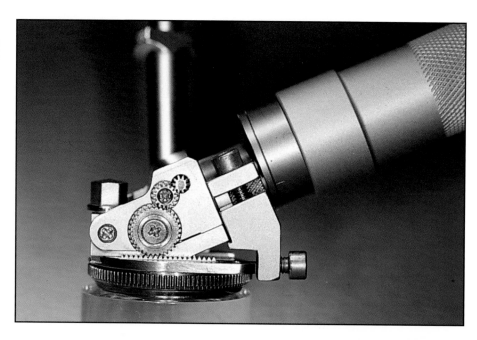

Figure 8-2a.
Schematic illustration of ALK demonstrating lamellar excision pattern of refractive pass with steep wound margins.

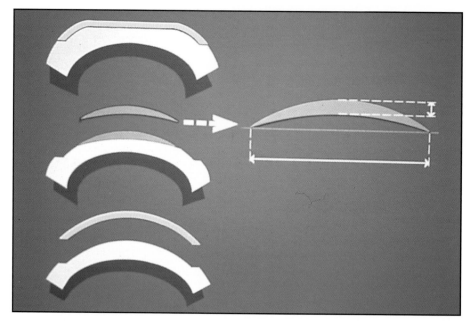

with tapered edges, whereas ALK creates a plano lamellar excision pattern with sharp margins. The induced topographical change on videokeratography with respect to the effective optical zone generated is markedly different between ALK and LASIK. The resected lenticle in ALK is only 4.2 mm, however, the corneal flap blends the plano excision pattern to create a 5.0- to 5.5-mm effective optical zone (Figures 8-1 through 8-2c). In direct contrast, the effective optical zone is smaller than the treatment zone with LASIK. The tapered wound edge profile of LASIK is

masked by both the corneal flap and the increased stromal hydration of the deeper stroma.

Like PRK, LASIK is subject to the development of central islands when larger optical zones of 6 mm or greater are utilized. In fact, the risk of central island formation is greater with LASIK because of the increased hydration status of the deeper stroma. Alterations in the technique or ablation profile are required to compensate for the central undercorrection anticipated with larger optical zones. Modifications in technique include drying the central stroma with a surgical

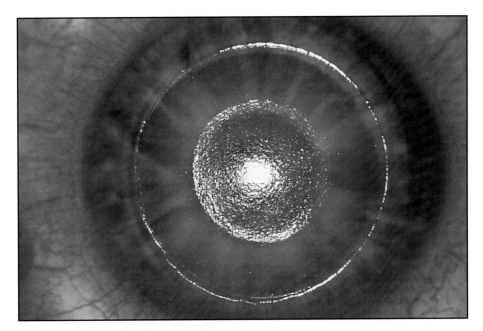

Figure 8-2b.
Clinical intraoperative view of ALK performed by Dr. Stephen G. Slade demonstrating steep 4.2mm wound margins.

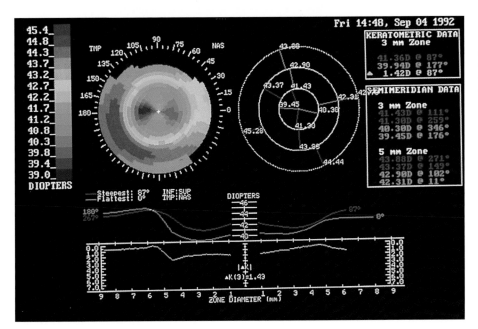

Figure 8-2c.
Post-operative videokeratography of ALK demonstrating enlarged 5.5-mm effective optical zone due to bending of corneal flap noted from topographical profile. Courtesy of Dr. Stephen G. Slade.

spear, air, or wiping with a blunt spatula. Ablation profile compensation would utilize a pretreatment approach; that is the application of additional pulses centrally beyond what is required for the refractive correction.

Original ablation nomograms for LASIK were based upon ALK concepts. Later nomograms were tailored after PRK, but LASIK requires a combination approach. PRK central treatment and blending combined with ALK wound margin profile. The central 3 mm of the ablation zone is responsible for daytime qualitative vision, whereas the peripheral 5 to 7 mm is responsible for nighttime qualitative vision. Most ablation nomograms are designed with respect to dioptric correction, which are essentially meaningless to the cornea. Ablation profiles must be designed with respect to micron depth and corneal contour produced. Each zone must have a minimum depth to be effective in producing a change in contour, overcoming the masking effects of the corneal flap and deeper stromal hydration. Each zone must also have a maximum depth to avoid steep contours, promote blending, and reduce the overall depth of ablation. The

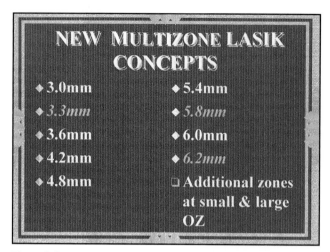

Figure 8-3.
Multizone pattern applies equal treatment at increasing optical zones. Additional zones at small and large optical zones (blue) to create profile depicted in Figure 8-4.

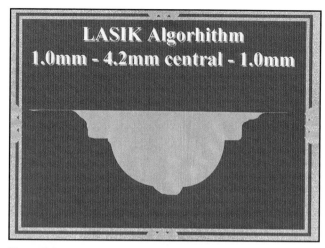

Figure 8-4.
Machat LASIK Ablation profile with increased central treatment to compensate for increased central hydration of deeper stroma to avoid central islands and improve qualitative vision. Peripheral knee also fashioned in ALK-like manner to reduce night glare and improve flap draping. Sharp contour will not induce haze under corneal flap. Small peripheral blend adequate intrastromally.

TABLE 8-1

LASIK NOMOGRAM FOR -13.00 D ATTEMPTED CORRECTION

Optical Zone	Dioptric Distribution	Percentage of Treatment	Micron Depth
3.0 mm	-5.40 D	Pretreatment 1 µm/D + 3 µm	16
3.6 mm	-3.63 D	27.9%	17
4.2 mm	-2.58 D	18.9%	17
4.8 mm	-1.90 D	14.6%	17
5.4 mm	-1.46 D	11.2%	17
5.8 mm	-1.23 D	9.5%	17
6.0 mm	-1.14 D	8.8%	17
6.2 mm	-1.06 D	8.15%	17

Eight zones of equal micron depth. Each zone 0.6 mm larger than the previous zone, with two additional zones within 0.2 mm of 6.0-mm optical zone to ensure adequate peripheral blend for reduced spherical aberration and night visual disturbances.

ideal micron depth of ablation per zone appears to be between 15 and 20 microns, with a 10 micron minimum depth needed within each zone.

Increased effectiveness for improved daytime and nighttime qualitative vision is created by increasing the number of zones, although each zone is an identical depth. Table 8-1 and Figures 8-3 and 8-4 show a LASIK nomogram comprised of nine zones of equal depth, blended in order of increasing size (Machat 1995). Six zones are divided between 3.0 and 6.0 mm equally at 0.6-mm intervals, meaning that each zone is 0.3 mm larger than the preceding zone circumferentially, which denotes excellent fixation. The treatment begins at 3.0 mm because 3.0 mm is the typical size of central islands produced and where daytime qualitative vision is derived. The sixth zone is 6.0 mm, the required minimum optical zone to ensure adequate quality night vision. The three additional zones highlighted represent additional zones interspersed between the standard six zones, designed to both counteract central island formation and achieve an effective 6.0-mm optical zone demonstrable on videokeratography. The peripheral blend is more closely crowded to create a more ALK-like effect and overcome the corneal flap masking effect. The same optical zone is never repeated in keeping with the blending principles of surface photoablation, creating a less abrupt wound edge profile and limiting the overall depth of ablation. Future scanning technology will create more complex ablation patterns and reproduce these profiles without pretreatment (Machat 1992) and multi-multizone (Machat 1993) techniques.

Excimer Laser Intrastromal Keratomileusis (ELISK): Comparison of the Technique On the Flap and In Situ

Lucio Buratto, MD

INTRODUCTION

Keratomileusis is a lamellar corneal technique for the correction of moderate and severe myopia. It can also be defined as a refractive autologous lamellar keratoplasty.

In this technique, a primary lamellar keratectomy of suitable diameter is performed, the corneal stroma is carved (on the flap or in situ) with the refractive keratectomy, then the flap is replaced in its original position. The objective of this procedure is to flatten the anterior corneal profile through the removal of a stromal lenticle with a positive dioptric value.

Less frequent, but also possible, is the treatment of moderate to severe hyperopia. In hyperopic keratomileusis, the anterior profile of the cornea is curved through the removal of a negative value stromal lenticle.

In myopic keratomileusis (MKM), the refractive keratectomy can be performed on the stromal face of the flap (MKM on the flap) or on the corneal bed (MKM in situ).

The techniques by which the refractive keratectomy is performed have seen rapid evolution over the past 15 years.

Barraquer's original technique, invented in 1964 and then perfected, used the cryolathe instrument—that is, a freezing microlathe (MKM on the flap). A refractive cut was performed on the flap once it was frozen.

On the other hand, Krumeich's technique, invented in 1982 with Swinger and Barraquer, uses the bench of the BKS 1000 and involves the refractive processing of the fresh corneal flap (Planar MKM on the flap).

Ruiz's technique, developed in 1988, uses the ALK and involves the refractive processing of the fresh corneal bed (MKM in situ).

In 1989, I developed a technique which used excimer laser for refractive keratectomy: intrastromal keratomileusis (ISK) or photokeratomileusis (PKM), or better still ELISK (excimer laser intrastromal keratomileusis).

But let's leave aside the first three, which can now be considered the historical variations of MKM, and describe my technique comparing the procedure of ablation on the lamella (ELISK on the flap technique) with the in situ technique (ELISK in situ). We will then compare ELISK to the other techniques of keratomileusis and the other procedures used for the correction of severe myopia.

SURGICAL TECHNIQUE ON THE FLAP→BURATTO'S ORIGINAL TECHNIQUE

Under pilocarpine-induced miosis and topical anesthesia, the cornea is marked in the centropupillary area with 30 to 40 excimer laser shots. The patient is asked to stare at the laser beam while this procedure is completed; the marking serves to identify the exact center of the area for ablation. The patient is then moved from the laser room to the operating room and lies on the operating bed. Using the operating microscope, marking is done along the horizontal corneal axis, from edge to edge with a gentian violet pen. The lines intersect on the central marking.

A second marking is done with the same pen, this time on one hemi-meridian (from the central marking to the edge) in the superior hemi-cornea. If astigmatic correction is also planned, this corresponds to the axis of astigmatism, measured topographically.

The markings permit the exact repositioning of the contact surfaces (stroma-stroma) of the refractive flap at the end of the operation, and the identification of the axis of astigmatism for the astigmatic treatment. The mechanical part of the operation follows; that is, the lamellar cut using a microkeratome.

THE PRIMARY KERATECTOMY

The lamellar incision, or the primary keratectomy, is performed using any microkeratome of modern design. I normally use the electromechanical microkeratome of the BKS 1000 set for planar MKM according to Barraquer-Krumeich-Swinger (Eye-Tech). The instrument and its accessories are assembled and prepared in such a way as to cut a flap with parallel surfaces, 300-micron thickness and 8.5-mm diameter.

For this reason, a 300-micron plate and a suction ring of suitable diameter are used. The thickness of the corneal flap depends on the plate, a device applied to the anterior part of the microkeratome's head which determines the required flattening of the corneal surface.

The diameter of the flap, on the other hand, depends on the diameter of the suction ring. This is applied to the perilimbal area of the eye bulb and guides the microkeratome. It is often chosen on the basis of the keratometric values of the cornea subjected to KM and on the dimensions of the bulb.

The suction ring is well centered on the patient's eye and after checking that the hold is optimal and that it has increased the ocular pressure to the required value, the lamellar incision is done using the microkeratome.

The primary keratectomy aims to obtain a flap of diameter between 7.0 to 9.0 mm and thickness of between 280 to 320 microns. These two measurements can be controlled intraoperatively with a compass and a micrometric thickness gauge.

The flap, with its parallel surfaces void of any refractive power, is placed on a Teflon support, epithelium-side down. It is then covered with a sterile cover and transferred to the excimer laser, where the refractive phase is completed.

PHOTOABLATION USING AN EXCIMER LASER

I use the Chiron Technolas Keracor excimer laser. The laser technician, prior to the lamellar incision, checks the correct functioning of the excimer laser; he or she then sets the values for correction by refractive photoablation, while the surgeon positions the flap under the laser. The laser beam is brought to target the preoperative markings in the prepupillary corneal area.

The computer can decide the number and diameter of the optical zones for the ablation on the basis of the dioptric values to correct. However, more often than not it is the surgeon who selects these parameters on the basis of the initial corneal thickness, that of the flap obtained through the lamellar incision and the total depth of the ablation planned.

Multizonal treatment is preferable to that with a single zone because the total surface of ablation is shallower and the peripheral ablation is more gradual.

Then the laser treatment is performed. It can be either myopic or combined, that is, myopic and astigmatic.

REPOSITIONING OF THE FLAP

Once the refractive photoablation of the stromal surface has been completed, the corneal flap is transported to the operating bed and positioned on the corneal bed with the help of a spatula.

The flap, which is now refractive, is replaced exactly in the original position by matching up the gentian violet markings on the flap and the peripheral cornea.

Following replacement of the flap, the edges are dried with a Merocel sponge and then with low-pressure compressed air, filtered through a micropore filter.

The slight dehydration of the flap is sufficient to make it adhere to the corneal bed, thanks to the slight suction force the stromal bed exerts on the stroma of the flap. Sutures are usually not required (sutureless technique). The flap is then tested in order to check the good adhesion to the bed. If adhesion is not good, the flap can be fixed to the corneal bed by way of an external triangular suture or of a single, anti-torsion running suture in 10-0 nylon. This will induce homogeneous traction around the cornea and thus limit the degree of postoperative astigmatism.

IN SITU SURGICAL TECHNIQUE

Buratto's technique using the refractive incision by excimer laser can be done with the refractive keratectomy on the stromal bed, as opposed to the stromal face of the lamella. In this procedure, the lamellar incision with the microkeratome is incomplete; a part is not cut, therefore, the flap remains attached nasally for about 1 to 2 mm of its circumference.

Another important difference in this procedure is the fact that a lamella cut performed initially by the microkeratome is thin. It will ideally have a thickness of between 140 to 180 microns.

AUTOMATIC MICROKERATOME WITH BLOCKING DEVICE

The primary keratectomy is performed using the Chiron-Steinway ALK microkeratome system. This electromechanical microkeratome slides automatically. The instrument has a toothed wheel on one side which engages perfectly in the complementary teeth on the runners of the suction ring; a motor controls the backward or forward movement of the microkeratome along the runners of the suction ring. This means that the microkeratome slides along the ring through the electromechanical progression of the microkeratome's toothed wheel along the toothed runners of the ring. The electromechanical device which rotates the microkeratome's toothed wheels can rotate in both forward and reverse directions. This means that the instrument can move in one direction, and once the primary keratectomy has been complete, return to the starting position.

The second important element is that the progression of the microkeratome can be regulated to a precise point, thanks to a variable blocking device fitted to one extremity of the head of the instrument. The microkeratome then moves along the ring to a precise, predetermined point and then it has to stop.

In brief, the microkeratome progresses along the toothed

guide, first from the temporal sector to the nasal one; once it reaches the blocking point, the direction of movement changes, and the instrument returns along the toothed runners from the nasal side to the temporal one, leaving the flap, obtained with the primary keratectomy, attached to the cornea for a small portion of the nasal periphery.

SURGICAL TECHNIQUE

The microkeratome is assembled with a plate suitable for obtaining a flap of around 160 microns; the blocking device is set in such a way as to leave at least 1 mm of tissue uncut (still attached to the cornea) at the end of the microkeratome's run. The incision with the microkeratome is done using an excimer laser microscope.

At the end of the primary laser keratectomy, the corneal flap is grasped delicately by the temporal edge with non-traumatic microsurgical forceps and flipped over nasally.

In the technique of keratomileusis in situ, a thin corneal flap is preferable (about 150 to 200 microns) because it is necessary to leave adequate corneal thickness in situ; the diameter must be at least 7.5 mm, although 8.00 to 8.5 mm or more is preferable. A large hinge would limit the laser ablation maximum optical zone size in cases with corneas of suitable thickness. A small hinge should not be targeted either, otherwise the lamella may be completely cut; that is, without leaving the nasal portion uncut.

PHOTOABLATION WITH EXCIMER LASER

The laser is aligned and centered on the stroma of the corneal bed. The refractive keratectomy is performed using the excimer laser (Buratto's technique in situ); during the ablation, the surgeon must carefully keep the lamella in the nasal sector so that it does not interfere with the laser emission. In addition, the patient must stare steadily at the laser so that the resulting ablation is well centered. If an astigmatic treatment has also been planned, the ablation axis must coincide with that of the astigmatism. The optical zone must be as wide as possible and compatible with the width of the stroma exposed by the lamellar cut. A multizonal ablation is preferable in the majority of cases.

REPLACEMENT OF THE LAMELLA

Once the ablation has been completed, the flap is closed and replaced in its original site. It does not require sutures. It is carefully dried with a Merocel sponge. The adherence of the flap to the cornea is checked by dabbing a dry sponge on the cornea just outside the keratectomized area. If the flap remains immobile, sutures are not required; otherwise, one or more single sutures may be preferable. Then the upper eyelid is lifted and positioned on the surface of the eye. If infiltration anesthesia was used, two or three steri-strips must be applied to prevent the eye from opening. Finally, an eyepatch and plastic protector are applied, all of which will be removed after 24 hours. If, on the other hand, topical anesthesia was used, the eye should be left open and unbandaged but protected by a pair of sunglasses.

COMPLICATIONS OF KERATOMILEUSIS

The historical keratomileusis techniques often had complications, and serious ones at that. Based on the surgical phase, they can be classified as follows:

- In the incisional phase with the microkeratome, there may be corneal perforation, an incomplete, superficial, or decentered incision, or an incision with irregular surfaces.
- In the refractive procedure, perforation of the free lamella is not uncommon when lasering the undersurface of the cap (error of calculation or insufficient thickness of the lamella), the destruction of the lamella due to its detachment during the refractive cut (because of insufficient freezing, inadequate fixing etc.); decentered refractive incision with the in situ technique; hypo or hypercorrection may be common to all.
- In the postoperative period, the complications are linked to the delay in keratocytic repopulation in Barraquer's freeze technique, surgical and physical trauma in Krumeich's technique, and irregular astigmatism in Ruiz's technique. In the various procedures, epithelial inclusions are common due to the transport of epithelial cells to the internal surfaces. In addition, inflammation and irritation and refractive disorders linked to the sutures are commonplace.

ADVANTAGES OF ELISK OVER OTHER TECHNIQUES

Photokeratomileusis using Buratto's technique, perfected in Milan in 1989, in addition to eliminating or strongly reducing the abovementioned complications, has some indisputable advantages over the other techniques. This procedure gives a better clinical outcome, the refractive result is more accurate, and the functional recovery, which is qualitatively superior, is more rapid.

If we go into more detail, when this technique is performed on the stromal face of the lamella it permits:

- Greater precision of the refractive cut, thanks to the possibility of micrometric ablations with the laser beam

- Real-time control of the centering of the refractive treatment in relation to the pupillary area
- Possibility of being able to perform a correct refractive cut even in the event of mistakes in the lamellar incision (incision which is decentered and/or irregular, thin, or reduced diameter)
- Possibility of adapting the depth of the ablation to the initial thickness of the cornea and/or the diameter of the pupil, possibility of adapting the optical zone in relation to the thickness of the flap obtained (smaller optical zones on thin flaps, wider on thicker flaps for equal refractive correction) without discarding the importance of producing the widest ablation possible in relation to the initial total thickness of the cornea
- Reduction of the operating times, which directly reduces the changes induced on the tissue by environmental factors (temperature, humidity, etc.)
- Less surgical trauma compared to the cryotrauma of Barraquer's technique, the procedure at the bench of Krumeich's technique, and the double resection in situ of Ruiz's technique
- Impossibility of irreversibly damaging the flap during the refractive phase, thanks to the fact that this procedure involves progressive tissue ablation under the direct visual control of the operator
- Possibility of associating a smoothing procedure to the refractive treatment in order to remove any irregularities of the flap or the corneal bed.
- Possibility of performing the refractive procedure in situ or on the flap.

COMPARISON OF THE TWO ELISK TECHNIQUES

The advantages of ELISK on the flap:
- The treatment is performed on an immobile free lenticle.
- Centering of the photoablative treatment is done independently of patient cooperation, and it is precise through marking done at the beginning of the operation.
- It allows the use of wider optical zones because the tissue to be treated is completely exposed; it is not limited by the nasal hinge.
- Endothelial damage caused by the excimer laser is impossible because the ablation is performed on the free lenticle.
- Errors, whether purely refractive or regarding the centering, can be corrected easily at a later stage through a lamellar keratoplasty with a homologous flap.

The disadvantages of the on the flap technique:
- There is a lower limit of the flap thickness (240 microns is a threshold value for an ablation of 140 microns or more). As a rough guide, about 100 microns of cornea must be left untreated to completely spare Bowman's layer, otherwise the ablation would be too close and damage to the membrane is possible (with consequent postoperative retraction).
- The photoablative treatment is completed on tissue which has been artificially distended. As a result, it may be presented incorrectly under the laser beam. In addition, it may be subjected to variations in hydration if any time is lost during the procedure.
- In the event of an associated astigmatic treatment, mistakes in the treatment axis are possible—the variation induced during repositioning of the lenticle must be taken into consideration.
- In the sutureless technique, rare cases where the flap has been lost have been described.

The advantages of ELISK with an in situ ablation:
- The surface subjected to the treatment is distended physiologically.
- The laser treatment is done immediately after the lamellar cut. As a result, the surface is subjected to minimal variations in hydration.
- The technique is faster and causes less trauma to the flap.
- The flap thickness is not of crucial importance for the amount of ablation; the flap can be very thin (100 microns) or quite thick (200 microns) but this does not change the result because the ablation is performed in situ on the stroma. If the lamella is very thick, treatment on the flap is necessary.
- The flap remains attached to the corneal tissues and it is impossible to lose it; anatomical recovery is quicker
- There is a smaller percentage of errors involving the axis in the astigmatic treatment.

The disadvantages of ELISK with an in situ ablation:
- The treatment is performed in a mobile area (the eye may move slightly); centering is therefore more difficult and less accurate. In addition, patient cooperation is required (the patient must stare steadily at the laser during the ablation)
- The diameter of the optical zone is limited by the nasal hinge

- The ablation is performed in the intermediate strata of the stroma, which may have repercussions on the deeper strata, possibly damaging the endothelium (considering that the ablation lasts longer in order to correct severe myopia).

COMPARISON BETWEEN KM AND THE INTRAOCULAR TECHNIQUES

Some surgeons also correct moderate to severe myopia by extracting the lens, with or without the implantation of the IOL in the posterior chamber. This procedure:

- Is an intraocular operation and presents all the risks common to intraocular surgery.
- Involves a loss of accommodation.
- Involves poor exploration of the peripheral retina due to peripheral opacification of the capsule and the visual difficulties following the optical passage—peripheral zone of the IOL.
- Involves a certain rhegmatogenic risk, particularly following a YAG capsulotomy.

Severe myopia can also be treated with an artificial lens implant of negative dioptric value in the anterior chamber. However, the technique involves some serious risks linked to the fact that:

- Repercussions on the endothelium are likely.
- There is a possible cataractogenic defect of the IOL in the anterior chamber.
- There is the possibility of long-term induction of glaucoma due to changes in the trabecular structures caused by the feet or loops of the IOL.
- The operation involves intraocular penetration (with all the inflammatory, infectious, and hemorrhagic complications connected to an operation of this type).

Implantation of a lens behind the iris, in front of the transparent human lens, is another method for correcting severe myopia. However, as this method is still in the experimental stages, it will not be dealt with here.

COMPARISON OF ELISK AND PRK

PRK gives a stable, precise outcome in the treatment of mild to moderate myopia (not more than 6 to 7 D). Nevertheless, there are several problems linked to its use for more severe myopia. In severe myopia, the fundamental problem with PRK centers around a deeper photoablation. It follows that in order to obtain an ablation with a peripheral smooth profile, a wider optical zone is required (transition zone). This brings about a further increase in the total depth of the ablation.

In contrast, by using smaller optical zones, the total depth of the ablation is smaller overall, but the lack of the transition zone results in a step being formed between the ablated area and the surrounding cornea. This is probably the reason behind the regression phenomena observed only a few months after treatment, more frequently in treatment of severe myopias following photoablation without the transition zone.

On the other hand, if treatment of a wider optical zone is not possible or not required, some functional problems linked to a smaller optical zone can be added to the anatomical problem—photophobia, glare, monocular diplopia, etc., which are more marked at twilight.

The extension of the ablation zone to the Bowman's brings about reactive and reparative phenomena which cause regression, which is sometimes marked, and haze, particularly in those patients classified as "responders."

In order to limit haze and the risk of regression, prolonged courses of cortisone therapy are often necessary, although this increases the risk of inducing glaucoma or cataract formation, and the patient must have frequent check-ups. The long-term effect of ablating Bowman's layer centrally is not known and must be considered when treatments are performed in younger patients. One should never underestimate the potential problems posed by an apparently simple treatment such as PRK, even when performed by an experienced surgeon.

In the event of hypocorrection with PRK, possibilities of retreatment are limited. First, retreatment in my opinion can only be performed a year after the primary PRK procedure, second, it may increase haze, and third, it does not guarantee that further regression will not occur. On the other hand, ELISK can be repeated. Even years after the first treatment with initial hypocorrection, the procedure can be repeated. The flap is easily removed from the remaining stroma, and it is possible to complete any undercorrection of the myopia or astigmatism by photorefractive ablation without running the risk of inducing haze.

Keratomileusis may appear to be more traumatic than PRK because it is more surgical; in fact, it involves the primary keratectomy with all the risks and complications that may involve. However, the developments made to the instruments used in the mechanical part and the stroma's lower reactivity to the ablation (compared to the Bowman's) make this technique an extremely promising one for even moderate myopia. Of particular importance is the marked stability of the refractive result. However, it goes without saying that this technique must be performed only by highly skilled ophthalmic surgeons.

INDICATIONS

If the corrective range for MKM using the historical techniques was between 10 and 18 D, with ELISK the range has been extended to cover myopias from 4 to 5 D (or less) to 25 D or more in very thick corneas.

MKM is indicated for the correction of myopic uni- or bilateral refractive defects when they are not correctable with the traditional optical or surgical methods. Another important indication is severe myopic anisometropia, not compensated by contact lenses. It is also indicated for improving non-corrected visual acuity in subjects with special professional or sporting requisites, or for other psychological reasons. The procedure is also extremely useful in severely myopic eyes for the treatment of superficial corneal opacities involving the first 300 to 350 microns; in this case a transparent homoplastic flap is required.

CONTRAINDICATIONS

The operation is not advisable if the refraction has not been stable for at least 2 years, in monocular subjects, or in those patients who eye conditions do not justify the procedure.

It is not indicated for patients affected by hypolacrymia (dry-eye), glaucoma, uveitis which is poorly controlled medically, other corneal pathologies such as dystrophy or degeneration, or vitreoretinal pathologies which carry with them a high risk of retinal detachment. Like other refractive procedures, this operation should be avoided in abnormally thin corneas.

Before the operation, pachymetric and topographical evaluations are obligatory.

CONCLUSION

In the treatment of severe myopia, the excellent functional results and the low frequency of complications obtained with ELISK (on the flap or in situ) have aroused widespread enthusiasm throughout the world, especially in the United States, Europe, and South America.

This is also because the continual evolution of refractive corneal surgery has presented us with increasingly sophisticated innovations. In fact, since the birth of keratomileusis, improvements in instruments and surgery have been constant and outstanding.

One important advance with the mechanical phase involved the automation of the microkeratome, which served to reduce human error at the hands of the surgeon to a minimum.

The use of the new automated microkeratome supplied with Chiron's ALK system permits a precise primary keratectomy. The flap has uniform thickness and the surfaces are perfectly smooth. This is because the instrument is not moved by the sur-

geon, but for the most part it is moved at constant speed and pressure through the advancement of the toothed wheel on the head of the microkeratome along the runners of the toothed suction ring.

The option of blocking the primary cut at the end of the lamellar incision represents a further small step toward perfecting the technique of KM. In fact, the blocking device permits a minimal part of the flap to remain attached to the remainder of the corneal tissue; this allows its precise, safe replacement at the end of the operation. The technique is therefore faster, and in the sutureless technique prevents the loss of the flap. As the microkeratome's direction of movement can be changed, it can be returned to its starting position with a steady, safe movement. This avoids damage to the flap following the primary keratectomy. In addition, there are all the advantages of an in situ photoablative treatment.

But undoubtedly the most important innovation is that of the intrastromal refractive ablation with the excimer laser. I feel this technique, despite being sophisticated and of recent invention, represents an enormous step in the evolution of the technique, through its precision, the possibility of varying the optical zone, and, above all, the site and depth of the ablation.

With the new excimer lasers, apart from a more homogeneous, constant laser beam, and a more gradual refractive ablation, there is the simultaneous treatment of preoperative astigmatism—something not to be dismissed lightly.

Elimination of the suture in the final stages of the operation is another step forward and has been made possible by the reduced trauma caused to the corneal tissue with this technique, all combining to give the surgeon a greater sense of security and avoiding the irritation of a suture.

Overall, MKM has become faster, safe, and precise, and the outcome is more predictable and encouraging for anyone using this technique of lamellar refractive surgery.

The indisputable advantages of keratomileusis, particularly in the two variations of ELISK (on the flap and in situ), compared to other intraocular techniques and PRK make this surgical procedure the most indicated for treating moderate-severe myopia.

Its superficial character (compared with the intraocular techniques), along with a better stromal response to the ablation using the excimer laser (compared to PRK where part of the Bowman's layer is also ablated), makes this a safe, predictable technique when performed by expert hands.

When the day comes that lamellar keratectomy can be performed using a laser system capable of resectioning tissue to the micron (both thickness and diameter) this procedure will be the elective technique for treating all types of myopia.

CHAPTER 9

Preoperative LASIK Patient Evaluation

CONSULTATIVE PROCESS

The consultative process for all refractive procedures is similar in concept. The risks, benefits, limitations, and reasonable expectations of the procedure are reviewed with each potential candidate. Laser in situ keratomileusis (LASIK) may offer candidates the ability to correct very high degrees of myopia with rapid visual rehabilitation, however, greater risk intraoperatively is associated and must be discussed. Patient management and expectations are facilitated and medical-legal responsibilities are fulfilled if a conservative approach is taken with each patient.

When the outcome is successful, the preoperative informed consent process has very little meaning; however, if a poor result is obtained, one always wishes he or she had ensured an adequate consent procedure preoperatively (see Appendix B). A surgeon who never has a complication is one who never performs surgery. Complications are an inherent part of any surgical procedure. Visual complications are emotionally traumatic, as the patient is reminded of the poor outcome during every waking hour. It is because the world is so visual that refractive surgery has the ability to dramatically improve the quality of a patient's life, and conversely, complications can be just as detrimental to that quality. Although no cases of blindness have ever been reported with photorefractive keratectomy (PRK) or LASIK worldwide, the potential for LASIK to produce real and irreversible harm to an eye cannot be overstated.

LASIK appears to share some of the benefits of both RK and PRK, with what I consider an intermediate risk and a greatly expanded refractive envelope of effectiveness.

> **A surgeon who never has a complication is one who never performs surgery.**

LASIK, unlike PRK, possesses the rapid visual recovery and minimal discomfort commonly associated with RK, but without the loss of corneal stability. LASIK similarly has greater refractive predictability associated with photoablation, but without significant risk of subepithelial haze formation.

In explaining to patients the LASIK procedure as compared to PRK, I state that both procedures are designed to change the curve of their eye to match that of their prescription, be it in glasses or contacts. It is unimportant whether the laser changes the curve on the surface of the eye or in the deeper layers, so long as the curve is changed. The surface of the eye is more sensitive and more reactive, requiring a longer healing time and more eye drops. Therefore, if we are performing a lot of surgery to correct moderate or high myopia, we prefer to treat the deeper layers with LASIK rather than superficially with PRK. PRK is associated with greater risk of infection, 1/1000 compared to 1/5000 with LASIK. PRK is also associated with more pain, 1/10 compared to 1/50 following LASIK. The risk of haze or scarring

Figure 9-1.
Dense confluent haze following attempted PRK correction of -10.50 D myope.

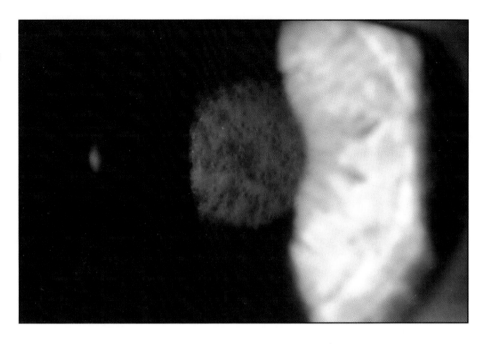

after PRK is only 1% or less for low degrees of correction but as high as 5% for higher degrees (Figure 9-1). The risk of scarring with LASIK is less than 0.2% for all degrees of correction. Visual recovery requires 1 to 4 weeks for PRK, compared to 1 to 4 days with LASIK. Steroid drops are needed for only 1 week with LASIK, compared to 4 months with PRK.

	PRK	LASIK
Pain	1/10	1/50
Infection	1/1000	1/5000
Scarring	1% to 5%	0.1%
Steroid drops	4 months	1 week
Visual recovery	1 to 4 weeks	1 to 4 days

The main disadvantage for LASIK is that a cut is involved, which adds the risk of a serious complication with LASIK, including corneal perforation. I explain the LASIK procedure and instrumentation by describing the microkeratome as a carpenter's plane which is used to create a corneal flap. The cornea is approximately 11 hairs thick, with the corneal flap about three hairs thick; I explain we must leave at least eight hairs (400 microns). I state that when a complication does occur, it is more serious with LASIK. I explain that I consider LASIK to be the best procedure, but that all procedures have to be considered in terms of their risk-to-benefit ratio for each patient. For mod-

erate and more severe degrees of myopia and astigmatism, above -4.00 to -5.00 D, LASIK is my procedure of choice. For low degrees of myopia, the predictability of PRK has been extremely high, and the risk of serious complication extremely low, making it the safer procedure in that range.

Bilateral simultaneous surgery is safer with LASIK than with PRK.

It is always safer to treat one eye at a time; bilateral simultaneous surgery with LASIK may even be safer than with PRK, since 95% of the complications with LASIK occur intraoperatively, compared to 95% of the PRK complications occurring postoperatively. Therefore, when the LASIK procedure has been completed, a good level of comfort has already been achieved prior to the fellow eye being treated, in direct contrast to bilateral simultaneous PRK. The major consideration with LASIK is to avoid overcorrections, as undercorrections are easily managed and enhancement surgery is very titratable.

The most important factors to patients contemplating LASIK have been the speed of recovery and the lack of pain. It appears that most patients, especially those with more moderate and severe degrees of myopia, still wish to have a procedure that disrupts their life as little as possible. Additionally, most people find it difficult to proceed with any procedure that produces pain, even if they place significant long-term value on a procedure associated with short-

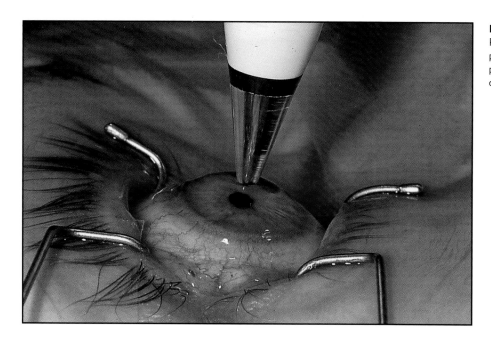

Figure 9-2.
Preoperative ultrasonic corneal pachymetry is performed for all patients prior to LASIK to ensure adequate corneal thickness.

term discomfort. It may very well be the image that eye surgery itself conjures up that keeps the majority of myopes from considering refractive surgery. As a general rule, female patients tolerate eye procedures better than male patients in my experience, perhaps because of years of applying eye makeup, perhaps for some completely different reason. All patients considering refractive surgery are fearful of losing their eyesight, which is why most patients, regardless of how motivated or affluent they are, will not proceed with any procedure. I surmise that only 5% to 10% of myopes will ever seriously contemplate any refractive procedure, and only 1% to 2% will proceed with what we consider to be highly evolved procedures utilizing the excimer laser, even when it becomes widely available.

CANDIDATE SELECTION

LASIK is capable of treating as much as 30.00 D of myopia, far in excess of what most potential candidates require for visual correction. The lower refractive limit for which LASIK is the preferred procedure is in dispute, primarily because of the variability in surgeon comfort and skill levels with this relatively new procedure. That is, if the surgeon achieves excellent results safely with PRK for mild and moderate myopia, the benefits of LASIK for these patients becomes more obscure. Some surgeons perform LASIK for all refractive procedures, even for corrections as low as 1.00 D of myopia, while others reserve LASIK for

patients with more than -10.00 D. The general consensus appears to be that the distinct advantage of LASIK over PRK (and RK) occurs over -6.00 D, with significant benefits occurring above -9.00 D. PRK toric ablations greater than 3.00 D and myopic ablations greater than 6.00 D are associated with a higher degree of clinically significant haze, in the range of 2% to 5% even with the best techniques. Although clinically significant haze is treatable, prolonged visual recovery and multiple procedures are required. Therefore, it appears reasonable to build a nomogram that considers RK and PRK the preferred procedures for myopia less than 3.00 or 4.00 D, PRK the procedure of choice from 4.00 to 8.00 D, and LASIK for refractive errors above that level. As surgeon comfort improves, LASIK replaces PRK as the preferred procedure above -4.00 D. Toric ablations may be performed within the stromal bed for the correction of several diopters of cylinder with LASIK, in direct contrast to standard automated lamellar keratoplasty (ALK). It should be noted, however, that new microkeratome designs encompass toric capabilities, and combined ALK-AK techniques remain quite effective for the treatment of severe myopia combined with astigmatism.

Candidate selection must also look at other elements independent of refractive error, specifically orbit configuration as well as ocular and general health considerations. Candidates with small or deep-set orbits should be avoided or forewarned that the procedure may have to be aborted if the microkeratome ring cannot be well positioned. Once surgical experience is adequate, these cases may be attempted,

TABLE 9-1
LASIK

Indicated	Caution	Contraindicated
High myopia	Flat corneas	Endothelial dystrophies (cell count <1500)
High astigmatism	Small orbits	Monocular patients
Keloid formers	Vitreal syneresis	Herpes zoster ophthalmicus
Long rigid gas permeable contact lens history	Anterior basement membrane dystrophy	Abnormal eyelid closure
Forme fruste keratoconus (normal corneal thickness age >35)	Post-RK	Active collagen vascular disease
Medication intolerance or noncompliance	Post-PKP	Systemic vasculitis
Steroid responders	Endothelial dystrophies (cell count >1500)	Keratoconus
Rapid visual recovery desired		Thin corneas

but initially they should be discouraged altogether. Similarly, narrow palpebral fissures may complicate placement of the suction ring, and may interfere with passage of the microkeratome. Any obstacles to smooth passage of the microkeratome will undoubtably compromise the success of obtaining a good corneal flap, and result in a higher complication rate. Patients with small orbits or narrow palpebral openings may experience increased discomfort intraoperatively and should be forewarned. Surgical techniques to deal with these patients will be discussed later.

Ocular conditions that should be specifically examined preoperatively include corneal neovascularization or macropannus, which may result in intraoperative bleeding following the lamellar cut. Although these patients are not contraindicated, measures to be discussed later may be taken to reduce intraoperative complications if noted preoperatively. Similarly, patients with flat corneas (mean keratometry <41.00) produce small corneal flaps and may result in a free cap, so the microkeratome should be adjusted to create a larger hinge to compensate and avoid this difficulty. Pachymetry should be performed on all patients, particularly high myopes, to ensure an adequate stromal bed thickness exists (Figure 9-2). Progressive corneal ectasia may be observed with a total corneal thickness of 300 microns or a stromal bed thickness of 200 microns. An absolute minimum corneal thickness of 360 microns, ideally 400 microns, must remain with a 250-micron stromal bed to ensure long-term stability. Alternatively, it is stated that no greater than 50% of the corneal thickness should be penetrated to ensure long-term corneal stability. For example, with a 540-micron

cornea and 160-micron flap, which leaves 380 microns, the maximum ablation depth is 110 microns, which will leave 50% or 270 microns. Patients with a history of prior ocular surgery, including vitreoretinal and cataract surgery, should be approached cautiously or avoided, as it is often difficult to achieve adequate suction pressure throughout the microkeratome cut and an irregular thin flap may be obtained. Once again, these are patients to avoid until considerable experience is obtained.

PRK may be preferable to LASIK in cases of recurrent corneal erosion syndrome, anterior basement membrane dystrophies, or superficial corneal scarring, in that surface photoablation offers these patients some specific benefits in improving epithelial adhesion or eliminating visual opacification. Furthermore, poor epithelial adherence complicates lamellar surgery significantly and increases the incidence of epithelial ingrowth dramatically. Any active ocular pathology, inflammation, or infection is contraindicated.

LASIK and RK should be considered preferable to PRK for any patient who requires rapid visual rehabilitation, although newer PRK techniques have reduced recovery time to as little as 1 week for many patients. LASIK should be considered, and perhaps may even be indicated, in cases where proper wound healing is critical or may be impaired, such as with keloid formers. PRK is absolutely contraindicated for autoimmune diseases and collagen vascular diseases, as the risk of stromal melt with an exposed stromal surface is significantly elevated. In LASIK, since the epithelium remains intact and the stroma only exposed intraoperatively, the concerns for precipitating a stromal melt are

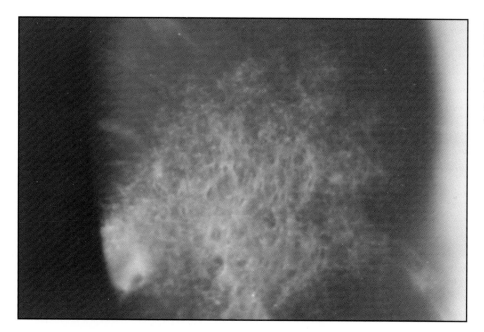

Figure 9-3.
High magnification view (40x) of dense central haze following attempted PRK correction of residual myopic astigmatism following RK 1 year previously. Note the areas of confluence developing from the coalescing areas of reticular haze.

unclear but likely minimal. I have performed LASIK on three patients with rheumatoid arthritis antibodies and two patients with lupus antibodies, all without active disease, with all five experiencing an uncomplicated recovery without any ocular sequelae. Active or severe vasculitic conditions should always be avoided for any refractive surgery procedure, as these procedures are always elective.

Another subset of patients who are preferably treated with LASIK rather than PRK are those who exhibit medication intolerance or non-compliance. Specifically, steroid responders observed from treatment of the first eye or those with a strong family history of glaucoma may do better with LASIK, since a steroid-induced pressure rise may seriously complicate the postoperative course or result in visual field loss. Patients with diagnosed glaucomatous field loss should be avoided for fear that raising, even briefly, the suction pressure intraoperatively with LASIK will further precipitate field loss. Patients living far away or traveling in the near future for prolonged periods of time, preventing adequate monitoring of steroid use, may also be better served with LASIK (Table 9-1).

CONTRAINDICATIONS

There are far fewer contraindications to LASIK than to PRK because of the dramatically reduced wound healing requirements. Systemic contraindications as outlined earlier are almost nonexistent, with only a few ocular contraindica-

tions. Monocular patients are always contraindicated for elective refractive surgery. Keratoconus is a specific absolute contraindication, although true forme fruste varieties may actually do better with LASIK than PRK. Corneal pachymetry to confirm adequate stromal thickness must be measured in all forme fruste patients, and young patients who may as yet develop clinical keratoconus are specifically contraindicated. As previously stated, autoimmune and collagen vascular disorders are not absolutely contraindicated with intrastromal ablation techniques, but caution is always advised and it is best to avoid any patients with active disease.

Although undercorrected RK is not a contraindication to LASIK, and may in fact be indicated, there is a risk that the flap will separate into pieces, especially in patients with greater than eight radial incisions. Surface photoablation may be preferable in specific multiple incision cases. Prior lamellar surgery is not a contraindication, however, prior penetrating keratoplasty may be relatively contraindicated because of risk to the endothelium and possible graft rejection, but has been performed accurately and successfully (Kritzinger, Ruiz). History of retinal detachment or retinal tears in themselves does not contraindicate LASIK.

Patients with anterior basement dystrophy and epithelial adherence problems should be avoided, although not contraindicated. If the epithelial surface becomes partially or fully denuded due to the microkeratome pass or perioperative medication, an increased risk of epithelial ingrowth is observed and slower visual recovery noted. Procedures

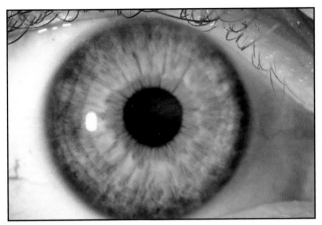

Figure 9-4a.
Bilateral LASIK correction of residual myopia following RK in right eye. LASIK procedure performed after 1 year to allow for full refractive stabilization and improved corneal integrity.

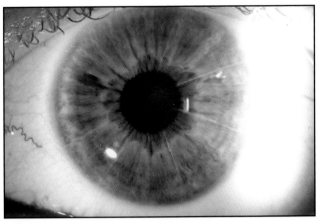

Figure 9-4b.
Bilateral LASIK correction of residual myopia following RK in left eye. LASIK procedure performed after 1 year to allow for full refractive stabilization and improved corneal integrity.

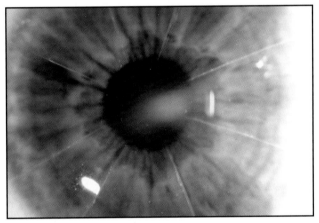

Figure 9-4c.
Biomicroscopic slit lamp clinical photo demonstrating small corneal flap misalignment under direct high magnification.

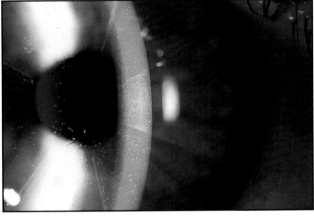

Figure 9-4d.
Biomicroscopic slit lamp clinical photo demonstrating small corneal flap misalignment under optical slit section.

which alter the conjunctiva significantly may interefere with the ability to obtain and maintain adequate suction during the lamellar cut, increasing the risk of a thin or perforated corneal flap. Similarly, any condition that results in significant vitreous syneresis, including pathogical myopia or procedures such as vitrectomy, may result in inadequate suction pressure intraoperatively. Once again, an experienced lamellar surgeon may attempt these more challenging cases, but complication rates are higher.

Clinical Note
LASIK and RK

Surface photoablation following RK is associated with a five- to ten-fold increase in haze formation and at least a 20% reduction in refractive predictability (Figure 9-3).

Patients may achieve the desired correction targeted, no correction, or triple the correction input; I have observed all three of these reactions. In counseling patients I explain that 2+2 does not always equal 4, but may equal 2 or even 8. It was for this reason that I attempted LASIK post-RK. LASIK post-RK should be performed following a minimum 1-year RK incision healing period. The two primary factors in producing regression following PRK enhancement of RK are haze formation and epithelial hyperplasia. The decided advantage of LASIK over PRK for this subset of patients is the virtual elimination of both of these regression factors. The elimination of haze as a significant complication should reduce the overall risk to these patients. The unaltered status of the epithelium should have a direct correlation with improved refractive predictability. The three primary surgical issues with LASIK post-RK are:

1. The application of suction to a destabilized cornea
2. Care of the RK-treated flap
3. Flap realignment

It has been stated that the suction ring may further destabilize the cornea and produce a dramatic overcorrection in 16- to 32-incision RK. Secondly, the corneal flap may split upon manipulation into multiple pie-like segments, especially if a small optical zone or greater than eight incisions had been performed. The final important aspect following delicate care of the flap is that of alignment, as the deeper stromal incisions must realign with those in the corneal flap. The patient from Figures 9-4a through 9-4d had bilateral LASIK for -3.00 D undercorrections post-RK with a successful outcome, but had notable misalignment.

I have performed only a handful of the 2000 LASIK procedures to date post-RK in light of these concerns. A number of experienced LASIK surgeons routinely perform LASIK post-RK and have not experienced any complications in hundreds of procedures. Two have experienced severe complications with fragmentation of the corneal flap. There is no ideal procedure as yet for the enhancement of undercorrected RK. LASIK, in certain refractive cases, becomes the only viable alternative, as indicated by the following two clinical examples.

Clinical Example 1

A 29-year-old female patient with an original refraction of -5.50 -2.00 x 180 had undergone two RK enhancement procedures prior to PRK referral for treatment of her residual refractive error of -2.00 -2.50 x 180. Unfortunately, following toric PRK, she developed dense haze requiring an additional phototherapeutic keratectomy (PTK/PRK) procedure to remove the corneal opacification. With retreatment, the patient obtained a clear cornea with 20/60 uncorrected visual acuity, correctable to 20/20, but with a residual refractive error of plano -2.50 x 180. For fear of reactivating haze formation once again, and in light of the fact that the corneal cylinder remained resistant to prior attempts with both RK and PRK, LASIK was performed. There were no corneal flap complications and the cylinder was reduced to 0.75 D, with 20/25 uncorrected visual acuity.

Clinical Example 2

A 32-year-old man with moderate myopia who was +1.50 D overcorrected post 16-incision RK, underwent

hyperopic ALK with a progressive myopic shift to finally stabilize at -14.00 D over 1 year later. The patient had intolerable anisometropia and was intolerant of his contact lens. LASIK was performed for -10.00 D to return the patient to -1.00 D and 20/60 uncorrected vision with surprisingly no loss of best corrected vision. The only alternative to LASIK in this case had been corneal transplantation.

PREOPERATIVE EXAMINATION

Preoperative evaluation is similar to that described in Chapter 2 for PRK and should be reviewed. In light of the greater range of correction with LASIK, evaluation of the higher myope becomes more important and high myopia considerations will be discussed below.

VISUAL ACUITY

Just as with all refractive procedures, documentation of uncorrected and best corrected visual acuity must be made. Severe and extreme myopia is associated with reduced best corrected visual acuity, which may differ between spectacle correction and contact lens correction. Higher myopes and astigmats may enjoy a level of visual acuity in rigid gas permeable contact lenses that may be impossible to replicate with refractive surgery. Documentation and discussion of these more challenging cases is important both medically in assessing postoperative outcomes, and in achieving high levels of patient satisfaction. Patients with reduced best corrected vision in one eye may not be suitable candidates, as complications in the good eye may preclude driving.

> Higher myopes and astigmats may enjoy a level of visual acuity in rigid gas permeable contact lenses that may be impossible to replicate with refractive surgery.

REFRACTION

A careful manifest and cycloplegic refraction must be performed with attention given to true vertex distance in cases of high myopia. Higher myopes often are overcorrected in their spectacle correction in an attempt to improve their quality of vision. In cases of extreme myopia, it may be necessary to fit the patient with a disposable contact lens for -8.00 or -9.00 D and overrefract the patient.

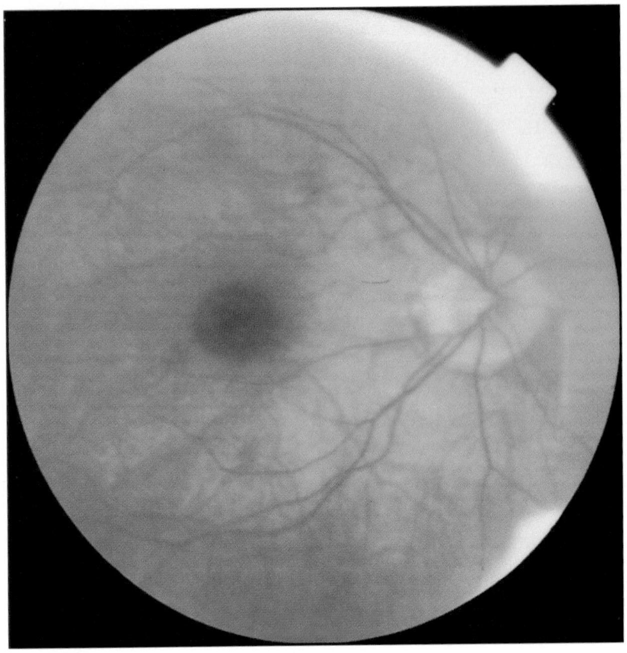

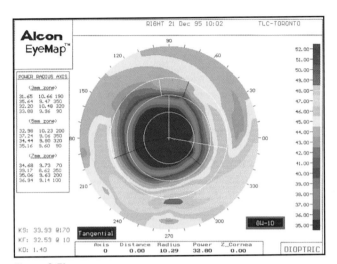

Figure 9-5a.
Fundus photography demonstrating superficial macular hemorrhage following LASIK in a highly myopic patient. Suction time was approximately 30 seconds. Role of procedure in precipitating hemorrhage unclear and surprisingly was felt to be coincidental by patient's retinal specialist, who observed macular changes several months preoperatively.

Figure 9-5b.
Corneal videokeratography demonstrating excellent central flattening following the LASIK procedure for -12.00 D. Patient remains 20/80 uncorrected at 6 weeks due to macular hemorrhage, although vision is slowly improving both subjectively and objectively.

ANTERIOR SEGMENT EXAMINATION

There is very little which differs from the evaluation performed prior to PRK. The orbit configuration, palpebral aperature, corneal diameter, and presence of corneal neovascularization should all be studied in evaluating each LASIK candidate in order to anticipate difficulties. Clinical keratoconus is contraindicated and ultrasonic pachymetry should be performed on all patients to assess the amount of correction obtainable. Endothelial changes should be ruled out, as Fuchs' endothelial dystrophy, traumatic breaks in Descemet's membrane, and other causes of endothelial dysfunction preclude intrastromal ablation.

> **Pachymetry should be performed on all patients to assess the amount of correction attainable.**

POSTERIOR SEGMENT EXAMINATION

Dilated retinal evaluation is of particular importance in high myopia, and any retinal tears or pathology requiring treatment should be referred preoperatively for management. Documentation of myopic macular degeneration and posterior staphylomas is important because postoperative deterioration of vision may be independent of the procedure.

Clinical Note

Retinal Hemorrhage Post-LASIK

A 27-year-old female patient with -13.00 D OS and -12.00 D OD underwent uncomplicated LASIK in her left eye, followed by surgery on her right eye 1 week later. Left eye visual acuity at 1 week was 20/40+2 with no loss of best corrected vision and good qualitative vision. Right eye recovery was complicated by development of a central scotoma, reducing visual acuity to 20/200 initially and 20/80 after 1 week. Anterior segment examination demonstrated bilateral corneal flaps in good position with clear interfaces. Fundus examination revealed a macular hemorrhage OD (Figures 9-5a and 9-5b). The LASIK procedure on the right eye was completely uncomplicated with a suction time in the range of 20 seconds and a total procedure time of less than 5 minutes. The etiology was determined to be related to her extreme myopia (Fuchs' spot) and was not considered by her retinal specialist to have been related to her procedure. Retinal pigment epithelial changes in her left eye were also appreciated.

One other reported case worldwide was a young man treated in South America who developed bilateral retinal hemorrhages following bilateral surgery. No surgical details are available. A review of over 10,000 LASIK procedures in South America failed to disclose any other cases. Considering that a number of surgeons routinely leave the suction pressure applied for 3 to 6 minutes, it is surprising that other cases have not been identified if a true causal relationship exists.

The coincidental nature is suspicious in that the macular hemorrhage was identified in the immediate postoperative period. It could well be that these patients had been predisposed to develop a break in Bruch's membrane with a secondary choroidal neovascular net, and that the surgery merely precipitated the occurrence at an earlier date.

CORNEAL TOPOGRAPHY

Corneal topography is important in assessing not only the target correction to be programmed, but the corneal curvature. Excessively flat corneas with mean keratometry below 41.00 D produce smaller corneal flaps unless associated with a small corneal diameter. The surgeon must anticipate that the presence of a flat cornea may result in a free corneal cap if no adjustments to the hinge size are made.

Patients with a long history of rigid gas permeable contact lens wear or forme fruste keratoconus patients over 30

> Excessively flat corneas with mean keratometry below 41.00 D produce smaller corneal flaps unless associated with a small corneal diameter.

with normal pachymetry are best treated with LASIK.

CANDIDATE PREPARATION

There is little difference in candidate preparation between surface photoablation and intrastromal ablation. Each patient not only requires a detailed understanding of the risks and benefits of each procedure, but also what to expect at each stage of the procedure and postoperative recovery.

Contact lenses must similarly be removed in advance with a re-establishment of the natural topography preoperatively. LASIK is the preferred procedure if corneal warpage persists for months or the patient is a longtime rigid gas permeable or PMMA hard lens wearer.

The immediate postoperative examination schedule is far simpler, with only one visit required the following day, as the epithelium typically remains intact. In fact, a baseline visual acuity and refraction can be performed. Fellow eyes are treated within days if bilateral simultaneous surgery is not performed, and should be tentatively scheduled as such. Repeat examination should then be scheduled at 1 week and at 3 weeks later, at which time assessment for enhancement surgery can be made.

CHAPTER 10

LASIK Procedure

OVERVIEW

Laser in situ keratomileusis (LASIK) involves the use of a microkeratome (similar to a carpenter's plane in concept) to create a 160-micron flap, about one third the depth of the cornea. A suction ring is used to both fixate the globe and increase the intraocular pressure (IOP) to 65 or 70 mmHg, which is necessary for a proper lamellar incision. Small and deep-set eyes are generally avoided until sufficient surgical experience is obtained, as exposure is needed for the suction ring and microkeratome. A hinge is typically created nasally to "hinge" the flap and secure it in position in the immediate postoperative period. The photoablation or photorefractive keratectomy (PRK) treatment is made in the stromal bed. The procedure takes several minutes to perform. The high IOP blurs the patient's view intraoperatively. The corneal flap is then laid back down, ensuring proper alignment.

PATIENT PREPARATION

It is useful to clean or irrigate the fornices preoperatively in order to help maintain a clean interface. There is a tremendous amount of debris and sebaceous material within the fornices and tear film of each patient, some significantly more than others. If the stromal bed is irrigated following the ablation, then it becomes far more critical to cleanse the fornices or aspirate the irrigating fluid.

Lid hygiene efforts are perhaps of even greater importance in reducing the risk of potential infection. Lid scrubs immediately preoperatively as used for PRK are recommended, but antibiotic ointment is contraindicated as it may invade the stromal interface. A periorbital antiseptic scrub is effective for sterilizing the surgical environment.

PREOPERATIVE MEDICATIONS

Preoperatively, each patient receives a topical anesthetic, topical antibiotic, and preoperative sedation. In general, it is wise not to pharmacologically manipulate the pupil preoperatively. Miotics may induce a superonasal shift, although they tend to reduce patient discomfort due to microscope glare. A topical non-steroidal anti-inflammatory drop such as Voltaren (diclofenac sodium 0.1%, CIBA) may be instilled preoperatively to help reduce any discomfort or inflammatory reaction.

Various topical anesthetics can be used; however, it is best not to utilize excessive amounts of topical anesthesia since it will disturb the surface epithelium. Proparacaine or xylocaine are probably preferable to tetracaine, which has a greater epitheliotoxic effect. Application of topical anesthesia with a soaked surgical spear to the upper and lower fornices is highly recommended (Figure 10-1), which is where

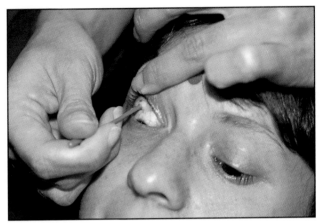

Figure 10-1.
Lidocaine 4% topical anesthesia applied directly to superior fornix with soaked surgical spear preoperatively to avoid direct epithelial toxicity of ophthalmic drops.

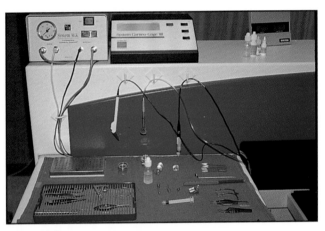

Figure 10-2.
LASIK operative set-up including Corneo-gage Ultrasonic Pachymeter, Chiron suction pump, Chiron Corneal Shaper, and additional fine instruments. Courtesy of Dr. Stephen G. Slade.

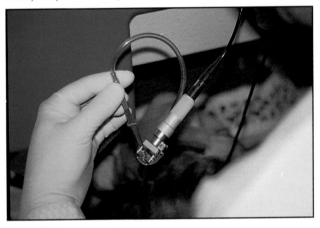

Figure 10-3.
Preoperative testing of Chiron-Steinway microkeratome. Prior to each lamellar procedure, the unit must be examined for proper assembly and function. The formalized concept of a Preflight checklist was advanced by J. Charles Casebeer, MD, to avoid potential serious lamellar complications due to microkeratome malfunction.

most of the discomfort from the eyelid speculum is created. The lamellar incision itself is virtually painless relative to the lid speculum, and the vacuum from the suction ring creates a well-tolerated mild pressure sensation. Therefore, by anesthetizing the fornices well, especially the upper fornix, patient comfort and cooperation are greatly enhanced. Apply anesthesia immediately preoperatively, and not 30 minutes prior, to reduce epithelial toxicity. Patients should also keep their eyes closed once anesthetized, as the blink reflex is diminished.

Topical antibiotic and betadine or other antiseptic preparations are utilized preoperatively to reduce the bacterial load in the conjunctiva. The choice of antibiotics is far less important than with PRK, as the risk of infection is greatly reduced. The choice is important insofar as antibiotics that are toxic to the epithelium, like the aminoglycoside gentamicin, should be avoided, although tobramycin has frequently been used successfully. Fluoroquinolones may be best suited, as they are not epitheliotoxic and are broad spectrum.

Preoperative sedation with a short-acting benzodiazepine such as lorazepam 1 to 2 mg is recommended for agitated patients, and all patients may benefit somewhat. Fixation may be ensured with the use of the suction ring, even without application of vacuum pressure, so that temporary sedation should not affect centration. Versed (Madazolam 0.3 to 0.5 mg/kg) has been used effectively to alleviate anxiety perioperatively, also providing an amnesic effect (Roy).

LASER CALIBRATION AND TESTING

There is no difference in the laser calibration technique required for LASIK compared to that for PRK. The only important differences lie in the software utilized and target correction attempted. In response to less wound healing than anticipated, lasers such as the Summit ExciMed and even the OmniMed with gaussian energy beam profiles require that a lower correction be targeted to avoid significant overcorrection. In general, other lasers require the use of the spectacle plane refraction, and may even add an additional diopter to the attempted correction because the mid-stroma is more hydrated, resulting in significant undercorrections. It is not important which nomogram is used, simply that the nomogram is conservative, since undercorrections are far more easily managed. Some surgeons leave the stroma naturally hydrated throughout the procedure, which may or may not improve corneal interface clarity. Other surgeons apply a fan across the entire surgical field, while some use a blunt spatula to wipe excessive stromal fluid away, or a surgical spear to dehydrate the stroma somewhat. Another technique utilized to control the hydration status of the deeper stroma and the ablation rate is to utilize a 23-gauge cannula which applies 3 liters of air per minute to the stromal bed for 2 seconds between each zone of ablation.

Additionally, not only does the increased hydration status of the mid-stroma relative to the superficial stroma result in undercorrections, but it is associated with a higher incidence of central island formation when optical zones greater than 5.0 mm are used with all lasers, including the Summit. Therefore, either a pretreatment step can be added prior to the refractive treatment, or an aspheric ablation pattern used, which concentrates the treatment within a small area of 4.5 mm or less with a 5.5- to 6.0-mm transition zone. Although night glare may be more apparent with the aspheric pattern, central islands are infrequent. Pretreatment can be applied with both single or multizone ablation patterns. Although wound contour and wound edge profile are far less important with LASIK than PRK, optical zone size and depth of ablation become critical factors to consider in the correc-

> **Wound contour and wound edge profile are far less important with LASIK than PRK.**

tion of severe myopia. Specifically, optical zones of at least 6.0 mm are required to avoid significant glare. It is impossible to use single zone techniques for severe myopes greater than -10.00 D because of the significant depth of ablation required. Therefore, it is best to use multizone techniques to reduce depth of ablation without sacrificing optical zone size. A pretreatment is necessary to avoid central island formation, the amount of which varies with the particular laser system. Larger optical zones also help to reduce regression in addition to night glare, which does occur even with LASIK.

OPERATIVE STEPS AND SURGICAL PRINCIPLES

The first step in the LASIK procedure, following fluence testing and programming of the laser, is patient alignment.

> **Optical zones of at least 6.0 mm are required to avoid significant glare.**

In addition, the microkeratome instrumentation must be carefully examined and tested. Preparation and care of the instrumentation is the most important element to a successful outcome (Figure 10-2). Staff training and expertise are of paramount importance and of equal significance to surgeon training. This single point cannot be overstated.

Five specific checks should be made prior to each and every procedure (Figure 10-3).

1. The first test involves listening to the microkeratome unit while in both forward and reverse motion. Each unit has a particular sound or pitch which often is altered when the unit is not functioning correctly. The unit should always be checked if the sound has changed.

2. The number and position of the microkeratome depth plate should be checked carefully (Figures 10-4a and 10-4b). The 160-micron plate is used routinely with the Chiron Corneal Shaper unit, and I feel produces less irregular astigmatism than the 130-micron plate suggested for higher myopes. The thicker flap may smooth any irregularities, but the 240-micron plate may mask too much of the ablative effect and is more difficult to manipulate. A 180- or 190-micron plate may be preferable for moderate and mild myopes. The plate, most importantly, must be in place, as failure will result in a cut depth of 900 microns, perforating the cornea and risking expulsion of the ocular contents. The plate must also be fully inserted, being flush with the end of the unit with no gap visible above the blade edge.

3. The blade must then be checked under the microscope, and ideally with a micron scope, for any blade edge irregularities. Movement of the blade must then be checked to ensure smooth back and forth motion. The gap between the plate and the blade should be clear of any debris or plastic filings.

4. The safety hinge must then be examined to ensure that it is attached and that the hinge screw is set according-

> **Preparation and care of the instrumentation is the most important element to a successful outcome. Staff training and expertise are of paramount importance and of equal significance to surgeon training.**

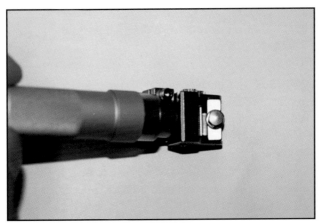

Figure 10-4a.
The microkeratome with depth plate in position should be compared with the appearance of the unit without the depth plate inserted (Figure 10-4b).

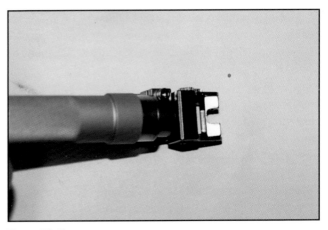

Figure 10-4b.
The microkeratome with depth plate in position (Figure 10-4a) should be compared with the appearance of the unit without the depth plate inserted.

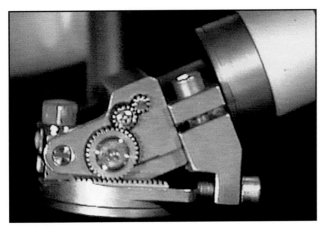

Figure 10-5.
Profile view of Chiron Corneal Shaper head during preoperative testing denoting action of hinge stop, preventing further advancement of unit. The hinge stop is set to create the size of hinge desired, but must take into account the preoperative keratometry.

ly if the stopper is not fixed into the unit (Figure 10-5).
5. The microkeratome is then inserted into the suction ring and the gears engaged. The foot pedal is depressed in the forward and reverse direction to ensure a smooth procession. Any difficulty engaging the microkeratome or lack of smoothness requires additional cleaning of the microkeratome and suction ring tract. The microkeratome should never be used unless the passage is smooth. The Corneal Shaper head should literally glide along the tract.

The entire testing process literally requires about 30 seconds when the unit is cleaned, prepared, and functioning properly.

SURGICAL PREPARATION OF THE OPERATIVE EYE

The patient is properly aligned with centration upon the pupil, which is preferred over the visual axis to avoid asymmetric night glare. If a large angle kappa exists, I routinely shift to the midpoint. The fellow eye is covered with an opaque shield and taped closed. Taping the fellow eye closed is helpful in preventing any drying effects of the epithelium.

An additional application of anesthesia is often effective as well as comforting to the patient, and is done by soaking a surgical spear with topical proparacaine 0.5% and placing it firmly on the bulbar conjunctiva in the upper and lower fornices. Some surgeons apply topical anesthesia at this point and not before. The eyelids are then dried and the eyelashes removed from the surgical field with surgical draping of the surgeon's preference. I have personally used surgical micropore tape with great effectiveness. Steri-strips can also be used. The objective is to clear the eyelashes from the surgical field and microkeratome gears, while covering the meibomian orifices of the lid margin.

OBTAINING ADEQUATE EXPOSURE

The ideal speculum will be a wire speculum to provide maximum exposure, rather than that of a solid blade variety, and will be adjustable. A titanium Lieberman speculum is my personal preference (Figure 10-6). I ensure that the draping is folded into the fornices so as to cover the upper and lower lid margins (Figure 10-7). If one looks carefully, an oily film

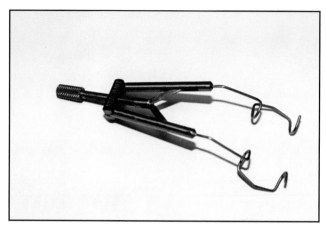

Figure 10-6.
Lieberman design adjustable wire eyelid speculum.

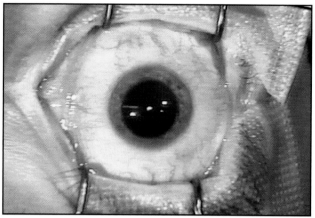

Figure 10-7.
Preparation of operative field for LASIK with wire eyelid speculum for maximal ocular exposure and draping of eyelashes and eyelid margins to reduce surgical field contamination. It is important to properly position head to obtain best centration, with equal amounts of sclera visible superiorly and inferiorly.

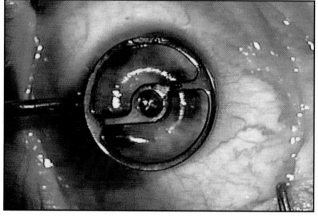

Figure 10-8.
Ruiz marker for lamellar surgery creating central and peripheral circular markings connected by a pararadial mark. Handle must be held temporally to correctly orient pararadial mark.

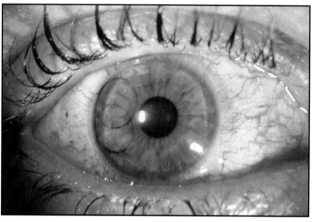

Figure 10-9.
Immediate LASIK postoperative clinical photograph demonstrating Machat alignment markings. Slight conjunctival injection and eyelid edema.

is sometimes evident in the tear film from the meibomian secretions; therefore, covering these orifices is important.

ALIGNMENT MARKINGS

Alignment markings are then placed on the corneal surface. There are two reasons for the markings: first for alignment with an intact hinge and second for alignment with an accidentally produced free cap. The importance of the latter is that the markings must not be able to align if a free cap is produced and is accidently placed epithelial side down. The classic alignment markings consist of a central 3-mm circular mark with a concentric 10-mm circular mark and a paraxial line radiating between the circles temporally

(Figure 10-8). However, there are two problems with this alignment system: the central marking disturbs the central epithelium, and the paraxial marking only provides a single point of alignment. I utilize two circular markings of 3.25 and 3.75 mm ideally. The circles are marked with gentian violet and placed peripherally and temporally (Figure 10-9). The circles extend from the limbus to leave the central 3 mm of epithelium untouched, improving visual recovery rate. Additionally, the circles provide four-point alignment with the different sized circles, preventing any chance that a free cap may be placed upside down. The size of the flap fashioned is variable from 7.2 to 9.0 mm, with a mean cap diameter of 8.5 mm, which is dependent upon the preoperative

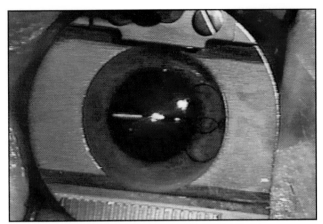

Figure 10-10.
Intraoperative clinical photograph demonstrating application suction ring on right eye. Note enlargement of pupil upon activation of suction pressure. Slight inferior decentration to avoid pronounced superior neovascularization from contact lens wear.

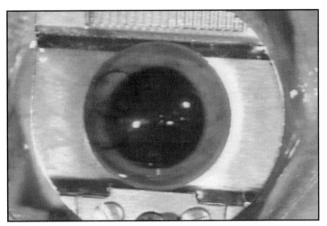

Figure 10-11.
Intraoperative clinical photograph demonstrating centration of suction ring with temporal alignment markings on left eye.

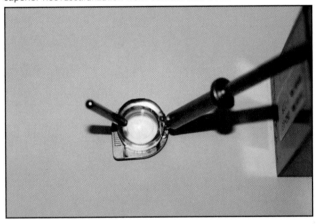

Figure 10-12a.
Applanation lens.

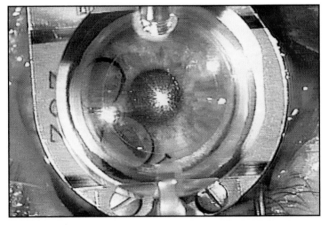

Figure 10-12b.
Intraoperative photo demonstrating assessment of corneal flap size with 8.5-mm applanation lens. Meniscus exceeds 8.5-mm demarcated ring indicating that corneal flap will be slightly larger. Applanation lens mimics microkeratome head, demonstrating the corneal tissue that will be presented to the advancing Corneal shaper head.

corneal curvature and suction pressure achieved. Smaller diameter corneas act like steeper corneas producing large corneal flaps. The diameter of the cornea also varies greatly between patients, and therefore the advantage of the circles is that they encompass the flap to a variable degree in all cases. Another recommended alignment marking system is that developed by Kritzinger and Updegraff.

CENTRATION OF THE SUCTION RING

The excimer LASIK ring, which is a non-adjustable suction ring, is then placed on the eye with the flat portion temporal (Figure 10-10). If it is difficult to obtain adequate exposure, a useful technique taught to me by Stephen G.

Slade, MD, is that the lid speculum can be depressed to help herniate the orbital contents and obtain better exposure for ring placement. The centration of the suction ring is another essential step, but far more so for automated lamellar keratoplasty (ALK) than for LASIK. With ALK, centration of the ring over the cornea for the initial or access pass for creating the lamellar flap is essential to allow for centration of the second refractive pass. With LASIK, however, centration of the flap is not essential for centration of the ablation within the stromal bed. There may actually be an advantage to slight nasal decentration of 1 mm or less. Slight nasal decentration allows the ablation to be centered (Figure 10-11) without concern that the ablation will ablate the undersurface of the flap, which would result in a doubling of the refractive effect along the hinge. Excessive decentration may, however, compromise smooth passage of the microkeratome. Inferior decentration is in fact indicated in cases of severe neovascularization related to contact lens wear to avoid the superior macropannus formation. The incision of these vessels intraoperatively may complicate the surgery, the management of which is discussed later.

The suction is activated once the suction ring is precisely positioned and seated firmly in place. If the suction is first initiated and then lowered into postion, two complications

> Centration of suction ring and corneal flap determines centration of ALK refractive pass but not centration of LASIK photoablation.

> The lid speculum can be depressed to help herniate the orbital contents and obtain better exposure for ring placement.

may occur: the centration may not engage as anticipated, and the conjunctiva may be pulled into the ring and interfere with obtaining or maintaining adequate suction pressure.

DETERMINING CAP DIAMETER

The ring is held perpendicularly to avoid breaking suction (Figures 10-12a and 10-12b). A stable surgical chair with armrests is recommended. The diameter of the corneal flap to be fashioned is then ensured to be adequate by inserting a 7.2- or 8.5-mm applanation lens. The last check before the microkeratome pass is the assessment of the IOP obtained using a Barraquer tonometer. It is important that the corneal surface be relatively dry for both diameter and pressure measurements, as excessive moisture will create a false meniscus. When measuring the diameter, a meniscus is visible to the surgeon (Figure 10-13), and should first be centered and symmetrical if the applanation lens is properly inserted. Within the applanation lens a ring is visible, the diameter of which is indicated by the applanation lens chosen. That is, the applanation lens acts like a transparent microkeratome, allowing the surgeon to visualize what will be presented to the microkeratome. Therefore, one can judge the anticipated diameter of the cap as well as centration.

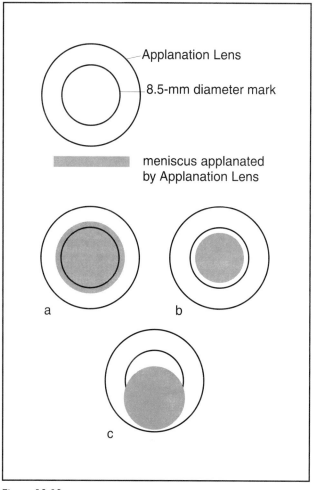

Figure 10-13.
Excellent/acceptable (a): Proceed to IOP measurement. Meniscus larger than 8.5 mm indicates that large corneal flap will be fashioned. Can also be produced if corneal surface is excessively wet.
Poor/acceptable (b): Do not proceed until check if keratometry less than 41.00 D. Indicates small corneal flap will be created. Increased risk of free corneal cap, adjust for larger hinge. Check pressure carefully.
Not acceptable (c): Remeasure as applanation lens not properly seated.

DETERMINING IOP OBTAINED

When measuring the IOP, the Barraquer tonometer is suspended by the ring vertically and perpendicularly over the pupil center, allowing the tonometer tip to applanate the corneal surface (Figures 10-14a through 10-14c). Pressure is defined simply as force over area. The weight of the Barraquer tonometer applies a given force which applanates a variable area, depending upon the pressure within the eye (Figure 10-15). If the eye is very soft, the area will be great, as the force is capable of compressing a larger surface area. If the pressure within the eye is very high, the force will not

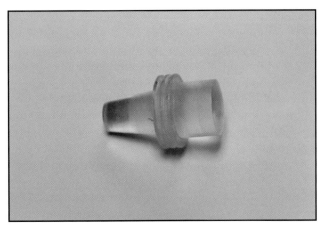

Figure 10-14a.
Barraquer tonometer for intraoperative IOP measurement during LASIK and ALK procedures prior to corneal flap resection.

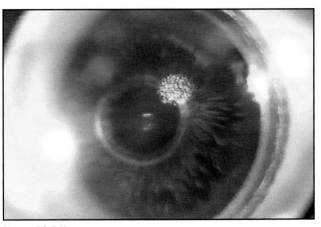

Figure 10-14b.
Intraoperative view of IOP testing with Barraquer tonometer. Note the applanation meniscus is smaller than the demarcated ring, indicating an applanation pressure greater than 65 mmHg.

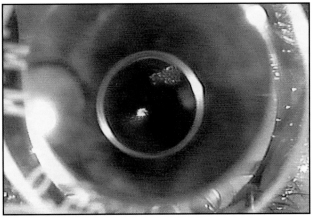

Figure 10-14c.
Intraoperative view of IOP testing with Barraquer tonometer demonstrating meniscus equal in size to demarcated ring, indicating a borderline applanation pressure.

be able to compress the eye very much, which will generate a small meniscus. The surgeon visualizes a ring within the tonometer, the diameter of which signifies 65 mmHg. If the meniscus observed is larger, the pressure within the eye is less than 65 mmHg; if the meniscus is smaller, the pressure is greater than the minimum allowable IOP of 65 mmHg. The smaller the meniscus, the higher the IOP, the safer the procedure, the better the quality and thickness of the flap. Under no circumstances should a surgeon ever attempt to

> **The smaller the meniscus, the higher the IOP, the safer the procedure, the better the quality and thickness of the flap.**

> **The tonometer measurement should always be the final maneuver prior to the microkeratome pass.**

perform a microkeratome pass with an inadequate pressure, as the integrity of the flap will be extremely poor, evidenced by a thin, torn, or perforated flap. The management of such complications will be discussed later. Excessive surface moisture of the cornea will increase the size of the meniscus applanated and indicate a falsely low IOP. Therefore, it is important not to rehydrate the epithelium immediately prior to checking the IOP, and to dry the epithelium and re-applanate if a large meniscus is observed, indicating a low pressure measurement. It is also useful to very gently digitally applanate the cornea to become familar with the feel of an adequate IOP, remembering that all manipulations should be performed prior to the tonometer reading. The tonometer measurement should always be the final maneuver prior to the microkeratome pass to help ensure that an adequate pressure is present for the critical microkeratome pass.

PNEUMATIC RING VACUUM PRESSURE

The pneumatic suction ring is placed differently for the right and left eyes, but always with the flat edge pointing temporally. Thus the handle is directed toward the surgeon for left eyes and away for right eyes (Figure 10-16). Once the suction ring is perpendicular to the eye and well seated, the microkeratome is then fully engaged into the tract grooves. When the vacuum pressure is activated, the surgical assistant should notify the surgeon of the vacuum pressure achieved. It is best to give control of the vacuum pres-

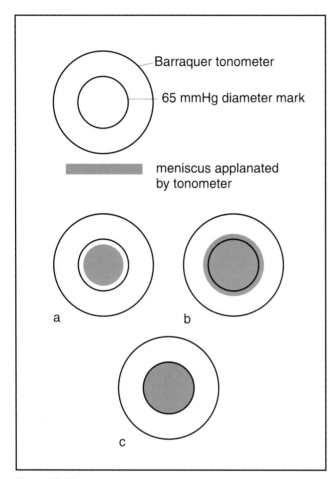

Figure 10-15.
Excellent/acceptable (a): Meniscus smaller than tonometer ring, indicating IOP above 65 mmHg. Proceed.
Poor/unacceptable (b): Meniscus larger than tonometer ring, indicating IOP below 65 mmHg. Do not proceed. High risk of thin or perforated corneal flap.
Fair/borderline acceptable (c): Meniscus equal size relative to tonometer ring, indicating borderline IOP. Confirm corneal surface dry and suction ring seated well, then retest. Higher risk of corneal flap problems, especially thin flap.

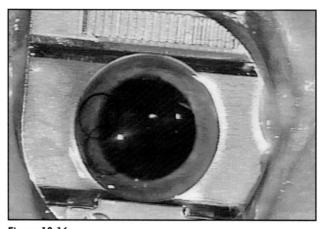

Figure 10-16.
Intraoperative clinical photograph demonstrating positioning of suction ring for left eye. Note the flat portion of the ring remains temporal and is the site at which the microkeratome is threaded.

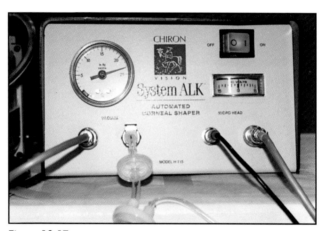

Figure 10-17a.
Chiron ALK System with adequate suction pressure of 23 mmHg.

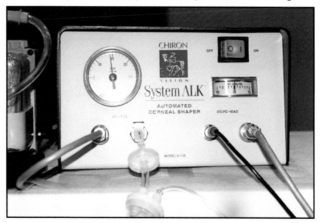

Figure 10-17b.
Chiron ALK System with inadequate suction pressure of <15 mmHg upon application of vacuum. Inadequate suction pressure may be secondary to pseudosuction of perilimbal conjunctiva into suction port or partial obstruction of suction ring from draping. The suction pressure should be identical each time full suction is applied; if lower assess for any obstacles which may affect seal.

sure to the surgical assistant, lest a surgeon accidently press the suction pedal rather than the microkeratome motor pedal, which could be disastrous to the flap. The maximum vacuum pressure produced by each unit is 23 to 28 mmHg. Each surgeon should note the precise reading for his or her unit (Figure 10-17a), as it is reproducible when full occlusion of the suction ring is created intraoperatively. If full occlusion is not achieved or is lost, the vacuum pressure typically reads a lesser value (Figure 10-17b). That is, if the maximum vacuum pressure is typically 25 mmHg and the assistant reads out 24 mmHg, then the suction ring should be

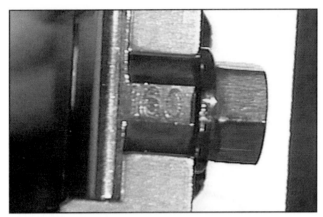

Figure 10-18a.
Preoperative testing of Chiron Corneal Shaper demonstrating 160 μm depth plate in proper position preventing corneal perforation and controlling corneal flap thickness. Gap between depth plate and blade must also be assessed to ensure no debris has inadvertently been introduced blocking flap passage.

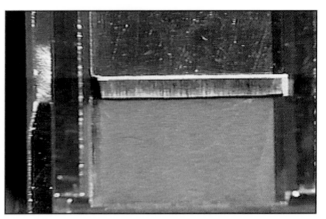

Figure 10-18b.
Preoperative testing of Chiron Corneal Shaper evaluating blade quality and demonstrating movement of blade. Blade can be stationary if blade block is assembled incorrectly or blocked with debris.

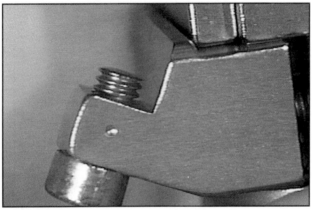

Figure 10-18c.
Preoperative evaluation of Chiron Corneal Shaper hinge stop setting. Adjustable screw setting can be varied for controlling corneal flap and hinge size based upon preoperative keratometry.

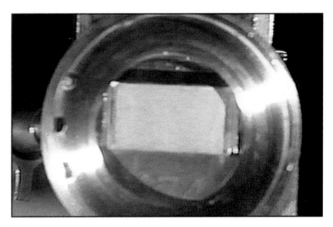

Figure 10-18d.
Preoperative testing of Chiron Corneal Shaper demonstrating hinge stop set too short, creating very small hinge. Newer hinge stops are fixed or preset to create the preferred hinge size automatically for the normal range of keratometry readings. Smooth passage of the microkeratome along the suction ring tract must also be assessed prior to the procedure.

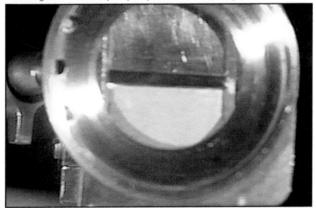

Figure 10-18e.
Preoperative testing of Chiron Corneal Shaper demonstrating hinge stop set too long, bisecting pupil. Newer hinge stops are fixed or preset to create the preferred hinge size automatically for the normal range of keratometry readings.

reapplied. However, even with full occlusion, adequate IOP is not guaranteed, as redundant or edematous conjunctiva can create a falsely high vacuum pressure without adequate IOP being achieved.

INSERTING THE MICROKERATOME HEAD INTO THE PNEUMATIC SUCTION RING

Although the cornea must be dry to properly assess the IOP, it must be wet for the microkeratome pass. Upon insertion of the microkeratome head into the suction ring, it is important to realize that the parallel tracts on the pneumatic suction ring have a triangular bevel or dovetail groove and a

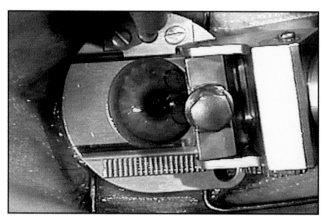

Figure 10-19a.
Insertion of the microkeratome head into the suction ring requires the unit to be tilted slightly away from the handle, thereby inserting the beveled guide first. The unit is then dropped into the parallel square guide and advanced, locking the unit into the tract. It is important to insert the unit properly into the parallel tracts, as the unit will still advance even if engaged into only one tract, thereby creating an uneven corneal flap.

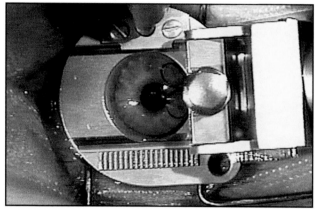

Figure 10-19b.
Intraoperative overview of Chiron Corneal Shaper unit being introduced into suction ring. It is important to ensure that there are no obstacles in the path of the microkeratome prior to engaging the unit.

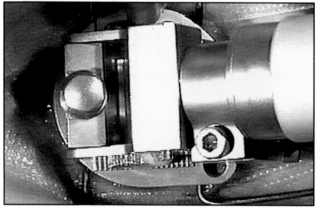

Figure 10-19c.
As the Chiron Corneal Shaper advances, the unit motor or wire must be delicately supported so as not to interfere with smooth passage, but maintain the unit within the parallel tracts.

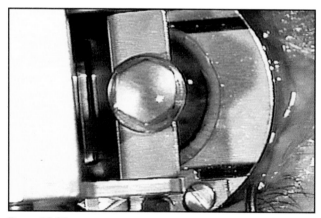

Figure 10-20.
Intraoperative view demonstrating engagement position of Chiron Corneal Shaper head. Note that for the fine gears to be aligned and engaged, the unit is advanced until it reaches the second screw on the suction ring. If the unit falls short of this point, the forward pedal will fail to advance the Shaper head. If this occurs, depressing the pedal briefly in either forward or reverse direction will rotate the gears and allow them to fully engage.

squared groove which accept the corresponding squared and triangular guides of the microkeratome head (Figures 10-18a through 10-18e). The microkeratome is tilted slightly, placing the dovetail guide in the triangular groove first, then dropped down into the squared tract, thus stabilizing it into position. The unit is then advanced along the tract until it is fully engaged (Figures 10-19a through 10-19c). The unit appears to be halfway across the cornea, but the cutting mechanism will be properly positioned. The end of the unit should be almost aligned with the forward screw (Figure 10-20). If the forward pedal, the one furthest away from the cord (Figure 10-21), is depressed and the unit does not

advance, it is likely that the teeth of the unit gears and those of the suction ring tract are not engaged. Depress the reverse or forward pedal for 1 second to spin the microkeratome head gears and advance the unit into position, as this may allow engagement. This process can be repeated and is usually effective. If the unit cannot be manually advanced, it should be pulled back and reinserted. Care should always be taken to avoid disengaging the suction pressure. If a considerable amount of manipulation is performed, the IOP should be reconfirmed.

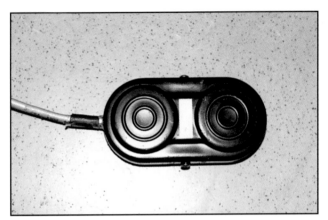

Figure 10-21.
Chiron Corneal Shaper system foot pedal. The forward pedal is positioned farthest away from the attached power cord.

CREATION OF THE CORNEAL FLAP

Immediately prior to depressing the forward pedal, the surgeon should scan the operative field for obstacles which could impede passage of the microkeratome, such as the lid speculum, lids, or draping. Medium or low magnification should be used on the microscope to have a full and adequate view. The suction ring should be supported, as should the microkeratome wire; however, pushing the suction ring down may result in redundant or edematous conjunctiva

> **The surgeon should scan the operative field for obstacles which could impede passage of the microkeratome.**

becoming trapped within the gears, producing an obstruction. The microkeratome forward pedal should be released just before, in a flat cornea, or at the microkeratome hinge stop, and the reverse pedal (closest pedal to the wire) depressed (Figure 10-22). The further along the microkeratome head travels, the narrower the hinge. The microkeratome unit will reverse and then can be readily disengaged from the suction ring once the gears have disengaged from the tract. The flap is visible just proximal to the plate. It is important not to disengage the suction pressure prior to reversing and removing the unit from its tract because of the potential danger of tearing the flap. Occasionally, it is difficult to reverse the unit completely. This is usually because the surgeon has tilted the microkeratome, which must remain perpendicular to the eye and parallel within the tract. Simply support the wire or motor lightly as the unit

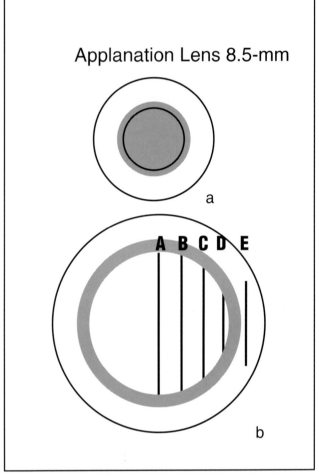

Figure 10-22.
Applanation lens meniscus larger than 8.5 mm (a) indicates large flap will be fashioned by microkeratome. The applanation lens demonstrates the corneal tissue presented to the microkeratome. As the microkeratome is advanced (b), the size of the hinge reduces from A to E, with E designating a free cap and A designating a flap bisecting the pupil. Although the size of the flap is dependent upon surgeon preference, larger and broader hinges are not only more stable, but easier to realign. The ideal hinge is likely C, outside the ablative zone but still broad for stability.

> **No vacuum recommended during ablation.**

> **Warn patients that their vision will be grayed during suction.**

advances and reverses rather than applying any pressure.

The unit should easily glide in and out of the suction ring into position. This maneuver should be practiced many dozens of times before attempting to perform the procedure, and should be tested with each unit once assembled and pre-

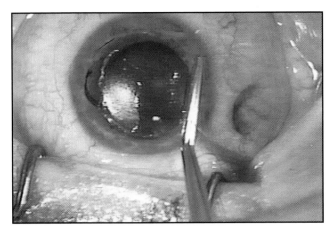

Figure 10-23a.
Intraoperative view demonstrating a somewhat small corneal hinge, ideal for hyperopic nomograms but more difficult to realign.

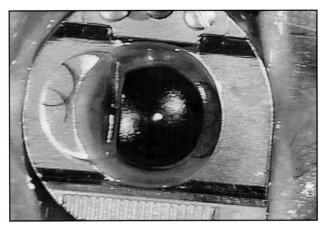

Figure 10-23b.
Intraoperative view demonstrating a somewhat large corneal hinge, ideal for alignment but encroaching on maximal ablation zone.

pared. If the microkeratome fails to slide easily into position, both the male and female aspects of the tract should be recleaned with dry brushing, as debris or more typically a film from the autoclave may have accumulated. The quality of the flap is entirely dependent upon the proper functioning and maintenance of the microkeratome unit. A very high level of caution is warranted, and recleaning the unit when the motion is not entirely smooth is rewarded with a dramatic reduction in flap complications.

ROLE OF PNEUMATIC SUCTION RING DURING INTRASTROMAL ABLATION

Once the microkeratome head has been removed, the suction ring may be left in place or removed. The approach is surgeon dependent, but I have found fixation far easier with the suction ring in place. The vacuum pressure need not be left on, and I caution against doing so, although many surgeons worldwide routinely do so. The suction ring will create an indentation within the sclera almost immediately; it will remain for some minutes after, thereby allowing the surgeon to control fixation during the intrastromal ablation by leaving the ring in place without vacuum pressure. A vascular occlusive accident of the retinal vasculature has yet to be reported worldwide; however, caution is prudent. It is felt that the vacuum pressure should be limited to less than 4 to 5 minutes, and many ALK surgeons have exceeded this by 1 or 2 minutes without incident to date. In patients who may be at greater risk for vascular occlusive events such as diabetics or hypertensives, the suction time can be reduced to less than 30 seconds. After an initial technique developed after visiting Luis Ruiz, MD, which left the ring and suction on, I now leave the vacuum off exclusively. It is very crucial to warn

patients that their vision will be grayed during suction. With the suction on, the pupil dilates secondary to ischemia and may result in decentration. I routinely prefer to leave the ring in position throughout the procedure after encountering patients who had severe difficulty maintaining fixation during the ablation. Drying the stroma excessively will require aiding a patient with his or her fixation, therefore, a more moist technique allows for patient self-fixation. Self-fixation has proven best for PRK and surgeons such as Richard Lindstrom, MD, feel the same is very likely true for LASIK.

EXAMINATION OF THE FLAP

Once the flap is created and the microkeratome head removed, the appearance of the cornea is deceiving, as it is often difficult to determine that a cut was made at first inspection. The flap is then reflected with the blunt side of closed fine tiers or cyclodialysis spatula to avoid damaging the flap. The epithelium should be hydrated with a wet surgical spear, not only before but after the microkeratome pass to help preserve the epithelium. Surgeons vary in their hinge size, with many preferring a small nasal hinge merely to secure it to the eye in case of cap displacement. The advantages to a small hinge are two-fold: it provides a larger ablation surface and it avoids inducing regular cylinder within the optical zone. I personally aim to create a broad hinge nasally (Figures 10-23a and 10-23b). The advantages to a broad hinge, especially when displaced slightly nasally, are three-fold and perhaps even more clinically relevant than those cited for small hinges. Broad hinges are clearly more stable both in preventing displacement and in securing the flap to the eye once displaced. Also, broad hinges extend a degree of resiliency, providing memory to the corneal flap for proper

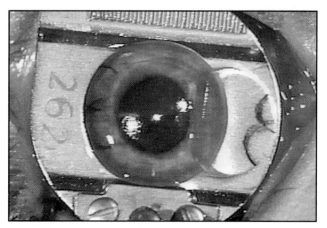

Figure 10-24.
Intraoperative photograph of naturally hydrated stromal bed immediately upon opening corneal flap. The suction ring can be left in position, but the suction pressure should be turned off. The ring sits nicely within the scleral indentation created to help patient fixation as can be assessed by the bright fixation reflex. Note the two half circle alignment markings on the corneal flap, which correspond to the two half circles on the uncut temporal corneal.

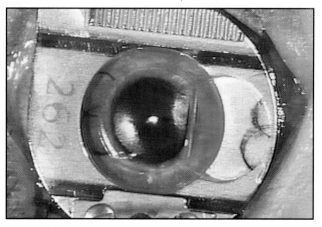

Figure 10-25b.
Intraoperative hydration pattern at conclusion of procedure, demonstrating encroachment upon corneal hinge and diffuse translucency. Peripheral taper of ablation pattern and increased hydration status of deeper stroma reduce effective optical zone created.

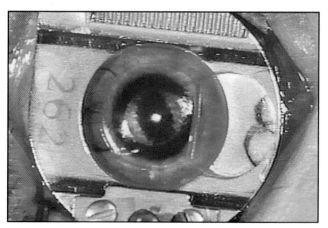

Figure 10-25a.
Intraoperative view of stromal bed ablation pattern during Chiron Technolas 6.6-mm multi-multizone technique, demonstrating central translucency denoting increased central hydration.

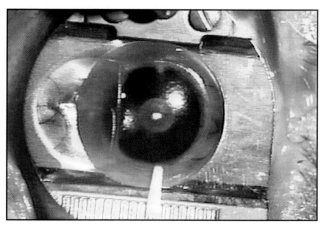

Figure 10-26.
Pretreatment technique with air application to prevent central island formation with Chiron Technolas 6.6-mm seven-zone multi-multizone technique for -10.50 D. Increased incidence of central islands is associated with LASIK due to increased hydration status of the deeper stroma, unless nomogram compensation or technique modifications are made. Amount of pretreatment depends upon beam profile, optical zone size, and nomogram. Scanning excimer lasers do not require pretreatment.

realignment. That is, it is far easier to realign the flap with a broad hinge than a narrow, more peripheral hinge. Perhaps most importantly, there is greater flap integrity maintained with a broad hinge, which seemingly reduces the degree of irregular astigmatism produced. The benefits of a broad hinge lessen with clinical experience gained.

INTRASTROMAL ABLATION AND NOMOGRAM FACTORS

The degree of mid-stromal hydration has a dramatic effect upon the ablation parameters required, both with respect to refractive predictability and with respect to induced topography (Figure 10-24). The mid-stroma is more hydrated, which results in an increased incidence of both undercorrections and central islands. The LASIK technique and ablation profile must reflect this fact. Typically, small optical zone sizes are utilized, particularly for high myopes, to reduce not only depth of ablation but also central island formation.

I have been developing multizone nomograms for the mid-stroma in order to minimize depth of ablation while maximizing optical zone size (Figures 10-25a and 10-25b).

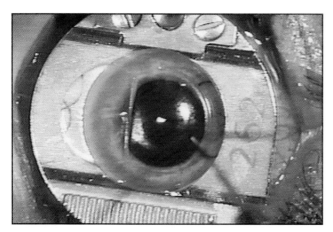

Figure 10-27.
Intraoperative photograph demonstrating use of air to control intraoperative hydration status of stromal bed. Nomogram can be adjusted to completely avoid the use of air.

I utilize the pretreatment technique (Machat 1992) developed for PRK on the inner stroma to remove stromal tissue within the central 3 mm, prior to the full refractive multi-multizone correction. The pretreatment step (Figure 10-26) is performed in anticipation of a central undercorrection evidenced on topography postoperatively as a central island. The central undercorrection is produced because of the naturally increased hydration of the central stroma (Lin 1994) and the acoustic shockwaves (Machat 1992) produced by each pulse which drive stromal fluid centrally. Additionally, I incorporate compressed air to dehydrate the stroma during the entire pretreatment step and preceding each zone of ablation, but further development of the algorithm will alleviate the need for air (Figure 10-27). I continue to use a variation of my PRK nomogram, dividing the refractive error into several steps, with each step performed at a successively larger optical zone, blending the preceding zone, and calculated to remove an equal ablation depth as the previous zone (Table 10-1 and Figure 10-28). I have noted that the optical zone size achieved is still smaller than that treated, due to the flap masking the peripheral blend zones or their reduced effectiveness in light of the increased hydration encountered. The use of air to control the increased hydration status of the inner stroma cannot be utilized for PRK in light of the increased association with haze formation, which is far less frequently observed with LASIK. Other

> The mid-stroma is more hydrated, which results in an increased incidence of both undercorrections and central islands.

TABLE 10-1
MACHAT NEW LASIK NOMOGRAM FOR HIGH MYOPIA

Important Points:

- No vertex distance correction
- Pretreatment 1 micron per diopter plus 2 to 4 microns total depth at 3.0 mm for Chiron Technolas Keracor 116 to compensate for central island formation
- All treatment zones of equal depth (not including pretreatment step)
- All zones ideally between 15 and 20 microns
- Goal is to achieve at least 6.0-mm effective optical zone
- Compressed air is used intraoperatively to control hydration

LASIK Nomogram for -13.00 D Attempted Correction

Optical Zone	Dioptric Distribution	Percentage of Treatment	Micron Depth
3.0 mm	-5.40 D	Pretreatment 1 µm/D + 3 µm	16
3.6 mm	-3.63 D	27.9%	17
4.2 mm	-2.58 D	18.9%	17
4.8 mm	-1.90 D	14.6%	17
5.4 mm	-1.46 D	11.2%	17
5.8 mm	-1.23 D	9.5%	17
6.0 mm	-1.14 D	8.8%	17
6.2 mm	-1.06 D	8.15%	17

Eight zones of equal micron depth. Each zone 0.6 mm larger than the previous zone, with two additional zones within 0.2 mm of 6.0-mm optical zone to ensure adequate peripheral blend for reduced spherical aberration and night visual disturbances.

methods to control hydration include wiping with a blunt spatula and drying with a surgical spear (Figure 10-29). A Merocel surgical sponge or other non-fraying spear is specifically recommended. Surgical spears, however, may leave debris on the stromal bed and within the interface and produce variable dehydration effects upon the stroma. The best option would be to develop an aspheric nomogram with an extensive peripheral transition zone to maximize optical zone size while leaving the stroma hydrated. An understanding of intrastromal recontouring is still developing (Table 10-2 and Figures 10-30 and 10-31).

Figure 10-28.
Corresponding corneal videokeratography with new LASIK ablation profile. Excellent central flattening and large effective optical zone.

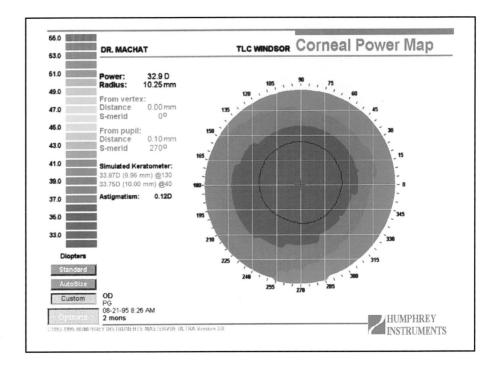

CREATING A CLEAR INTERFACE

Following intrastromal ablation, replacement of the flap may be preceded by cleaning of the stromal interface. There are two schools of thought, one in which the stromal bed is irrigated and the cap replaced onto the wet stromal bed, and one in which the stromal bed remains dry and is left untouched. In both schools, the cap must be rehydrated.

Simply stated, the stromal bed can be wet or dry, but the cap must be wet or hydrated to allow for manipulation during realignment. The potential advantages of irrigating the stromal bed prior to flap replacement are two-fold: first, to obtain a cleaner interface, and second, to assist with realignment floating the cap back into position. Irrigating may increase interface debris within the interface. The difficulty lies in the fact that as one irrigates the ablation particles and other such accumulated debris, irrigation fluid may wash debris from the fornices back onto the stromal interface. Care must be taken to either aspirate the irrigation fluid or clear debris that floats to the top of the meniscus which forms over the stromal bed. Filtered balance salt solution (BSS) may be used to irrigate the stromal bed, and a sable brush as used by Luis Ruiz, MD, or other instrument used to wipe debris away prior to closing the flap (Figure 10-32). Preferably, the interface is irrigated beneath the flap and excess fluid simultaneously aspirated, as described in the Kritzinger-Updegraff method. Irrigation and cleaning the interface may potentially reduce the incidence of epithelial

ingrowths by clearing any trapped epithelial cells. With the stromal bed and cap moist, alignment is easier, as the cap literally floats into position and irregular astigmatism may be reduced. The primary disadvantage is that the cap may take several minutes to lock into position unless the flap is wiped or compressed air is used, which may shrink the cap and may increase irregular astigmatism. In general, a surgical spear is used along the flap edge to promote a more rapid seal. In practice, not irrigating the stromal bed may still leave a clear interface, as the ablation plume is composed of virtually invisible particles that are clinically insignificant.

Current personal technique is a delicate balance of rehy-

> It is important to ensure that the reflected flap has not adhered to the suction ring prior to disengaging the vacuum, as patients may occasionally move and risk tearing the flap.

drating the cap while keeping the stromal bed devoid of any hydration. Rehydration of the inner flap involves placing drops of filtered BSS on the cap and along the hinge. The suction ring is left in place, although the suction is arrested immediately following the ablation. It is important to ensure that the reflected flap has not adhered to the suction ring prior to disengaging the vacuum, as patients may occasionally move and risk tearing the flap. The suction ring at this

TABLE 10-2
CHIRON TECHNOLAS PRK AND LASIK NOMOGRAM

Degree of Myopia (D)	Number of Zones Pretreatment (pretx) Cylinder	%	Optical Zones (mm)
-1.00 to -1.50	1+	1 μm/D + 2 μm	3.0 pretx
		100	6.00-6.60
-1.60 to -3.00	2+	1 μm/D + 2 μm	3.0 pretx
		60	5.6
		40	6.6
		1 μm/D + 2 μm	3.0 pretx
		55	6.0
		45	6.5
-3.10 to -5.50	3+	1 μm/D + 2 μm	3.0 pretx
		45	5.0
		29	6.0
		26	6.6
-5.60 to -10.00	4+	1 μm/D + 2 μm	3.0 pretx
		40	4.0
		25	5.0
		19	6.1
		16	6.6
-10.10 to -12.00	6+	1 μm/D + 2 μm	3.0 pretx
		31.6	3.6
		22.4	4.2
		15.3	5.0
		11.0	5.8
		10.3	6.0
		9.4	6.2
>-12.00	7+	1 μm/D + 2 μm	3.0 pretx
		27.9	3.6
		18.9	4.2
		14.6	4.8
		11.2	5.4
		9.50	5.8
		8.80	6.0
		8.15	6.2

An important concept to appreciate is that rehydration of stromal tissue is a measure of time exposed to fluid, rather than the quantity of fluid used to irrigate.

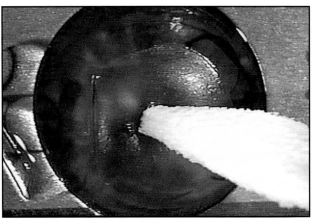

Figure 10-29.
Intraoperative photograph demonstrating use of a dry, non-fraying surgical spear to control intraoperative hydration status of stromal bed. Nomogram can be adjusted to completely avoid the use of a spear.

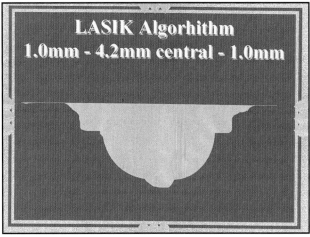

Figure 10-30.
Machat LASIK algorithm ablation profile.

Important Points of Ablation Profile

- Increased central treatment to compensate for increased hydration of deeper stroma. Compensation prevents central islands with LASIK and improves qualitative vision.

- Peripheral shoulder at 6 mm to ensure adequate effective optical zone. ALK-like knee improves peripheral flattening with better induced topography.

Figure 10-31.
Key points of ablation profile.

LASIK Operative Steps

1. Calibrate and program excimer laser system.
2. Assemble and test microkeratome function.
3. Prepare eye with topical anesthesia, antibiotics, and non-steroidal.
4. Clean eyelashes and fornices.
5. Drape eye covering eyelid margins.
6. Obtain adequate exposure and center eye within operative field.
7. Place alignment markings.
8. Apply pneumatic suction ring, seat firmly, and activate vacuum pressure.
9. Assess cap diameter with 8.5 mm applanation lens.
10. Ensure adequate IOP with Barraquer tonometer.
11. Insert microkeratome head into tract and advance.
12. Check operative field for obstacles.
13. Depress forward pedal until hinge stop reached, then reverse.
14. Remove microkeratome head alone or with suction ring.
15. Open corneal flap with fine tiers or cyclodialysis spatula.
16. Ablate stromal bed with desired refraction.
17. Control hydration of deeper stroma with air, spatula wiping, surgical spear drying, pausing between steps or through nomogram itself.
18. Irrigate corneal flap and hinge with filtered BSS and close flap.
19. Irrigate beneath flap for a few seconds to clean interface debris.
20. Wipe corneal flap into alignment with wet surgical spear.
21. Dry along edges of corneal flap with dry surgical spear to promote flap adhesion.
22. Wait 2 to 3 minutes, apply diffuse low flow air for a few seconds if desired to promote more rapid adhesion.
23. Insert antibiotic-steroid preparation, viscous lubrication, and tape eyelid shut for 15 to 30 minutes.
24. Recheck corneal flap alignment prior to discharging.

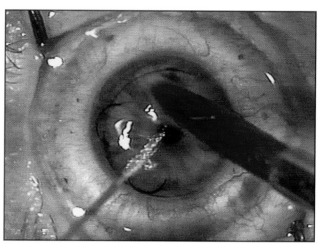

Figure 10-32.
Intraoperative photo demonstrating cleaning of stromal interface with sable brush and copious amounts of filtered BSS. Simultaneous aspiration is important with this technque to prevent washing debris from fornices back beneath corneal flap. Current preferred technique is to irrigate within interface after corneal flap closure to prevent debris from becoming re-introduced.

fornices with anesthetic-soaked surgical spears to clean the fornices and reduce potential interface debris. Lint fibers from gauze or the air may still be found within the interface (Figures 10-33a and 10-33b). Once the corneal flap is repositioned, a 27-gauge cannula is inserted beneath the flap for a few seconds to irrigate out any debris.

An important concept to appreciate is that rehydration of stromal tissue is a measure of the time it has been exposed to fluid rather than the quantity of fluid used to irrigate. A small amount of fluid is also placed at the hinge, which will help lubricate the interface, forming a fluid wedge as the stromal bed and flap come together. This fluid is important in potentially reducing irregular astigmatism.

CLOSING THE FLAP

Fine closed tiers or a cyclodialysis spatula of some variety should be inserted the full length of the hinge nasally. The flap should be replaced in one smooth, even motion in an effort to minimize irregular astigmatism once again

> **Avoidance of irregular astigmatism is the greatest challenge in lamellar surgery.**

> **Most surgeons remove the pneumatic suction ring immediately following the lamellar incision.**

point has a dual purpose in that it continues to afford a measure of fixation, and it prevents debris from the conjunctival fornices from reaching the interface. Many surgeons advocate irrigating the fornices preoperatively or even wiping the

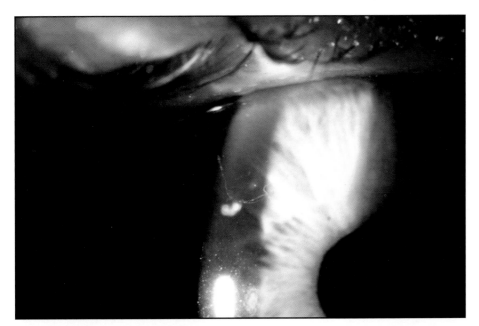

Figure 10-33a.
Clinical photograph of postoperative LASIK demonstrating a lint foreign body within the interface that was not cleared.

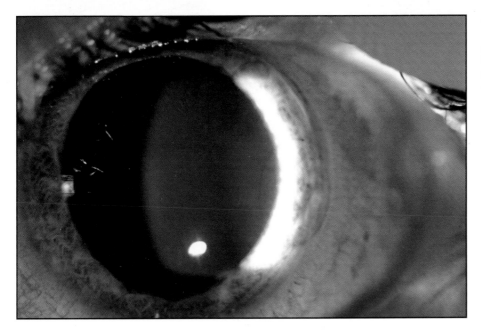

Figure 10-33b.
Immediate postoperative clinical photograph demonstrating clear interface with proper technique irrigating beneath a closed corneal flap.

(Figures 10-34a through 10-34e). Avoidance of irregular astigmatism is the greatest challenge in lamellar surgery. Replacement of the cap can be performed with the suction ring still in position, as the dual advantages of maintaining fixation and preventing contamination of the interface are still helpful until the flap is closed. For the left eye, the suction ring may be twisted clockwise to allow room for the maneuver with the right hand. Left-handed surgeons must remove the ring to access the nasal hinge. Most surgeons remove the pneumatic suction ring immediately following the lamellar incision. Patients do not require a fixation device if the stroma is left relatively moist during the ablation. Self-fixation is compromised with excessive drying of the stromal bed during the ablation.

Once the flap is replaced, and the interface irrigated, the correct position of the flap is confirmed through two primary methods. First, the alignment markings (Figure 10-35) are examined to ensure that the ends are approximated, and second, that an even and well-approximated gutter exists between the cap edge and the peripheral cornea (Figure 10-36).

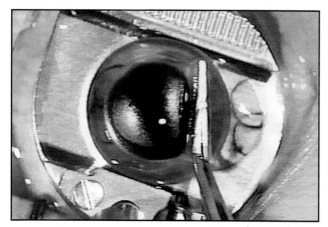

Figure 10-34a.
Intraoperative series of views demonstrating closure of the corneal flap following ablation.

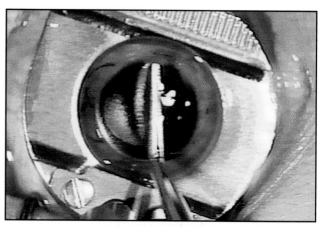

Figure 10-34b.
Closed fine forceps or a fine spatula can be inserted along the entire hinge length and used to reflect the corneal flap in one smooth motion.

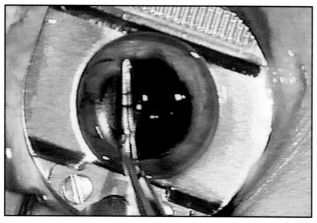

Figure 10-34c.
Use closed fine forceps or a fine spatula to insert along the entire hinge length and reflect the corneal flap.

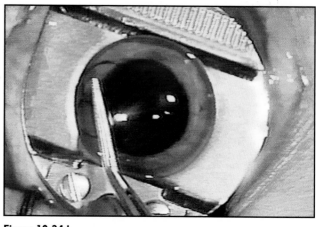

Figure 10-34d.
Filtered balanced saline is used to irrigate the corneal flap and hinge prior to repositioning of the corneal flap.

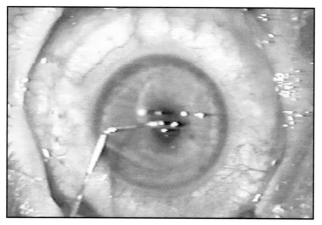

Figure 10-34e.
A cannula can then be inserted beneath the closed flap if desired to irrigate out debris and epithelium from within the interface.

If correct placement is not achieved, the cap can easily be lifted once again, as this is the easiest time to achieve good alignment. With a small hinge, alignment may be difficult to achieve, as the flap is more mobile and multiple attempts may sometimes be required. Occasionally, a slower movement may be helpful when reflecting the flap back into position, allowing for better control. When the flap is reopened, the bed may be dry and it may be helpful to rehydrate the inner flap and hinge interface before attempting to close the flap again, or irrigate the stromal bed and float the flap into position.

Once the flap is closed and properly aligned, a wet surgical spear may be used quite effectively to smooth the flap and maintain the health of the epithelium. The surgical spear is moistened with BSS and the spear is always passed tem-

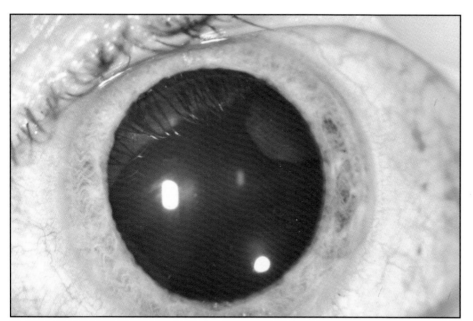

Figure 10-35.
Clinical photograph of eye treated with LASIK in the immediate postoperative period, demonstrating clear cornea, absence of corneal flap edema, and excellent four-point alignment as indicated by matching circles.

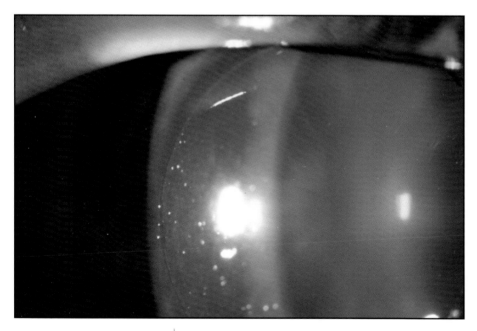

Figure 10-36.
Clinical photograph of LASIK treated eye in immediate postoperative period, demonstrating excellent flap apposition as indicated by smooth corneal flap edge and appearance of fine symmetrical peripheral gutter.

Figure 10-37.
Clinical photograph of retroilluminated corneal flap during immediate postoperative period to assess for corneal striae. Retroillumination is the best technique to detect fine corneal striae secondary to flap misalignment, which may be associated with irregular astigmatism.

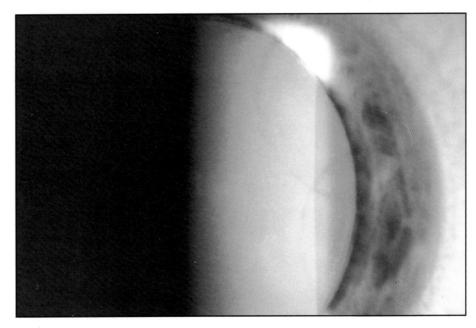

Flap Adhesion
- Wait 2 to 5 minutes
- Dry surgical spear dabbed along flap edge
- Air drying flap edge

porally, starting at the nasal hinge each time. Minor misalignments are often corrected with this technique; however, flap rotations cannot be corrected, as flap striae will be produced and irregular astigmatism increased. That is, do not try to twist the flap if rotated, but lift the flap and reclose to avoid striae. If striae are evident postoperatively, the cap is always misaligned and typically rotated several degrees and must be realigned as soon as possible, as striae become quite difficult to eliminate within days (Figure 10-37).

ENHANCING FLAP ADHESION

Compressed air at 1 to 2 liters per minute can be used to dry the flap and peripheral gutter along the cap edge to enhance flap adhesion time. Many surgeons avoid air drying the flap and wait 2 to 5 minutes for adhesion of the flap. Another technique is to use a dry surgical spear and lightly dab the gutter. The central cap epithelium is maintained moist with the wet surgical spears passed temporally over the flap. The air helps the peripheral flap form a seal, which allows the small amount of fluid within the interface to literally be pumped out by the negative internal pressure created by the endothelial cell pump. The disadvantages of air

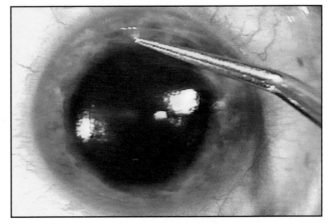

Figure 10-38.
Reverse corneal striae test. Peripheral corneal flap is depressed and massaged outward, demonstrating strength of peripheral flap adhesion and smoothing flap to approximate peripheral gutter. Peripheral cornea must be dry for striae tests. Side of fine forceps or blunted spatula can be used.

are that the cap often contracts, increasing the peripheral gutter and possibly inducing irregular astigmatism. Epithelial defects are more common with the use of air, and the flap edges may not be as smooth. One technique is to use the blunt side of fine tiers or a similar tool to stretch or iron the flap edges away from the cap center toward the peripheral gutter if the flap margins contract. The cap must be relatively dry. If too much force is used, the entire flap will move.

Surgical Technique

Maria Clara Arbelaez, MD

PREOPERATIVE EXAMINATION

- Visual acuity (standard procedure)
- Refraction (subjective, manifest, cycloplegic)
- Best corrected visual acuity measurements
- Keratometry
- Corneal topography
- Glare testing
- Contrast sensitivity test (bright-dim)
- Specular microscopy (central-peripheral)
- Central pachymetry (optic and ultrasonic)
- Axial length measurement
- Slit lamp examination
- IOP
- Dilated fundus

INCLUSION CRITERIA

- Myopia -1.00 to -25.00 D
- Astigmatism -0.50 to -10.00 D
- Hyperopia +1.00 to +5.00 D (now in clinical study)
- Presbyopia (now in clinical study)
- Stable refraction for last 12 months
- Patients who are contact lens users must discontinue wearing hard lenses for at least 4 weeks and soft lenses for 3 weeks prior to the preoperative evaluation
- Patients must sign a written informed consent form

EXCLUSION CRITERIA

- Patients with active pathology anterior or posterior segment
- Signs of early or clinical keratoconus
- Patients who are blind in one eye
- Patients who are pregnant

SURGICAL PROCEDURE

SURGICAL SCHEDULE

- Only one eye at a time, the fellow eye 1 week later according to the evolution

ROOM CONDITIONS

- Sterile surgery room (ultraviolet lights 12 hours before treatment)
- Particle-free environment
- Temperature 59° to 77°F
- Humidity 20% to 50%

PATIENT PREPARATION

- Face cleaned with surgical scrub
- Surgical clothes
- Pilocarpine 1% one drop
- Proparacaine four drops
- Midazolam 2 mg orally
- Acetaminophen 500 mg orally
- Diclofenac IM

EYE CLEANING

- Povidone two drops and saline solution

ANESTHESIA

- This procedure may be performed under topical anesthesia (general anesthesia only in very special cases of very anxious patients)

PROCEDURE

- The laser system is switched on. Following the steps of gas change and fluence test, I perform fluence test for every case.
- The calculations have to be introduced in the computer before starting the procedure based upon manifest refraction.
- Microkeratome is prepared for use:
    It has to be perfectly cleaned and sterilized
    I use the ALK-E suction ring and the two kinds of stoppers
    The keratome head is assembled with a new blade for each procedure
- I use 160 microns and 130 microns only in myopia >15 D or corneal thickness <530 microns
- After the laser and microkeratome have been checked out, the patient can come to the surgery room.
- No gloves or powderless gloves are employed.
- It is good to explain to the patients every surgery step; they feel more comfortable.
- Place the surgical fields and a plastic drape to hold the eyelashes out of the surgery area. The marker has two concentric circles: one internal 3 mm in diameter and one external of 10.5 mm with a pararadial mark.
- Next, the pneumatic fixation ring is placed with the eyeball as exposed as possible; the handle of the ring should be

placed inferiorly on the right eye and superiorly on the left eye. The pneumatic ring allows slight manual adjustment of the position of the eyeball. The corneal surface has to be lubricated with BSS to facilitate the passage of the microkeratome.

- If the disk is still in place you have to move with the cannula to the nasal side as far as you can to avoid any damage in the excimer keratectomy.

- Dry the exposed corneal stroma with filtered air, refocus the laser and start the ablation according to the calculations that you had introduced in the computer prior to initiating the procedure, leaving the suction ring in place, without active suction pressure (I still use pressure in hyperopic eyes). It is normal to observe water during ablation. For this reason, it is better to dry the surface with filtered air in every step of multizone treatment.

- Once the ablation has been completed, maintain the ring in place to avoid eye movements and the risk of uncleaned interface. The interface is then irrigated with filtered BSS, using a marta hair brush and the suction tube at the same time. At that point, the flap is then gently laid back onto the eye. The cannula is then inserted beneath the flap to clean the interface. Dry the borders with filtered air. It is critical that the disc be centered and aligned with the pararadial maker line.

- Retire the suction ring without touching the disc borders.

- After that you can see a striae sign.

- You can now remove the speculum, being careful to avoid touching the disc.

POSTOPERATIVE CARE

- At the end of the surgery, one drop of tobramycin 0.3% will be administered.

- A shield is taped over the eye (for 24 hours), and no eye drops can be used for the first 12 hours following the procedure.

- Acetaminophen is administered every 6 hours if necessary.

- At the first visit, remove the shield and check the visual acuity and eye in the slit lamp, and start fluorometholone 0.1% + terizolin, one drop three times a day for a week.

EXAMINATION SCHEDULE

- Day 1 (slit lamp and visual acuity)
- 1 month (slit lamp, corneal topography, visual acuity, refraction)
- 3 months (same preoperative examination)
- 6 months (same preoperative examination)
- 1 year (same preoperative examination)

ENHANCEMENTS

- Can be performed 3 months postoperatively (if the refraction is stable) like a new procedure.

TESTING FLAP ADHESION

There are multiple methods of assuring adequate cap adhesion. The primary method is known as the Slade Striae Test, and involves depressing the peripheral cornea with fine tiers or forceps and observing for striae transmission onto the cap itself (see Figure 10-35). If the epithelium is too moist, it will be impossible to determine if corneal striae are evident on the cap. The second essential test is known as the lid or "blink" test, and involves re-examination of the integrity of flap adhesion after allowing the patient to blink several times. If there is any movement of

the edges of the flap, the eyelid speculum must be reinserted, and the flap edges smoothed with a wet surgical spear and air dried repeatedly. It is important to insert and remove the eyelid speculum carefully to avoid engaging the flap

Primary test for corneal flap adhesion is the Slade Striae Test, which involves depressing the peripheral cornea with fine tiers or forceps and checking for striae transmission onto the cap itself.

Factors Responsible for Securing the Flap

Four factors are believed to secure the flap in position:

1. The natural capillary attraction of the tissues and mucoproteins (rapid, seconds to minutes)
2. Endothelial pump action (minutes to hours)
3. Epithelial covering along the margin (12 to 24 hours)
4. Scarring along the cut edge of Bowman's layer (weeks to months)

In some cases, interface fibrosis occurs, which binds the central flap tightly.

Kritzinger/Updegraff Technique for Lamellar Surgery

Michiel S. Kritzinger, MD, and Stephen A. Updegraff, MD

The most common sight-threatening complication following lamellar corneal surgery is irregular astigmatism.[1,2] Although earlier studies attributed this problem to the suturing required for myopic keratomileusis, irregular astigmatism can still be a major complication of LASIK, or ALK in which no sutures are used,[3] especially when compared to surface ablation techniques. When a corneal flap or cap is returned to the stromal bed, micro-irregularities can exist, resulting from folds on the epithelial surface. Another complication of lamellar surgery which, with time, can be sight-threatening is the presence of debris, such as meibomian secretions or epithelial nests within the interface (Figure A-1). We have designed instrumentation and developed techniques which incorporate low flow irrigation with repositioning of the corneal flap or cap, which we call low flow tectonic keratoplasty. The goal is to minimize irregular astigmatism and reduce or eliminate debris in the interface.

The original Ruiz marker was designed primarily to prevent the surgeon from inverting a free corneal flap by having a single pararadial temporally (Figure A-2). Some alignment of the corneal cap was obtained by making sure that this pararadial was symmetrically aligned across the gutter. We have developed a marking system that utilizes seven radials and one pararadial (Figure A-3). The radial marks ensure proper orientation of the entire cap/flap. Each of the blades on this marker is very short, so as to minimize the amount of ink that is placed on the corneal surface. The surface area of ink is actually less on this marker than on the original Ruiz marker, which reduces the incidence of visually significant epitheliopathy from the ink marks, which can lead to disappointing visual acuities in the immediate postoperative period. The broad cross hair marks on the peripheral cornea, outside the bed, are used to maintain laser ablation centration by aligning with the reticule of the laser microscope.

When the cornea is marked, the frontal plane of the patient's head should be 90° to the point of fixation. Centering the marker over the cornea light reflex of a normally constricting pupil will ultimately accurately center the laser ablation.

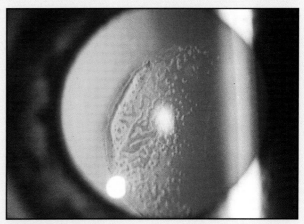

Figure A-1.
Epithelium in the interface.

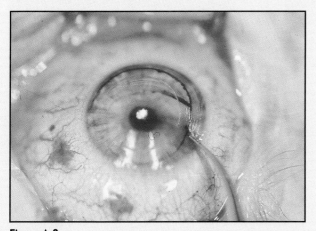

Figure A-2.
Ruiz corneal mark and Slade Striae Test. Note one pararadial.

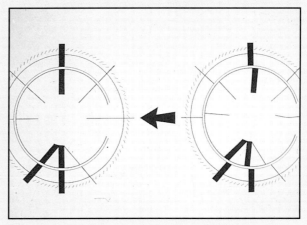

Figure A-3.
KU marker.

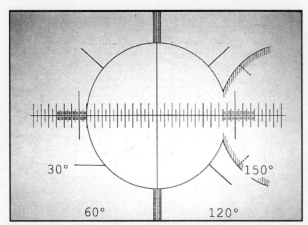

Figure A-4.
Reticule alignment with marks on cornea.

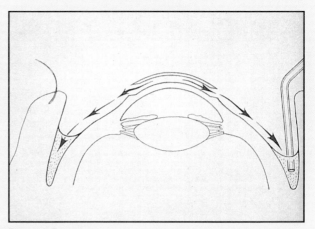

Figure A-5.
Irrigation under flap.

The suction ring is centered over the concentric circular mark of the KU marker. After the keratectomy is performed, the flap is folded back nasally. The peripheral markings of the KU marker are still visible. Thus, these are used as a visual cue to line up the cross hair of the reticule which corresponds to the exact fixation prior to the keratectomy (Figure A-4). It is very important not to chase the patient's eye by moving the bed. Rather, move the patient's head gently to achieve centration if they have drifted. Improper alignment of the patient's head does not mean the bed has moved but rather the patient's head has moved and thus must be oriented back to the position you had initially worked so hard to achieve. We use the KMZ (Kritzinger Multi Zone) nomogram, which is as follows:

KRITZINGER MULTI ZONE PROGRAM

Low to moderate myopia

Zone 1   47%

Zone 2   27%

Zone 3   17%

Blend Zone 9%

Add 12% to the sphere of the spectacle correction.

Note:

1. The lower the myopia, the better the visual outcome.
2. Be cautious for patients with over 15 D of myopia—less predictable outcome.

Cylinder: 4-mm wide ablation

Hydration state essential by wiping bed

1 D=one wipe

2 D=two wipes

3 D=three wipes, etc.

Note: Relationship of clinically significant hyperopic shift.

Hyperopic shift with astigmatism correction

2 D=0.5 D

3 D=0.75 D

4 D=1.00 D

5 D=1.50 D

Note: Do not add 10% to sphere when treating ≥2 D of cylinder.

The technique for repositioning a lamellar flap or cap is based upon the dilution principle and plate tectonics. A steady flow of fluid is more effective in removing debris than short bursts and smaller volume with a syringe or bulb delivery. We use BSS from an IV set-up. The flow is adjusted so that it is constant and does not "jet" the cap/flap but rather "floats" the flap with fluid steadily exiting from under the entire edge of the flap. The KU irrigation cannula creates fluid flow patterns that aid in the removal of interface debris (Figure A-5). The surgeon uses a two-handed technique by irrigating with one hand and aspirating with the other (Figure A-6). A 19-gauge cannula is used for aspiration. The patient is fixating so that the apex of the globe is in line with the microscope. This will allow the fluid to flow from underneath the cap or flap peripherally and out past the limbus into the fornices. The fornices are aspirated first. This removes debris and meibomian secretions that have flowed downhill. After approximately 15 to 20 seconds of central irrigation, the irrigating cannula can be moved toward the hinge and gently swept back and forth from the hinge and then held centrally again. This allows any epithelium entrapped by the blade at the hinge to be freed and irrigated out. Once the fornices are cleared of fluid and debris, the aspiration cannula can be moved towards the gutter and with a low flow irrigation, the cap can be nudged with smooth tying forceps so that the radial

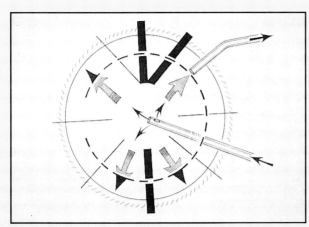

Figure A-6.
Aspiration and irrigation maneuvers.

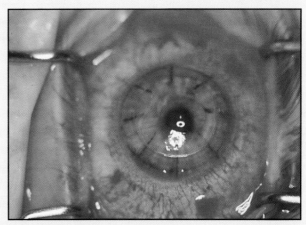

Figure A-7.
Alignment of flap.

marks are fairly aligned. This is like plate tectonics, where the earth's crust constantly moves on a bed that is more fluid. However, this is a controlled repositioning, so that as the flap floats into position, the peripheral marks are aligned. Once this is achieved, the gutter should be aspirated for 270°, while there is steady irrigation. This again removes debris that could have become lodged at the edge of the keratectomy. Aspiration of the gutter is continued as the irrigating cannula is gently withdrawn, taking note of the approximation of the radial and pararadial marks. We are presently using a curved tying forceps to smooth the flap from the center to the periphery in making sure the radial and pararadial marks are aligned. If alignment is not achieved, the irrigating cannula is once again reintroduced and the aspiration is performed in the gutter, and the cap is allowed to be adjusted on a bed of fluid (Figure A-7).

To date, we have not experienced any dislocation of caps/flaps postoperatively. We discourage the use of air blown on the corneal surface and believe it can cause cracks in Bowman's membrane, as well as push debris accumulated in the gutter back under the flap. Aspiration or Merocel sponges that wick fluid from the gutter in an outward motion from under the flap work well to ensure cap adherence. A drop of BSS is placed on the central cornea during these maneuvers to prevent epitheliopathy. We always utilize the Slade Striae Test to confirm adherence and then remove the speculum. Once again, adherence and alignment of the flap is reconfirmed with the "blink test" prior to placing clear shields over the patient's eyes.

We have demonstrated, in a prospective study, the usefulness and safety of low flow tectonic keratoplasty.[4] We do notice an early hyperopic shift because the irrigating fluid creates stromal edema at the edge of the keratectomy, thus effectively creating more central flattening. This resolves in 2 to 3 days.

Another major advantage of this technique is that it allows the surgeon to safely and predictably retreat patients by lifting the corneal flap. Many experienced LASIK surgeons have always created another keratectomy when retreating patients, due to the risk of introducing debris and irregular astigmatism when lifting a flap. These risks are higher when lifting a corneal flap because the overlying epithelium at the edge of the keratectomy tears and does not have a sharp edge as with the primary keratectomy. Utilizing the marking and irrigating techniques, the corneal flap can be realigned and the torn edges tend to "float" into position. We have developed a corneal flap elevator that creates a sharper edge and aids in lifting flaps that are more than 3 months after surgery. We do not recommend lifting flaps that are older than 6 months. This application is particularly useful in treating penetrating keratoplasty corneas, in which we have demonstrated that waiting 2 to 3 months after the primary keratectomy to perform the ablation significantly reduces retreatment for these patients.[5]

References

1. Updegraff SA, Ruiz LA, Slade SG. Corneal topography in lamellar refractive surgery. In: Sanders DR, Koch DD, eds. *Corneal Topography.* Thorofare, NJ: SLACK Inc; 1994.

2. Nordan LT, Fallor MK. Myopia keratomileusis: 74 corrected non-ambloypic cases with one year follow-up. *J Refract Corneal Surg.* 1986;2:124-128.

3. Arenas-Archila E, Sanchez-Thorin JC, Naranjo-Uribe JP, Hernandez-Lorano. Myopic keratomileusis in situ: a preliminary report. *J Cataract Refract Surg.* 1987;17:424;435.

4. Updegraff SA, Kritzinger MS. *A Prospective Evaluation of Flow Tectonic Lamellar Keratoplasty: A New Technique fo LASIK and ALK.* International Society of Refractive Surgery (ISRS); October 1995; Atlanta, Ga.

5. Updegraff SA, Kritzinger MS, Slade SG. *Therapeutic Lamellar Surgery: ALK Homoplastic Grafting and LASIK.* International Society of Refractive Surgery (ISRS); July 1995; Minneapolis, Minn.

The second essential test is known as the lid or "blink" test, and involves re-examination of the integrity of flap adhesion after allowing the patient to blink several times.

Consistency of technique is more important than speed.

edge. If the flap edges are retracted significantly by more than 1 mm and fail to smooth out with the wet spear, a dry technique can be used. The epithelial surface is allowed to dry or air is applied locally, and the side of fine tiers used to iron the edges out toward the peripheral gutter. If the irregularity or retraction is significant, the flap should be lifted and the flap replaced. There are a few other non-specific techniques to assess flap adhesion which involve maneuvering the flap itself. The peripheral flap, when dried, can be wiped toward the peripheral gutter to not only smooth the edges but to assess how much resistance is evident in what I term the "iron test." A more definitive but controversial maneuver would be a "reverse iron test," attempting to pull or depress the flap centrally, away from the peripheral gutter. I have on occasion been able to produce corneal striae on the flap only to have the flap move once the patient was allowed to blink. However, the flap never moves if a "reverse striae test" (Figure 10-38) is negative for movement. I prefer to use low air flow for 5 to 10 seconds and test the flap after 3 minutes of settling so that if the flap has any tendency to become displaced, I know immediately. The wet cap and dry bed technique produces much faster cap adhesion, which is often noted within the first minute, but waiting an additional minute or two is prudent. Some surgeons, including myself, advocate having the patient wait 15 to 30 minutes or so following surgery with their eyes closed, and rechecking their flap position at the slit lamp prior to discharging them.

IMMEDIATE POSTOPERATIVE MEDICATIONS

Another helpful recommendation is lubrication with a viscous preparation, which aids not only epithelial health but in reducing friction over the flap with blinking. I personally instill Celluvisc and TobraDex into the eye immediately postoperatively and have the patient keep his or her eyes closed for 15 to 30 minutes. A viscous agent should be avoided intraoperatively, as this will inhibit and delay flap adhesion. The eyelids can be taped closed for minutes or hours to prevent blinking, which reduces shearing forces. Taping the eyelid is especially useful in unilaterally treated patients, and I usually leave them taped until the next morning. I found that when I performed unilateral surgery, patients squinted the operative eye while looking through their non-operative eye. With taping the eyelid shut, no shearing forces are produced, no pressure from a patch is required, and patients can open the fellow eye easily. Taping does not replace the eyeshield, which affords protection from trauma.

The entire LASIK procedure is typically less than 10 minutes in duration, and can take as little as 3 to 5 minutes with flap adhesion once proficiency is achieved. Consistency of technique is more important than speed to maintain a similar hydration status of the tissues intraoperatively. Each step must be executed properly to ensure a safe outcome.

CHAPTER 11

Postoperative LASIK Patient Management

The need for postoperative care of laser in situ keratomileusis (LASIK) patients varies considerably, from virtually none to intensive treatment of severe flap complications. Most LASIK patients require minimal follow-up care and improve over time, even when flap irregularities exist. Postoperative medications and examination schedules vary considerably between surgeons, with the common element being that most patients do well with very little intervention (Figures 11-1 and 11-2).

MEDICATION REGIMEN

Antibiotic preparations are used for 5 to 7 days, and intensive lubrication for 3 days. No additional medications are required beyond the first week. There may be a role for short-term topical steroids to reduce inflammation and possibly even control myopic regression in specific patients who exhibit pronounced wound healing. Topical steroid and nonsteroid anti-inflammatory agents during the first few days may be helpful in improving comfort.

Although most patients exhibit good stability by 1 month, a subset of patients, particularly higher myopes, will regress an additional 1.00 to 3.00 D over the proceeding 3 months. Larger optical zones appear to regress more. A 4- to 6-week tapering regimen of topical steroids may have a role, although retreatment has been the rule to date. Intrastromal ablation has far less tendency for regression than surface ablation because of less wound healing activity of the deeper stroma, but wound healing, although reduced, is still quite evident in some individuals.

In general, topical steroids are not recommended beyond the first week postoperatively, and their need within the postoperative regimen at any stage remains unclear. My standard regimen includes an antibiotic, tobramycin 0.3% or ofloxacin 0.3%, combined with a full-strength steroid, dexamethasone 0.1%, for 1 week. Diclofenac 0.1% is used immediately postoperatively and is only continued for 1 to 2 days in patients with epithelial defects. All medications are qid regimen, except for eye lubricants.

FOLLOW-UP EXAMINATION SCHEDULE

LASIK patients are typically examined on day 1 to specifically examine the flap, then at 1 week and 1 month to measure the visual and refractive performance of the eye. The eyes are then re-examined at 3, 6, and 12 months to check refractive stability. The first day visit is the most important, as it represents the first opportunity to assess the corneal flap position and alignment. It is far easier and safer to intervene with corneal flap displacement or alignment problems at this early stage (Figures 11-3 and 11-4). At the

Postoperative LASIK Schedule Examination

- 1 day
- 1 week
- 1 month
- 3 months
- 6 months
- 1 year

Figure 11-1.
Clinical photograph of LASIK treated left eye in early postoperative period demonstrating preserved corneal clarity with minimal conjunctival injection. Patient treated for -6.00 D sphere with 20/20 -2 vision recorded from first postoperative day.

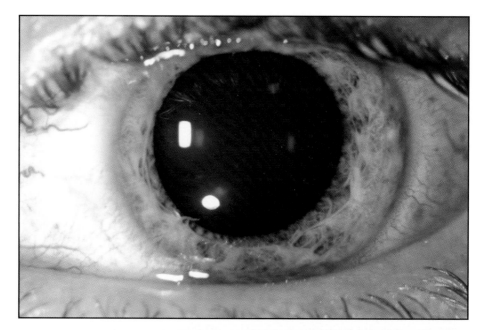

Figure 11-2.
Clinical appearance of left eye treated with LASIK in early postoperative period demonstrating clear cornea and minimal inflammation.

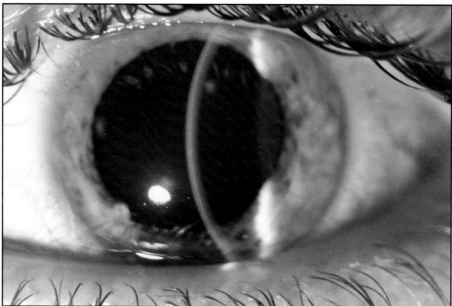

1-week visit, temporary glasses or disposable contact lenses may be fit, and at the 3-month visit, enhancement planned and performed.

REFITTING WITH CONTACT LENSES

Patients requiring enhancement surgery due to undercorrection or myopic regression may be fit with temporary glasses or contact lenses. It is important to wait at least 1 week prior to fitting a patient with contacts to ensure that the flap is secure. Disposable contacts are preferable, as the prescription may be quickly updated at little expense and have

> The first day visit is the most important, as it represents the first opportunity to assess the corneal flap position and alignment.

> At the 1-week visit, temporary glasses or disposable contact lenses may be fit, and at the 3-month visit, enhancement planned and performed.

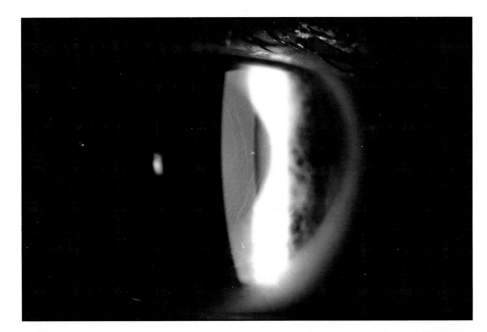

Figure 11-3.
Clinical detection of fine corneal flap striae during slit lamp biomicroscope examination with optical section during early postoperative period. Uncorrected vision was 20/60 with best corrected vision reduced by one line with qualitative blur.

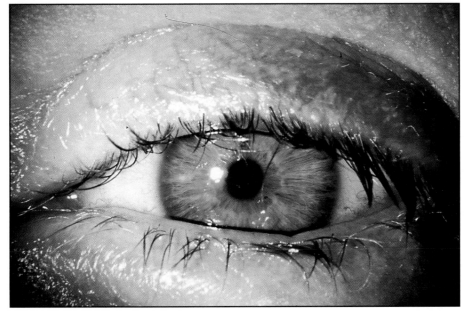

Figure 11-4.
Clinical appearance of LASIK treated eye on first postoperative day demonstrating quiet white eye with no corneal edema but slight eyelid edema. Uncorrected visual acuity was 20/40 despite -10.50 D preoperative spherical equivalent.

the least effect upon the recovering cornea. Rigid gas permeable lenses should not be used, as they will alter corneal topography pending treatment. Early visual rehabilitation of patients is essential for improving overall patient satisfaction, as even 1.00 D of undercorrection following treatment of a -10.00 D myope will result in blurred vision. Although the undercorrected vision postoperatively greatly exceeds the uncorrected visual acuity preoperatively, it will not compare to the best corrected vision preoperatively. A stronger disposable contact lens prescription may be required postoperatively, as there may be excessive central clearance. The fit is on the mid-peripheral cornea and tends to be similar to the preoperative fit or steeper. Disposable contact lenses are well tolerated, and lubrication should be encouraged.

IMMEDIATE POSTOPERATIVE CARE

MEDICATION

At the conclusion of the procedure (Figures 11-5 through 11-7), lubrication and an antibiotic-steroid preparation are instilled. I instill one or two drops of diclofenac

Figure 11-5.
Clinical appearance of LASIK treated eye during immediate postoperative period with visible alignment markings.

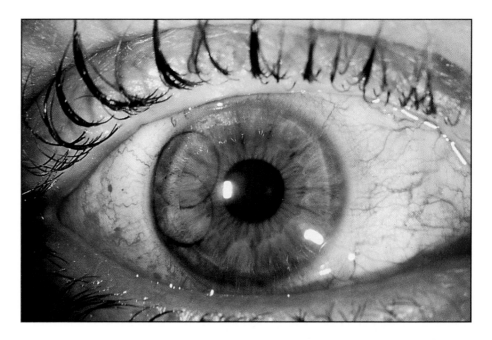

Figure 11-6.
Clinical appearance of LASIK treated eye during immediate postoperative period demonstrating immediate return of a good corneal reflex because of preservation of surface epithelium.

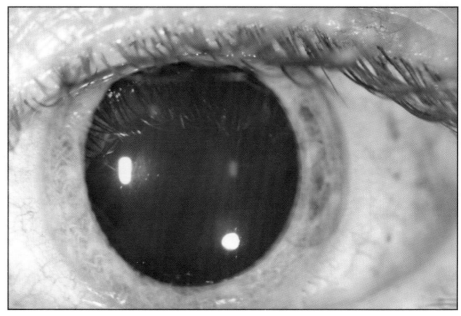

0.1%, but no additional topical non-steroidal is required unless an epithelial defect is evident and NSAIDs can be used along with a bandage contact lens. A topical steroid may be helpful in reducing postoperative inflammation and I will routinely place the patient on an antibiotic-steroid regimen. Many surgeons advocate topical non-steroid usage for the first few days to avoid any steroid adverse effects. I feel that the short-term use of steroid agents is safe and their effectiveness unequaled for inflammation control.

EYESHIELD USE

During the immediate postoperative period, great care must be taken to avoid displacement of the flap. Patients are instructed to absolutely avoid rubbing their eyes or squeezing their eyelids forcefully for the first week. An eyeshield is placed over the operative eye or eyes in cases of simultaneous bilateral surgery. The eyeshield should be clear, as patients often have good functional vision although still quite blurry; one patient described this accurately as "Vaseline vision," reducing qualitative vision while quanti-

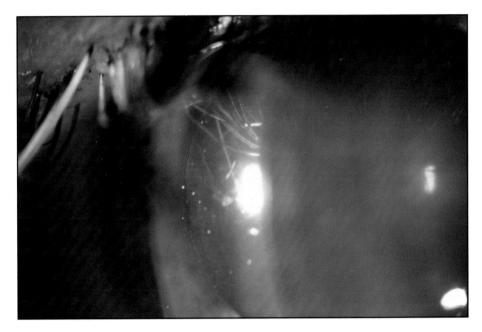

Figure 11-7.

Clinical appearance of LASIK treated eye during immediate postoperative period demonstrating intact epithelium, with well-positioned corneal flap and clear corneal interface. Corneal flap status with respect to epithelial defects, edema, displacement and interface opacities are assessed 15 to 60 minutes postoperatively prior to discharging patient.

tative vision is dramatically improved. The eyeshield should remain in place for the first 24 hours, then nightly for 1 week. Sunglasses should be worn during the day initially to reduce light sensitivity and ensure that the patient does not touch his or her eyes. Patients instill an antibiotic-steroid preparation daily for the first 5 to 7 days. This is a conservative regimen, although some surgeons do not utilize any medications or eyeshields whatsoever.

> **The eyeshield should remain in place for the first 24 hours, then nightly for 1 week.**

> - The eye should never be pressure patched
> - Taping the eyelid shut is both allowable and indicated in cases where a free corneal cap is produced

It is important to recognize that the eye should never be pressure patched even with an epithelial defect, as eye movement may dislodge the flap. A light pressure patch, or more preferably, taping the eyelid shut is both allowable and indicated in cases where a free corneal cap is produced. Although ointment is avoided preoperatively because of the possibility of it becoming entrapped within the interface, it is acceptable to utilize ointment postoperatively once the epithelium is intact.

CLINICAL FINDINGS

Pain is uncommon unless an epithelial defect is encountered; however, a foreign body or eyelash sensation is not uncommon. Some patients, particularly those with small orbits, will complain of an orbital ache or bruising sensation which dissipates rapidly.

Vision immediately postoperatively is usually quite blurry and improves rapidly over the first 12 to 24 hours. It is not surprising, however, that the occasional patient will sit up immediately after surgery and be overwhelmed at the dramatic subjective and even objective improvement in his or her uncorrected visual acuity (Figures 11-8a and 11-8b).

Conjunctival injection and edema that is evident at the conclusion of the case disappears rapidly, leaving only the occasional conjunctival hemorrhage (Figures 11-9 and 11-10). The corneal cap alignment markings are barely visible within minutes to hours (Figure 11-11). The corneal cap may be a little edematous, appearing somewhat gray and thickened. This corneal cap edema is especially common if the stromal side of the flap is too well hydrated, that is, the flap stroma was left immersed in balanced salt solution (BSS) too long. Fortunately, it clears within 12 to 24 hours in most cases. A traumatic procedure or an excessively long or complex procedure will also leave the flap more edema-

> **Vision immediately postoperatively is usually quite blurry and improves rapidly over the first 12 to 24 hours.**

Figure 11-8a.
Clinical appearance of LASIK treated eye on first postoperative day demonstrating common pattern of excellent corneal clarity associated with a subconjunctival hemorrhage. Reduced suction ring manipulation and suction time diminish both inflammation and incidence of subconjunctival hemorrhages. Patient was treated for -7.75 D with mild astigmatism, reading 20/30 on first day examination.

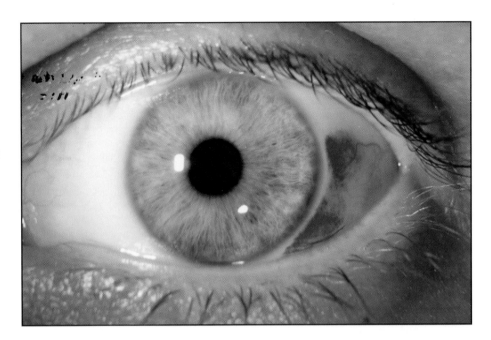

Figure 11-8b.
High magnification appearance of corneal flap demonstrating clear interface.

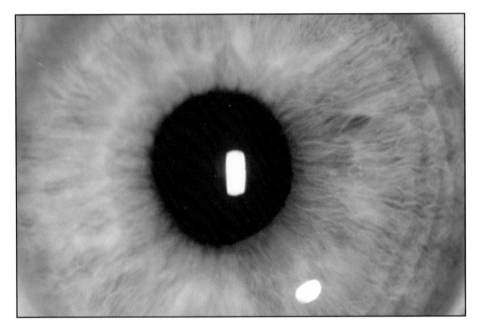

tous. An edematous corneal flap will be less adherent and may become displaced more easily, requiring greater care. Increasing topical steroid use may help reduce corneal flap edema more rapidly.

displaced. Typically, cap displacement occurs during the first 24 to 48 hours, particularly within the first few hours, and rarely without trauma thereafter. If the cap is displaced, simply keep the flap well hydrated with hourly preservative-free lubrication and both eyes closed until it can be replaced.

EARLY POSTOPERATIVE CARE

The patient is examined the following morning (see Figure 11-10) to ensure that the corneal cap has not become

Cap displacement occurs during the first 24 to 48 hours, particularly within the first few hours, and rarely without trauma thereafter.

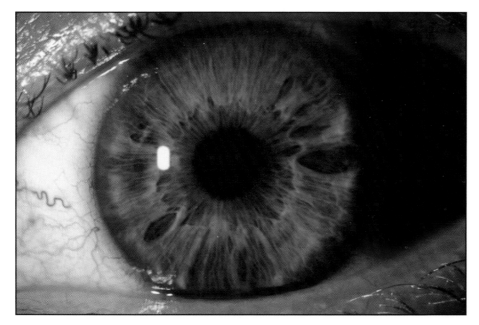

Figure 11-9.
Clinical appearance of LASIK treated eye on third postoperative day demonstrating large subconjunctival hemorrhage. Unaided vision was 20/50 on first postoperative day with a manifest refraction of -0.25 -1.00 x 175, improving from -4.00 -3.00 x 180 preoperatively.

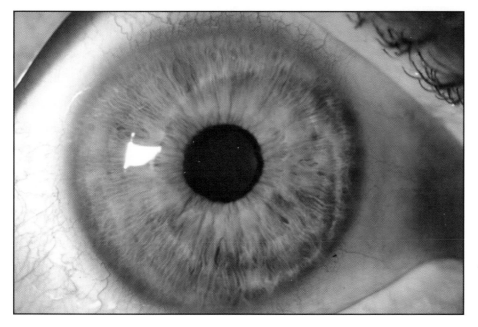

Figure 11-10.
Clinical appearance of LASIK treated right eye during early postoperative period demonstrating minimal inflammation, no subconjunctival hemorrhage formation or evidence of corneal edema. Unaided visual acuity improved to 20/80 with -1.25 D residual myopia, reduced from -10.50 -2.00 x 175.

Once again, although not necessary, tape the eyelid rather than pressure patching in any form. It is said that if the cap is significantly displaced, it can be discerned from the doorway of the exam room, as the patient will be in severe discomfort, which is quite unlike other first postoperative day LASIK patients (Figure 11-12).

The uncorrected visual acuity should be checked prior to any examination. Although the quantitative visual acuity may be impressive on the first postoperative day, it should be recognized that the qualitative vision is often still poor.

The vision will also fluctuate greatly over the first few days. Typically, patients will read 20/100 or better, with most in the 20/40 to 20/60 range and a number of patients will be 20/30 or better. It is not surprising to have mild to moderate myopes 20/20 the first day. The preoperative refractive error has a direct correlation with not only the final outcome, but the speed of visual acuity recovery quantitatively and qualitatively. Patients with less than 9.00 D of myopia do exceedingly well, with near perfect results reported for moderate myopes. Above -10.00 D, the results are more variable, with

Figure 11-11.
Clinical appearance of -13.00 D LASIK treated eye 10 to 15 minutes postoperatively demonstrating rapid clearing of alignment markings, rapid clearing of residual corneal flap edema, intact epithelium, and absence of corneal striae on retroillumination.

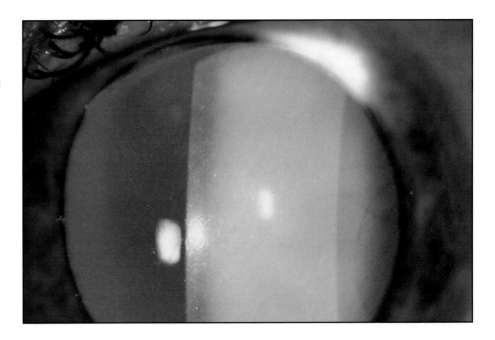

Figure 11-12.
Clinical appearance of LASIK treated right eye for -6.50 -1.00 x 180 during early postoperative healing phase demonstrating white eye with clear corneal interface.

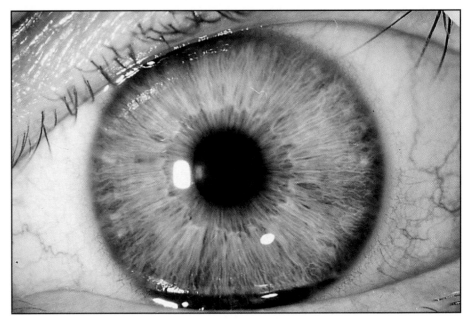

anticipation that virtually all the extremely severe myopes above 15.00 D will require two procedures. Preoperative cylinder also greatly affects immediate postoperative visual recovery, as treatment of spherical corrections is more predictable. It is important to counsel patients preoperatively with respect to both anticipated quantitative and qualitative vision expected. It must be recognized that patients never complain if they see better than expected, but always if the vision falls short of their expectations. In general, severe myopes have the same expectations as mild myopes, despite

appropriate preoperative counseling. Patients also have tremendous difficulty remembering what their uncorrected preoperative vision was like.

A baseline refraction can usually be measured on the first postoperative day, although best corrected vision is often still reduced by one to three lines. Lower myopes retain and regain their best corrected vision better. Manifest refraction is typically within 1.00 D for moderate to severe myopes and within 2.00 D of emmetropia for severe myopes. Extreme myopes are typically grossly undercor-

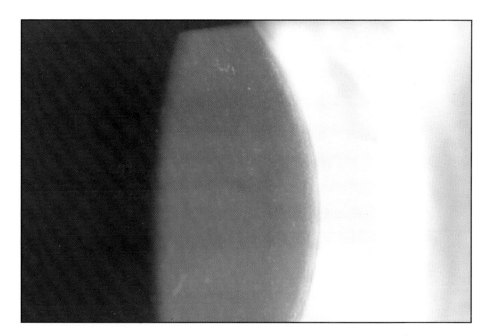

Figure 11-13.
High magnification clinical appearance of corneal flap during immediate postoperative phase demonstrating almost imperceptible flap edge. Corneal flap edges are notably smooth and flat, with an evenly symmetrical peripheral gutter indicating excellent flap apposition.

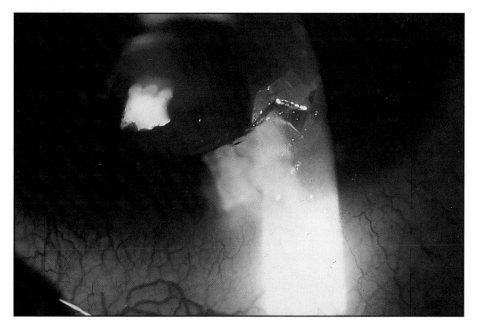

Figure 11-14.
Clinical appearance of LASIK treated eye immediately postoperatively demonstrating small epithelial defect along flap edge. Epithelial disruption is most common along flap margin and increases the incidence of epithelial ingrowths.

rected. Severe myopes often have manifest refractive errors disproportionately high relative to their uncorrected visual acuity. That is, they may have an uncorrected visual acuity of 20/40, but have a noncycloplegic refraction of -2.00 D,

rather than the expected -1.00 D. This is due to multiple factors, from accommodative spasm even in older presbyopes to a central island formation. The topographical change induced by the intrastromal ablation can often result in a somewhat multifocal cornea.

Corneal examination reveals an almost imperceptible flap edge (Figure 11-13) in most instances, as the peripheral gutter has been filled in by epithelium. There is often slight stippling or punctate keratitis in the area of the alignment markings because gentian violet dye is epitheliotoxic.

> **A baseline refraction can usually be measured on the first postoperative day, although best corrected vision is often still reduced by one to three lines.**

Figure 11-15.
Postoperative clinical appearance of irregular epithelium following LASIK with focal areas of keratitis related to intraoperative drying of surface epithelium, gentian violet marking dye, and topical perioperative medications (topical anesthetic and aminoglycoside antibiotics). Interface clear with the exception of minimal fine particle dusting. Corneal flap clarity restored with preservative-free lubrication.

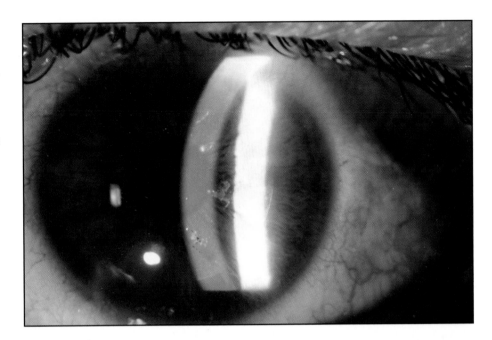

Figure 11-16.
Clinical appearance of left eye following LASIK for -8.00 D demonstrating minimal eyelid edema with 20/25 unaided vision at 1 week.

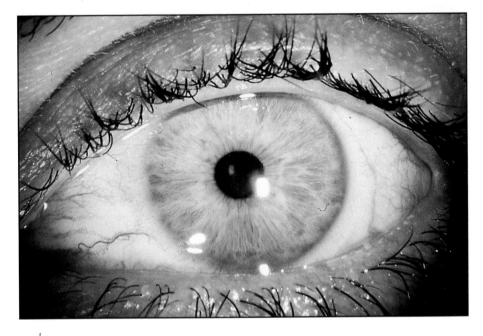

There may also be small epithelial defects apparent (Figure 11-14), typically along the flap edge but also centrally if excessive drying occurred intraoperatively (Figure 11-15). Stromal edema of the cap may persist for 24 to 48 hours, but rarely longer, and is an uncommon finding with good technique (Figure 11-16).

Interface clarity is dependent upon technique and the amount of debris within the patient's tear film. Small amounts of debris and lint fibers may be observed (Figure 11-17), however, these are clinically insignificant both visu-

ally and physiologically, as the stroma is quite inert and an inflammatory reaction will rarely ensue (Figures 11-18a and 11-18b). In general, interface debris bothers the doctor more than the patient. Removal of foreign particles is only performed if clinically significant, and should be done early or at the time of enhancement (Figure 11-19).

CLINICAL FINDINGS AFTER 3 TO 4 WEEKS

The uncorrected visual acuity has typically reached the maximal level expected, and the eye has usually regained its

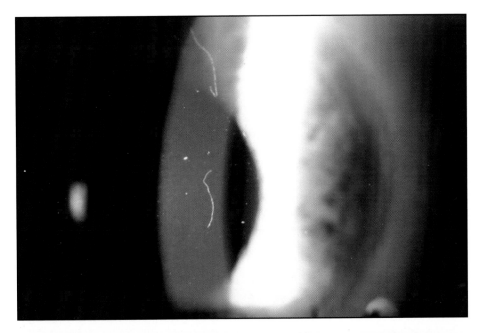

Figure 11-17.
Clinical appearance of lint fibers with interface postoperatively. Interface opacities of limited clinical significance, as patient is subjectively unaware of them and inflammatory reactions to foreign matter are very infrequent.

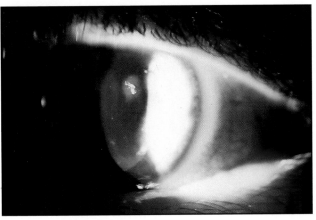

Figure 11-18a.
Clinical appearance of localized interface inflammatory reaction surrounding foreign matter under low magnification. Lint fibers are one of the most commonly encountered and frustrating interface opacities. Patient was monitored closely, but not treated as there was no associated patient symptoms, no clinical progression, and discernible visual sequelae.

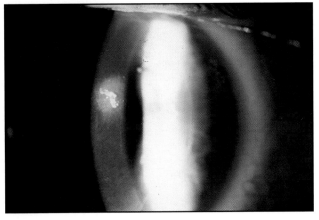

Figure 11-18b.
Clinical appearance of localized interface inflammatory reaction surrounding foreign matter under medium magnification.

best corrected visual acuity level, although very severe myopes greater than -12.00 D may require months. The eye requires about 1 month to begin stabilizing, with subjective complaints of glare and ghosting beginning to dissipate (Figures 11-20 through 11-22).

The refractive error can be measured and determined quite accurately at this time. Some patients who achieved better than 20/25 vision initially with near plano refractive errors may have regressed by 1.00 D or more. The healing

> **The uncorrected visual acuity has typically reached the maximal level expected and the eye has usually regained its best corrected visual acuity by 3 to 4 weeks.**

> **The healing pattern and stabilization occurs about three to four times faster than with PRK.**

Figure 11-19.
Peripheral interface opacity, consisting of lint fibers in this clinical example. It is important to keep all gauze and eyepads which can produce lint away from operative field and surgical instruments.

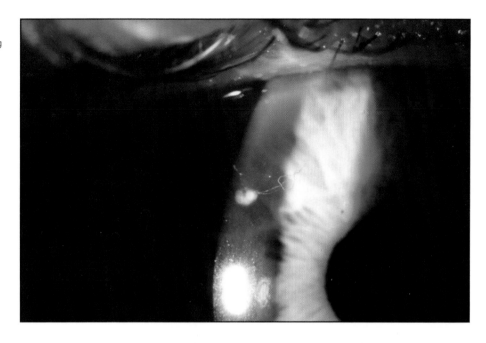

Figure 11-20.
Clinical appearance of LASIK treated left eye 1 month postoperatively demonstrating excellent preserved corneal clarity. Unaided vision was 20/50 on the first postoperative day with a preoperative cycloplegic refraction of -7.25 -1.00 x 005, improving to +0.50 -0.75 x 180 with 20/25+1 uncorrected visual acuity at 1 month.

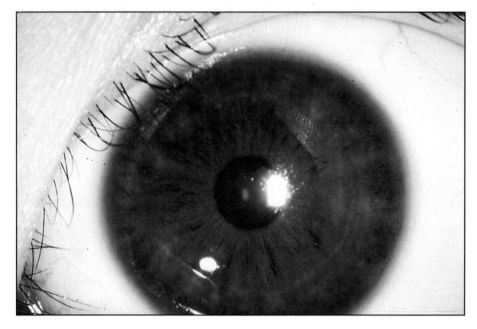

pattern and stabilization occurs about three to four times faster than with PRK. Consideration of repeat surgery for enhancement of the refractive and visual result is performed after 4 to 12 weeks and can be planned at this visit, with retesting performed the day of the procedure, ideally after 3 months (Figure 11-23).

Corneal examination reveals a clear interface, although a small amount of interface debris is not unusual (Figures 11-24 through 11-26). The flap edges are well healed and a faint white ring along the cap edge may become apparent. The white ring represents scarring along the cut surface of Bowman's layer and is about 0.5 mm in diameter (Figures 11-27 and 11-28). In a small number of patients, epithelium is observed to be invading the interface along one edge or circumferentially (see Chapter 12).

Corneal topography demonstrates central flattening, although the optical zone size often appears smaller than attempted (Figures 11-29a and 11-29b). There are two

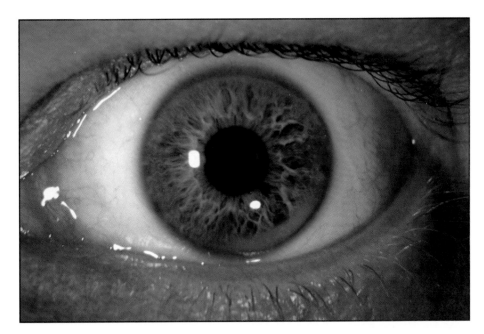

Figure 11-21.
Clinical appearance of LASIK treated left eye 2 months postoperatively demonstrating clear corneal interface. Unaided vision was 20/30 on the first postoperative day, following -7.25 D spherical correction, with gradual improvement to 20/20 by 1 month and slight regression back to 20/30, but with improved qualitative vision.

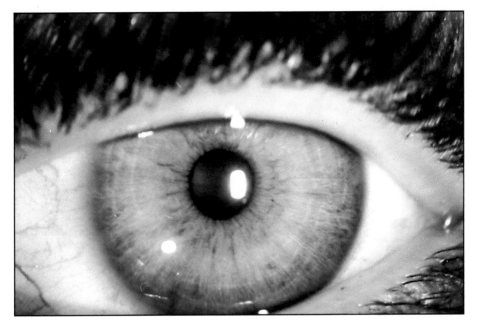

Figure 11-22.
Clinical appearance of LASIK treated left eye 3 months postoperatively demonstrating clear cornea. Unaided vision was 20/40 on the first postoperative day following -4.25 -2.50 x 10 toric ablation, with gradual improvement to 20/25 by 1 week and no regression of effect observed.

parallel explanations for this:

1. The hydrated stroma makes the peripheral blend zone less effective.
2. The corneal flap may mask the ablation pattern somewhat.

LASIK appears to quite unlike ALK in this regard, as the ALK flap aids the small 4.2-mm typical refractive resection creating a 5.5-mm effective optical zone. With RK, the effective optical zone is far greater than the surgical optical

RK	effective optical zone > surgical optical zone
ALK	effective optical zone > surgical optical zone
PRK	effective optical zone = surgical optical zone
LASIK	effective optical zone < surgical optical zone

zone. As noted above, the same is true for ALK, with the effective optical zone exceeding the surgical optical zone. With PRK, however, the surgical optical zone and the effec-

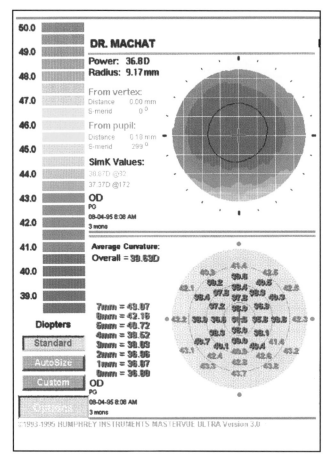

Figure 11-23.
Postoperative videokeratography following LASIK for -9.00 D with multizone technique. Postoperative refraction -1.00 D at 3 months. No night glare.

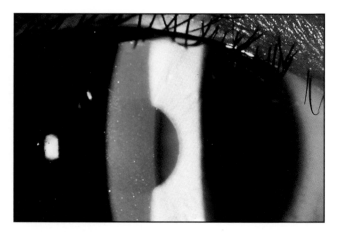

Figure 11-24.
Clinical appearance of LASIK treated right eye 3 months postoperatively demonstrating clinically insignificant trace interface haze. Unaided vision was 20/40 on the first postoperative day following -11.25 -2.75 x 170 high myopia toric ablation with rapid regression to 20/200 uncorrected vision requiring retreatment for -2.00 -1.00 x 177.

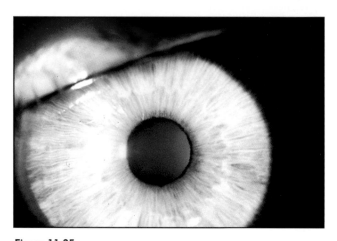

Figure 11-25.
High magnification clinical appearance of clear corneal interface 3 months following LASIK correction of -8.75 D. Patient regressed to -1.25 D by 3 months, requiring retreatment despite +0.50 D refraction day 1.

tive optical zone are equivalent, and with LASIK, the effective optical zone appears to be smaller than the surgical optical zone. Transition zone blending may actually act to diminish the effective optical zone observed on topography, accounting for symptoms of night glare with LASIK (Figures 11-30 and 11-31).

> A large broad hinge may induce cylinder if not adequately decentered nasally.

Corneal videokeratography (Figures 11-32a through 11-32c) after LASIK may demonstrate a number of patterns, aside from central circular or elliptical flattening (Figure 11-33) with adequate or inadequate optical zone size as discussed above, specifically decentration (Figures 11-34a through 11-36), nasal steepening (Figures 11-37a through 11-38b), and central island formation. Decentration of the ablation and appearance of videokeratography is unrelated to centration of the flap. If the ablation is performed with a dilated pupil or with suction active, the ablation may be decentered superotemporally due to the shift in pupil alignment. That is, the center of the pupil appears to be more superior and more temporal than is actually the case. A non-pharmacologically manip-

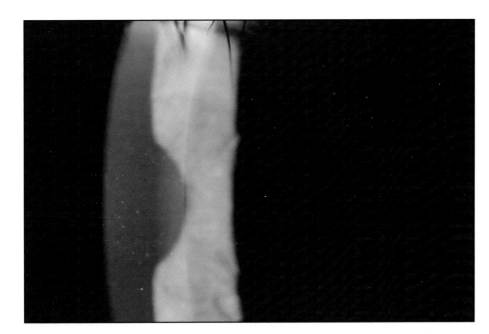

Figure 11-26.
Clear cornea post-LASIK with barely perceptible interface even under high magnification.

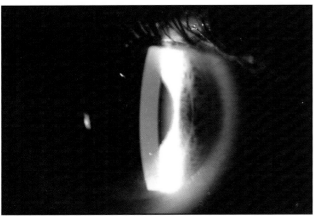

Figure 11-27.
Low power clinical appearance of LASIK treated eye 6 months postoperatively demonstrating clear corneal interface centrally with peripheral flap scarring along cut edge of Bowman's layer.

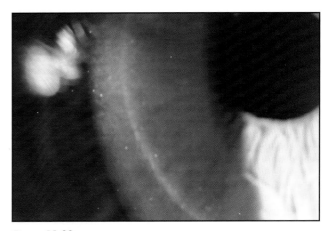

Figure 11-28.
Clinical appearance of LASIK treated eye 12 months postoperatively demonstrating 0.5 mm white peripheral scarring along corneal flap edge. No clinical significance noted.

> **If irregular astigmatism and night glare persist beyond 6 months, they may very well be permanent.**

ulated pupil without suction applied provides the most ideal circumstance for achieving good centration. Additionally, the centration toward the visual axis and not the pupillary center may be preferable in some cases in which a large angle kappa exists, as is the case for radial keratotomy (RK). A large broad hinge may induce cylinder if not adequately decentered nasally. Fluid accumulation along the hinge or a short flap may result in inadequate treatment nasally, resulting in a nasal step. Typically, a nasal step does not possess any clinical symptoms. Central island formation, both the clinically dramatic and clinically subtle, should be appreciated, and retreatment planned in accordance. Central islands post-LASIK appear to be more stable and less likely to resolve (Figure 11-39).

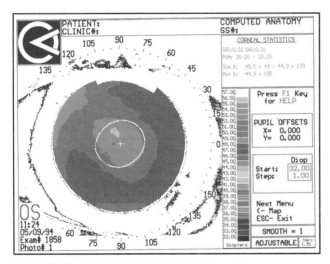

Figure 11-29a.
Preoperative videokeratography prior to LASIK for -13.50 D.

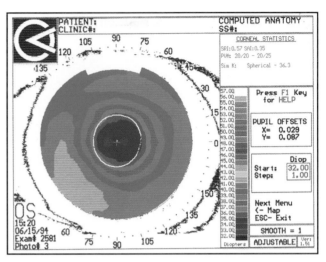

Figure 11-29b.
Postoperative videokeratography demonstrating central flattening following multizone LASIK. Effective optical zone smaller than anticipated due to corneal flap masking effect of peripheral taper. Postoperative uncorrected vision 20/60, preoperative best corrected vision 20/25.

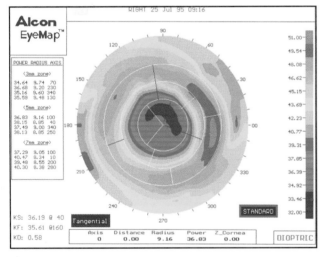

Figure 11-30.
Videokeratography post-LASIK demonstrating small effective optical zone despite 6.6-mm attempted optical zone.

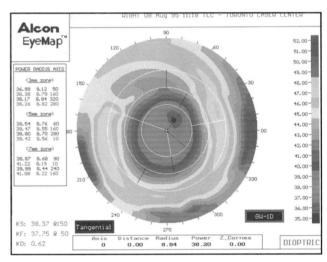

Figure 11-31.
Postoperative videokeratography demonstrating small effective optical zone post-LASIK for high myopia.

CLINICAL FINDINGS AFTER 3 MONTHS

The uncorrected and best corrected visual acuity has stabilized in virtually all patients. A number of extremely high myopes and complicated patients may continue to demonstrate improvement over an entire year, as with all forms of lamellar surgery. Qualitative vision and night visual disturbances dramatically improve over the first 3 months, but continue to improve over 6 months or longer.

The refractive error is measured with cycloplegia to accurately quantify the residual refractive error. Myopic regression of severe myopes usually ceases after 3 months, and retreatment of these performed between 3 and 6 months.

Corneal examination may reveal interface haze in a very small number of patients centrally, and in a greater number of patients peripherally. There is definite haze for-

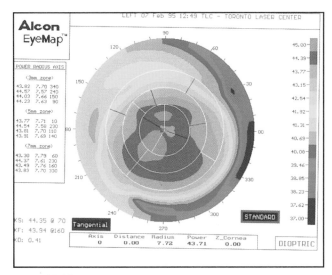

Figure 11-32a.
Preoperative videokeratography of left eye with refraction -9.50 +1.00 x 80.

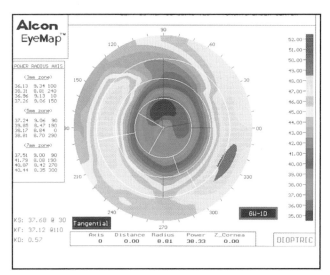

Figure 11-32b.
Postoperative LASIK videokeratography of well-centered ablation. Postoperative refraction -0.75 +1.00 x 17 at 1 month.

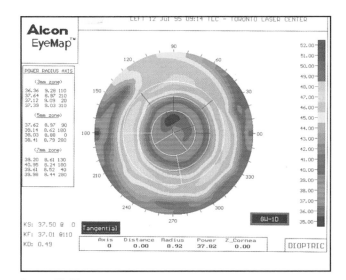

Figure 11-32c.
Postoperative videokeratography at 4 months with myopic regression to -2.50 +1.00 x 10. Note the smaller optical zone.

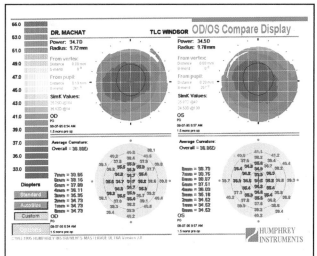

Figure 11-33.
Postoperative videokeratography of bilateral primary elliptical LASIK for extreme myopia and astigmatism.
OD: -10.50 +1.50 x 100
OS: -11.75 +2.50 x 80
Postoperative refraction
OD: -1.00 +0.50 x 96
OS: -1.50 sphere
Uncorrected visual acuity
OD: 20/30
OS: 20/80
Patient desired repeat LASIK OS and decided against monovision despite presbyopic age group.

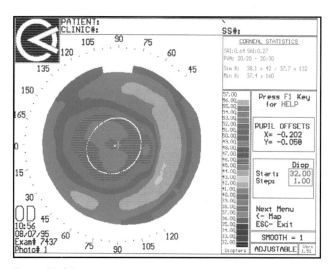

Figure 11-34a.
Right eye with mild temporal decentration following bilateral LASIK for -8.00 D OU. Right eye 20/30 uncorrected visual acuity with -0.50 D refractive error. Patient asymptomatic OU. Nasal step evident on videokeratography OU.

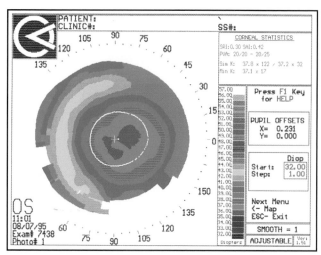

Figure 11-34b.
Left eye with mild temporal decentration following bilateral LASIK for -8.00 D OU. Left eye plano with 20/20 uncorrected visual acuity. Patient asymptomatic OU. Nasal step evident on videokeratography OU.

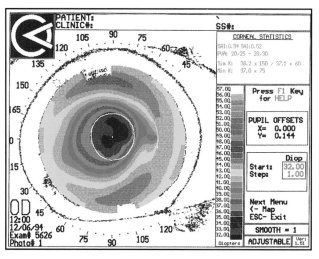

Figure 11-35.
Small optical zone evident following LASIK for extreme myopia. Minimal decentration.

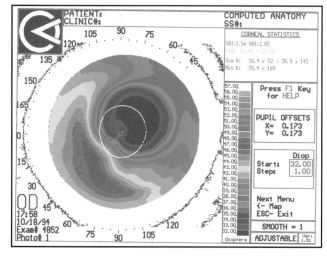

Figure 11-36.
Clinically significant decentration following LASIK for high myopia. Greater than 2 mm decentration. Etiology related to performing LASIK with dilated pupil. Elevated SRI indicating irregular astigmatism. Preoperative refractive error -15.00 D, decentration resulted in gross undercorrection with induced cylinder. Correction involves reablation centrally with residual error beneath corneal flap. No concerns with blending zones as with PRK.

mation in a select number of high myopes who undergo LASIK and have a propensity toward aggressive wound healing. Interface fibrosis makes lifting the flap extremely difficult for reablation. Interface debris remains unchanged from prior examinations. The white ring which demarcates the flap edge may increase in intensity over the first 3 months, but is not readily apparent in many patients (Figures 11-40 and 11-41). It is unclear whether the size of the peripheral gutter contributes to the width and density of the peripheral ring, but I suspect this to be the case. A direct cor-

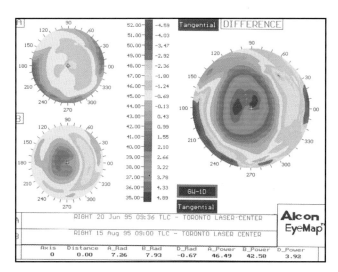

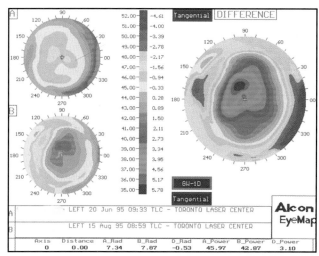

Figure 11-37a.
Nasal hinge creates nasal step on videokeratography (right eye map). Although difference map demonstrates central flattening, postoperative videokeratography, subset B map, demonstrates nasal area of steepening secondary to LASIK hinge.

Figure 11-37b.
Nasal hinge creates nasal step on videokeratography (left eye map). Although difference map demonstrates central flattening, postoperative videokeratography, subset B map, demonstrates nasal area of steepening secondary to LASIK hinge.

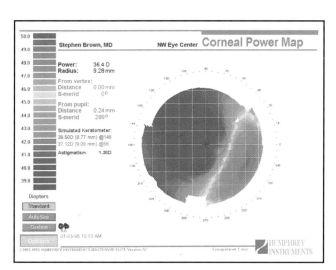

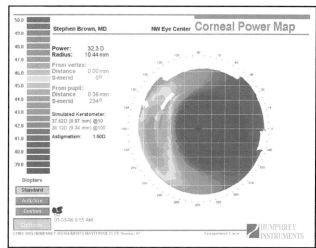

Figure 11-38a.
Postoperative right eye videokeratography of highly myopic patient with large nasal steps evident OU. Patient was well-centered OU, but large nasal hinge gives appearance of temporal decentration.
Preoperative refraction
OD: -13.00 -3.00 x 90
Postoperative refraction
OD: -1.00 -3.00 x 95
No loss of best corrected visual acuities observed.

Figure 11-38b.
Postoperative left eye videokeratography of highly myopic patient with large nasal steps evident OU.
Preoperative refraction
OS: -16.00 -3.00 x 100
Postoperative refraction
OS: -3.75 -1.75 x 105
No loss of best corrected visual acuities observed.

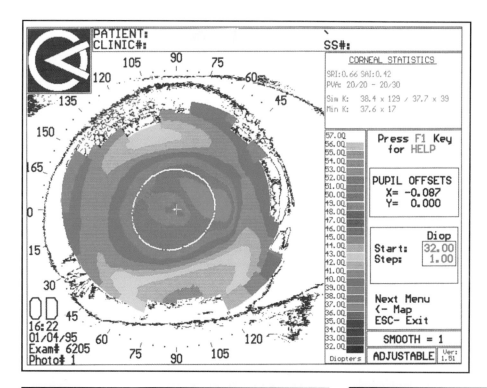

Figure 11-39.
Small 2 D central island following LASIK for -8.00 D.

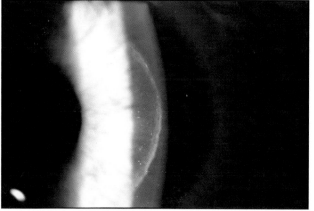

Figure 11-40.
Clinical appearance of LASIK treated eye 9 months postoperatively, demonstrating white peripheral scarring along corneal flap edge. Width and presence of peripheral scarring may be related to size of peripheral gutter at conclusion of procedure.

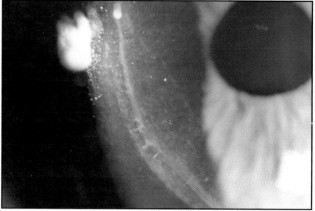

Figure 11-41.
Peripheral corneal flap edge may thicken and retract over 3 to 6 months. This may be in association with epithelial ingrowth, or not. Must observe closely, especially if epithelial ingrowth evident.

relation likely exists, but patient variability plays a factor.

Corneal topography typically demonstrates little change from the first month examination, although slight regression may be observed in patients.

LATE POSTOPERATIVE CARE

Examination of patients at 6 and 12 months is important primarily to ensure that stability of cycloplegic refraction has been maintained. These are also the most essential visits to monitor return of best corrected visual acuity and subjective reduction of night glare. If irregular astigmatism and night glare persist beyond 6 months, they may very well be permanent. The clinical appearance of the cap is typically unchanged over the first year beyond the 3-month examination (Figures 11-42 and 11-43).

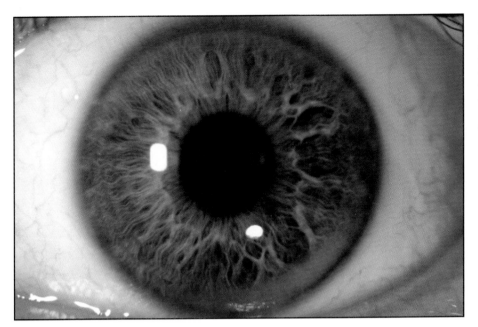

Figure 11-42.
Clinical appearance of LASIK treated eye 14 months postoperatively demonstrating naturally clear cornea with no change in refractive stability from 6 weeks following -7.00 D correction. Patient achieved -0.75 D refractive endpoint with 20/30 visual acuity.

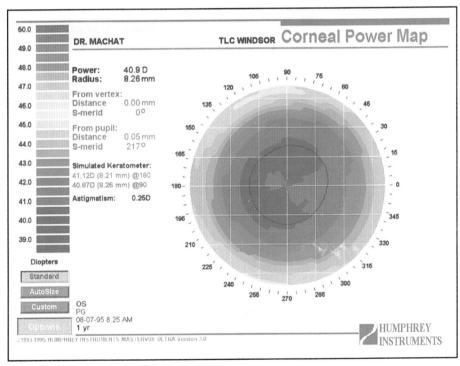

Figure 11-43.
Postoperative videokeratography PRK for -7.00 D with pretreatment multizone technique. Uncorrected visual acuity 20/20 with +0.75 D refraction in 27-year-old patient 1 year postoperatively.

CHAPTER 12

LASIK Complications and Their Management

There is a definite surgical learning curve to laser in situ keratomileusis (LASIK), one filled with many nuances that require hundreds of procedures to fully grasp. Experience with automated lamellar keratoplasty (ALK) and other lamellar procedures are clearly beneficial in shortening the learning curve. In fact, radial keratotomy (RK) surgeons will fair better in the short-term, as they will not only have a better appreciation of how to select and counsel candidates for LASIK, but they also will have acquired the discipline required for any elective refractive procedure. I feel experience with photorefractive keratectomy (PRK) is an important prerequisite to fully understanding all that encompasses LASIK. With respect to photoablation dynamics, it has been said that LASIK is 90% keratectomy and 10% laser (Slade) and I believe this is true. The number of procedures required to feel completely comfortable with LASIK to handle truly difficult cases is dependent upon the individual surgeon. I myself have found that I continue to learn at a rapid pace, despite having performed over 2000 LASIK procedures. The first 40 procedures were associated with a 25% complication rate, varying from minor problems to those quite serious. After 2000 LASIK procedures, the complication rate has dwindled to 1% to 2% for minor complications, such as epithelial ingrowths and irregular astigmatism, and 0.2% or 0.3% for severe complications relating to loss of flap integrity from microkeratome performance and stromal melts.

> **Incidence of LASIK Complications**
> 1% to 2% for minor complications (ie, epithelial ingrowths and irregular astigmatism)
> 0.2% to 0.3% for major complications (ie, loss of corneal flap integrity from microkeratome performance and stromal melts)

With proper training, education, and caution, LASIK complications should not be feared, but understood. Understanding the mechanisms that produce LASIK complications is the first step in prevention, followed by the second step of complication management. Most complications are related to the lamellar dissection or cap management. Errors in refractive predictability and topographical abnormalities are a result of the LASIK nomogram, and ablation profiles are still evolving. Controlling hydration, however, remains the greatest enigma. The greater standard deviation encountered in higher myopes must be shifted toward undercorrections until the range of predictability is improved.

Complications can be divided into those which occur intraoperatively, in the early postoperative period, and in the late postoperative period beyond the first month.

> "LASIK is 90% keratectomy and 10% laser."
> —Stephen G. Slade, MD

LASIK Complications

Stephen G. Slade, MD

Lamellar refractive surgery and LASIK have the advantage over some forms of refractive surgery in that fewer overall complications are produced. This is the main advantage of lamellar surgery, the reduction of the effects of wound healing. There is the potential for a more serious group of complications however. Fewer complications mean less postoperative pain, less haze, and fewer over- and undercorrections due to variable epithelial regeneration. More serious complications include displaced flaps, epithelial ingrowth, and stromal melt, and the rare but real possibility of entry into the anterior chamber. These complications, along with severe irregular astigmatism from poor quality cuts, are extremely difficult to repair and can require a deep therapeutic lamellar graft done by hand or a penetrating keratoplasty. In short, compared to PRK, LASIK with the addition of the microkeratome can produce surgical rather than wound healing problems.

Complications with LASIK tend to be immediate and must be detected early in the postoperative course. The appearance of the eye at postoperative day 1 is crucial. The patient should see 20/80 or better uncorrected, assuming 20/20 or better corrected preoperative vision. There should be minimal discomfort and the eye should be quiet externally. The cornea flap should be in place and there should be no edema present. Basically, it should be difficult to detect that anything has been done to the eye (Figure A-1). Cases done early in the learning

curve may have decreased early uncorrected vision due to drying and roughening of the epithelium. This is not permanent and will improve over the first few days. It is important to avoid excess manipulation of the epithelium, a minimum of marking and handling is desirable.

The potential for serious complications that are difficult to fix makes prevention the main focus with the set-up and performance of LASIK. First is the training of the surgical team. All members of the team should attend a course that includes didactic and hands-on wet lab instruction. A further course or mini-fellowship where live surgery observation is combined with more didactic instruction and wet lab training is desirable. Finally the presence of a trained surgeon or technician at the student's first cases is extremely helpful. Once the surgeon has begun performing lamellar surgery, continuing education in the form of user group meetings and other traditional meetings is recommended.

The set-up for the actual surgical case is vital. Most of LASIK complications can be related to the preoperative set-up (Figure A-2). The preparation of the equipment is critical. It is likewise important to avoid the misuse of the nomograms or LASIK algorithms. A poor or inaccurate refraction or poor pachymetry can also cause problems. When the depth of the cut is critical as in thin corneas, it is helpful to know the relationship between the plate and the blade to know the gap and thick-

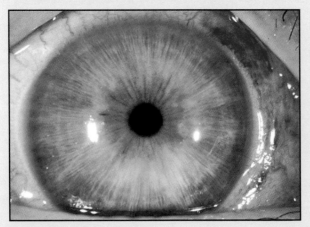

Figure A-1.
A normal LASIK case at postoperative day 1. Note the clarity of the cornea and the hemorrhage from the application of the suction ring.

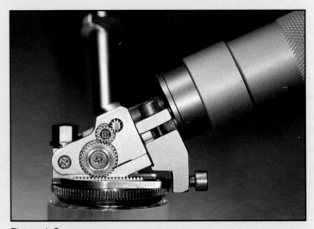

Figure A-2.
The Chiron Ruiz keratome set up with the three-piece suction ring.

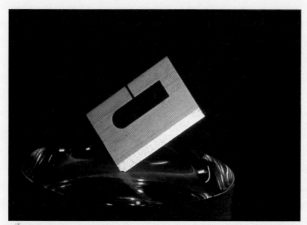

Figure A-3.
A perfect blade, ready to be installed.

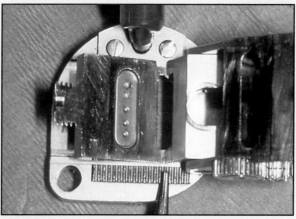

Figure A-4.
The keratome opened, demonstrating the point to check for proper setting of the stopper.

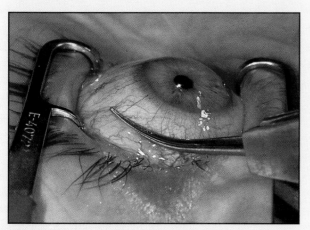

Figure A-5.
Chemosis with the curved tyers set just before the edema.

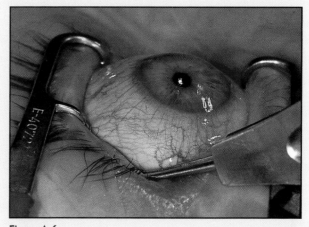

Figure A-6.
The chemosis has now been milked posterior and tucked beneath the lid speculum.

ness the keratome will cut. The keratome scope is vital for this purpose. The blade must be pristine and the stopper set perfectly (Figures A-3 and A-4). Of course the patient must be examined thoroughly and all contraindications ruled out. A checklist or Preflight list which has all the points to set up the equipment can help avoid many mistakes for the beginning and expert surgeon. LASIK has the disadvantage of much more equipment than other refractive operations. The laser and keratome must both be prechecked before the surgery.

GENERAL COMMENTS ON LASIK COMPLICATIONS

Complications can arise from the surgeon, keratome, and the laser. There are also the individual wound healing charac-

teristics of the individual patient. The laser must be at peak efficiency. This is difficult as the optics are continuously being degraded from use. Some method must be used to determine the fluence of the beam and the purity or homogeneity. A poor beam or variable power can result in gross to fine irregular astigmatism and over- and undercorrection. The proper ablation for the individual patient must be entered and rechecked. This includes the axis of astigmatism, spherical power, and the correct diameter profile.

Most of the serious complications of LASIK will be related to the use of the keratome. The aspects of the keratectomy cut that are critical are several. Exposure is vital to the keratectomy. This is largely dependent on orbital anatomy. The deepset eye with an overhanging brow is best avoided in the early

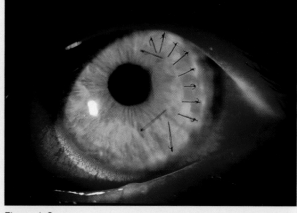

Figure A-7.
The suction ring in proper postion with the cornea marked.

Figure A-8.
A penetrating injury from the keratome as the plate was not properly inserted. The wound has been repaired with interrupted sutures.

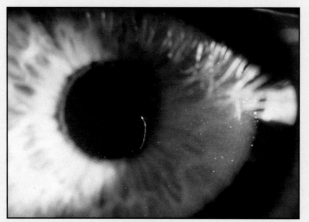

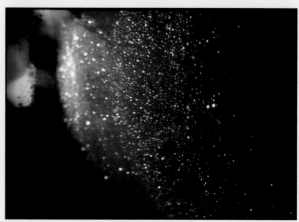

Figure A-9.
A fiber in the interface, showing the lack of inflammation.

Figure A-10.
Talc from gloves that has been introduced into the interface.

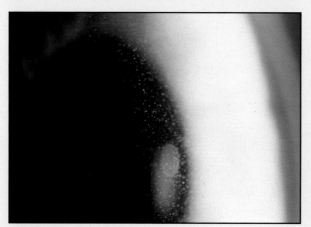

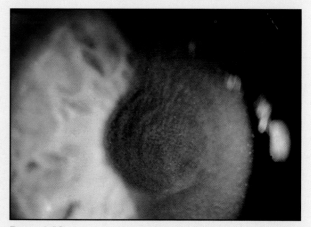

Figure A-11.
Oil from the keratome that has been introduced into the interface. The keratome was sticking and so oil was applied instead of properly cleaning the unit.

Figure A-12.
Instrument that has been introduced into the interface. The milk was used to lubricate the keratome and was not completely irrigated off.

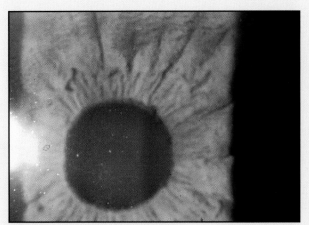

Figure A-13.
Blood from a superior pannus that has layed out in the interface.

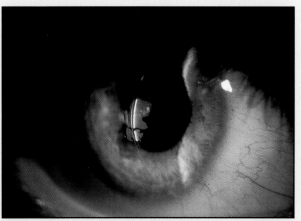

Figure A-14.
Epithelium in the interface, in a central location.

cases. Proper anesthesia and sedation will aid in achieving good exposure. The use of a retrobulbar block, while not desirable, will give good proptosis and exposure in difficult settings. The main goal is to provide a clear path and gear track. Fluid management is important to avoid a false meniscus in the measurement of the cap diameter and IOP. The cornea should be wet for the pass but a little dry for the applanation. Always take a moment to inspect the eye before the placement of the suction ring. There should be no chemosis and the pupil should be centered between the speculum. If chemosis is present the fluid should be milked out with curved tiers down beneath the lid speculum (Figures A-5 and A-6). A speculum that provides maximum exposure with reasonable patient comfort is desirable. The pupil should be constricted only with the light from the microscope. The case should be set up for maximum exposure, good suction must be present, good centration is desirable although not as important as in ALK, a slow controlled pass of the keratome and a sharp, accurate blade (Figure A-7). The keratome must be checked for smooth operation, a perfect blade, and good suction. Failure to check the plate, for example, can result in the keratome entering the anterior chamber and even penetrating the lens into the vitreous (Figure A-8). The patient's eye must be set up properly for maximum exposure and a clear path for the keratome. Sterile field and overall clean technique must be followed.

INTERFACE PARTICLES

Common complications include decentered ablations and keratectomy, over- and undercorrections, and infiltrates in the interface. The most common complication seen at day 1 is

debris in the interface (Figure A-9). Most of this is harmless particles that have no visual consequences. Most often the surgeon is more concerned from an aesthetic viewpoint. Much of this particulate matter can be avoided by the use of powderless gloves or no gloves (Figure A-10). There is a continuous debate about whether to wear gloves. Many of the surgeons that trained with Barraquer by tradition do wear gloves. There are advantages in the no glove method in less debris and some ease in handling the keratome to assemble it. The disadvantage is to possible infections control. There has been a very low infection rate with lamellar surgery in general, however. At present, approximately 60% of surgeons in the US do not wear gloves. Particles in the interface can be avoided by careful draping and preparation of the field. Irrigation of the patient's eye prior to surgery reduces meibomian secretions in the field and debris. Draping the eyelashes out of the field further reduces debris. Careful irrigation at the end of the case can wash out particles.

There are some unusual forms of debris in the interface. If ever one mistakenly uses dome form or lubrication for the keratome this can be seen the next day. We have seen oil in the interface as well as instrument milk (Figures A-11 and A-12). Both were stable and did not affect the visual outcome. Of course lubrication should never be used on the device. Blood can also be seen beneath the cap flap. Often in high myopes there is a pannus present and vessels that are transected by the keratome. While the cut ends will ooze heme during the case, it is a mistake to take too much time and attention to try to stop the flow as replacing the flap will tamponade the blood. However with this method blood can occasionally be seen at day 1 (Figure A-13). This will resolve over the next few weeks and does not

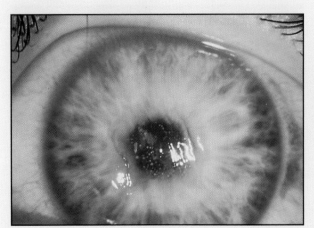

Figure A-15.
Epithelium has grown completely across the interface and melting and wrinkling has resulted.

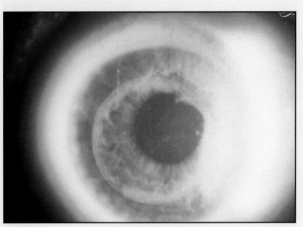

Figure A-16.
A decentered keratectomy with the edge very close to the visual axis.

require treatment. Another source of fine particles is a misused or over used blade which can produce fine metallic debris that is also inert. Single large filaments are usually inert and also do not require treatment. A mild feathering over the filament is all that we have noticed with interface fibers. If they are in the visual axis or if the surgeon feels they must come out they can be removed at the slit lamp with a Sinskey hook under topical anesthesia. One does run the risk of inducing irregular astigmatism or epithelium in the interface with this treatment. In summary, most debris is technique dependent. As the speed and ease of technique increases less debris is usually noted.

EPITHELIUM WITHIN INTERFACE

The most significant material in the interface is epithelium (Figure A-14). Epithelium may be introduced in the interface by three different methods. The most common is in growth. A solid sheet of host epithelium grows beneath the flap rather than meeting the epithelium on the flap and merging. Poor technique and adhesion of the flap is the most common cause of this type. Epithelium can also occur in rest of cells that are presumably implanted during surgery from the blade as it cut across the bed or contamination by cells that are dislodged and washed or implanted on the stromal bed. A third more unusual way occurs with lamellar surgery over previous incisional corneal surgery. When a flap is cut across incisions that have epithelial plugs the epithelium can spread from the plug laterally into the interface. There are four reasons for attempting to repair epithelium in the interface:

Epithelium can range from 30 to 70 microns in thickness

and so can create astigmatism or undercorrection.

Epithelium in the interface can even be picked up with topography showing astigmatism where the thickness of the epithelium raises up the edge of the flap. Another good diagnostic technique for epithelium is to dilate the pupil and retroilluminate the cornea. Often epithelium will stand out better with this method. One can see the full extent of the spread and the clear halo of epithelium beyond the foamy central islands that are easier to see. Stroma sandwiched between two layers of epithelium can melt (Figure A-15). A sheet of epithelium can actually block the visual axis. Finally in any case where the epithelium is observed to be progressing, repair should be considered.

Epithelial removal can be simple and quick. It should not be attempted though, unless one of the above reasons is present. With a quiet, small rest of epithelium that does not affect vision, the patient is safer with no treatment. Photos should be used to document the position of the epithelium and placed in the chart to be reviewed at subsequent examinations. There is a risk of irregular astigmatism and failure to remove all the epithelium with any surgery. To remove epithelium, first the full extent and location should be noted. The visible foamy cell or islands of epithelium often are surrounded by a clear halo that extended further and is difficult to visualize. It is easiest to lift the flap although small amounts or rests that are peripheral can be squeegeed out with blunt forceps. If the extent of the epithelium is such that the flap must be creased across the visual axis it is best to lift the entire flap to avoid inducing fine wrinkles and irregular astigmatism. Scrape the epithelium out with a 69

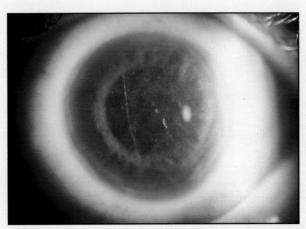

Figure A-17.
A truncated flap from a suction break. The vertical line is where the keratome surfaced after the eye fell away from the suction ring.

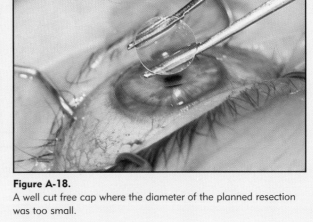

Figure A-18.
A well cut free cap where the diameter of the planned resection was too small.

Beaver blade or comparable instrument. Always check the undersurface of the flap although most epithelium is present on the bed. When lifting the flap, try to cut the epithelial edge to avoid large tears or flaps. Replace the flap with the standard technique of fluid control and minimal handling. Finally, in some cases where the epithelium has grown completely across the bed and there is a good deal of wrinkling and stromal melt present, the best course might be to remove the flap and allow the epithelium to heal over as in PRK. While the surface of a LASIK ablation is not as smooth as one in PRK where smooth Bowman's layer is mirrored down into the stroma, good results can be obtained. There is now downside to trying before it is decided a homoplastic graft is needed.

IRREGULAR ASTIGMATISM

One of the main causes of loss of best corrected vision with lamellar surgery is irregular astigmatism. A decentered or uneven resection caused by a suction break can cause induced irregular astigmatism (Figure A-16). Centration or the ability to lace the keratome where one desires is very important. It is the placement of the ring and the first few seconds of suction that determine this. Slight pressure on the ring and speculum before the suction is applied will help the ring stay seated. One should also avoid torque or rotation of the globe in the first few seconds of suction. Simply watch the setting for a few seconds and come off suction if the globe rotates. Avoid leaving the ring on too long during this test or a ridge will be formed that will make it very difficult to place the ring properly. If this happens it is better to abort the case and perform surgery another day.

Always eliminate chemosis as described above to avoid psuedosuction where the conjunctiva occludes the suction port and causes the suction gauge to rise but good suction is not obtained. Always abort if not satisfied with the situation.

Irregular astigmatism can be caused by a poor keratectomy, poor replacement of the flap, or a poor or decentered ablation. If the ablation is on the bed as in in situ LASIK, a decentered ablation will be very difficult to fix. Scanning lasers that are coupled to real-time topography are in the future, but now choices are limited to less sophisticated masked ablations or therapeutic lamellar surgery. Topography is indispensable to detect subtle decentrations which are suspected on patient complaints or poor quality of vision. Especially with higher myopes, small zones need to be well centered. Complications due to poor keratectomy can cause major visual problems. Keratectomies can be poor by being incomplete, decentered, or uneven. A bad or damaged blade can cause a grossly irregular keratectomy. An incomplete keratectomy is usually caused by a suction break (Figure A-17). It is critical to have good suction for the duration of the keratome pass. If the keratome stops before the pass is complete, there might not be room to place the ablation. The keratectomy can be extended by hand but will not be of the same quality of the microkeratome section. If the keratome is allowed to go too far, a free cap can result (Figure A-18). This in itself is not a problem; with extra care a proper technique is used to replace the flap. Depending on the keratome used an irregular section can result. If a keratectomy has an irregular surface there is an important safety feature of lamellar surgery that should be known. No matter how irregu-

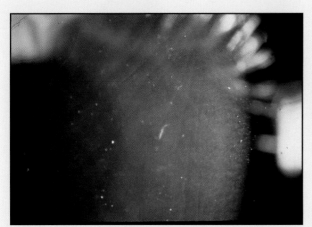

Figure A-19.
Subtle wrinkles radiating out from the edge of the flap where the flap has been torqued from an imperfect placement.

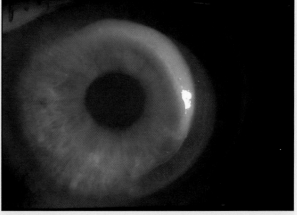

Figure A-20.
A loose flap edge that is demonstrated by fluorescein leakage beneath the lifted edge.

lar the surface of the bed might be, there is a perfect match in the underside of the flap. Therefore, if the flap is simply replaced the patient will return to the preoperative refraction and best corrected vision by the next morning. Problems are created when the bed is altered with an attempted ablation which so that the flap no longer matches. This is important to remember with incomplete resections also. When in doubt put the flap back and do not ablate. One of the more pleasant features of lamellar surgery is that the eye can be back to the exact preoperative state the next day, and then re-operated on in the next few weeks or months depending on the situation. If an incomplete resection is present and there is room for the ablation one can proceed.

With resections that stop short of the needed diameter, surgeons have extended the flap by hand but this is dangerous and will not give as smooth as a surface as the microkeratome. Remember that incomplete resections, can also be caused by a blade that has been damaged, dulling the cutting edge so that a lunette, vertically incomplete resection is produced. With severe suction breaks and very small eccentric resections never attempt to ablate, just try to replace the cap as best as possible.

MICROKERATOME ISSUES

The stopper should always be double checked to attempt to produce a flap. While the flap will not stick down any easier than a free cap with the same handling, the attachment will ensure that the tissue is still there if it does stick. The flap also makes the operation easier and more elegant. There are several reasons for a free flap. Of course the main reason is a miss-set

stopper. A suction break or loss of IOP can also cause the problem. In some eyes with very flat K readings the flap might not be possible. The use of a diameter applanation lens to check before the cut, while not mandatory, will at lease warn the surgeon of the situation. The best preparation for a free cap is to always have the antidessication chamber set up with a small drop of BSS to place the epithelium side on. While the cap is stored in this chamber the goal is to keep the epithelium moist but the stroma at a dryer state. This is the same reason to avoid the flap to be placed in a nasal cul de sac that is flooded so the flap is hydrated during the ablation and harder to stick down. The most vital check of the keratome is to insure the correct plate is placed and placed correctly. If the plate is not pushed all the way back, or if it is not present at all the anterior chamber can be entered and the lens and iris can be damaged. Make sure this is checked and double checked. If the anterior chamber is entered repair with sutures may be needed. If the lens is damaged a PC IOL should be considered at the time. Proper preoperative K readings and axial length to pick the lens is helpful in this situation. (It is good to have the axial length on record for all cases for the eventually that they develop cataracts.)

CORNEAL FLAP PLACEMENT

Poor flap placement and adhesion can take many forms from the obvious flap that is slid out of position at day one the more subtle form of wrinkles in the layer (Figure A-19). These wrinkles can be caused by poor placement at surgery or be induced by the patient rubbing the eye. Wrinkles can also be seen radiating from the hinge if the flap is twisted. The flap

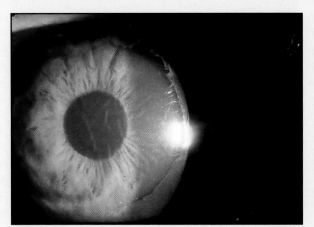

Figure A-21.
A flap that was not adherent at day one and has been repositioned. Note the cut epithelial edge.

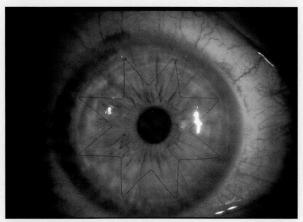

Figure A-22.
An eight bite anti-torque suture, typically another would be placed interspersed with the first.

must be placed exactly so that no such torque is present. Subtle wrinkles can be seen with careful high magnification or better in retro-illumination. If these cross the visual axis they can cause significant irregular astigmatism. If this is noted, early intervention is possibly helpful. The longer the wrinkles are present the harder they are to fix. They may be treated by lifting up the entire flap and massaging them out, then replacing the flap. Subtle poor adherence can be difficult to detect. If there is any question of poor adherence, it must be ruled out. If there is any edema present one should suspect non adherence of the flap. Examine the edge of the flap at high magnification and look for a fluid line. Further put a drop of ophthaine in the eye and try the striae test around the edge of the flap. If still in doubt it is better to actually test the flap itself by attempting to move the layer by placing forceps on the flap. Another helpful method when there is only subtle signs of poor adhesion is to use fluorescein. One should place the dye and then examine the eye some minutes later. Often in this case the dye can be seen to seep beneath the loose edge (Figure A-20).

If it is determined that the flap is to be repositioned, the patient should be taken back to the operating area. The flap should be laid back with care to disrupt the epithelium as little as possible. Avoid the creation of flaps of epithelium. It may be necessary to actually cut the epithelium along the edge of the flap. Lay the flap back as a whole so that the epithelium is moist and the stroma is dry as always. Avoid inducing wrinkles. Carefully remove the epithelium that has grown over the edge onto the bed. Incise it with a beaver blade and cut it centrally (Figure A-21). Avoid stacking up heaps of epithelium at the edge of the bed. Clean the bed, one might even fire a few shots of the laser to lyse any cells and then replace the flap carefully. Watch the flap for a longer time, test for striae and if not intact consider sutures. Usually if the patient returns the next day with the flap off sutures are called for.

Proper suturing is vital (Figure A-22). The best technique is to place one or two anti-torque sutures. Do not use a running as this will torque the flap and create striae. Interrupted sutures can be used, but use at least 12. Do not use overlay sutures as these might cause stromal melt and actually damage the bed which would make a homoplastic impossible and result in a PKP. Place these symmetrically around the edge including the area of the hinge for equal tension. Poor or loose placement can result in the flap not adhering and the sutures loosening early. With a free cap it must be certain that the flap is oriented and right side up. This mistake will result in a cap that might stick but will not properly epithelialize. Cases where the flap is lost and poor healing results call for a homoplastic graft. Without a flap to cover the ablation severe haze can result (Figures A-23 and A-24). This is more common in deep ablations, brown eyes, and younger patients. In patients with preexisting pathology such as pterysium, scarring can be more common. These cases must be clear of the scar and redone before the flap is replaced with a homoplastic graft. Even so with a lost cap or flap first allow the eye to attempt to epithelialize, good results have been obtained and one does not stand to lose much if any final result. This is a much more difficult learning than LASIK and as very few cases will be encountered one should consider referring these to a center that has experience.

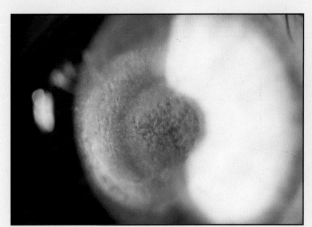

Figure A-23.
Corneal haze resulting from a missing flap in a lamellar case.

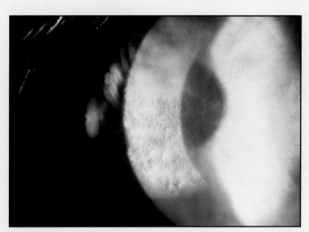

Figure A-24.
Severe haze and scarring resulting from a lost flap in a lamellar case.

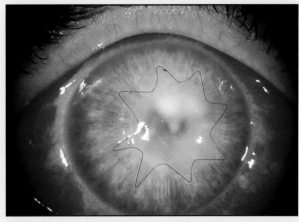

Figure A-25.
An infection within the layers of the cornea.

INFECTION

Perhaps the final but most devastating complication is that of infection. Luckily these are rare and can usually be avoided. Proper technique and postoperative antibiotic coverage is needed. The infection rate is low with lamellar surgery. We have seen one infection present as a superficial corneal ulcer at 2 months that resulted in several lines lost of best corrected vision. This can not be attributed to the surgery however. In referral we have seen an extreme case of intralamellar infection that presented at day 2 postoperative, after the loose flap was sutured at day 1 postoperative (Figure A-25). In this situation the best course is to remove the flap so that maximum penetrations of the antibiotics can be obtained. A penetrating graft was needed in this case.

CONCLUSION

One can expect fewer overall complications with LASIK. The tradeoff is that a new set of very serious complications can present. These can be largely avoided with proper set-up and well treated if present by aggressive careful therapy. Extreme cases should be referred if possible. Rapid visual recovery and diminished pain will make LASIK the operation for most, but not all, myopes. LASIK does have disadvantages. There is a fairly difficult learning curve. More equipment must be mastered and paid for. There is the potential for a more serious type of complication to occur, such as entering the anterior chamber, which does not exist with PRK. However, with LASIK there are fewer overall PRK complications such as haze, regression, and discomfort. One is reminded of the comparison between phacoemulsification and extracapsular cataract surgery. Phaco, like LASIK, has more of a learning curve, requires more equipment and money, and has the risk of a more severe type of complication. But it is the ability of phaco to deliver rapid results in a more elegant fashion that motivated patients to seek this new form of cataract surgery and drove surgeons to adopt the technique. I believe that LASIK and PRK will take a similar course, with patients learning about and requesting LASIK over PRK. LASIK will become, by virtue of patient demand, the preferred procedure for most myopes for the immediate future.

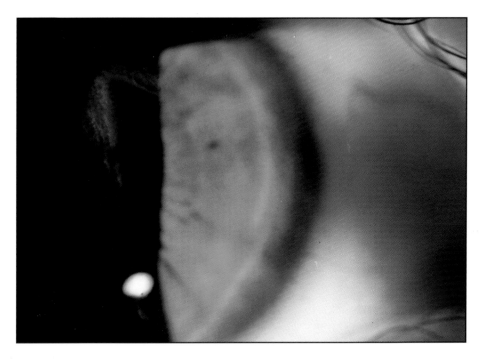

Figure 12-1.
Clinical appearance of corneal flap complication following automated lamellar keratoplasty during initial access pass of microkeratome. Pupil was bisected with short corneal flap by referring surgeon due to either an encountered obstacle or unit malfunction, resulting in linear vertical scarring across the visual axis which was more pronounced superiorly. Refractive error remained unchanged at -8.00 D with reduced best corrected vision of 20/25 with qualitative visual distortion. Patient was treated with multizone PRK with 7.0-mm blend zone with transepithelial approach to remove scarring and re-establish smooth contour. Patient required two surface ablation procedures achieving 20/25 uncorrected vision and improving best corrected vision back to 20/20 with elimination of scar.

LASIK Complications

First step: Education and training for prevention of complications

Second step: Education and training for management of complications

INTRAOPERATIVE COMPLICATIONS

The primary intraoperative complication is that related to creation of the corneal flap. The proper assembly and preparation of the microkeratome is fundamental to avoiding corneal flap complications. Training of the surgeon and staff in nuances of the care of the unit is the cornerstone to achieving high quality lamellar incisions reproducibly. The corneal flap complications can essentially be divided into five major problems—simply stated, they are a lamellar incision that is too short, too long, too superficial, or too deep. The cut can also be of poor quality or irregular.

PUPIL BISECTION

Clinical: If the microkeratome is stopped too early because of the surgeon lifting the pedal prematurely, the shaper stop set incorrectly, or because an obstacle has has been encountered, an inadequate size flap will be fashioned. The hinge will bisect the pupil and make it impossible for an

adequate ablation size to be fashioned (Figure 12-1). The point at which the hinge is fashioned determines whether the procedure can be continued safely and without clinically significant glare nasally. Even if the hinge is more temporal than anticipated and encroaches upon the pupil, the procedure can often be continued and a wet surgical spear that has been expanded and dried out can be used to protect the hinge. If the undersurface of the flap is ablated, two problems occur: first, that area locally will be overtreated disturbing normal topography and second, it is possible to damage the integrity of the flap and hinge.

Management: There are two approaches to a short flap

Training of the surgeon and staff in nuances of the care of the unit is the cornerstone to achieving high quality reproducible lamellar incisions.

Five Primary Corneal Flap Complications

1. Pupil bisection: lamellar incision too short
2. Free cap: lamellar incision too long
3. Thin or perforated flap: lamellar incision too superficial
4. Corneal perforation or amputation: lamellar incision too deep
5. Irregular flap: lamellar incision of poor quality

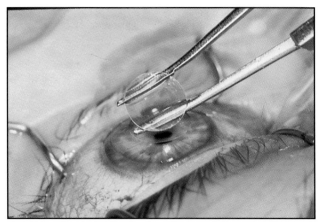

Figure 12-2.
Free corneal lenticle from inadvertent resection of the corneal flap hinge. Most commonly associated with flat corneas. Increased risk of irregular astigmatism, delayed visual recovery, epithelial ingrowth, and lost corneal caps. Must maintain hydration status of lenticle within anti-desiccation chamber then tape eyelid shut postoperatively once flap adherent. Sutures not required.

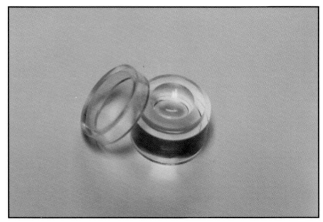

Figure 12-3.
Anti-desiccation chamber used in cases of free corneal caps to maintain hydration status of lenticle. A drop of filtered BSS is dropped in the chamber and the lenticle is placed epithelial side down. The stromal side is not rehydrated until it is replaced on the ablated stromal bed. Placement of the lenticle in excess fluid or stromal side down will result in considerable swelling of the cap.

bisecting the pupil. The first is to close the flap and wait 3 months for the corneal flap to adequately solidify then repeat the procedure. Once the eye has healed, a PRK may be indicated if there was a specific difficulty for the problem such as a small, deep-set, or crowded orbit. The second, more complex approach is to extend the flap manually with a free-hand lamellar dissection. The former approach is recommended for all but the most experienced lamellar surgeons. I highly recommend closing the flap and waiting a minimum of 3 months at which time a repeat keratectomy can be fashioned safely.

FREE CAP

Clinical: In theory, free flaps should not occur if the shaper head stop screw is assembled and set properly to create a hinge, but this is not a complication in the true sense, since free caps were the standard method by which LASIK was performed when developed. The clinical findings which increase their incidence and their proper management once one obtains a free cap are the more important aspects to this intraoperative occurrence. Patients with flat corneas with mean keratometry below 41.00 are at a higher risk of encountering a free cap. Insight into the mechanism is important as it allows the surgeon to anticipate and therefore avoid surprises. A flat cornea will protrude relatively less into the suction ring compared to a steep cornea, thereby presenting a smaller cap diameter to the microkeratome blade. The applanation lens meniscus will appear smaller

with flat corneas. If the shaper head stop is set for a narrow or small hinge, a free flap may result.

An eye that is flat with a small diameter cornea may be suspect for developing a free cap, however, when the eye is placed within the suction ring, the cornea sits higher as the ring is seated on the surrounding limbus. This placement essentially presents an effectively steeper and larger cornea for the microkeratome blade, typically producing a relatively large flap relative to the corneal diameter. Peripheral neovascularization may in fact be encountered.

Patients with flat corneas with mean keratometry below 41.00 are at a higher risk of encountering a free cap.

Management: Free caps occur to most if not all surgeons at one time or another, typically earlier in the learning curve (Figure 12-2). Anticipation and preparation are the first steps in management. Once a free cap is inadvertently produced, the cap must be placed within an anti-desiccation chamber. The key principle to managing a free cap is to prevent excessive drying and swelling of the cap, while preserving the epithelium. The cap is therefore placed epithelial surface down on a drop of balanced salt solution to help preserve the epithelium (Figure 12-3). No fluid is placed upon the stromal surface as corneal edema is a function of time rather than a function of the amount of fluid. Therefore, even

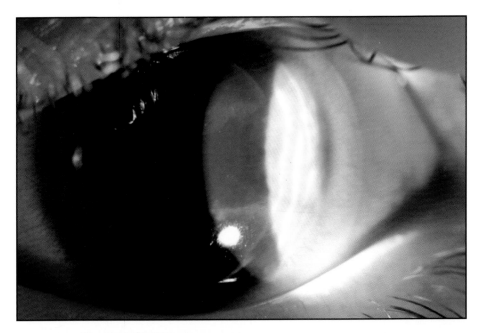

Figure 12-4a.
Clinical appearance of a perforated corneal flap under low magnification following LASIK for -14.00 D myopia correction. Patient retreated with LASIK 3 months postoperatively achieving 20/70 uncorrected vision with surprisingly no loss of best corrected vision. Patient enhanced for -1.25D residual myopia achieving stable 20/30 uncorrected vision, equivalent to preoperative contact lens vision with 9 months follow-up.

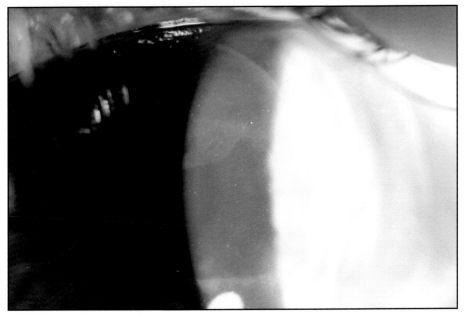

Figure 12-4b.
Clinical appearance of a perforated corneal flap under high magnification. Most likely cause is plastic filings from blade packaging within gap between depth plate and blade centrally preventing central corneal flap tissue from being resected.

a small amount of fluid left on the stroma during the procedure will result in considerable edema. The anti-desiccation chamber will prevent excessive drying of the cap. Once the cap is prepared, the ablation is performed and the stromal bed is kept dry. The free cap is then removed from the chamber and at this point the stroma can be rehydrated. The cap is then placed on the stromal bed, stromal surface down and with the alignment markings coinciding. The importance of the alignment markings is most easily recognized when one encounters a free cap, as the markings not only become paramount to correct placement but in distinguishing the epithelial side from the stromal undersurface of the cap. It can be more difficult to assess the epithelial surface from that of the stroma with a free cap than one would expect, especially if stromal swelling or loss of the epithelium occurs. The classic alignment marking is the paraxial line extending from the central cap to the peripheral cornea. It is impossible to align the paraxial line unless the corneal cap is oriented properly, however, the double circle markings provide easier four-point alignment. The two different sized circles only coincide if the correct orientation is achieved with the epithelial side up. Even minor misalignments are

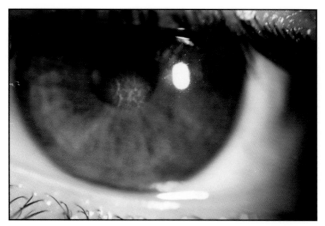

Figure 12-5a.
Postoperative LASIK flap with central thinning and irregularity.

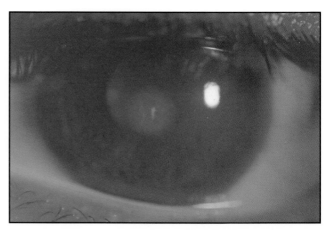

Figure 12-5b.
Fluorescein staining demonstrates central uptake of dye.

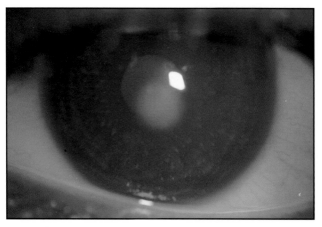

Figure 12-5c.
Migration of fluorescein within interface indicating exposed stroma and infection risk.

more readily observed with the four-point alignment system with hinged flaps. The Kritzinger-Updegraff marking system with multiple radial and pararadial lines is another excellent system. Therefore, the beginning surgeon must always prepare the anti-desiccation chamber and place alignment markings for orientation.

THIN AND PERFORATED CORNEAL FLAPS

Clinical: The incidence of clinically significant corneal flap problems is 0.5% or less once the initial learning curve is passed (Figures 12-4a and 12-4b). Although thin flaps may be produced from a lack of blade sharpness, perforated flaps occur as a result of inadequate intraocular pressure or a poorly functioning microkeratome (Figures 12-5a through 12-5c). Each patient should be treated with a new blade. LASIK results, unlike ALK, are dependent upon laser ablation rather than the resection, therefore, bilateral cases may be performed safely with one blade.

Theoretically, and in some countries routinely, several or more procedures can be performed with the same blade, but this practice is discouraged as flap complications clearly increase. Even after one procedure if the flap appears thinner or even displays any unusual irregularity, it should not be used again. The blade should always be inspected preoperatively for any irregularities under the microscope. As well, the gap should be examined as debris or plastic filings may become entrapped between the blade and the depth plate and must be removed.

Thin or perforated corneal flaps are related to:
- Poor blade quality or sharpness
- Inadequate suction pressure
- Microkeratome malfunction

Perforated flaps can be avoided primarily by ensuring an adequate pressure is achieved and not manipulating the eye once it has been confirmed prior to the cut (Figures 12-6a and 12-6b). Maintaining adequate suction pressure is the single most important ingredient to preventing a perforated flap. Eyes with loose or redundant conjunctiva and eyes with extensive vitreous synersis are at greater risk for losing vacuum pressure once achieved. Patients with a history of cataract surgery or vitreoretinal surgery may be at higher risk. Beginning LASIK surgeons should avoid these cases as

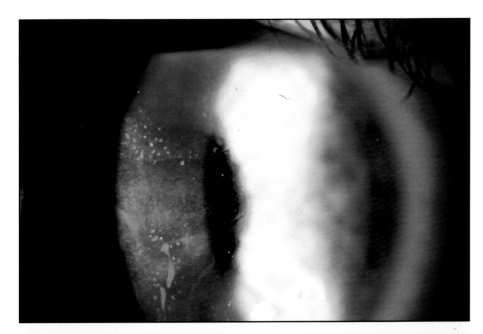

Figure 12-6a.
Central perforated corneal flap following unsuccessful LASIK procedure 3 months earlier demonstrating stromal haze formation where surface epithelium in contact with exposed stromal bed. Epithelial ingrowth centrally through site of central perforation expanding area of perforation. Best corrected vision reduced by three lines.

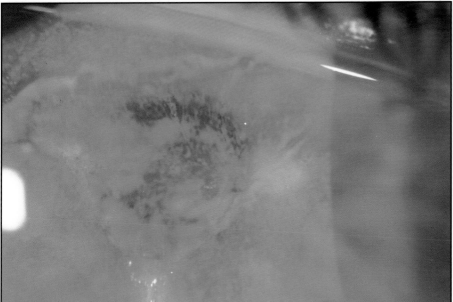

Figure 12-6b.
Central perforated corneal flap of 12-6a demonstrating irregular fluorescein staining. Patient treated with removal of the non-viable flap and surface PTK for haze removal followed by PRK at 6 months post-operatively for refractive error improving best corrected vision to 20/25 and uncorrected vision to 20/40. Most likely cause is loss of suction pressure intraoperatively as temporal flap thickness good.

they should avoid patients with small orbits. Microkeratome functioning must be flawless as any impediment to the microkeratome advancing at a steady speed and a smooth rate may result in flap irregularities. Staff preparation and surgeon testing of the microkeratome unit are integral steps

> Maintaining adequate suction pressure is the single most important ingredient to preventing a perforated flap.

in preventing a perforated flap (Figure 12-7).

Management: If a perforated and thin flap is produced, the integrity of the flap determines the management. A corneal flap that is essentially thin and irregular and may have a small peripheral perforation can still be treated with care. The visual rehabilitation may be slower, requiring weeks rather than days for functional vision. The second eye should be postponed if not already treated and the specific cause for the complication determined before proceeding. A corneal flap that is perforated centrally or a flap that has been severed into horizontal strips must be replaced and let

Figure 12-7.
Linear horizontal fluorescein staining of corneal flap representing fine flap perforation. Most likely cause is focal blade abnormality. Patient was -7.75 D OU malpractice attorney who achieved 20/20 uncorrected vision 1 week prior on his fellow eye from day 1. Patient did observe subjective blur for 3 to 4 weeks, with unaided vision gradually improving from 20/40 on day 1 to 20/20 by 1 month. Both eyes have remained 20/20 for 11 months with no enhancement procedures required. Preoperative informed consent is paramount in these situations, as patient not only understood risks, but variable recovery times between eyes. In general, etiology of perforated flap related to: 1) inadequate suction pressure, 2) obstruction of gap between depth plate and blade with foreign matter, or 3) poor blade quality, with non-cutting portion.

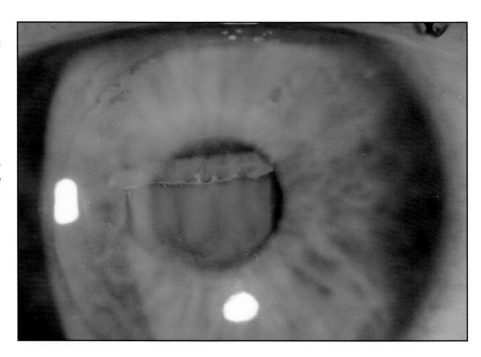

heal for 3 months before retreatment. Late management involves retreatment with either LASIK or PRK utilizing a transepithelial approach. Immediate management involves realigning the flap as best as possible. The procedure may turn into a jigsaw puzzle with missing pieces in the worst case scenario.

Once the flap is laid down, air at 1 liter per minute or less can be used to secure the flap pieces into position. Strong air will often displace the flap fragments. Compressed air is not necessary but it is important to ensure that the flap fragments are adherent before removing the lid speculum. Alternatively wait 5 to 10 minutes or longer. A bandage contact lens is inserted until the epithelium is healed. Patients are more comfortable with a bandage contact lens which is somewhat snug but not tight allowing less than 1 mm of movement; a base curve of 8.4 works well in most cases. Despite the clinical appearance when first observed, once the flap fragments are aligned and positioned, the appearance improves and by the time at which the eye has epithelialized in 24 to 48 hours, there has been tremendous improvement in the clinical appearance. Unfortunately, not every patient returns to his or her preoperative best corrected visual acuity following flap perforation, but surprisingly many do. Once the eye integrity has been re-established, the approach is variable from non-surgical, rigid gas permeable, or soft lens fitting, to removing and discarding the flap altogether. Ideally, a PRK with a transepithelial approach can be utilized to re-establish a smooth surface and correct the refractive error, however,

epithelium and stroma ablate at different rates and this may not be the best approach or even suitable in some cases. If central irregularity is absent, repeating LASIK after 3 months is preferable. If central irregularity is present, then a decision must be made with respect to flap viability. If viable, perform PRK with transepithelial approach; if non-viable, remove the flap and ablate. Since the flap has no refractive power, removing the flap should not alter the baseline refractive error. The only problem is dealing with a very high myope who will likely regress with haze formation and thus have a substantially thinner cornea. Recognize that an irregular flap fits precisely into the irregular stromal bed. Ablating the bed alters this fit. Allowing the eye to settle for 3 months is recommended prior to repeat LASIK or transepithelial PRK.

As stated, LASIK can be repeated successfully but only after 3 months and only when the specific cause has been recognized and remedied. In certain cases, the eye problems become more severe as the eye settles, as epithelium may invade the interface from any site of perforation, as well as the flap edges. In such a case, it is impossible to lift the flap and clean the interface, and eventually the flap stroma melts. The treatment, therefore, must be to remove the flap altogether. Despite the fact that tissue has been removed, the flap constitutes lamellar tissue with a plano refractive effect. The eye can then be allowed to re-epithelialize or a surface ablation can be performed immediately and then allowed to epithelialize. The most important aspect in the removal of the

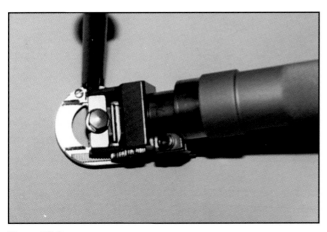

Figure 12-8a.
The microkeratome can be inserted into the pneumatic suction ring and the gears engaged whether or not the depth plate is inserted. Appearance of unit with depth plate inserted contrasted with Figure 12-8b.

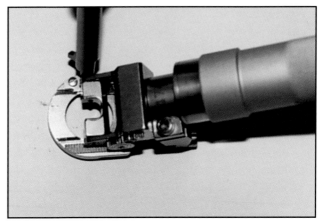

Figure 12-8b.
The microkeratome can be inserted into the pneumatic suction ring and the gears engaged whether or not the depth plate is inserted. Without the depth plate the cornea will be perforated as the unit cuts at 900 microns.

flap is to flatten the hinge, in order to allow for a smooth transition zone for epithelial growth. The hinge can be smoothed with a surgical blade or even focal phototherapeutic keratectomy (PTK) to blend the tissue edge. If the eye is treated, the

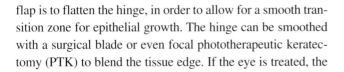

Recognize that an irregular flap fits precisely into the irregular stromal bed. Ablating the bed alters this fit. Allowing the eye to settle for 3 months is recommended prior to repeat LASIK or transepithelial PRK.

removal of the flap essentially converts the case into a surface ablation and should be treated as such with a tapering regimen of topical steroids as in any PRK case.

PERFORATED CORNEA

Clinical: Although the perforated flap is the most clinically significant intraoperative complication I have encountered to date, the most significant potential intraoperative complication is perforation of the cornea. In reality, despite the natural fear one encounters when first utilizing the microkeratome, this complication is impossible when adequate training and preparation of the surgeon and staff occurs and a preoperative checklist is followed without exception. In fact, most corneal flap problems can be avoided and the risks dramatically minimized when adequate training and testing of the microkeratome are carried out. The major errors which result in a perforated cornea are the absence of the depth

plate altogether or failure to insert the depth plate fully. The microkeratome unit immediately cuts at a depth of 900 microns when the depth plate is absent (Figures 12-8a and 12-8b), which exceeds the thickness of the cornea, resulting in corneal perforation or even amputation. Failure to insert the plate fully leaves a greater gap between the blade edge and depth plate, allowing a greater amount of corneal tissue to enter the cutting mechanism, producing a deep or perforating cut. Perforation of the cornea is far more serious with LASIK than RK since the globe pressure exceeds 65 mmHg and perforation may result in an expulsion of the globe contents. This complication has been reported with ALK in a dozen or so cases and twice worldwide with LASIK. Both cases of LASIK corneal perforation occurred with novice surgeons who did not complete formal LASIK training.

ALK involves two passes with the microkeratome: first, the access pass for the formation of the lamellar flap and second, the refractive pass. The error occurs in ALK when the 160-micron depth plate used for the lamellar flap is exchanged for a new depth plate corresponding to the desired refractive resection. The surgical assistant or surgeon either forgets to insert the new plate or inserts it incompletely without recompleting the mandatory checklist. The problem is in part due to the fact that some surgeons leave the vacuum pressure elevated and in position during the replacement of the depth plate and therefore the time element for exchanging the depth plate is more critical. Although perforation with ALK has occurred with the second refractive pass rather than the initial pass, perforation and severe penetration of the cornea can occur with LASIK. Despite the fact that only one pass is performed for the lamellar flap with LASIK, if the microkeratome instrument is not assembled properly to begin with and the depth plate is absent or not fully inserted, perforation will occur immediately upon advancing the shaper head. Therefore, the surgeon is immediately aware if any significant intraoperative complications have occurred once a flap of good quality is produced, thus ensuring at least the safety of simultaneous bilateral surgery. Almost all the significant risk associated with LASIK occurs with the microkeratome cut, unlike PRK whereby postoperative risks of haze and infection remain unknowns when bilateral simultaneous surgery is performed. Therefore, in many ways, LASIK performed bilaterally is safer than simultaneous bilateral PRK with its prolonged risk period.

An irregular flap can be produced if the blade quality is inadequate or the rate of advancement of the microkeratome is not consistent. Poor placement of the flap can also lead to irregular astigmatism.

> **Corneal perforation is impossible when adequate training and preparation occur and a preoperative checklist is followed without exception.**

> **Failure to insert the depth plate results in corneal perforation or even amputation with the expulsion of ocular contents.**

> **Causes of irregular astigmatism:**
> - Poor blade quality
> - Poor microkeratome function
> - Thin corneal flaps
> - Poor flap alignment

OTHER FACTORS CAUSING COMPLICATIONS

CORNEAL SHAPES AND ORBITAL CONFIGURATIONS

Various corneal shapes and orbital configurations have an effect upon the interaction of the microkeratome and the eye. It is important to understand both how to anticipate, avoid, and adjust for these variants to avoid complications.

> **LASIK performed bilaterally is safer than simultaneous bilateral PRK with its prolonged risk period.**

SMALL AND DEEP-SET EYES

Small, deep-set eyes are more difficult to treat in that little space exists to properly apply the suction ring, the narrow palpebral aperture may obstruct the microkeratome pass, or the flap created may encroach upon blood vessels from previous contact lens wear. When still gathering clinical experience, these patients are best avoided until one becomes proficient with the procedure. The most useful technique to applying the suction ring in these cases is to push down on the eyelid speculum, thus causing the globe to further protrude (Slade). In addition, an adjustable wire eyelid speculum maximally expanded is necessary. Some surgeons will even perform a lateral canthotomy to increase access to the globe. A retrobulbar injection will dramatically improve exposure but adds its own set of complications, from retrobulbar hemorrhage to globe perforation, which is more common in higher myopes. The presence of chemosis will prevent proper suction pressure from being achieved. LASIK can, however, be performed much more easily than ALK on patients owing to both the smaller pneumatic suction ring and the less surgical manipulation requirements. Another technique for the highly experienced lamellar surgeon is to remove the lid speculum altogether (Suarez). In this way, the suction ring keeps the eyelids apart. Obtaining adequate exposure is one of the most fundamental elements to performing an uncomplicated procedure and PRK may be indicated for such cases. It must always be remembered that there is no one procedure ideal for every patient.

> **Obtaining adequate exposure is one of the most fundamental elements to performing an uncomplicated procedure.**

LARGE, BULGING EYES

Eyes which are large and exophthalmic are ideal first cases to perform as exposure is maximal and obstacles are non-existent. There are a few considerations, however, most importantly of which is that highly myopic patients may have extensive vitreous synersis and obtaining adequate pressure can be problematic in the rare individual.

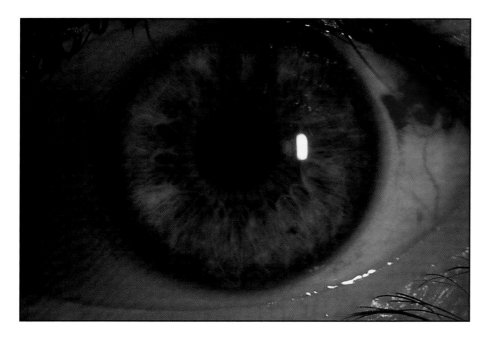

Figure 12-9.
Subconjunctival hemorrhage observed following uncomplicated LASIK procedure. No clinical or visual significance.

Additionally, there is often considerable orbital fat which allows for a certain amount of spring or ballottement to these eyes when applying the suction ring. This excessive movement can make both fixation with the suction ring and the microkeratome pass slightly more difficult as there remains a certain degree of play. The conjunctiva can also be loose or redundant in these eyes. The risk with redundant conjunctiva is that the conjunctiva will occlude the suction ring without elevating the intraocular pressure, giving false impression of adequate suction.

CORNEAL SHAPE
Curvature

The shape of the cornea both in curvature and diameter has an impact upon the size of the flap that will be fashioned and potential complications which may occur. Essentially flatter corneas produce smaller flaps and steeper corneas produce larger flaps. As described earlier, flatter corneas with mean keratometry less than 41.00 D present less corneal tissue to the microkeratome blade and, therefore, care should be taken to avoid producing a free cap by stopping the microkeratome 1 mm earlier or extending the shaper hinge screw. If a patient has a very steep cornea, with mean keratometry greater than 47.00 D, first, it may occasionally make advancing the microkeratome into position slightly more difficult by obstructing the depth plate, and second, it may result in a large flap encroaching on peripheral blood vessels. One may wish to decenter the flap inferiorly up to 1 mm in the case of prominent blood vessels but

a very steep cornea may preclude excessive decentration for fear of encountering limbal vessels inferiorly.

Diameter

Small corneas are more similar to steep corneas in that the pneumatic suction ring is seated on the limbus or limbal conjunctiva, thereby placing the corneal vertex at a much higher plane relative to the suction ring. Occasionally, the greater height can impede engaging the microkeratome into position so that the gears are engaged. Large corneas have no specific problems associated except that the suction ring adheres to the peripheral cornea and can create abrasions and even break limbal blood vessels. It is seldom more difficult to obtain adequate occlusion and consequently adequate pressure.

It is important to be able to apply alignment markings appropriately, especially in cases of flat corneas, so that if a free cap is produced proper alignment can be achieved. Alignment markings on large and steep corneas may remain on the flap and be of no help. Care must be taken to mark out to the limbus.

SUBCONJUNCTIVAL HEMORRHAGES

The pneumatic suction ring produces considerable vacuum pressure which can produce subconjunctival hemorrhages (Figure 12-9). There are no sequelae typically and the most important aspect is to explain to the patient that these changes are common, may get worse before they get better, may change color, and clear over 3 to 4 weeks.

Figure 12-10a.
Management of conjunctival edema by milking the edema away from the perilimbal area and toward the fornices so that adequate suction can be obtained. Pseudosuction may be obtained if the conjunctiva occludes the suction ring without elevating the intraocular pressure resulting in potentially serious corneal flap complications. If clinically borderline pressure, delay surgery by 1 to 24 hours and apply frequent topical steroids to reduce inflammation during interval. Courtesy of Dr. Stephen G. Slade.

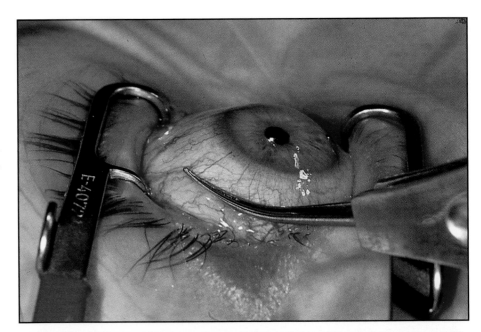

Figure 12-10b.
Management of conjunctival edema by milking the edema toward the fornices, away from the perilimbal area, so that adequate suction can be obtained. Courtesy of Dr. Stephen G. Slade.

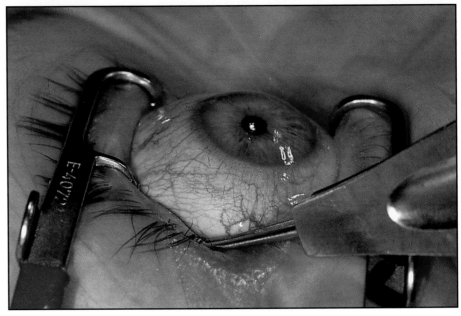

The only clinical note of significance is that a large subconjunctival hemorrage or significant conjunctival edema during manipulation of the suction ring may prevent adequate suction pressure from being achieved and/or maintained. There are two means by which this may be managed: the blunt side length of forceps may be utilized to milk the edema or subconjunctival heme into the fornices (Figures 12-10a and 12-10b), or the procedure may be postponed for several hours to days. It is important to recognize that any question of achieving adequate pressure should always be treated conservatively and surgery canceled.

IMPROPER POSITIONING

If the pneumatic suction ring is improperly positioned, the vacuum pressure must be released immediately or repositioning is impossible. Within seconds, a scleral ridge is formed from the vacuum pressure and reapplication of the suction ring regardless of the new position chosen will immediately return to the initial application site. Therefore, it is essential to align the suction ring carefully and seat it firmly in position prior to application of the vacuum pressure and to immediately determine if the position is correct. The surgical assistant should be in position to control the vacuum

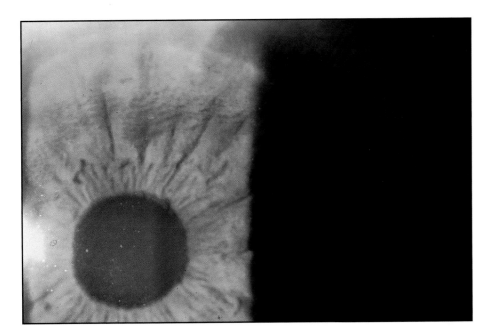

Figure 12-11.
Interface blood observed during early postoperative period from corneal neovascularization bleeding intraoperatively. Interface heme cleared gradually over months without treatment. There were no visual sequelae associated. Courtesy of Dr. Stephen G. Slade.

pressure both to engage and disengage suction at the time the pneumatic ring is positioned. If the suction ring is more than 1 mm decentered or improperly decentered and the scleral indentation precludes proper placement, the procedure should be postponed by hours or to the following day.

Neovascularization

Clinical: Many patients have a history of extensive contact lens wear and have developed superior and occasionally inferior macropannus. Bleeding from the area of neovascularization may occur when the corneal flap involves the vessels, which is common with either large corneal flaps or extensive corneal neovascularization. Preoperative examination should specifically note not only the presence but the extent to which the vessels encroach upon the peripheral cornea so that technique modification may be considered. Intraoperative bleeding complicates the procedure both with respect to intraoperative visualization and postoperative interface opacification (Figure 12-11). Bleeding can be very extensive and difficult to control if the neovascular vessels are numerous and lysed proximally. It is also important to remember that the excimer laser beam consists of far ultraviolet radiation and is essentially non-thermal in nature and therefore is incapable of coagulating the vessels. Fortunately, despite the clinical appearance of bleeding blood vessels at the edge of the flap, the sequelae are minimal.

Management: The most important aspect to management of intraoperative bleeding during LASIK from corneal

neovascularization is that of prevention. The pneumatic suction ring should be placed on the eye such as to avoid the vessels upon creation of the corneal flap. If the suction ring is somewhat decentered inferiorly, superior macropannus can be avoided with the lamellar incision. There are two risks with this approach:

1. The inferiorly decentered corneal flap will involve inferior vessels
2. Excessive decentration will result in a poor quality flap.

Another alternative is to either use an adjustable ALK ring and create a smaller corneal flap. As well, an argon laser can be used to preoperatively to coagulate the vessels in preparation. In general, no precautions need be taken with corneal neovascularization as closing the flap with active bleeding will typically result in bleeding externally and not within the interface. As well, interface blood that has been entrapped will clear over weeks to months spontaneously and is outside the visual axis.

If bleeding from corneal neovascularization does occur, management involves a host of options. The suction pressure utilized during the lamellar cut if left on during the ablation will arrest blood flow until the treatment is complete. Once the vacuum pressure is stopped, bleeding will begin and can be profuse unless sufficient pressure is applied manually to the ring. Air can be used to constrict the blood vessels and promote coagulation of blood within the vessels. As well, pharmacologic agents can be used to reduce or arrest blood flow, including phenylephrine, topical steroids, and tissue thromboplastin. Phenylephrine can be

Figure 12-12.
Videokeratography of decentered LASIK ablation.

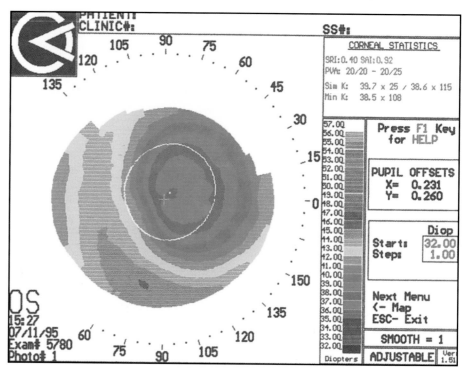

used in concentrations ranging from 2.5% to 10%, however, the 10% formulation should be used cautiously if at all, and only for young patients with no cardiac histories or patients with a history of beta-blocker use, such as that for migraines or hyperthyroidism. Only phenylephrine 2.5% is recommended. Phenylephrine is best applied with a surgical spear locally for maximum effectiveness and safety. Topical steroids are known vasoconstrictors and can be used as well. I have not used tissue thromboplastin and do not feel it necessary in the management of intraoperative bleeding. Occasionally, bleeding cannot be arrested or pharmacologic agents are not available and management involves closing the flap after the interface has been cleaned of heme. As well, any disruption of the vessels, even if bleeding has been controlled, will cause them to rebleed and it is often a matter of obtaining control for several seconds to close the flap, knowing that they may bleed shortly thereafter. Fortunately,

the cut edge of the vessels is along the cap edge and rebleeding will ensue within the peripheral gutter and externally and not within the interface beneath the flap.

DECENTRATION

Clinical: This intraoperative complication is usually not apparent until the patient is examined in follow-up (Figure 12-12). Pupil centration is more appropriate than visual axis fixation as symptoms occur chiefly from an expanded pupil in dim light extending beyond the treatment area. If there is a large angle kappa, the treatment should be shifted toward the visual axis. The incidence increases when the pupil is pharmacologically altered. Topographical appearance is that of a superior ablation if the patient looks down in an effort to get away from his or her surgeon during the procedure, an inferior ablation if the patient squeezes his or her eyes inducing a Bell's phenomenon. Nasal decentration is more common with the use of miotics and temporal decentrations with attempts to avoid hitting the nasally hinged flap. Dilatation makes centration more difficult and may obscure proper centration, usually resulting in superotemporal decentrations. Self-fixation is optimal, but drying measures of the stroma obscure adequate target fixation.

Decentration may produce asymmetric night glare or ghosting of images and tilting or distortion of images related to induced cylinder. Decentration may produce both a

---

Management of LASIK Intraoperative Bleeding Secondary to Corneal Neovascularization
- No treatment required
- Reapply suction immediately prior to closing flap
- Phenylephrine 2.5%
- Air applied locally
- Topical steroids
- Tissue thromboplastin

reduction of best corrected vision secondary to irregular astigmatism and a reduction of uncorrected visual acuity from the associated undercorrection, since the maximally treated area is not aligned.

Management: There is very little in the form of treatment to offer these patients when fully corrected other than artistic attempts to reconfigure the ablation pattern. If the patient is undercorrected, which is common in these cases, the patient can be retreated with proper centration with emphasis on correcting the original topography simultaneously. That is, the untreated area may be kept more dehydrated to increase the refractive effect in that area. In general, treating the undercorrection and expanding the optical zone maximally with the enhancement procedure reduces patient symptoms dramatically. Most patients improve with time and bilateral treatment.

Patients who do not improve and remain significantly symptomatic require innovative treatment plans based upon topography and symptoms. The most difficult case to correct would be one with a significant decentration, asymmetric night glare but plano refractive error and excellent daytime visual acuity. The corneal flap is lifted and the adequately treated area protected with a surgical spear which has been wet then dried so as to remain expanded. The calculated ablation is then centered properly and performed, leaving only the previous untreated area to become ablated. The amount of treatment required would be 25% to 50% of the

> If there is a large angle kappa, the treatment should be shifted toward the visual axis.

> If the patient is undercorrected, he or she can be retreated with proper centration with emphasis on correcting the original topography simultaneously.

original refraction at the largest optical zone, or the last two zones of a multizone ablation. Unlike PRK, where there is significant concern for creating an edge effect inducing haze, the essentially inert stroma can be manipulated more safely to improve corneal topography. It remains to be seen if similar cases of poorly centered PRK treatments can be corrected intrastromally as well. Kritzinger has described surface PTK for the correction of decentered intrastromal ablation with significant improvement observed upon videokeratography.

> Unlike PRK, where there is significant concern for creating an edge effect inducing haze, the essentially inert stroma can be manipulated more safely to improve corneal topography.

EARLY POSTOPERATIVE COMPLICATIONS

PAIN

Clinical: Most patients remarkably do not experience any discomfort, however, a foreign body or gritty sensation is commonplace. Some patients complain of both eye pain and orbital discomfort, which may be related to the pressure exerted by the eyelid speculum and suction ring rather than the lamellar incision itself. Most patients do not require any postoperative narcotic analgesia, although sedatives and non-narcotic agents may be helpful. Infrequently, some complain of severe pain and a short differential diagnosis consisting of a displaced corneal flap or an epithelial defect are examined for. As with all procedures, patient variability plays a large role as to the amount of discomfort experienced.

> Complaints of severe pain indicate a displaced corneal flap or epithelial defect.

Management: The most important aspects are ensuring that the flap and epithelium are intact. Most patients are simply concerned that any pain or discomfort is indicative of a healing complication and therefore simple reassurance is an essential part of management. Non-narcotic agents and sedatives are routinely prescribed postoperatively for LASIK patients. Narcotic agents are rarely indicated. Topical non-steroidals and bandage contact lenses may be useful adjuncts to control pain. Lubrication is another important element as these eyes may have an associated superficial punctate keratitis.

DISPLACED FLAP

Clinical: Patients with a displaced corneal flap can typically be diagnosed upon entering the examination room in direct contrast to most LASIK patients who have white, quiet eyes; these patients have their eyes covered, are tearing profusely, are quite photophobic, and are in considerable pain. The vision is extremely blurry, in the counting fingers range as would be expected.

Figure 12-13.
Epithelial ingrowth following inadvertent resection of corneal flap hinge during LASIK procedure resulting in a free cap. Preoperative mean keratometry was 40.0. Induced irregular and regular astigmatism. Irregular astigmatism gradually resolved over 11 months, improving best corrected vision from 20/50+ to 20/25+ without treatment. At 11 months, astigmatic keratotomy performed for regular mixed astigmatism reducing cylinder from 1.75 to 0.75 D.

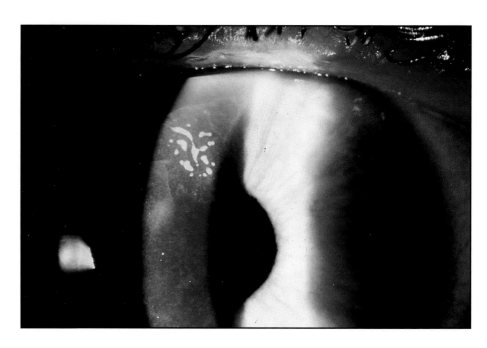

The introduction of the hinged flap technique by Ioannis Pallikaris, MD, dramatically improved the safety and even the results of LASIK. The corneal flap reduced the concern of a free or lost corneal cap. It is highly unusual for the corneal flap to displace if the striae and lid test is normal without incurring trauma. Occasionally, however, the corneal flap will displace postoperatively, especially during the first 12 to 24 hours. Typically, displacement is 1 mm or less, producing corneal striae peripherally or centrally.

> **The best technique to detect fine striae is to dilate the patient and examine the flap with retroillumination.**

Rarely will the flap become completely free and attached only by the hinge. If the procedure had been complicated or a wet stromal bed technique utilized, then the risk of displacement is greater. Movement of the flap to smooth or extend the flap edges during intraoperative positioning can break the adhesion created and can increase the chance of displacement if not allowed to re-adhere properly. The utilization of Celluvisc (Allergan) or other viscous agent to coat the epithelium intraoperatively increases the time required for full adhesion and the vulnerability for displacement. Free caps are also not only more likely to become dislodged but require that the eyelid be taped shut so that if dislodged the loss of the cap would not further complicate management. Even if the cap is lost, it is important to recognize

that it has no refractive effect upon the eye and that it should be managed with a topical steroid regimen as with PRK.

Management: Once again, prevention of corneal flap displacement is the primary form of management by ensuring the flap is secure at the conclusion of the procedure. Testing the flap with the striae and lid test are essential steps in the procedure. The iron test is a technique I employ to place the flap under increased stress and assure adequate adhesion. The iron applies force to the corneal flap rather than the peripheral cornea, along the flap edge and serves to smooth the flap edges as well.

If the corneal flap becomes displaced either completely or partially, it must be replaced as soon as possible to not only avoid infection and reduce pain but avoid permanent striae and damage to the flap. The incidence of epithelial ingrowth increases with both displacement and free caps (Figure 12-13). If the flap has been displaced anesthetize the eye for examination. Management until flap replacement involves frequent lubrication, every 30 minutes with sterile preservative-free artificial tears. It is important to keep the displaced flap well hydrated as the flap is more vulnerable to damage when desiccated. As well, striae and various irregularities will form more easily in the flap and be more difficult to remove when repositioning the flap if the flap dries.

The technique by which the flap is replaced involves the same principles by which the flap is first secured. Exposure and fluid management are important elements to all lamellar procedures. Once the stromal bed and flap are cleaned of

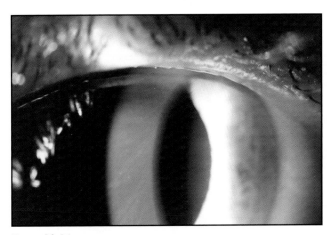

Figure 12-14a.
Corneal flap striae secondary to displacement.

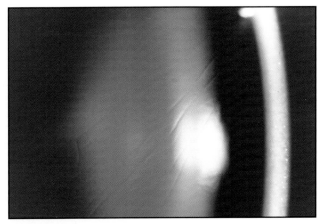

Figure 12-14b.
High power view demonstrating corneal striae with reduced best corrected and uncorrected visual acuity.

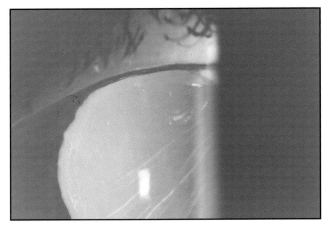

Figure 12-14c.
Retroillumination of corneal flap with dilated pupil is the best technique to assess striae.

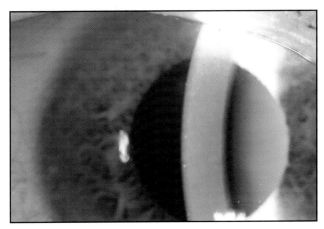

Figure 12-14d.
Three days postoperative view following correction of flap striae.

debris, the stromal bed can be dried with compressed air, or the cap can be floated into position, depending upon surgeon preference. Second the corneal flap must remain rehydrated. If there are any striae (Figures 12-14a through 12-14e), the cap should be ironed while wet using the blunt side of forceps and then placed into position on the stromal bed. Residual striae may still be evident and the cap should be ironed as smooth as possible. It is helpful to dry the epithelial surface of the cap with air and with dry forceps carefully continue to smooth out any irregularities. It may be apparent that the peripheral gutter is asymmetrical and the flap should be lifted and replaced if unable to realign properly. If the flap is well postioned but contains persistent striae, it may be necessary to lift and re-iron the flap (Figure 12-15). It is not essential to completely eliminate all the striae, however, surprisingly many of the striae will clear by the next

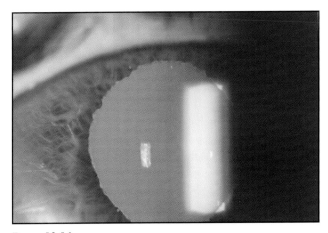

Figure 12-14e.
Day 3: no striae visible on retroillumination.

Figure 12-15.
Late corneal flap striae evident in association with mild interface haze after LASIK for extreme myopia correction. It is difficult if not impossible to correct misalignment at this late stage, several months postoperatively. Best corrected vision was reduced from 20/25 to 20/30 postoperatively, with minimal subjective qualitative visual disturbance.

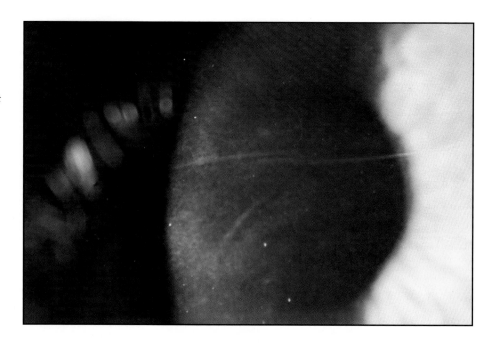

morning if the flap is taut. That is, as the corneal flap is drying over 5 to 15 minutes, iron the edges of the flap outward to fill the peripheral gutter and remove corneal striae. This is tedious but very successful, even months postoperatively.

> Operative exposure and fluid management are important elements to all lamellar procedures.

EPITHELIAL DEFECTS

Clinical: Epithelial defects only occur in a small percentage (<3%) of patients with large defects being more common early in the surgical learning curve secondary to drying of the flap surface. The most frequent site of epithelial defects is along the flap incision edge related to manipulation of the flap or the microkeratome pass. Certain patients have very loose epithelial adherence and the microkeratome head may pull the epithelium rather than incise it cleanly. Central epithelial defects may occur with excessive use of topical anesthetic related to epitheliotoxicity or in second eyes of bilaterally treated cases owing to dehydration. It is not uncommon for a superficial punctate keratitis to be observed in the area of the alignment markings associated with the use of gentian violet. Avoiding markings of the central 3 mm of epithelium provides for faster visual recovery.

Maintaining the epithelial integrity improves comfort, safety, and visual rehabilitation. Epithelial defects can be associated with tremendous pain, especially when large. Photophobia and tearing are commonly associated. There are two potential complications which may ensue with epithelial effects: the risk of infection is increased and the incidence of epithelial ingrowth is also higher. The theoretical advantages of LASIK over PRK are reduced when an epithelial defect is produced.

> There are two potential complications which may ensue with epithelial effects: the risk of infection is increased and the incidence of epithelial ingrowth is also higher.

Management: The importance of maintaining adequate hydration of the epithelium and reducing manipulation of the flap is immediately apparent from the preceding clinical discussion in order to reduce the incidence of epithelial defects. Patients with anterior basement dystrophy should be avoided. Topical anesthesia should be applied sparingly with direct application to the conjunctiva, with an anesthetic-soaked surgical spear preferred.

If an epithelial defect occurs, however, there are several principles to maintain. First, the patient must be observed daily as with PRK for evidence of infection. Second, although routinely recommended, a prophylactic antibiotic should be used postoperatively in cases of an abrasion and some surgeons recommend double coverage

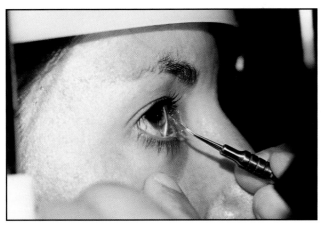

Figure 12-16.
Removal of bandage contact lines with fine non-toothed forceps. Therapeutic lens is hydrated and topical anesthetic instilled. Patient gaze is elevated and inferior aspect of lens is grasped and drawn down and away from the eye.

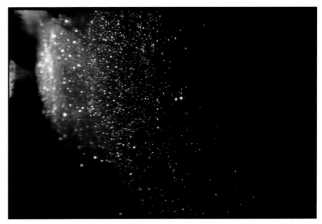

Figure 12-17.
Interface talc related to use of powdered gloves. Greater risk involves microkeratome malfunction secondary to talc within gears and oscillating blade mechanism. In general about half of all surgeons use powderless gloves and half perform the procedure without gloves. Courtesy of Dr. Stephen G. Slade.

such as a fluoroquinolone (Ocuflox, Allergan) and an aminoglycoside (tobramycin). Third, pain management is quite variable and dependent both upon the patient and the size of the epithelial defect. For small epithelial defects, it may simply involve reasuring the patient that he or she will experience some discomfort associated with a foreign body sensation. Frequent lubrication is always advocated. For larger epithelial defects, a bandage contact lens may be inserted and the patient placed on a topical non-steroidal anti-inflammatory preparation such as ketorolac tromethamine 0.5% (Acular, Allergan) or diclofenac sodium 0.1% (Voltaren, CIBA). The bandage contact lens must be carefully inserted so as not to disturb the flap. A bandage contact lens with a base curve of 8.4 or fit on preoperative mean keratometry is recommended as excessive movement will increase patient discomfort and slow epithelial healing. The fit of the contact and re-examination of the flap should be performed after instillation of the lens. If observed to be tight, the contact must be replaced with a flatter base curve of 8.8. Topical non-steroidals can delay epithelial healing and should not be used beyond 48 to 72 hours. Patients are maintained on a topical steroid in addition to antibiotic and non-steroidal anti-inflammatory agents, with a four times daily regimen. Oral agents such as a sedative, non-narcotic, and even a narcotic agent may all have a role in maintaining patient comfort during the epithelial healing process. Pressure patching is contraindicated as patient eye movement against the firmly applied eyelid may create excessive shearing forces and displace the flap. The bandage contact lens should be removed in

the same manner as that for a patient following PRK, ensuring that the contact lens is well lubricated with artificial tears or even a topical anesthetic such as proparacaine 0.5%, which is the least epitheliotoxic. The technique preferred is to have the patient look up while at the slit-lamp biomicroscope; in this manner the inferior aspect of the bandage lens is visible and may slide down. Using fine non-toothed forceps, the inferior aspect of the contact lens is firmly grasped and the lens pulled down and away from the eye (Figure 12-16). This is the most gentle and precise technique for bandage contact lens removal with least risk of flap displacement. It is important to copiously lubricate the contact lens and anesthetize the eye first.

INFECTION

Clinical: The incidence of infection is rare, likely in the order of 1 in 5000, based upon international experience. The nature of the procedure when properly performed with an intact epithelium makes the stroma only vulnerable to bacterial inoculation for a very brief period of time intraoperatively. However, operative trauma or breakdown of the epithelium increases the risk of surface infection. Prophylactic antibiotics and sterilization of the microkeratome between procedures reduces the risk dramatically. The risk can further be reduced with proper lid hygiene and an antiseptic eyewash such as poviodine preoperatively. Gloves are used by roughly half the surgeons performing the procedure, and, if utilized, are of the talc-free variety, as the talc can damage the microkeratome gears and be found within the interface (Figure 12-17).

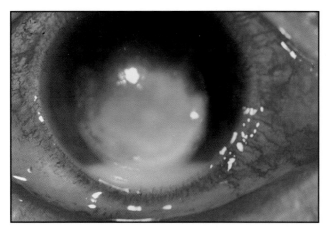

Figure 12-18a.
Acute *Serratia marcescens* corneal ulcer following superficial infection of corneal flap. Postoperative inferior corneal abraision on second postoperative day with rapid deterioration and infection of corneal flap. High magnification clinical appearance of corneal ulcer and hypopyon observed less than 24 hours after focal infiltrates first noted.

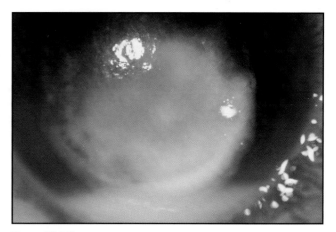

Figure 12-18b.
Severe conjunctival injection and chemosis associated.

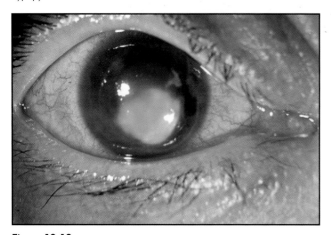

Figure 12-18c.
Low magnification clinical appearance of treated corneal ulcer after three weeks with loss of corneal flap. No hypopyon evident and ocular inflammation reduced.

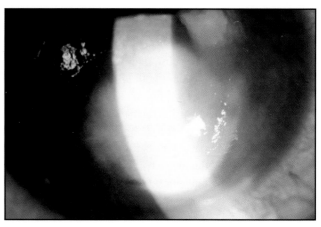

Figure 12-18d.
High magnification view of necrotic stromal bed following intensive antibiotic therapy at 3 weeks.

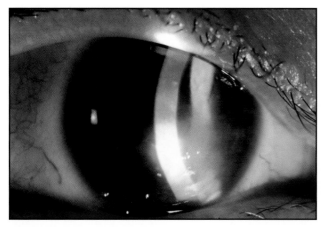

Figure 12-18e.
Clinical appearance of corneal ulcer after 9 weeks demonstrating residual stromal scarring.

Clinical Note

Infiltrates can rarely be observed within the interface and may be in response to infection but may also be inflammatory in reaction to foreign matter. The stromal interface is typically inert and does not elicit any reaction to foreign debris entrapped. One such case I encountered I managed by lifting the flap and debriding the infiltrates, then irrigating the infiltrates with antibiotics. The patient had remained pain-free postoperatively and was observed to have two pinpoint infiltrates on routine follow-up on the first postoperative day. The patient was placed on frequent fluoroquinolone and aminoglycoside topical antibiotics and within 24 to 48 hours of this course of therapy had a clear and quiet interface with no sign of infection or infiltration.

Another much more unfortunate postoperative course involved a 35-year-old woman who underwent LASIK for extreme myopia correction of -14.00 D. On the first postoperative day the patient was completely comfortable with a quiet white eye and clear cornea with intact epithelium. Uncorrected vision was a remarkable 20/40. On the second postoperative day, the patient returned late in the afternoon complaining of pain and tearing. Examination revealed two small epithelial defects at 5 and 6 o'clock, just within the area of the flap. Both denuded areas contained small infiltrates and the patient was cultured and placed on hourly tobramycin and Ocuflox (Allergan) by her ophthalmologist, a corneal specialist, and referred back the following morning for follow-up at our facility. No bandage contact lens was placed. Despite an acute increase in the pain, redness, and swelling of the eye within hours, the patient did not seek further assistance until her appointment the following morning. Copious purulent discharge was evident in the morning although frequent antibiotics had been instilled. From 5:00 pm to 9:00 am the following morning the eye had dramatically worsened. The two 0.5-mm superficial infiltrates described by the comanaging physician had increased to 3-mm arcuate infiltrate along the inferior aspect of the flap with a 2-mm hypopyon. There was a mild to moderate degree of conjunctival injection and chemosis. Vision had reduced to counting fingers and the patient was quite photophobic. A tentative diagnosis of Pseudomonas aeruginosa or possibly pneumococcus was made. The patient was started immediately on hourly fortified cefazolin 50 mg/cc alternating with fortified tobramycin 14 mg/cc in addition to hourly ocuflox. Cycloplegia was maintained. After discussion with the comanaging ophthalmologist, it was decided to admit the patient to hospital for the initial management of the corneal ulcer in light of the rapid deterioration. The patient returned to the corneal specialist for subconjunctival injections of tobramycin and cefazolin and in preparation for hospital admission closer to her home. Within hours, the flap had become necrotic and dislodged with the stromal bed infiltrated also (Figure 12-18a). The flap was removed and treatment in hospital continued (Figure 12-18b). Initial culture indicated a gram negative organism, possibly hemophilus, sensitive to cefazolin. After 48 hours of hourly broad spectrum coverage with topical fortified antibiotics and twice daily subconjunctival antibiotic injections, final cultures yielded *Serratia marcescens* sen-

sitive to tobramycin. After 5 days, the patient was discharged as the infection appeared under control with a reduction of the hypopyon. The surface epithelium healed over 3 to 4 weeks (Figures 12-18c and 12-18d) and the corneal scarring reduced over months (Figure 12-18e).

There are a few unusual features of this case in that the infection was incredibly virulent and occurred 2 days postoperatively. The epithelium was initially intact. The postoperative prophylactic antibiotic was tobramycin. The infection was superficial rather than within the interface. No other patients had developed an infection. The only conclusions to draw are that the procedure had merely made the patient vulnerable to an epithelial breakdown. The inoculation of bacterium had likely occurred postoperatively. The patient's only risk factor was a history of very dry eyes for many years with an intolerance to contact lens wear. Lindstrom describes three cases of *Serratia marcescens* seen in consultation and determined infected make-up (eyeliner) to be the underlying etiology (personal communication). The primary conclusion is that the epithelium provides an important barrier to infection and measures such as frequent postoperative lubrication are critical elements in preventing infection.

IRREGULAR ASTIGMATISM

Clinical: Virtually all patients immediately postoperatively have some degree of irregular astigmatism and will complain of poor qualitative vision despite excellent quantitative vision. Patients should be counseled that this is a normal part of the healing process, especially those requiring higher degrees of myopia correction. High myopes typically complain of what can best be termed "Vaseline vision." The qualitative disturbance is compounded by any residual refractive error. Most irregular astigmatism clears over 2 to 4 weeks, with some cases requiring as long as 6 to 12 months. Approximately, 1% to 2% of patients have a significant degree of irregular astigmatism resulting in a permanent loss of best corrected visual acuity of two or more lines. During the early stages of the surgical learning curve and in complicated cases such as those resulting in a free cap, the incidence of irregular astigmatism resulting in loss of best corrected vision is likely in the order of 5% to 10%.

Management: Surgical technique is important in reducing the incidence and severity of irregular astigmatism. A certain degree of irregular astigmatism, however, is unavoidable with lamellar surgery. Specific aspects of flap replace-

Figure 12-19.
Corneal videokeratography demonstrating small effective optical zone following LASIK procedure. Clinically significant night glare is generated postoperatively, especially in high myopes secondary to spherical aberration.

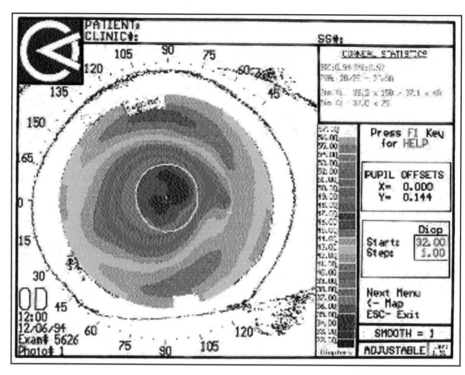

ment constitute the greatest step at which the eye is vulnerable to the creation of irregular astigmatism. The corneal flap must be floated back into position in as smooth a maneuver as possible. The size of the hinge may also have relevance in that a broader hinge typically has greater memory and resiliency to return to the natural alignment and placement with least effort. Smoothing the flap into position with a wet surgical spear helps to reduce any flap irregularities and gently stretch the cap into postion. The amount and force of the compressed air may also play a role in that the cap will shrink and contract irregularly to high volume air flow. It is unknown what impact various ablation profiles have upon the development of irregular astigmatism, however, central island formation may produce irregular astigmatism in itself.

> 1% to 2% of patients have a significant degree of irregular astigmatism resulting in a permanent loss of best corrected visual acuity of two or more lines.

NIGHT GLARE

Clinical: Night glare is another seemingly unavoidable side effect experienced by many corrected high myopes. Night glare is a result of a pronounced form of spherical aberration, with the pupil diameter in dim light exceeding that of the effective optical zone created (Figure 12-19). Efforts to increase the diameter of the optical zone utilized are complicated by the greater depth of ablation and the formation of central islands. Patients complain of halos, starbursts, and a general reduction of qualitative vision in conditions of reduced illumination. Night glare can virtually disable extremely myopic individuals both preoperatively but especially postoperatively for night driving. The longer daylight hours of summer reduce complaints during that season and is a favorite of patients and surgeons alike. Any residual refractive error will exacerbate the night glare, especially residual myopia.

Management: Fortunately most patients improve with time and bilateral treatment as a result of cortical integration. Simply stated, they learn to ignore the visual disturbances that surgery produces under low light conditions. Various ablation algorithms have been attempted to achieve superior visual results both quantitatively and qualitatively, but almost all sacrifice diameter for reduced depth of ablation or reduced central island formation. With broad beam excimer delivery systems, a multizone technique or aspheric profile can be utilized to reduce depth of ablation in high myopia correction while maximizing the effective optical zone. Just as with the PRK nomogram, a pretreatment must be performed as the risk of central island formation is not only equal but greater when ablating within the stroma.

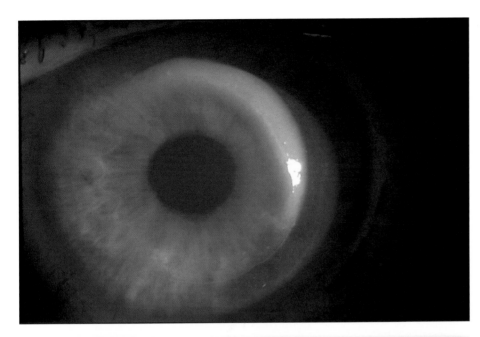

Figure 12-20.
Postoperative clinical appearance of advancing epithelial ingrowth detected with fluorescein staining 10 days postoperatively, demonstrating nonadherent flap edge. Advancing edge or wave border of epithelium commonly visible without staining. Epithelium within ingrowth can be thick, easily observed, and possibly commonly requiring treatment or very thin, more difficult to detect and usual stable without treatment.

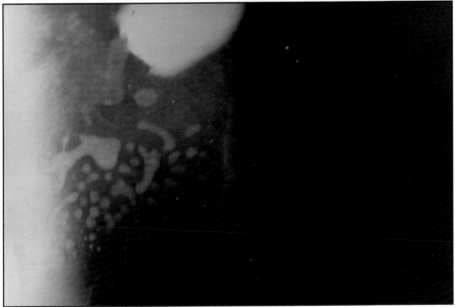

Figure 12-21.
Epithelial ingrowth growing within corneal interface, usually extending from periphery although can have implanted nests of epithelium. Gray clinical appearance with white pearls forming whorl pattern within the epithelial pennisulas. The thicker the epithelial ingrowth the darker gray in appearance and the more likely it will be associated with white geographic patterns or pearls. These white areas most likely represent necrotic islands of epithelium within the ingrowth.

Another essential principle is that unlike ALK, whereby the corneal flap actually acts to increase the effective optical zone relative to the resected area, in LASIK, the corneal flap acts to decrease the effective optical zone. That is, the second refractive pass of ALK removes a plano lenticle but the corneal flap drapes over the area of excision enlarging the effective optical zone. In LASIK, the tissue removed is a myopic lenticle with tapered edges which allow the flap to actually mask the peripheral area of ablation. In addition, not only does the flap appear to mask the extent of the treatment area, but the increased hydration of the deeper stroma reduces the effectiveness of the peripheral ablation curves. In PRK, one requires well-blended peripheral curves to avoid inciting haze formation, such is not the case within the stroma. A new approach must be conceived to ablate within the stroma and improve qualitative and quantitative vision. This fact becomes readily apparent when one examines the postoperative LASIK topography and compares it to that of PRK performed with the same nomogram. The circular area of flattening representing the treatment area of LASIK is reduced indicating a smaller effective optical zone than that programmed.

Figure 12-22a.
Epithelial ingrowth clinical appearance under low magnification revealing vacuoles and pearls within migrating epithelium associated with mildly irregular flap edge.

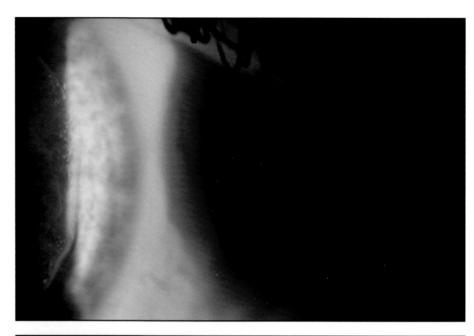

Figure 12-22b.
Epithelial ingrowth clinical appearance under high magnification revealing vacuoles and pearls within migrating epithelium associated with mildly irregular flap edge.

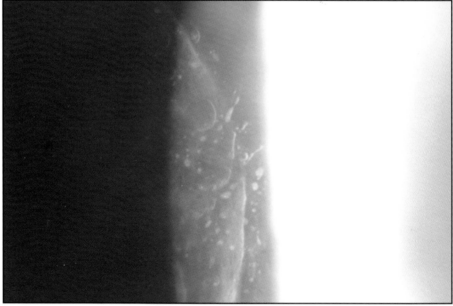

New LASIK nomograms will further evolve with multizone or aspheric generated profiles to reduce depth of ablation, with additional treatment centrally to reduce central island formation and additional peripheral treatment to reduce night glare. Not only can the ablation profile be altered but air can be used to decrease the hydration of the stroma peripherally during the last few seconds of treatment, increasing the effectiveness of the peripheral blend. It must be understood that increased peripheral treatment must be compensated for with even greater central treatment, and therefore greater overall depth of ablation.

EPITHELIAL INGROWTHS STROMAL MELTS

Clinical: The incidence of epithelial implantation and ingrowths is roughly 2% and usually is observed within the first few weeks of surgery. Epithelium within the interface may occur in nests that have been implanted and are usually non-progressive or grow in peripherally beneath the cap edge. The epithelial ingrowth may be progressive in nature or self-limited, rapid in onset or slow in development. The natural history is variable in that the epithelial ingrowth may be static or precipitate a stromal melt of the overlying cap. The stroma is sandwiched between epithelium within the

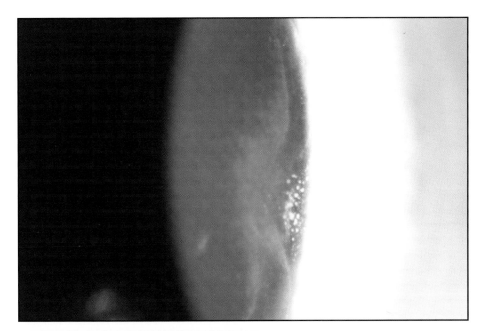

Figure 12-23.
Corneal flap edge may appear clinically gray, rolled, eroded, or even necrotic in association with epithlial growth beneath the lamellar flap. The epithelium will be both on the undersurface of the flap and on the stromal bed. It appears that the corneal flap edge is pulled or rolled underneath with the advancing epithelium, giving the darker gray clinical appearance with blunted raised and uneven flap margins. In my clinical experience, the most common site for an ingrowth is likely temporally followed by inferiorly.

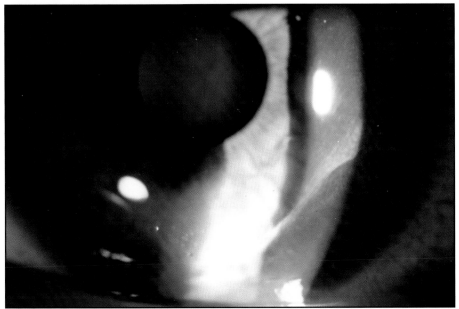

Figure 12-24.
Epithelial ingrowth producing peripheral stromal melt of corneal flap edge inferotemporally. Stromal melts are precipitated by sandwiching the corneal flap stroma with both the surface epithelium and the interface epithelium.

interface and on the surface and therefore may experience necrosis. The primary risk factors for an epithelial ingrowth are a peripheral epithelial defect, poor flap adhesion, and a perforated corneal flap. Poor or improper adhesion of the corneal flap will encourage migration of epithelial cells into the interface (Figure 12-20). The clinical appearance of an epithelial ingrowth is typically a tongue or peninsula extending from the cap edge with a whorl-like pattern (Figures 12-21 through 12-22b). The flap edge may be gray and rolled or necrotic (Figures 12-23 through 12-25). The visual acuity, topography, and refraction may all be affected

The incidence of epithelial implantation and ingrowths is roughly 2% and usually is observed within the first few weeks of surgery.

as the epithelium extends beneath the flap. Regular and irregular astigmatism may be induced reducing best corrected and uncorrected visual acuity even if a stromal melt is not clinically evident.

Management: An epithelial ingrowth of 2 mm or greater

Figure 12-25.
Peripheral corneal flap erosion secondary to epithelial ingrowth. Corneal flap edge appears gray, rolled, and contracted. Exposed stromal bed responds with arcuate confluent haze because of epithelial-stromal interaction associated with steep peripheral contour. No visual symptoms reported by patient.

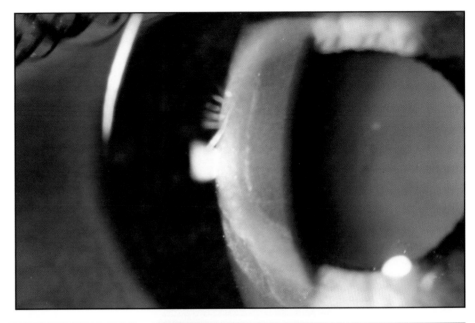

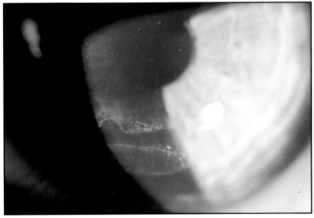

Figure 12-26a.
Epithelial ingrowth following LASIK resulting in linear stromal melt of inferior corneal flap.

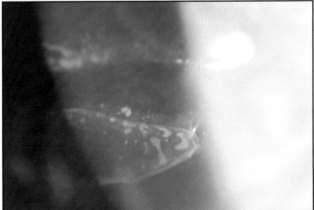

Figure 12-26b.
High magnification appearance demonstrating whorl pattern of migrating epithelium within interface.

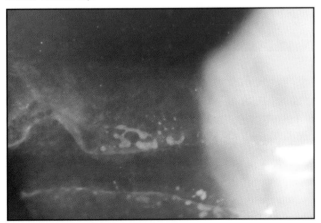

Figure 12-26c.
High magnification appearance demonstrating erosion of corneal flap edges with associated interface haze.

usually requires treatment to prevent a stromal melt. The presence of epithelium itself does not indicate that treatment is warranted, but size, progression, altered residual refractive error, induced astigmatism, and reduction in best corrected and uncorrected vision are all factors to be considered. An epithelial ingrowth greater than 2 mm in diameter, especially if associated with rapid onset and progression, should be treated. If localized epithelium within the interface is observed, it should be followed closely to ensure that no progression or accompanying stromal melt is occurring. A schedule of 1 week, 2 weeks, 1 month, 2 months, and 3 months is usually adequate. An epithelial ingrowth requiring treatment should be performed as soon as possible to avoid progression with stromal melting which complicates treat-

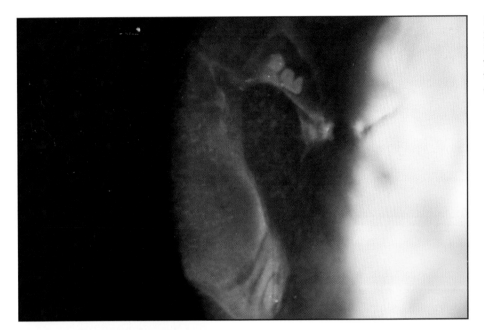

Figure 12-27a.
Stromal melt secondary to epithelial ingrowth encroaching upon central visual axis. Qualitative vision reduced with significant glare inferotemporally and monocular diplopia.

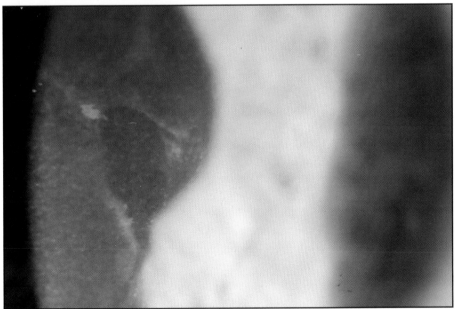

Figure 12-27b.
Management consisted of debridement of the interface and smoothing of the corneal flap. Subsequent flap removal failing stabilization. Removal of the corneal flap increases haze formation but does not alter refraction.

ment and usually results in a worse prognosis. Treatment involves lifting the flap and removing the epithelium from within the interface. Typically, these flaps are much easier to lift due to the presence of the epithelium itself within the interface and the fact that management usually occurs within the first month. The corneal flap edge should be marked preoperatively and an alignment marking placed as described later for retreatments. The flap edge should be lifted with a Suarez spreader or equivalent to expose the undersurface of the flap and stromal bed. Many times a spreader is not required and the flap edge can be grasped temporally

with non-toothed forceps and gently reflected back. Although epithelium is typically adherent to the undersurface of the flap, both stromal surfaces should be debrided. Sharp debridement is preferable, to improve the probability that all the residual epithelial cells have been removed. The epithelium often can be dissected off in a single sheet. A dry surgical spear is useful to scrub the stromal surfaces but must be discarded after each pass to avoid re-implanting epithelial cells. The edges of the corneal flap and along the periphery of the stromal bed are the primary sites to clear of epithelial remnants. Do not use alcohol or cocaine within the

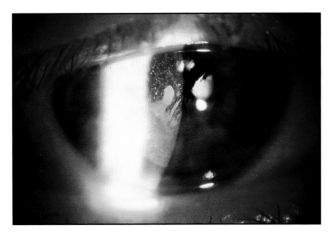

Figure 12-28a.
Clinically aggressive epithelial ingrowth.

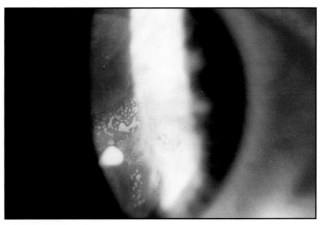

Figure 12-28b.
Epithelial ingrowth resulting in rapid deterioration with corneal flap melt necessitating flap removal in a secondary procedure.

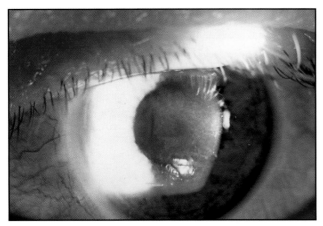

Figure 12-28c.
After topical steroid treatment and repeat PRK, uncorrected visual acuity returned to 20/40 after 9 months, although best corrected vision remains reduced at 20/25 with residual stromal haze.

> **The removal of the flap can elicit a wound healing response producing haze and regression.**

STROMAL MELTS

Clinical: The patient with an aggressive epithelial ingrowth, especially if associated with a thin corneal flap, will develop a stromal melt. These are often very rapid in onset with blurred vision, photophobia, and occasionally pain being associated. The flap is seen to lose its integrity and alter its shape, with flap edges becoming blunt and squared off or eroded (Figures 12-26a through 12-26c). The flap edge itself usually appears gray and rolled. Small focal nests of epithelial cells are often visible in the area of the stromal melt (Figures 12-27a and 12-27b). An epithelial erosion may be evident as well placing the patient at risk for infection. The appearance is radically different from a normal flap with scarring along the cut edge of Bowman's layer at the periphery of the flap, which appears white with smooth flap edges.

Management: Management is difficult at best and involves determining first if the flap is viable. An attempt should be made in all but the most damaged flaps to preserve the tissue as best as possible. The earlier these flaps are treated, the more likely they will remain viable. The initial steps of surgical management are to lift the flap, even if fragmented, and debride the undersurface and stromal bed. Care should be taken to remove all the epithelial nests without further damaging the flap. The flap should then be replaced and allowed to settle. A bandage contact lens can provide comfort if the surface epithelium is not intact both preoperatively and postoperatively. Residual epithelium

stromal bed or other such toxic agents as they will cause irreparable damage. If there is any concern for additional epithelial nests, irrigation and brushing can be used. Epithelial cells will also fluoresce in a dark room with no microscope illumination, if five to 10 pulses of PTK are placed over the bed and flap. This is not routinely recommended. Once the epithelium has been adequately debrided, the flap is replaced as for any retreatment with the stromal bed dry and the stroma of the flap wet. It is advocated to irrigate beneath the flap to clear any residual epithelial cells from the interface. Wet surgical spears are used to smooth the flap into alignment and air used to seal the edges of the flap securely. A bandage contact lens may be required if the surrounding epithelium has been denuded during the debridement.

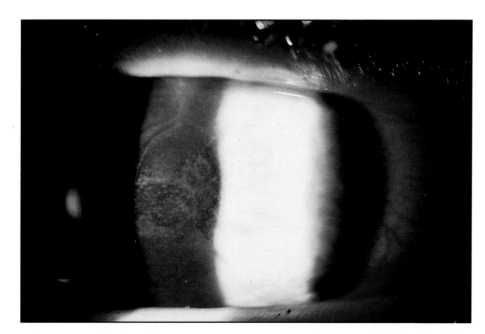

Figure 12-29a.
Central corneal flap perforation with central epithelial ingrowth and haze formation. Intraoperative loss of suction experienced.

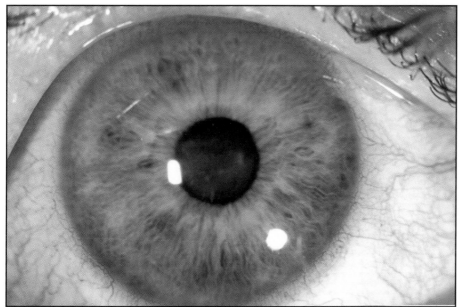

Figure 12-29b.
Following removal of non-viable corneal flap, PTK retreatment was performed to reduce central scarring. Residual haze and myopia required further PRK enhancement after 6 months. Best corrected vision still reduced to 20/30, with uncorrected vision of 20/60 and +0.25 -1.25 x 60 refraction. Time will likely restore one additional line of best corrected vision and no further surgery would be attempted for the residual refractive error.

with further progression of necrosis and with loss of flap integrity necessitates removing the flap completely.

One of the fundamental principles concerning the lamellar aspect of LASIK is that the flap has no refractive power. Therefore, removal of the flap should have no effect on the refractive predictability of the initial procedure. The removal of the flap can elicit a wound healing response producing haze and regression. Therefore, topical steroid regimens such as that used for PRK are indicated. As well, although the cap has zero refractive power, epithelial hyperplasia peripherally may result in increased myopia.

Clinical Note

Stromal Melting Associated With Epithelial Ingrowth

Bilateral LASIK was performed on a 40-year-old woman for -8.00 D correction with excellent and immediately good results in her right eye but rapid onset of aggressive epithelial ingrowth in her left eye following an epithelial defect. Epithelium within the interface produced edema of the left flap, with persistent surface epithelial erosion. The patient was fit with a bandage contact lens for comfort. Although vision in her right eye was 20/20 with near emmetropia, vision in the left fluctuated between

Figure 12-30a.
Sunrise holmium laser thermokeratoplasty for hyperopic overcorrection following LASIK procedure for severe myopia. The patient measured +1.75 D 6 months postoperatively with a very stable refractive pattern observed from 3 months. Following LTK application, no corneal flap shrinkage was observed.

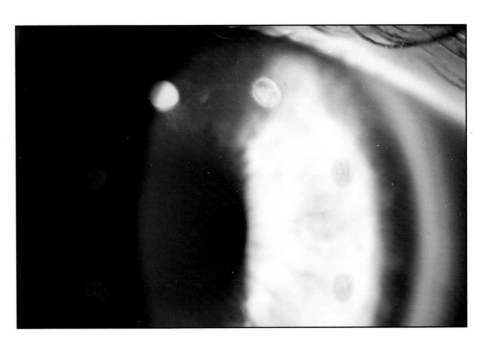

20/50 and 20/400. Within 2 weeks stromal melting of the left corneal flap was observed from the 4 o'clock postion toward the central axis (Figures 12-28a and 12-28b). The corneal flap was lifted and the epithelium debrided. The patient experienced significant clinical improvement within days of cleaning the interface, only to have the epithelial ingrowth reoccur with further stromal melting necessitating cap removal (Figure 12-28c).

Cases of rapid and progressive onset epithelial ingrowths must be treated not only aggressively but without delay to avoid stromal melting of the corneal flap.

Clinical Note

Central corneal flap perforation occurred in the right eye of a 42-year-old man who underwent LASIK in his left eye. The cause of the flap complication was unclear, but assumed to be a loss of adequate suction intraoperatively. The corneal flap was replaced and the patient allowed to heal for 3 months with best corrected visual acuity gradually improving from 20/100 initially to 20/25. The postoperative course was complicated by the development of an epithelial ingrowth centrally which expanded the small defect substantially, exposing the stromal interface. Although the stromal interface was covered with surface epithelium, central confluent haze developed reducing best corrected vision to 20/60 (Figure 12-29a). The treatment performed was carried out in two steps. The central haze was first ablated using a transepithelial approach centrally. The corneal flap was lifted and found

to be clearly nonviable and resected along the hinge edge. Focal PTK was utilized to smooth the hinge edge. The surface epithelium healed over 72 hours with a bandage contact lens and the patient started on a 2-month tapering course of topical fluoromethalone 0.1%. A small amount of mild reticular haze remained which is scheduled to be treated with his myopia during his enhancement procedure after 3 months (Figure 12-29b).

LATE POSTOPERATIVE COMPLICATIONS

Late postoperative complications are ones which either occur over time or are independent of time, typically observed at or after 1 month. Errors in refractive predictability are included in this section in concert with regression and central islands.

ERRORS IN REFRACTIVE PREDICTABILITY
Overcorrections

Clinical: An overcorrection with any refractive procedure is difficult to manage, however, LASIK represents a greater challenge than overcorrected PRK, which is more easily managed with pharmacologic manipulation and the holmium laser. Although hyperopia ablation patterns can be fashioned within the stromal bed with LASIK without concern for haze and regression, nomogram development is still

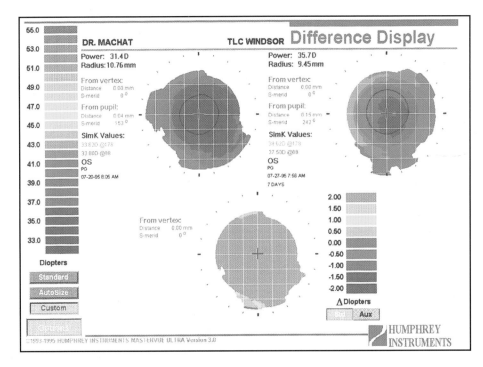

Figure 12-30b.
Humphrey MasterVue Ultra corneal videokeratography demonstrating corneal steepening effect of holmium LTK. Preoperative mean keratometry was 31.4 D, which improved to 35.7 D 1 week following Sunrise LTK. Refractive error measured -0.75 D at 1 week regressing to +0.25 D at 5 months following LTK for LASIK overcorrection.

in its infancy. Patients with PRK experience a slow and gradual visual recovery with a slight hyperopic overcorrection anticipated early during the healing process and resolving with steroid withdrawal. LASIK patients conversely experience rapid visual rehabilitation without an intended hyperopic overcorrection as regression is much less common and variable. Unlike LASIK patients, it is usually possible in fact to manipulate the refractive error somewhat in post-PRK patients through steroid titration. Therefore, an overcorrected LASIK patient not only has less pharmacologic options available but is subjectively much more aware of the refractive miscalculation. As always, although younger patients may cope well with mild hyperopia, pre-presbyopic and presbyopic patients are immediately disconcerted by the loss of reading ability and distance blur imposed. Some patients will gradually improve with regression but a subset of these overcorrected LASIK patients must be treated.

Management: The management of an overcorrected LASIK is a continuum of approaches with no clearly preferred method. Although the technique I currently prefer involves performing a Sunrise holmium ablation at 6 or 7 mm on the corneal flap after 6 months. It may even be possible to lower the energy and perform the procedure directly upon the stromal bed after 2 or 3 months if no regression has occurred. The holmium settings currently used are six pulses directed at eight spots with 30 mJ/cm² of energy per spot (240 mJ/cm² total). It should be noted that performing the laser thermokeratoplasty (LTK) with the holmium laser invites potential flap problems and irregular astigmatism which may be refractory to treatment. It should also be clearly understood and anticipated that if one performs the LTK on the stromal bed a dramatically greater effect will be achieved, in the order of three-fold or greater, as Bowman's layer is avoided and the stroma is more than 100 microns thinner at this level. I have treated five overcorrected LASIK patients on the corneal flap surface after at least 6 months recovery with remarkable predictability, all within 0.50 D of attempted plano correction and without complications (Figures 12-30a and 12-30b).

Other approaches include PTK on the surface epithelium or on the stromal bed at 1 month to produce a relative central island centrally. The surface ablation may also reduce any peripheral epithelial hyperplasia decreasing any hyperopic effect from the surface contour (F. Tayfour, MD). A PTK ablation within the stroma will flatten the periphery greater than the central 3 mm. The corneal flap will smooth most stromal bed irregularities and the refractive effect gained or lost is based upon the final contour of the flap. The primary problem with these approaches is that they are not predictable with respect to the refractive effect achieved.

The most appropriate approach would be to perform a hyperopic LASIK procedure after 3 months once stable, either by lifting the flap or with a second microkeratome pass at the same or greater depth. Nomogram development is rapidly progressing in this area and will soon be a viable option with minimal risk of irregular astigmatism.

Undercorrections

Clinical: Undercorrections are common in higher attempted corrections, especially those above -10.00 or 12.00 D. Creating a tight nomogram is optimal, however, reality dictates that overcorrections will occur with greater frequency as the standard deviation of the refractive outcomes increases with increasing correction. Since it is far easier to correct residual myopia than a hyperopic overcorrection, the nomogram should always be developed conservatively and undercorrections anticipated as the attempted correction increases. Undercorrected patients complain of poor distance vision and night glare, but have functional vision at near.

Management: Patients should be prescribed temporary glasses by the end of the first week of surgery or fit with disposable contact lenses after 1 to 2 weeks. Patient symptoms dramatically reduce once some form of temporary correction is obtained pending additional surgical treatment.

> **Regression also appears to occur much more rapidly than with PRK and seems much less responsive to topical steroid manipulation.**

Fluctuating vision and loss of best corrected vision experienced frequently by highly myopic patients early in their healing are much better tolerated. Night visual disturbances, although reduced, continue to remain a problem for most patients. Additional refractive surgery options are discussed in Chapter 13.

Regression

Clinical: Somewhat surprisingly, some LASIK patients experience myopic regression despite the fact that the deep stroma is considered to be virtually inert with respect to wound healing. It is unclear precisely what occurs physiologically, but there appears to be multiple factors in regression observed with LASIK. The fact that more severe degrees of myopic correction have a greater likelihood of myopic regression is of little help in determining the cause of myopic regression in LASIK patients as both epithelial hyperplasia and stromal remodeling are affected by deeper ablations. Regression also appears to occur much more rapidly than with PRK and seems much less responsive to

topical steroid manipulation.

It may very well be that the initial baseline refraction and unaided visual acuity measured on day 1 or 2 is not representative of the achieved refractive endpoint but is altered by early edema, irregular astigmatism, and dehydration effects of the procedure. A hyperopic refraction can mean irregular astigmatism and a myopic refraction the presence of a central island. The multifocal nature of the corneal contour produced can create a poorly defined refractive endpoint.

Although there are multiple problems in defining the true residual refractive error early in the healing process, it does appear that a certain amount of myopic regression is inevitable in the correction of severe myopia. Myopic regression in moderately severe myopes (-6.00 to -9.00 D) may be as great as 1.00 or 2.00 D, and in severe myopia (-9.00 to -15.00 D) as high as 3.00 or 4.00 D. Regression of several diopters may seem to occur in patients treated for over 15.00 to 20.00 D of myopia. Excluding poor refractive predictability of the procedure for severe myopia producing various degrees of undercorrection, the cause of such apparent regression is a combination of epithelial hyperplasia and stromal remodeling. It is evident that the epithelium will increase in thickness in response to a significantly flattened cornea. Stable central mean keratometry below 33.00 D is difficult to achieve and below 30.00 rarely obtained. Larger optical zones blending into the periphery may reduce or eliminate the cause for epithelial hyperplasia centrally by creating a smoother, more acceptable contour to the anterior corneal curvature. Despite the amount of tissue removed centrally with PRK, epithelium will increase in thickness or haze formation will occur to re-establish a more blended contour when a small optical zone is used. As LASIK flattens the anterior corneal curvature without inciting a stromal reaction at the epithelial-stromal interface, epithelial hyperplasia alone must reconfigure a more gradual contour.

> **Principles in Maintaining Long-Term Corneal Stability**
> - 50% Rule: total depth of ablation + corneal flap thickness should not exceed 50% of the preoperative total corneal thickness
> - Total corneal thickness of 400 microns or greater advocated
> - Residual stromal bed thickness of (at a very minimum) 200 microns and preferably 250 microns is advocated

A pachymetric evaluation of the epithelium and stroma following LASIK is underway to determine their role in regression. In certain cases of LASIK, a significant stromal reaction at the site of the ablation becomes evident with reticular haze or fibrosis observed within the interface. The incidence of such cases is 0.3% or less. The only association observed in these rare cases is severe myopia correction of at least 10.00 D and excessive drying of the interface intra-operatively. These patients have an aggressive healing course with myopic regression, but elevation of the flap for retreatment is very difficult even early in the healing process once the clinical appearance is noted. The aggressive wound healing response of PRK is centered about an epithelial-stromal interaction which is absent from the reaction observed with LASIK. It is unclear to what degree stromal remodeling may occur within the stroma and to what extent it may contribute to myopic regression in LASIK. Stromal remodeling that is deemed clinically significant does, however, appear to play a role in at least a minority of LASIK cases experiencing myopic regression.

One particularly disturbing cause of myopic regression is iatrogenic keratoconus, when an inadequate amount of stromal tissue remains after the primary procedure. It is vital to maintain the 50% rule, and not allow the depth of ablation and corneal flap thickness to exceed 50% of the preoperative corneal thickness. As well, leaving a stromal bed of at least 250 microns is definitely advocated.

Management: Management for myopic regression is unchanged from that for myopic undercorrection and is discussed in Chapter 7 on LASIK retreatments. Rarely, patients post-LASIK will develop interface fibrosis, which appears as reticular and even somewhat confluent haze and may reduce quantitative and qualitative vision. These very rare cases occur in extremely severe myopes with aggressive wound healing responses. Treatment of myopic regression and ablation of the fibrosis must occur early if the flap can be elevated and the interface ablated and cleared. Excessive force will result in tearing or damaging the flap. If the flap cannot be elevated, clearing the interface is virtually impossible short of a free-hand lamellar dissection or automated lamellar dissection at a level immediately above the scarred interface if at all possible. Fitting with contact lenses for the residual refractive error or glasses may be preferable to a PRK procedure which may result in additional scarring. Repeat LASIK may be performed with the addition of a postoperative steroid regimen similar to that used for PRK.

> The most common topographical abnormality observed postoperatively with LASIK patients is central island formation. Unlike central islands observed with PRK, the topographical abnormalities observed with LASIK do not seem as likely to resolve with time

ABNORMAL INDUCED TOPOGRAPHY
Central Islands

Clinical: The most common topographical abnormality observed postoperatively with LASIK patients is central island formation. The incidence of central islands is actually increased unless nomogram and/or technique alterations are made to compensate for the pronounced hydration of the deeper stroma. Although small optical zones are not associated with central island formation, optical zones of 6 mm or greater have an extremely high incidence approaching 100% if no compensation is made. Symptoms of central island formation include blurred vision, ghosting, and monocular diplopia. Objectively, they are difficult to refract and have a disproportionately high degree of residual myopia relative to their uncorrected visual acuity. For example, a typical central island patient post-LASIK may have an uncorrected visual acuity of 20/30 with a measured refraction of -2.00 D, far greater than would have been predicted based upon the unaided vision. Unlike central islands observed with PRK, the topographical abnormalities observed with LASIK do not seem to resolve with time. Topographically, a central island appears as a central steepening appearing as red or a lighter shade of blue-green, 2 to 3 mm in diameter, relative to the surrounding area, which is notably a darker green or more typically blue. Clinically, it is impossible upon corneal examination to determine the presence or absence of a central island.

Management: The management of central islands focuses on both prevention through modification of software algorithms and techniques and retreatment, the latter of which will be covered in the chapter on LASIK retreatments. Understanding the cause of central islands is essential in developing appropriate measures to prevent their formation. Central islands are related to differential hydration of the corneal stroma which is both naturally occurring (Lin) and related to acoustic shockwave (Machat) effects of photoablation. Although the cornea itself is 70% water, the distribution is not homogeneous with the central stroma being more hydrated than the peripheral cornea making the central tissue more resistant to photoablation and less compact. Scanning lasers, however, do not produce central islands unless related to other factors and therefore a second mechanism peculiar to broad beam lasers must be operational. Broad beam laser pulses produce circular acoustic shockwaves during myopic correction which drives stromal fluid both centrally and peripherally. Although peripheral fluid has limited clinical effect beyond possibly decreasing effective optical zone size and increasing night glare, central fluid produces a relative central undercorrection or central island. The increased incidence of central island formation at the deeper layers of the stroma are simply related to the increased hydration level of the deeper stroma.

Intraoperatvely, it is very evident that central fluid accumulation occurs during the ablation process, as the iris diaphragm expands for myopia correction. The central stroma appears translucent or black relative to the expanding gray ring demarcating the extent of the treatment zone. Management, therefore, centers about compensating for the central undercorrection and controlling stromal hydration. Compensation for the central undercorrection is made by altering software algorithms and hydration is controlled through the application of compressed air, drying with surgical spears, or wiping fluid accumulation with a spatula.

As discussed in earlier sections of PRK and LASIK, the pretreatment technique is the application of pulses to the central 2 to 3 mm above and beyond what is required for the full refractive effect. The pretreatment technique compensates for the central undercorrection produced when applying a theoretical lenticular curve to the hydrated stroma. Pretreatment not only reduces the incidence and size of central islands but improves qualitative vision. The amount of pretreatment required is increased for both higher degrees of correction and for intrastromal ablation as the deeper layers are more hydrated. The pretreatment nomogram for PRK and LASIK is dependent upon the laser system utilized, the specific technique, and the number and size of the optical zones. In addition to pretreatment, some means of controlling the hydration status must be employed.

Although excessive drying, especially with air, will produce haze with PRK, there is much less concern with LASIK. Compressed air at a fixed flow rate, cannula size, and specific duration can standardize the hydration status of the stromal bed. Use of a surgical spear to dry the stromal bed is variable and may leave debris within the interface. Wiping with a spatula is only partially effective as the fluid accumulation is too rapid, occurring with each pulse, multiple times per second. Air via a 23-gauge cannula at 3 liters per minute for 1 to 2 seconds between zones is a useful starting point. Excessive air will produce significant overcorrections especially if left on the stroma during the ablation process.

All broad beam excimer laser systems produce central islands when a large optical zone is utilized unless a very gaussian energy beam profile is used. The gaussian beam profile being much hotter or of higher energy centrally will both remove a greater proportion of tissue centrally and/or drive fluid peripherally. Although the Summit OmniMed series has a gaussian beam, it will produce a central island if the optical zone is 6 mm or greater. The aspheric multizone program of the Summit OmniMed series places the majority of the treatment in the central 4.5 mm and blends out to 6.0 or 6.5 mm, thereby reducing the incidence of central island formation. The Chiron Technolas aspheric LASIK program concentrates the treatment within 4.2 mm with a 5.5-mm transition zone. Chiron Technolas multizone programs have a pretreatment step within the software to reduce central island formation. The Chiron Technolas and Summit excimer laser systems are the two most frequently used lasers worldwide for LASIK, although many other systems have been utilized including Schwind Keratom II, Nidek EC 5000, CIBA—Autonomous Technologies Corporation Tracker-PRK laser, LaserSight Compak-200 Mini-Excimer, and VisX 20/20. Scanning excimer laser delivery systems do not require pretreatment as they produce minimal acoustic shockwave. Treatment of a central island is fully explained in the next chapter but involves lifting the flap and concentrating the treatment in the area of the topographical island. Compressed air is used to control hydration and care is taken to avoid overcorrection as the degree of undercorrection reduces dramatically with treatment of the central island itself.

CHAPTER 13

LASIK Retreatment Technique and Results

PRINCIPLES OF LASIK RETREATMENT

Although there are a number of retreatment options, there are two primary alternatives: repeating the entire laser in situ keratomileusis (LASIK) procedure with a second microkeratome cut, or lifting the flap and reablating. The microkeratome incision can be performed at the same depth as the original procedure, typically 160 microns or another depth, usually deeper. Other techniques for treating residual myopia and astigmatism include both photorefractive keratectomy (PRK) and radial keratotomy (RK).

> **Retreatment Options**
> - Repeat LASIK at same depth
> - Repeat LASIK at different depth
> - Lifting flap and reablating
> - RK
> - PRK

The advantage of performing a second microkeratome pass is that the procedure dynamics and nomogram remain unchanged. The depth of the second pass is dependent upon the surgeon, with the majority using the identical depth plate. Even with the same depth plate, the previous interface is not usually recut, but several microns away. There may be a theoretical advantage to performing the lamellar dissection 30 microns deeper, as it prevents problems with creating a free lamellar wedge of tissue, which I encountered with one patient 10 weeks postoperatively. The other potential disadvantages are those encountered with the primary LASIK procedure with a flat cornea, subjecting the patient to flap complications once again. Repeat LASIK should be performed after 3 months to allow the original flap to restabilize. If a second lamellar pass is performed too early, the original flap may be damaged with the microkeratome.

Lifting the flap within 6 months is not technically challenging and avoids potential flap complications. LASIK patients appear to stabilize, typically between 1 to 3 months postoperatively, although some patients continue to display a small amount of regression between 3 to 6 months. The primary disadvantages are that the procedure creates an epithelial defect along the flap edge which must heal, increasing the risk of epithelial ingrowth and postoperative discomfort. Following repeat LASIK, the risk of epithelial ingrowth is unchanged and postoperative discomfort remains minimal with recovery.

Combining LASIK with PRK or RK, although effective, adds complexity in that the techniques and nomograms are altered. Performing RK following LASIK requires careful pachymetry to avoid corneal perforation, and requires delaying retreatment by a minimum of 3 months, typically 6 to 9 months, to ensure that the flap is fully adherent and will not move with the formation of incisions. PRK can be performed earlier if a transepithelial approach is utilized, as

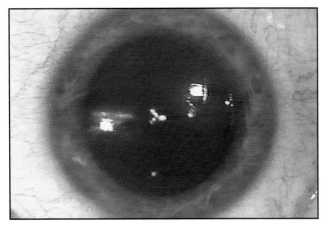

Figure 13-1.
Intraoperative view of prepared right eye for retreatment of residual myopia after primary uncomplicated LASIK procedure 3 months earlier. Centration of eye important.

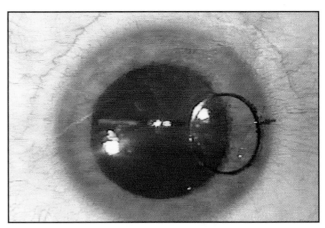

Figure 13-2.
Single circular alignment mark along temporal peripheral cornea is sufficient, as there is no risk of creating a free flap with a lift and reablate retreatment technique.

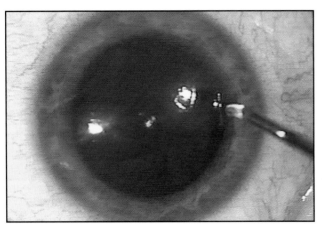

Figure 13-3a.
Intraoperative series of clinical photographs demonstrating preferred LASIK retreatment technique performed 3 to 6 months postoperatively. A repeat LASIK procedure is performed after 6 months or in cases of strong corneal flap adherence. Intraoperative view of LASIK retreatment performed with lift and reablate technique. A Suarez spreader or similar dissector is inserted along the corneal flap edge, which has been marked at the slit lamp biomicroscope pre-operatively.

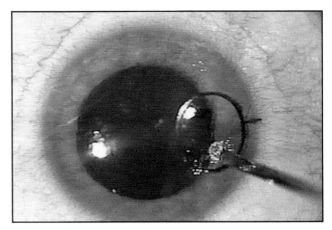

Figure 13-3b.
Once inserted, the spreader is passed in an arcuate fashion along the flap edge.

mechanical debridement may displace the flap, unless retreatment is performed after 3 to 6 months to ensure the flap is secure. In addition, even if PRK is performed 1 year postoperatively and the epithelium is debrided, the stromal surface of the flap is often irregular. PRK is a viable alternative, but introduces the inherent complications and recovery of surface ablation. Patients undergoing PRK enhancement would require months of topical steroids and potentially develop subepithelial haze. RK is preferable in that it avoids the need for topical steroids and is associated with

rapid visual recovery. The nomogram for PRK and RK may well be altered as one combines different procedures.

Therefore, lifting the flap and reablating appears to be the safest procedure for performing LASIK enhancement without introducing a myriad of clinical variables. Any debris or epithelium trapped beneath the epithelium could be cleared and any topographical abnormality addressed while the flap is raised. Surgeons who perform a very high volume of LASIK will feel comfortable in performing all enhancements with a second LASIK procedure, so this option remains at the discretion of the surgeon. The technique for repeat LASIK remains unchanged. My preferred technique for retreatment remains lifting the flap and reablating, which will be described in detail.

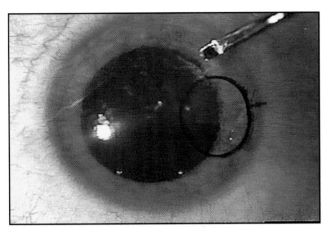

Figure 13-3c.
The greatest adhesion occurs along the resected margin of Bowman's layer. The Suarez spreader is used to free the temporal margin. Once the lamellar plane is determined, dissection of the corneal flap follows easily.

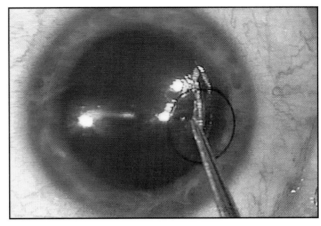

Figure 13-3d.
Fine forceps are used to lift the temporal flap edge, which has been dissected.

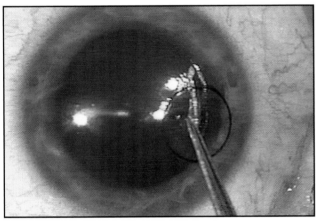

Figure 13-3e.
It is important to raise the flap both slowly and carefully, as focal areas of strong adherence may occasionally be encountered.

TECHNIQUE OF LASIK RETREATMENT

Patients should be taken to the biomicroscopic slit-lamp and the edge of the flap marked with fine forceps for 1 to 2 clock hours. The reason for this maneuver is that the flap edge is difficult to discern once the patient is beneath the surgical microscope (Figure 13-1).

The patient should then be aligned beneath the microscope and the lid speculum inserted as for any primary procedure, once prepped and anesthetized. Once again, it is important to anesthetize the fornices with an anesthetic-soaked spear.

A single circular optical zone marker with gentian violet can be placed temporally, encompassing the flap and

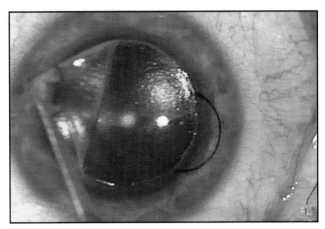

Figure 13-3f.
Adhesion of the central flap to the stromal bed is minimal, especially if the flap is elevated before 3 months. After 6 months, although usually possible, it is easier to repeat the lamellar resection as was performed for the primary procedure.

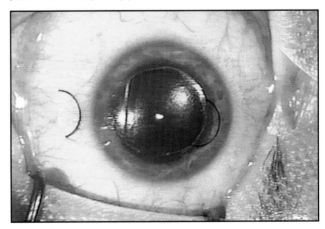

Figure 13-3g.
The corneal flap is reflected back to expose the stromal bed for reablation. It is important not to allow excess tears to accumulate nasally and swell the flap.

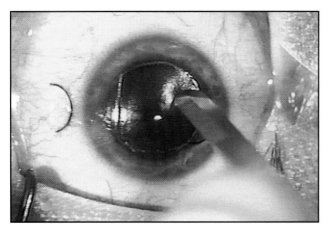

Figure 13-4a.
Intraoperative photograph demonstrating cleaning of epithelial debris from stromal bed margins with sharp blade.

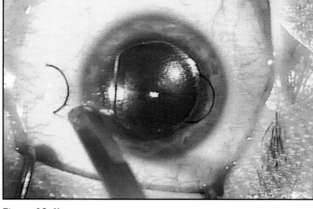

Figure 13-4b.
Intraoperative photograph demonstrating cleaning of epithelial debris from corneal flap margins with sharp blade.

peripheral cornea. A double ring is not required as there is no risk of obtaining a free flap, and a single ring is sufficient for cap alignment (Figure 13-2).

A Suarez spreader or similar instrument is then inserted within the interface at the demarcated flap edge. The marking helps delineate the point of entry into the interface, reducing the trauma to the surrounding epithelium. Once the flap interface is identified, the spreader is passed along the flap edge circumferentially. The primary site of flap adhesion is along the cut edge of Bowman's peripherally. It is along this peripheral 1 mm that the spreader must separate the flap and stromal bed. The tip of the spreader should be pulled along the flap edge peripherally and centrifugally to avoid inserting epithelium beneath the flap (Figures 13-3a through 13-3g). Depending on how early postoperatively that the flap is lifted, the most temporal edge of the flap can be grasped with non-toothed forceps and reflected back without any dissection. This should only be attempted if no resistance is encountered, and should be performed slowly.

The strength of the adhesion peripherally is highly dependent upon the amount of time passed since the primary procedure was performed, and the patient wound healing characteristics. Once the flap edge is opened, the adhesion centrally is virtually non-existent within the first 3 months and the flap is easily lifted. In specific patients with aggressive wound healing characteristics, and patients retreated after several months, the adhesion of the central flap may be greater. In those cases, a spatula or blunt edge of forceps can be used to gently dissect the established interface and separate the corneal flap and stromal bed. Some surgeons advocate the use of filtered balanced salt solution (BSS) to

dissect the interface, however this alters both the hydration status of the stroma during ablation and the re-adhesion rate. If there is excessive debris, irrigation of the interface may be indicated.

Once the flap is reflected back, care should be taken to ensure that no epithelium has been introduced. A dry surgical spear or preferably a surgical blade can be used to debride the peripheral corneal flap and the peripheral stromal bed (Figures 13-4a and 13-4b). This procedure can be performed before or after the ablation, but should be consistently performed at that point in the procedure to standardize stromal hydration for the reablation nomogram.

The ablation performed is similar to the primary LASIK procedure in that a pretreatment is required and stromal hydration must be controlled. In general, the ablation attempted is planned not only with respect to a cycloplegic refraction, but with respect to both uncorrected visual acuity and topography. For example, the patient may refract at -2.00 D, but the uncorrected vision is in the 20/50 to 20/60 range, indicating that the expected refraction would be -1.00 to -1.25 D. In this example, the attempted correction should be -1.25 D maximally. Topography in this example may demonstrate a small central island, which would account for the disproportionate refraction. In such a case with a central island, additional treatment may be applied centrally or the central stroma dried additionally. Air may be applied during the pretreatment step to increase the efficacy of the central pulses, and between each zone to control intrastromal hydration (Figure 13-5). Alternatively, the stromal bed may be wiped with a spatula or dried with a surgical spear.

Following the ablation, the flap is rehydrated for

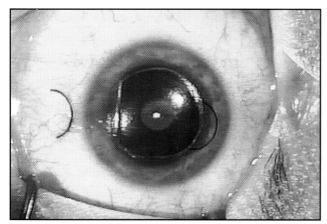

Figure 13-5.
Intraoperative photograph of photoablation technique demonstrating application of low flow air with 3-mm pretreatment to prevent or treat central island formation.

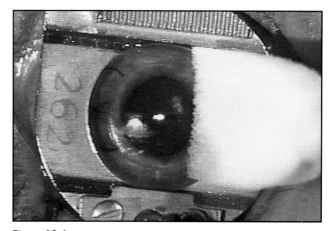

Figure 13-6.
Protection of underface of corneal flap during photoablation when maximal optical zone or toric pattern encroach upon flap hinge.

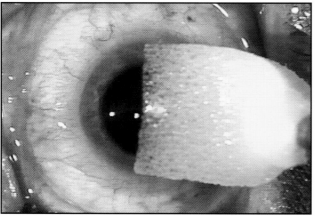

Figure 13-7.
Intraoperative appearance of smoothing the reflected corneal flap back into alignment with a wet, fully expanded surgical spear. Each pass must always be from the nasal aspect toward the temporal aspect, away from the hinge in smooth continuous and deliberate brush strokes. The surgical spear must always be well hydrated to prevent damage to the surface epithelium.

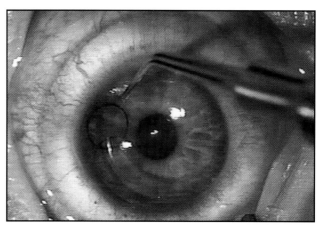

Figure 13-8.
Slade Corneal Striae test for assessment of corneal flap adhesion. The peripheral cornea just external to the corneal flap margin is depressed, generating corneal striae. If the striae extend onto the corneal flap, a relatively good adhesion has already been generated and the eyelid speculum can be removed after an additional 30 to 60 seconds.

replacement, and the stromal bed left dry to enhance flap adhesion or wet to float the cap into position. The principles of the technique are the same as those outlined for the primary LASIK procedure. Filtered BSS is dropped slowly onto the corneal flap and hinge to allow the flap to glide back into position on a fluid wedge to hopefully reduce any irregularities and promote realignment (Figure 13-6). Excess fluid in the fornices is removed with a surgical spear or sponge. Any visible foreign particles or fibers which typically fluoresce with photoablation should be removed prior to flap closure with fine-tipped forceps. A cannula may be inserted beneath the flap and the interface irrigated for sev-

eral seconds to clear debris and residual epithelial cells. Once the corneal flap is closed, surgical spears that have been soaked in BSS are passed temporally from the nasal aspect to aid flap adhesion and repositioning and reduce flap irregularities. Care is taken to ensure adequate reapposition with the circular alignment markings (Figure 13-7).

After 2 to 5 minutes, the corneal flap is tested to ensure adequate adhesion using the striae and lid tests described with respect to primary LASIK procedures (Figure 13-8). Air can be used to help seal the peripheral flap, although this is not mandatory. A dry surgical spear dabbed along the flap edge promotes rapid adhesion without disturbing flap

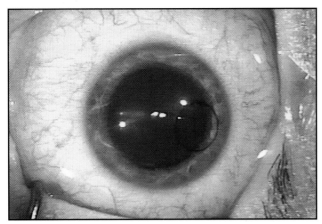

Figure 13-9.
Clinical appearance of corneal flap at conclusion of LASIK retreatment using lift and reablate technique demonstrating restored corneal flap alignment. Eye remains quiet. Occasionally, the epithelium along the corneal flap edge is disrupted considerably, resulting in postoperative pain for several hours.

smoothness.

The postoperative regimen is identical to that following the primary LASIK procedure, with 2 days of rest and copious lubrication in conjunction with 5 to 7 days of a combination topical steroid-antibiotic agent being the cornerstone of the postoperative care (Figure 13-9). It is not uncommon to produce small peripheral epithelial defects along the flap edge, which may create increased discomfort following repeat LASIK when the corneal flap is lifted, compared to a second lamellar cut. A bandage contact lens-topical NSAID combination for 24 to 48 hours is helpful in reducing pain in cases of large defects if necessary.

The surgical plan for LASIK enhancements is based upon videokeratography and cycloplegic refraction. Patients may be dispensed temporary spectacles, or more ideally, disposable contact lenses after 1 to 2 weeks, which can be more easily changed if further regression is observed. It is important to rehabilitate these patients early, as even 1 D of uncorrection in a patient who measured -10.00 D preoperatively will reduce the degree of expected satisfaction and increase apprehension, as postoperative blur and night glare are exacerbated. Most postoperative patients have stabilized within 1 to 3 months following LASIK. There is a balance between performing the enhancement early to simplify raising the corneal flap, and delaying the secondary procedure to ensure stability. Two to 3 months following the primary procedure is more than adequate for all but the most severe cases, which may have a more prolonged recovery. Mild to moderate myopes can probably be safely enhanced after 1 to

2 months, and some extreme myopes may require 3 to 6 months to fully stabilize. Since myopic regression rather than hyperopic shift is the rule, premature enhancement will only necessitate an additional procedure.

> **Most postoperative patients have stabilized within 1 to 3 months following LASIK.**

There are various opinions with regards to the total amount of stromal tissue that can be safely removed without compromising the structural integrity and long-term stability of the cornea. In general, there are two approaches: one which involves leaving a minimum absolute amount of corneal tissue, and the other is not exceeding removal of a certain percentage. The absolute minimum amount of total corneal tissue required to ensure corneal stability is stated to be 350 microns, with a stromal bed of not less than 200 microns. Similarly, other surgeons will never ablate more than 50% of the preoperative measured corneal thickness. I personally use a total corneal thickness minimum of 400 microns, which translates directly to a stromal bed thickness of 240 microns, since I always use a standard corneal flap thickness of 160 microns. I believe the 130-micron corneal flaps may increase irregular astigmatism and prolong visual recovery. In fact, I utilize a 180- or 200-micron corneal flap for mild to moderate myopia treatment. Patients with thinner or inadequate corneal thickness following their primary LASIK procedure may be fit with contact lenses or thin glasses.

I tell all my patients that I will perform an enhancement if they desire and are less than or equal to 20/40 uncorrected or -1.00 D or higher once they are stable, unless it is unwise or unsafe. I have each patient initial this statement specifically, as one of my patients remained surprisingly dissatisfied after being reduced from -25.00 to -3.00 D with a 380-micron residual corneal thickness. The patient

> **I routinely attempt to leave 400 microns of corneal tissue to provide a greater comfort zone for patient and surgeon alike.**

regressed from plano on day 1 and could not understand why I could not retreat him, despite having this specific discussion prior to surgery. Other refractive surgery options such as PRK and RK are viable, but may also destabilize the cornea. I routinely attempt to leave 400 microns of corneal

The Martines Enhancement Technique for Correcting Residual Myopia Following LASIK

Eduardo Martines, MD, and Maurice John, MD

LASIK was developed in its present "Flap & Zap" form by Pallikaris[1-3] in 1991 and has rapidly gained popularity abroad as a procedure for correcting both moderate and severe levels of myopia.[4] In this procedure, a partial lamellar dissection is followed by in situ photoablation of the stromal bed before repositioning the flap back.

Buratto[5-8] described another laser-assisted keratomileusis technique in which the excimer was used to photoablate the posterior surface of the cap following a complete lamellar dissection. By combining the most advantageous aspects of ALK and PRK, higher levels of myopia may be quite accurately corrected while avoiding the haze associated with PRK. Bowman's layer is left intact. LASIK is highly effective. Visual recovery is swift and there is significantly less pain than with a PRK procedure. This results in fewer postoperative drops and much easier postoperative management.

Reported predictability of LASIK has been promising. Nevertheless, as with any refractive procedure, enhancement will be indicated in some cases. One of the advantages of the LASIK procedure is that a repeat procedure may be readily and accurately performed.

For several years, we have carried out some joint studies of LASIK, more recently at the Instituto de Oftalmologia in Sao Paulo, Brazil. I (EM) developed a laser enhancement technique for undercorrected LASIK cases, which was first done in April 1992. The visual and refractive results of 14 laser-enhanced LASIK cases, using the Martines technique, are reported herein.

MATERIALS AND METHODS

All patients who received laser enhancements to correct residual myopia following a LASIK procedure were evaluated. Initially, only patients with larger levels of residual post-LASIK myopia were enhanced. Subsequent good results led us to offer enhancement procedures to patients with lower levels of residual myopia. Refractive and visual data prior to the primary LASIK procedure were abstracted from the medical chart along with the final pre-enhancement data. Following enhancement, patients were seen at 1 day, 1 week, 1 month, 3 months, and 6 months postoperatively. Thereafter, patients were asked to

return at yearly intervals. A Summit ExciMed UV 200 laser was utilized. Data were abstracted onto case report forms and entered into a statistical software package[9] for tabulation.

Surgical Technique

The Martines enhancement technique is based on the residual myopia with adjustments for the Summit gelatin calibration numbers and the vertex distance. Laser enhancement of undercorrected LASIK should not be done prior to 3 months after the primary LASIK procedure. Prior to surgery, the cornea is marked at the slit lamp wherever the exact point is on the original microkeratome cut. This is done due to the difficulty in finding the surgical plane through a surgical microscope. Under topical anesthesia, a cyclodialysis spatula is used to locate the plane and to dissect open the cap. Because of the irregular surface, some patients will complain of difficulty in seeing the fixation light. Therefore, the surgeon may need to hold the eye steady with forceps to keep the eye centered. Prior to beginning the surgery, the gelatin block has been tested with the laser according to standard Summit protocol. Depending on how the gelatin responds, and adjusted for the vertex distance, 60% and 80% of the intended correction is programmed into the laser according to the enhancement plan shown in Table A-1. One case received a multiple zone ablation. Generally, the photoablation is the simplest part of the procedure. After completion of the ablation, the bed is irrigated with BSS, the cap is replaced, and the edges are dried. After about 4 minutes the case is completed.

TABLE A-1 PRELIMINARY ENHANCEMENT PLAN	
Residual Myopia	**Percent of Intended Correction Programmed**
<-3.0 D	80%
-3 to -6 D	70%
>-6 D	60%

TABLE A-2
PATIENT DATA

Case/ Eye	Sex	Age	Last Exam	Pre-LASIK Myopia	Pre-LASIK VAcc	Pre-Enh VAsc	Pre-Enh VAcc	Residual Pre-Enh Myopia	Final Spherical Equivalent	Final VAsc	Final VAcc
1	M	28	2 years	-11.50	20/30	20/60	20/25	-3.00	-1.00	20/30	20/25
2	M	23	2 years	-20.25	20/100	20/400	20/70	-10.50	0.00	20/50	20/50
3	F	32	2 years	-19.00	20/40	20/80	20/30	-3.88	-1.12	20/40	20/25
4	F	22	2 years	-18.75	20/30	20/100	20/40	-6.75	0.00	20/50	20/40
5	F	28	2 years	-14.25	20/25	20/400	20/30	-5.75	-1.25	20/100	20/40
6	F	29	2 years	-17.25	20/70	20/200	20/50	-5.75	-0.88	20/60	20/40
7	F	35	2 years	-11.62	20/40	20/200	20/50	-4.50	0.75	20/60	20/50
8	F	22	6 months	-8.50	20/20	20/40	20/25	-1.50	-0.75	20/30	20/25
9	M	21	6 months	-25.62	20/80	20/200	20/60	-8.25	-1.25	20/80	20/70
10	F	22	6 months	-14.50	20/30	20/50	20/30	-3.00	-1.00	20/30	20/25
11	F	21	6 months	-13.12	20/30	20/60	20/25	-2.62	0.00	20/30	20/30
12	F	25	6 months	-11.50	20/50	20/70	20/50	-2.75	-0.25	20/50	20/50
13	F	29	6 months	-9.12	20/20	20/50	20/20	-2.25	0.50	20/20	20/20
14	F	38	6 months	-9.75	20/30	20/70	20/20	-2.25	-0.38	20/20	20/20

RESULTS

From April 1992 through August 1995, 297 LASIK procedures were performed. Intended corrections ranged from 8 to 24 D of myopia. Since April 1993, 14 (5%) have been enhanced using the Martines technique. All 14 cases have been followed for at least 6 months; 7 cases (50%) have been followed for 2 years. Patients were 21 to 38 years of age (mean=27 years) and 11 of the 14 were females.

Refractive and visual data prior to the primary LASIK procedure, just prior to enhancement, and at the final examination are listed in Table A-2. Mean pre-LASIK myopia was -14.6 D (SD=49). Residual mean myopia for these patients was -4.5 D (SD=2.6) ranging from -1.5 to -10.5 D. Mean spherical equivalent was -0.28 D at 3 months postoperatively and -0.22 D at 6 months postoperatively. The first seven cases were followed for 2 years. Mean spherical equivalent at 2 years for these cases was -0.50 D (SD=0.28). However, this mildly more myopic mean is attributable to the fact that these earlier cases with longer follow-up were those with higher residual myopia following the primary LASIK procedure. Mean post-LASIK residual myopia for these seven cases was -5.73, which was higher than that for the group as a whole. Mean post-LASIK residual myopia for the last seven cases was -3.23 D. In these more recent cases, the surgeons were more willing to operate on lower levels of myopia.

All cases were targeted for plano refractions. Mean deviation from target was -0.65 D. Eleven of the 14 cases (78%) were with 1 D of target and all cases were within 1.25 D. Only two cases were at all overcorrected: one at +0.5 D and the other at +0.75 D.

Uncorrected vision was substantially improved in all cases. Fifty percent of cases had uncorrected vision 20/40 or better; median uncorrected vision was 20/30 with a mean improvement of three and a half lines of vision.

Best corrected vision was 20/25 or better in six of the 14 cases (43%) and 20/40 or better in 10 cases (71%) at the final visit. All patients had either improved or remained within one line of the pre-enhancement best corrected vision. However, one case went from 20/25 pre-LASIK to 20/30 pre-enhancement, and 20/40 at the final visit at 2 years. Three-month topography on this patient showed an irregular, mildly decentered ablation. This patient had started with -14.25 D of myopia and was improved to -5.25 D prior to enhancement and -1.25 D at 2 years following enhancement. Nevertheless, uncorrected visual acuity was improved from 20/400 before enhancement to 20/100 at 2 years.

There were no other surgical complications among these 14 cases and no postoperative complications. The quality of vision has been good except for one patient who occasionally saw mild ghost images at night.

DISCUSSION

Laser enhancement of undercorrected LASIK cases is efficacious. All patients had substantially improved refractions and uncorrected visions. Best corrected visual acuity was not compromised in 13 of the cases. However, the occurrence of a decentered ablation did not result in a 20/40 best corrected vision after the enhancement in one case. The patient had lost a single line (20/25 to 20/30) after the original LASIK procedure. The loss of an additional line of vision following enhancement was troubling, despite the great improvement in uncorrected visual acuity. Enhancing refractive procedures should always be considered in terms of the benefit to risk ratio of improving uncorrected vision vs. compromising best corrected vision. Technique is important here; during the enhancing ablation, some patients experience difficulty in fixating. The surgeon should be cognizant of this potential problem and use forceps to steady the eye.

The Martines plan using the residual myopia level adjusted for vertex distance and calibration numbers, then programming a percent as the ablation target, has worked quite well. The procedure has been predictable in our hands with all patients within 1.25 D of the target refraction and 11 of 14 within 1 D.

In the current refractive surgery environment, there are suddenly several options which may be offered to a patient both for the primary procedure and to enhance and optimize the refractive and visual outcome. Patients with higher levels of myopia may now expect better results. In our opinion, LASIK is an effective procedure for moderate and severe myopes, and any undercorrected patients may be enhanced quite readily and predictably using this technique to obtain the best outcome possible.

References

1. Pallikaris IG, Siganos DS. Excimer laser in situ keratomileusis and photorefractive keratectomy for correction of high myopia. *J Refract Corneal Surg.* 1994;10:498-510.

2. Pallikaris IG, Papatzanaki M, Stathi EZ, Frenschock O, Georgiadis A. Laser in situ keratomileusis. *Lasers Surg Med.* 1990;10:463-468.

3. Pallikaris IG, Papatzanaki ME, Siganos DS, Tsilimbaris MK. A corneal flap technique for laser in situ keratomileusis. *Arch Ophthalmol.* 1991;145:1699-1702.

4. Salah T, Waring GO, El-Maghraby A, Slade SG, Updegraff SA, Brint S. Excimer laser keratomileusis. In: Salz JJ, McDonnell PJ, McDonald MB, eds. *Corneal Laser Surgery.* St. Louis, Mo: Mosby; 1995.

5. Buratto L, Ferrari M, Rama P. Excimer laser instrastomal keratomileusis. *Am J Ophthalmol.* 1991;113:291-295.

6. Buratto L, Ferrari M. Excimer laser instrastromal keratomileusis: case reports. *J Cataract Refract Surg.* 1992;18:37-41.

7. Buratto L, Ferrari M, Genisi C. Myopic keratomileusis with the excimer laser: one year follow-up. *Refract Corneal Surg.* 1993;9:12-19.

8. Buratto L, Ferrari M, Genisi C. Keratomileusis for myopia with the excimer laser (Buratto Technique): short term results. *J Corneal Refract Surg.* 1993;9(Suppl):5130-5133.

9. *Statmost version 2.5 for Windows.* Salt Lake City, Utah: Datamost Corp: 1994-1995.

tissue to provide a greater comfort zone for patient and surgeon alike. Ultrasonic pachymetry and a thorough discussion of possible endpoint correction is mandatory in all severe and extreme myopes. One fear is that the intrastromal ablation of excessive tissue will result in a destabilized cornea with progressive ectasia. There is the potential that most regression in extreme myopes is related to posterior corneal ectasia (Assil).

TREATMENT OF LASIK OVERCORRECTION

The management of the overcorrected LASIK patient presents additional challenges, as the nomogram for hyperopic LASIK is still evolving. The primary problem with hyperopic PRK programs is regression, which is dramatically minimized by intrastromal correction, but the algorithms are still being developed and refined for routine use. In addition, placing a hyperopic ablation pattern over a prior myopic ablation pattern may not only reduce the refractive predictability, but increase the amount of irregular astigmatism encountered. Even a phototherapeutic keratectomy (PTK) at 6 mm or larger will induce a central island in the stromal bed and reduce hyperopia. The strategy in the near future will be hyperopic LASIK, but holmium:YAG thermokeratoplasty may well be the likely short-term solution and presents us with new possibilities for hyperopic correction in general (Figure 13-10). Laser thermokeratoplasty (LTK) is discussed in detail Chapter 4.

Figure 13-10.
Sunrise holmium LTK for LASIK overcorrection.

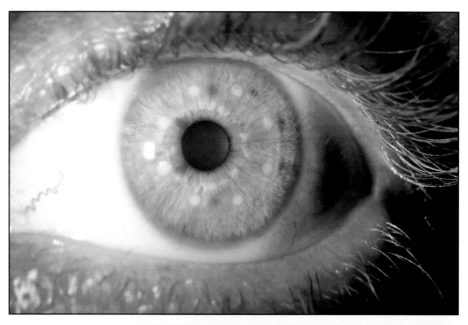

Figure 13-11.
Single LTK ring with Sunrise holmium laser for +1.25 D of overcorrection following LASIK for -8.00 D in a 52-year-old man 7 months postoperatively.

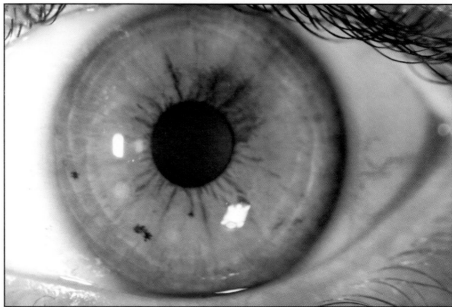

LTK has an increased effect in patients who have been treated with PRK. The possible mechanisms for the increased effect are:

- Thinner cornea
- Absence of Bowman's layer
- A combination effect

A cornea that has been treated with LASIK is not only thinner in the true sense, but has an interface separating the anterior one third from the posterior two thirds. The interface also allows for a separation of the posterior two thirds from Bowman's layer, which may reduce the resiliency of the cornea to return to its natural contour. Nonetheless, most LASIK overcorrections are in the +1.00 to +2.00 D range and are amenable to the Sunrise holmium non-contact LTK system. Patients should be treated after 6 months to ensure an adequate flap healing time has passed (Figure 13-11). The theoretical risk of an LTK application prior to adequate healing is contraction of the anterior corneal flap without a concomitant reaction by the posterior stroma, resulting in irregular astigmatism. Clinically, in the handful of patients treated for hyperopic overcorrections post-LASIK, no corneal flap irregularities were produced after

> Most LASIK overcorrections are in the +1.00 to +2.00 D range and are amenable to the Sunrise holmium non-contact LTK system. Patients should be treated after 6 months to ensure an adequate flap healing time has passed.

allowing several months of healing.

Treatment should be titrated, as an increased effect may be experienced with 1 LTK ring at 7 mm providing approximately 1.00 to 1.50 D of steepening effect. Cylinder can be treated with a four-spot application along the minus cylinder axis at 6 to 7 mm. The pulse energy is 220 to 240 mJ/cm^2 and five to eight pulses per LTK ring application programmed. Cylinder treatment is less predictable.

One theoretical and untested extension of this application is to perform LTK following LASIK beneath the corneal flap to increase the range of hyperopia correctable in congenital hyperopia. That is, creating a corneal flap at 160-

> The stability of thermokeratoplasty is typically poor, as collagen fiber contraction reverses with time.

micron depth without myopic photoablation to potentially increase the hyperopic corrective effect in holmium:YAG LTK candidates. Contrary to automated lamellar keratoplasty (ALK) for hyperopia, where a lamellar incision is made at an approximate depth of 70% to produce what is presumably "controlled ectasia" of the posterior cornea, corneal stability would remain excellent. An overall corneal steepening effect would occur as a result of the LTK application and not ectasia of the posterior cornea. The risk associated with

hyperopic ALK procedures of producing iatrogenic keratoconus because of cuts at depths beyond 80% are avoided, as depths are limited to 30%. The effect of performing LTK on the peripheral stromal bed may well be dramatic for the correction of very severe hyperopia, as the posterior corneal thickness is far reduced and Bowman's layer is altogether avoided. A greater risk to the endothelium and Descemet's membrane may be incurred, and this aspect will have to be investigated and the nomogram and energy levels adjusted. The stability of thermokeratoplasty is typically poor, as collagen fiber contraction reverses with time. The impact of having an intact and undisturbed Bowman's layer overlying the treated posterior stroma may well have a stabilizing effect as the flap becomes adherent.

RETREATMENT CONCLUSION

In conclusion, retreatment to improve refractive predictability can be performed with a variety of techniques, including a repeat performance of the initial LASIK procedure and alternatively, lifting the flap and reablating. Lifting the corneal flap between 3 and 6 months is not technically difficult, but repeating LASIK with a 180- or 200-micron corneal flap may become the preferred technique when surgical experience is gained. Repeat ablation is planned with the help of videokeratography to determine whether adequate central treatment and optical zone size were achieved, or compensation should be made during repeat ablation. That is, the ablation can be adjusted to improve not only quantitative vision with respect to refractive error, but qualitative vision with respect to induced topography. Correction of other non-refractive indications for retreatment such as epithelial implantation and ingrowth were discussed in Chapter 12.

CHAPTER 14

LASIK Clinical Issues and Results

The clinical results of laser in situ keratomileusis (LASIK) are impressive, but despite the dramatic reduction of wound healing effects and the precision of excimer laser technology, corneal hydration continues to have a significant impact upon clinical results. The control of stromal hydration and the development of specific LASIK nomograms will likely enable the highest level of refractive predictability possible with the least risk of adverse effects. Further development of the microkeratome will reduce the risk of serious complications. As our understanding into LASIK expands, our results will improve. Although more technically challenging than photorefractive keratectomy (PRK), the rapid and virtually painless visual rehabilitation combined with reduced risk of stromal scarring, infection, and topical steroid complications will allow LASIK to develop as the predominant refractive procedure of the next decade.

Clinical results are most accurate for lower degrees of spherical myopia, as was true for PRK. The primary difference between PRK and LASIK clinical results are that the significant fall-off in refractive predictability begins to occur around -6.00 D for PRK, but above the -10.00 to -12.00 D range for LASIK. Although the refractive envelope of PRK may extend from -1.00 to -15.00 D, with even -20.00 D corrections possible, the predictability and complication rate beyond -9.00 D clearly make LASIK preferable. The LASIK refractive envelope is far more encompassing, extending from -1.00 to -25.00 D with corrections up to -35.00 D possible. It always must be understood that simply because a procedure has certain refractive capabilities, it need not make it the procedure of choice, or even a viable procedure at that range. Radial keratotomy (RK) is highly effective for mild to moderate myopia, but increasing the number of incisions and decreasing the surgical optical zone for the treatment of higher degrees of myopia only serves to reduce corneal stability and invite complications. Additionally, PRK for extreme myopia can no longer be considered the standard of care. Although PRK is effective in the majority of these highly myopic candidates, the risk of complications, slower recovery, and dependence upon topical steroid usage define LASIK as the procedure of choice. Conversely, LASIK for -1.00 or -2.00 D invites potentially serious complications relative to RK and PRK, and, in my opinion, cannot be considered the procedure of choice at this end of the refractive spectrum in my opinion. The lower range of the LASIK envelope is therefore artificially limited to -4.00 D by most surgeons. That is, there is no single refractive procedure which can be all-encompassing, but rather a number of refractive tools must be available and combined to maximize clinical results while minimizing potential adverse effects and complications. I personally combine astigmatic keratotomy (AK), PRK, LASIK, and holmium:YAG LTK to provide a wide range of refractive options for potential candidates. In addition, and perhaps most importantly, I offer patients time for technology to improve, avoiding surgery for those I believe are beyond the scope of my armamentarium. As refractive surgeons, we constantly focus on providing refractive solutions for our patients, but simply because a patient is +6.00 or -30.00 D with reduced corneal thickness does not mean we possess the necessary techniques or technology at present.

> The primary difference between PRK and LASIK clinical results are that the significant fall-off in refractive predictability begins to occur around -6.00 D for PRK, but above the -10.00 to -12.00 D range for LASIK.

> The LASIK refractive envelope is far more encompassing, extending from -1.00 to -25.00 D.

> PRK for extreme myopia can no longer be considered the standard of care.

MILD MYOPIA

The clinical results of mild myopia are equivalent to those of PRK in most published and unpublished series, with the overwhelming majority of patients achieving near emmetropia with a single procedure. All but two low LASIK myopia treatments below -3.00 D in our series were performed for enhancing previous LASIK procedures for higher degrees of myopia. The two primary cases were one patient with known keloid formation, and one eye for monovision in a schoolteacher with rheumatoid arthritis. For the 59 residual myopia cases between -1.00 and -3.00 D, 100% (61/61) of patients achieved better than 20/40 uncorrected visual acuity and 64% (39/61) achieved 20/25 or better. Visual recovery is most rapid for this group of candidates, with excellent preservation of best corrected vision. Although corneal flap problems occur in roughly 0.2% of procedures and epithelial implantation with stromal melt in approximately the same percentage, overall I feel PRK and RK remain the procedures of choice for congenital myopia under -3.00 D (Table 14-1).

MODERATE MYOPIA

LASIK correction of moderate myopia between -3.10 and -6.00 D is highly effective, with 94% (31/33) of eyes measuring 20/40 or better uncorrected after one procedure, with roughly half (18/33) reading 20/25 or better. The retreatment was performed in three patients or 9% (3/33), with one patient achieving a final visual result of 20/30 and both others attaining 20/25 uncorrected visual acuity. All three patients who needed retreatment required correction of cylinder greater than 1.00 D in combination with moderate myopia. With one or more procedures, 100% of patients with moderate myopia treated with spherical and toric abla-

TABLE 14-1
MACHAT LASIK VISUAL AND REFRACTIVE RESULTS

	<-3.00 D	-3.10 to -6.00 D	-6.10 to -9.00 D	-9.10 to -15.00 D	-15.10 to -30.00 D
n=561 primary	61 (2 primary, 59 secondary)	33	250	228	48
Cylinder cyl>1.25 D (#)	10% (6)	31% (10)	52% (130)	54% (123)	69% (33)
20/25 or equivalent (#)	64% (39)	55% (18)	42% (105)	22% (50)	0%
20/40 or equivalent (#)	100% (61)	94% (31)	78% (195)	65% (148)	23% (11)
Percent of retreatments that achieve 20/40 or better	—	100%, n=3	100%, n=26	89%, n=36	66%, n=9
Loss of best corrected visual acuity after 6 months of two or more lines	0% (0)	0% (0)	1.2% (3)	2.2% (5)	4.2% (2)

tions achieved 20/40 or better unaided visual acuity with the majority distributed within one line of 20/20. Moderate myopes benefited from a rapid visual recovery, without long-term steroid usage and with no patient losing two lines of best corrected vision.

SEVERE MYOPIA

The correction of severe myopia (-6.10 to -9.00 D) with LASIK provides not only more rapid visual rehabilitation, but more stable results. Uncorrected visual acuities of 20/40 and 20/25 were achieved in 78% (195/250) and 42% (105/250), respectively. Retreatment was performed in approximately 10% (26/250) and improved refractive results dramatically, with 100% (26/26) reading 20/40 or better uncorrected. The reduced need for topical steroid therapy is important, as PRK steroid requirements and complications are increased for this highly myopic population. Severe myopes continue to do almost equally well compared to lower myopes in direct contrast to PRK and RK. Night glare is more prevalent in this group, as spherical aberration is more pronounced. Central islands are encountered with increased frequency when larger ablation zones are introduced to compensate for poor night vision and halos. Visual recovery is still quite rapid. Loss of best corrected vision of two lines or greater occurred in just over 1% (3/250) of patients in our series (see Table 14-1).

EXTREME MYOPIA

The treatment of extreme myopia greater than -9.00 D presents new challenges, as ablation algorithms are evolving and the influence of stromal hydration increases in direct proportion to attempted correction. An increasing number of these extremely myopic candidates will require retreatment, which is directly dependent upon the severity of the prescription. In general, a small undercorrection of 1.00 to 3.00 D is typically observed between -9.00 and -15.00 D of attempted correction, with 4.00 to 8.00 D of undercorrection observed between -15.00 and -30.00 D. Since residual myopia is much more easily managed than consecutive hyperopia, and since retreatment of residual myopia is quite accurate, it is best not to be overly aggressive in the treatment of extreme myopia. It is not uncommon to record near plano refractions with excellent uncorrected vision on the first postoperative day, only to observe myopic regression within

the first 1 to 2 weeks. The cause of myopic regression in these patients is unclear. The possible mechanisms for myopic regression include:

- Alteration of the postoperative stromal hydration status
- Epithelial hyperplasia in response to an excessively flattened corneal curvature
- Stromal remodeling

As the stromal bed is dried intraoperatively with air, a surgical spear, or through evaporation and ablation, there may well be some re-establishment of natural state hydration in the immediate postoperative period to account for the rapid initial myopic regression observed. Epithelial and stromal wound healing are the mechanisms known to produce PRK regression of effect and likely play some role, although much more limited. Even with RK, epithelial hyperplasia can occur in response to an altered corneal contour. LASIK for extreme myopia can produce corneal flattening with measured keratometry in the 31.00 to 37.00 D range, with a mean of 34.50 D. This profound flattening can induce epithelial hyperplasia, and clinical studies to examine alterations in epithelial thickness are underway. Although the deeper stroma is stated to be inert, some patients treated for higher attempted corrections with more aggressive wound healing patterns exhibit haze or fibrosis within the interface. Myopic regression is likely associated with a wound healing reaction at the level of the interface.

The percentage of extreme myopes achieving 20/40 or better visual acuity is always somewhat misleading, as many of these patients had reduced best corrected vision preoperatively. A more useful equivalent measure is the percentage of patients achieving an uncorrected visual acuity within three lines of their best corrected vision. For patients with preoperative myopia greater than -9.00 D but less than -15.00 D, 65% (148/228) achieved 20/40 or equivalent with one procedure, and of those patients that were retreated, 89% (32/36) achieved that same level of uncorrected visual acuity. Only 22% (50/228) achieved 20/25 or equivalent uncorrected visual acuity.

The most impressive and long-term clinical result I have achieved in high myopia is reducing a patient from -27.00 to -4.00 D bilaterally, followed by bilateral enhancement procedures which further reduced the residual refractive error to -0.75 D bilaterally. Best corrected visual acuity increased by one line and stability has been remarkably good with no regression observed over several months following retreatment. I have treated several patients between -25.00 and -30.00 D, with all patients requiring retreatment for 3.00 to

LASIK Clinical Results

Enrique Suarez Cabrera, MD

Between February and August 1995, 1460 eyes were treated with LASIK for various degrees of ametropia, which are divided into five groups for statistical analysis based upon their preoperative refractive error. Minimum follow-up was 3 months and clinical results were based upon assessment as of the last examination.

- **Group I:** **EKM**
  Spherical myopia (cylinder 0.50 D or less), n=332 eyes (Figures A-1a through A-1d)
- **Group II:** **EKMA**
  Myopic astigmatism (cylinder 0.75 D or more), n=666

eyes (Figures A-2a through A-2e)
- **Group III:** **EKH**
  Spherical hyperopia (cylinder 0.50 D or less), n=109 eyes (Figures A-3a through A-3c)
- **Group IV:** **EKAH**
  Hyperopic astigmatism (cylinder 0.75 D or more), n=140 eyes (Figures A-4a through A-4e)
- **Group V:** **EKA**
  Astigmatism (myopic), n=213 eyes (Figures A-5a through A-5e)

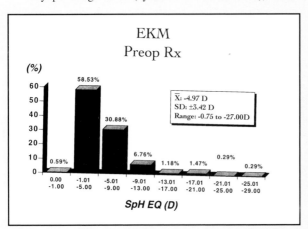

Figure A-1a.
Group I: preoperative refraction for spherical myopia.

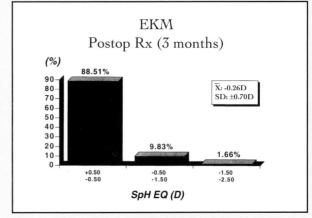

Figure A-1b.
Group I: postoperative refraction for spherical myopia.

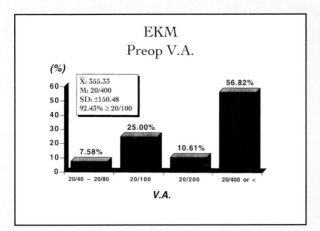

Figure A-1c.
Group I: preoperative uncorrected visual acuity for spherical myopia.

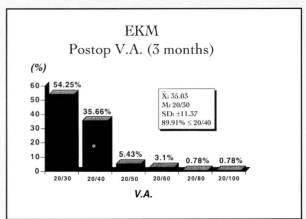

Figure A-1d.
Group I: postoperative uncorrected visual acuity for spherical myopia.

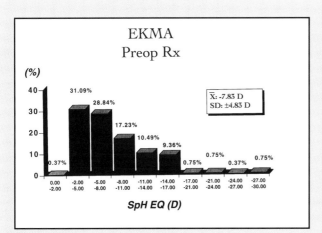

Figure A-2a.
Group II: preoperative refraction for myopic astigmatism.

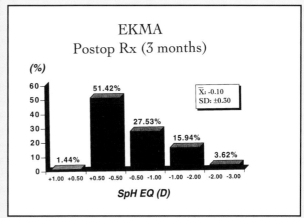

Figure A-2b.
Group II: postoperative refraction for myopic astigmatism.

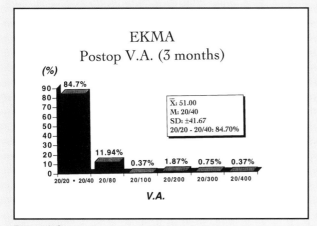

Figure A-2c.
Group II: postoperative uncorrected visual acuity for myopic astigmatism.

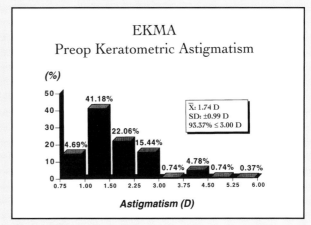

Figure A-2d.
Group II: preoperative keratometric astigmatism for myopic astigmatism.

INSTRUMENTATION

The Chiron Automated microkeratome Coherent-Schwind Keratom II excimer laser was used.

TECHNIQUE

Under topical anesthesia, partial resection of an anterior stromal flap, 8.5 mm in diameter and 130 to 160 microns in thickness, is carried out using the microkeratome. The flap remains adherent along the nasal margin hinge, measuring no greater than 30° in arc length. Following eversion of the flap, mid-stromal surface ablation is performed with the laser. For hyperopic corrections, an annular ablation pattern is performed, beginning at an optical zone periphery which varies between 5.0 to 6.0 mm in diameter, and ablating centrally. Once the laser

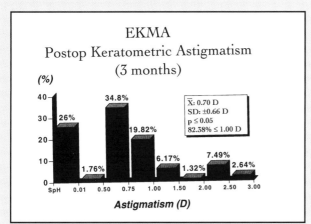

Figure A-2e.
Group II: postoperative keratometric astigmatism for myopic astigmatism.

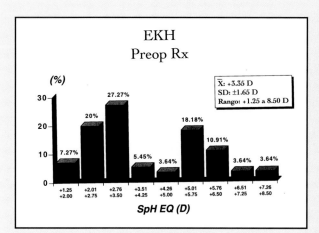

Figure A-3a.
Group III: preoperative refraction for spherical hyperopia.

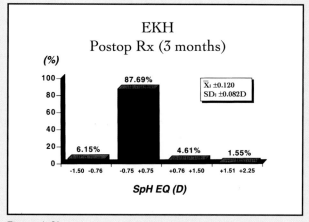

Figure A-3b.
Group III: postoperative refraction for spherical hyperopia.

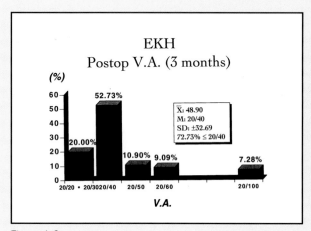

Figure A-3c.
Group III: postoperative visual acuity for spherical hyperopia.

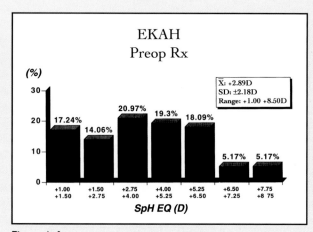

Figure A-4a.
Group IV: preoperative refraction for astigmatic hyperopia.

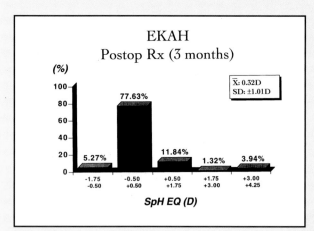

Figure A-4b.
Group IV: postoperative refraction for astigmatic hyperopia.

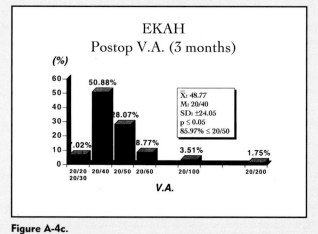

Figure A-4c.
Group IV: postoperative uncorrected visual acuity at 3 months for astigmatic hyperopia.

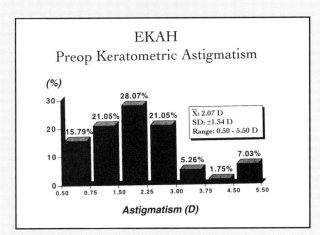

Figure A-4d.
Group IV: preoperative keratometric astigmatism distribution for astigmatic hyperopia.

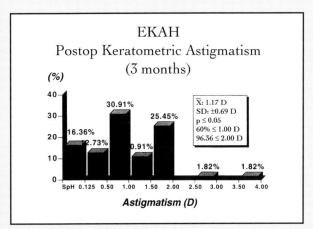

Figure A-4e.
Group IV: postoperative keratometric astigmatism distribution for astigmatic hyperopia.

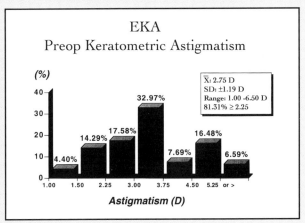

Figure A-5a.
Group V: preoperative keratometric astigmatism.

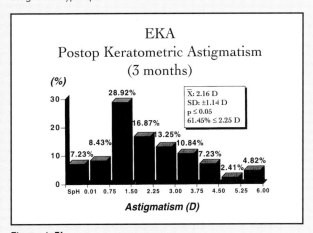

Figure A-5b.
Group V: postoperative keratometric astigmatism.

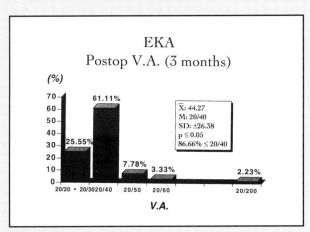

Figure A-5c.
Group V: postoperative uncorrected visual acuity for astigmatism group.

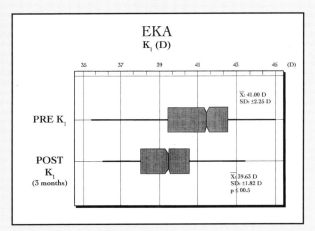

Figure A-5d.
Group V: change in K1 and K2 values with treatment.

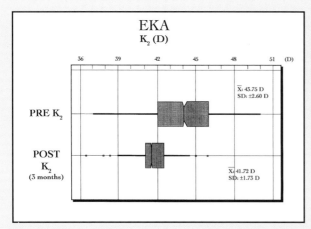

Figure A-5e.
Group V: change in K1 and K2 values with treatment.

photoablation has been completed, the interface is irrigated and the flap is repositioned, secured, and dried using compressed air for a few seconds over the epithelial surface.

POSTOPERATIVE REGIMEN

Eyes were not occluded postoperatively, but an eyeshield is applied for 24 hours. A mixture of gentamicin and betamethasone is used three to four times per day for 1 to 2 weeks.

We have moved away from other refractive techniques for myopia, astigmatism, and hyperopia. While data on long-term safety and stability are lacking, we are becoming increasingly convinced that, due to its broad capability for treating high degrees of all categories of refractive error, fast visual rehabilitation, reduced dependency on wound healing, and low complication incidence, LASIK is now the single most versatile and powerful refractive technique.

5.00 D of residual myopia. Two patients had inadequate corneal thickness (discussed in Chapter 6) to proceed with further surgery. The minimum acceptable total corneal thickness postoperatively is 350 microns or stromal bed thickness of 200 microns, although 380 microns is the minimum residual corneal thickness I have left, with 400 microns being my standard minimum thickness.

ASTIGMATISM

The correction of cylinder is always more challenging with all refractive procedures and is just as true for LASIK as PRK (discussed in Chapter 7). Axis and magnitude of cylinder must be accurately targeted, with errors in axis resulting in a significant reduction of efficacy, both with respect to increased residual cylinder magnitude and the induction of cylinder at a different axis. Any torque applied to the eye during LASIK can therefore be detrimental with respect to achieved refractive results. LASIK, however, is superior to toric PRK in two respects: less regression of effect is observed and haze is not encountered. Photoastigmatic refractive keratectomy (PARK) for the correction of cylinder greater than 3.00 D is associated with an increased incidence of both confluent haze and regression. The correction of higher degrees of cylinder with PRK often requires intensive or prolonged topical steroid therapy. LASIK is the preferred technique for high cylinder correction. I have successfully treated 6.00 D of cylinder with

PRK and 7.50 D of cylinder with LASIK in a single procedure with less than 0.50 D of residual cylinder. Predictability, reproducibility, and stability are superior with LASIK when higher degrees of cylinder are attempted. The production of steep edges intrastromally is not associated with haze and regression, as it is with surface photoablation.

It is possible to combine both PRK and LASIK with AK to correct associated cylinder, but toric ablation patterns allow for the entire refractive error to be corrected in a single step. Postoperative residual cylinder with residual

LASIK, however, is superior to toric PRK in two respects:
- Less regression of effect is observed
- Haze is not encountered

LASIK is the preferred technique for high cylinder correction.

myopia is still best treated with a second toric ablation beneath the corneal flap, but residual cylinder without myopia is best managed with AK. AK is also indicated in postoperative PRK patients with mixed astigmatism. AK can be performed under the corneal flap or after several months once the corneal flap is quite secure. Most surgeons wait 6 to 12 months before performing any incisional procedures on the corneal flap.

Laser-ALK: Results of 202 Cases

Frederic B. Kremer, MD, and Georgietta R. Gdovin, OD

There have been many anecdotal reports and much conjecture concerning LASIK or ALK-E or Laser-K, the refractive procedure that combines the automated microkeratome and the 193-nm excimer laser. But until now, to the best of our knowledge, there have been no well-controlled study results with at least 6 months to 1 year follow-up showing the performance of the procedure in practice. What follows is just such a report, covering the primary treatment of low, medium, and high myopia.

PATIENTS AND METHODS

Under protocol, we performed Laser-K on 202 consecutive eyes of 59 male and 54 female patients in a certified ambulatory surgical center. The mean age of the 113 patients was 37.1 years.

We included eyes with dry-eye syndrome, map-dot-fingerprint dystrophy, and corneal scars, as long as the pathology did not affect best corrected visual acuity. There were no other preexisting corneal diseases and the patients had never undergone a refractive procedure.

Preoperative spherical equivalent refraction ranged from -1.00 to -23.00 D, with a mean spherical equivalent of -6.31 D. Preoperative astigmatism ranged from 0 to +4.75 D, with a mean astigmatic error of +.94 D. Broken into groups, the mean preoperative spherical equivalent refraction ranged from -3.61 D for the low myopia group (-1.00 to -5.00 D), -6.39 D for moderate myopes (-5.01 to -8.00 D), and -11.24 D in the high myopia group (-8.01 to -23.00 D).

Prior to the procedure, we measured uncorrected and best corrected visual acuity and performed manifest and cycloplegic refractions. We performed slit-lamp exams and tested pupillary function and diameter in bright and dim light. We conducted dilated fundus exams, brightness acuity tests, and Schirmer tear tests. We also determined eye dominance and performed keratometry, tonometry, pachymetry, and topography. We made sure patients stopped wearing soft contact lenses 2 weeks prior to surgery and that they discontinued rigid contacts 3 weeks before the operation.

On the day of the procedure, we calibrated the laser and tested beam quality. We prepped each patient with a Betadine lid scrub prior to draping. We then administered topical anesthetic, placed a lid speculum, then simultaneously vacuumed the globe and irrigated it with BSS. The surgeon placed the microkeratome's suction ring on the eye, then used the microkeratome to create a corneal flap 160 microns thick and approximately 8 mm in diameter. The incision started at the temporal side and stopped 90% of the way across, leaving a hinge on the nasal side. The surgeon then swung the cap nasally to expose the stromal bed.

While the patient fixated on a light coaxial with the laser beam, the bed was ablated with a 193-nm wavelength excimer laser, typically using a fluence of about 140 mJ/cm^2.

If there was greater than 0.75 D of astigmatism present, the surgeon placed the astigmatic ablation in a lenticular fashion prior to the myopic one.

When figuring the spherical ablation depth using a computerized algorithm, the depth (figured as the depth of the corneal cap plus the depth of the ablation) was kept to less than one half of corneal thickness. The largest portion of the treatment zone was typically 6 mm. Multizone approaches were used with portions of less than 6 mm, if needed, to keep the maximum depth of ablation at less than one half corneal thickness. We are confident this keeps the endothelium safe, for if the excimer beam does not penetrate 130-micron sections of corneal stromal tissue, as we have demonstrated with a fluence meter, it cannot penetrate 250 microns.

Following the ablation, the surgeon placed the corneal cap in its original position without sutures.

Postoperatively, we fit a clear shield over the eye and had the patient keep it closed for the rest of the day. We instructed patients to wear the shield constantly for the first 24 hours and then only while sleeping throughout the first week. We also prescribed prednisolone acetate 1% twice daily for 1 week and gentamicin four times daily for 1 week.

We scheduled follow-up visits at 1 day, 1 week, 1 month, 3 months, 6 months, and 1 year. We responded to missed visits with a postcard reminder and then by telephone. The surgeon examined all patients postoperatively; however, all measurements were taken by optometrists or ophthalmologists other than the surgeon. We entered all the preoperative, intraoperative, and postoperative data into a computer data base.

THE RESULTS

Patients showed a large immediate reduction in myopia with an initial slight overcorrection at 1 week, which gradually decreased over the next 4 weeks. We also found that the higher the preoperative refractive error, the longer the eye requires to stabilize.

Six months after the first Laser-K procedure, 79% of eyes in the low myopia group, 77.8% of eyes in the moderate myopia group, and 51.1% in the high myopia group achieved a result between +1.00 to -1.00 D of the desired spherical refraction.

The mean spherical equivalent refraction of the patient group dropped from -6.31 D preoperatively to -0.31 D postoperatively. Mean astigmatism dropped from +0.94 to +0.53 D.

Patients who did not fall within ±1 D of the desired result had the option of a second stage Laser-K procedure/enhancement; 17.3% elected to have this done. Broken down by group, 12.9% of those with low myopia, 18.6% of those with moderate myopia, and 24% of those with high myopia eyes underwent enhancements.

After the second procedure, 88.9% of the eyes in the low myopia group, 81.5% in the moderate myopia group, and 74.5% of those in the high myopia group showed a result between +1.00 and -1.00 D of the desired spherical refraction. Uncorrected distance visual acuity was 20/40 or better after all procedures in 97.4% of eyes in the low myopia group, 90.2% in the moderate myopia group, and 83.7% in the high myopia group. These percentages do not include eyes corrected for near (monovision). Of 42 eyes at 1-year follow-up, 47.62% achieved +.50 to -.50 D, 80.95% achieved +1.00 to -1.00 D, and 97.62% achieved +2.00 to -2.00 D.

Complications were minimal. The procedures induced no stromal haze of the type that occurs with PRK. Some patients had minor foreign bodies in the interface, including tear components and lint. However, in no case did the foreign bodies appear to be of clinical significance, and they were absorbed over time. None of the patients in this study exhibited epithelial cells in the interface, but this may occur and needs to be removed in less than 0.5% in our cases. Pain and discomfort were minimal. Ten percent of patients complained about a transient foreign body sensation, and 15% reported transient halos around lights at night. There were no cases of significant irregular astigmatism in this series.

CONCLUSION

In our experience, Laser-K compares very favorably with other refractive surgical procedures.

Postoperatively, we have found that we do not need to prescribe strong pain medications, drops with anesthetic effects, or a bandage contact lens, all of which are typical with PRK. None of the patients sustained postoperative infections, and none required extension of their steroids.

Though PRK is relatively accurate for low myopia, high myopes are much more successful with Laser-K than with PRK. About 51% of the highly myopic eyes in this study achieved +1.00 to -1.00 D residual error after a single procedure. In another study in which patients underwent surface ablation, only 18.8% of high myopes achieved this refractive range. This may be due to the preservation of Bowman's membrane. As mentioned earlier, there is no need for extended use of postoperative steroid drops (needed in PRK). This eliminates the associated risks of cataract formation and glaucoma.

Though RK is relatively accurate for low myopia, Laser-K's benefits, when combined with evolving technological improvements, have led us to choose it over RK for low myopia as well as moderate and high levels. Compared to RK patients, postoperative Laser-K patients are more comfortable and have less of a problem with fluctuations in their vision. Also, the larger optical zones of Laser-K diminish starbursts and halos in dimly lit conditions.

Compared to patients undergoing mechanical ALK, Laser-K patients have better vision at night and less ghosting, possibly due to better centering of the refractive phase of the procedure and a smoother transition at the optical zone effected by the laser. Laser-K is also much more accurate than mechanical ALK, which, in our experience, requires second-stage procedures approximately 40% of the time.

Laser-K's smoother postoperative period and other benefits have made it our procedure of choice for all levels of myopia.

Though our results with this study were very good, we have since updated our computer algorithm and are achieving a higher level of accuracy with Laser-K. Our overall enhancement accuracy has dropped below 10%. With newer algorithms, 90% of eyes with less than -8.00 D of myopia are within 1.00 D of the desired spherical refraction after only one procedure, and more than 70% are within 0.50 D. Refinements in fixation, surgical technique, and technology will undoubtedly further enhance accuracy. Based on our experience with the procedure, we strongly believe Laser-K will be the procedure of choice for both primary and secondary refractive operations. Since we began using Laser-K in 1993, we successfully used it for hyoperia and second-stage procedures following RK, AK, ALK, KM, PRK, Laser-K, PK, cataract extraction, and retinal detachment.

Bibliography

Buratto L, et al. Excimer laser intrastromal keratmileusis. *Am J Ophthalmol.* 1992;113:291-295.

Buratto L, Ferrari M, Genisi C. Myopic keratomileusis with the excimer laser: one year follow-up. *J Refract Corneal Surg.*1993;9:12-19.

Gomes M. Keratomileusis in situ using manual dissection of corneal flap for high myopia. *J Refract Corneal Surg.* 1994;10:255-257.

Kremer FB, Dufek M. Excimer laser in situ keratomileusis. *J Refract Surg.* 1995;11:5244-5247.

Kremer FB, Suscavage P. Radial keratotomy—improved predictability. *Annals of Ophthalmology.* 1992;24:299-302.

McDonald MB, Frantx JM, Klyce SD, et al. Central photorefractive keratectomy for myopia. The blind eye study. *Arch Ophthalmol.* 1990;108:799-808.

Pallikaris IG, Siganos DS. Excimer laser in situ keratomileusis and photorefractive keratectomy for correction of high myopia. *J Refract Corneal Surg.* 1994;10:495-510.

Rogers CM, Lawless MA, Cohen PR. Photorefractive keratectomy for myopia of more than -10 diopters. *J Refract Corneal Surg.* 1994;10:171-173.

Seiler T, Wollensak. Myopic photorefractive keratectomy with excimer laser: one year follow-up. *Ophthalmology.* 1991;98:1156-1163.

Sher NA, et al. 193-nm excimer photorefractive keratectomy in high myopia. *Ophthalmology.* 1994;101:1575-1582.

Slade SG, Brint SF. Excimer laser myopic keratomileusis. In Rozakis G, ed. *Refractive Lamellar Keratoplasty.* Thorofare, NJ: SLACK Inc; 1994.

Tong PP, Kam JT, Lam RH, et al. Excimer laser photorefractive keratectomy for myopia: six-month follow-up. *J Cataract Refract Surg.* 1995;21.

Reprinted with permission from *Review of Ophthalmology*, August 1995.

CYLINDER RESULTS

Associated cylinder of greater than 1.00 D reduces refractive predictability and visual results of LASIK by only 2% to 3%, and appears to have a greater impact on attempted versus achieved results with surface ablation.

Vector analysis improves astigmatism results and produces more comparable spherical PRK and toric PRK visual outcomes with 90% of the spherical equivalent and 90% of the astigmatism corrected in the Melbourne series (see Table 7-1). Irregular epithelial healing, however, was felt to be responsible for much of the variability in astigmatism correction, a problem not encountered with LASIK. Higher degrees of myopia are associated with a greater amount of cylinder correction. It is not uncommon to have 1.50 to 2.00 D of accompanying cylinder in a 10.00 D myope. LASIK is very accurate in cylinder correction in this range, as is PRK, however, the patient with -1.00 -5.00 x 180 is where LASIK truly excels over PRK (Table 14-2) as the steep toric contours are not associated with haze or regression, as they would be in surface ablation and frequent topical steroids are not required. I have been amazed at the ability of LASIK to correct as much as 7.50 D of cylinder in a single treatment in two patients treated bilaterally with as little as 1.50 D of accompanying sphere to as great as 6.50 D.

In general, we have found 88% mean cylinder correction with LASIK, compared with roughly 80% mean cylinder correction with PRK utilizing the same laser system and same toric ablation program. This difference is clinically significant and can be attributed to the reduction in both epithelial and stromal healing encountered with LASIK.

> Advances in excimer laser delivery systems and refinements of PRK techniques have allowed greater PRK predictability within a greater range of myopia with less associated adverse effects.

> LASIK is a marriage of the precision of excimer laser technology with the control of wound healing provided by lamellar surgery techniques.

> All procedures have limitations and risks and the recognition of this statement is the first and last principle of refractive surgery.

Even more importantly, residual cylinder can be easily managed with retreatment.

OVERVIEW

As stated in the beginning of this chapter and this book, excimer laser refractive surgery is a rapidly evolving field which is still in its infancy. It is not so much the clinical results we have achieved, but that we have achieved so much in so little time. It is not the details or the numbers, but the principles and the patterns.

Advancements in excimer laser delivery systems and refinements of PRK techniques have allowed greater PRK predictability within a greater range of myopia with less

TABLE 14-2
COMPARISON OF REFRACTIVE PROCEDURES: RK, PRK, ALK, AND LASIK

	RK	PRK	ALK	LASIK
Range of Correction in 30-Year-Old Male	-1.00 to -6.00 D	-1.00 to -9.00 D	-4.00 to -30.00 D, +1.00 to +4.00 D	-1.00 to -30.00 D, +1.00 to +6.00 D
Corneal Penetration Depth	90% to 95%	10%	30%	30%
Procedure Time	3 to 5 minutes	3 to 5 minutes	10 minutes	5 to 10 minutes
Ocular Integrity	good	excellent	excellent	excellent
Predictability	very good	excellent	good	excellent
Stability	very good	very good	excellent	excellent
Safety	very good	excellent	good	very good
Surgical Skill	moderate	low	very high	high
Patient Procedure Ease	very good	excellent	very good	excellent
Postoperative Pain	low (1%)	moderate (10%)	low (1%)	low (1%)
Patient Recovery Time	1 to 2 days	3 to 4 days	1 to 2 days	1 to 2 days
Visual Rehabilitation	rapid	gradual	rapid	rapid
Enhancement Rate	high	low	high	moderate

associated adverse effects. The limitations of PRK, however, will forever remain those associated with wound healing, pain, infection, slower visual recovery, stromal scarring, and topical steroid dependency. LASIK is a marriage of the precision of excimer laser technology with the control of wound healing provided by lamellar surgery techniques. By leaving the anterior cornea and Bowman's layer intact, epithelial-stromal interaction is avoided and wound healing effects dramatically minimized. Optical performance of the cornea following refractive surgery is often compromised and, although improved with time, is subject to permanent potential alteration. Although all refractive procedures operating on the cornea alter the anterior corneal curvature, intrastromal ablation may allow for improved optical performance through new ablation algorithms, while leaving the anterior corneal structures undisturbed. Controlling wound healing is the greatest hurdle to overcome in achieving linear refractive predictability for all degrees of myopia. The introduction of hydration as yet another poorly understood variable has limited our understanding to date.

LASIK provides equal clinical results to PRK at mild to moderate degrees of myopia, but with the improved visual rehabilitation, commonly observed with RK. For severe degrees of myopia, LASIK and PRK utilizing advanced technology and techniques achieve comparable clinical results but PRK complications such as haze and steroid usage make LASIK the procedure of choice. Further refinements in LASIK nomograms and techniques will produce even better clinical results in the higher degrees of myopia.

Automated lamellar keratoplasty (ALK) is associated with rapid visual recovery, minimal discomfort, and little, if any, need for topical steroids. ALK is highly effective at correcting higher refractive errors but does not parallel the predictability of either LASIK or PRK. LASIK for extreme myopia is the refractive procedure of choice. Clinical results are clearly superior with LASIK compared to all other refractive procedures, with a lower associated incidence of complications. Visual recovery, retreatment rates, and loss of best corrected vision are not as optimal for higher myopes as for lower myopes but are still better than those associated with other refractive procedures.

In reviewing my clinical experience with LASIK and PRK, it is clear that narrowing the standard deviation for refractive predictability for higher degrees of myopia correction remains an ever-present challenge. Those patients who can truly benefit the most are those who we appear to be able to help the least. The observation that we have improved so dramatically in such a short span of time is encouraging and somewhat overwhelming. I explain to all may patients that technology and techniques will improve, but never will I be able to guarantee clinical results or completely prevent complications. No patient needs refractive surgery, although the benefits are in many ways unimaginable. The most important principle that I have learned is instinctual, learning when to simply say no to a potential candidate. All procedures have limitations and risks and the recognition of this statement is the first and last principle of refractive surgery.

Appendices

TLC - THE LASER CENTER INC.

Informed Consent Form for Excimer Laser Photorefractive Keratectomy

Please read the following consent form very carefully. Please initial each page where indicated. Do not sign this form unless you read and understand each page.

PATIENT'S NAME: _____

SURGEON'S NAME: _____

DATE OF PROCEDURE: _____

TREATMENT: (circle) Left Eye Right Eye Both Eyes

Patient Initials_____

SURGEON WILL REVIEW:

SUCCESS RATE FOR 20/ OR BETTER _____%

RETREATMENT RATE _____%

MONOVISION (circle) Yes No Slight

SURGEON COMMENTS:_____

_____

INTRODUCTION:
It is our hope to fully inform you concerning the side effects, limitations, and complications of surgery. We continually struggle to balance the benefits of laser surgery with the known and unknown risks. The first important message to understand is that it is impossible to perform any form of surgery without the patient accepting a certain degree of risk and responsibility.

This consent form in combination with the extensive educational materials provided and the entire consultation procedure is designed to enhance your understanding of the potential for the difficulties which may be encountered during both the procedure and the healing process.

Many of our patients are surprised and some are upset by the extent to which we attempt to inform them of the potential for complications. It is not our intention to frighten or dissuade someone from pursuing laser surgery, as most of our patients will never encounter any serious complications and the vast majority are pleased with the improvement they achieve. It is our intention, however, to accurately outline the associated risks to all candidates so that they may either elect not to accept the risks associated or be better prepared to deal with any unexpected complication or side effects which may arise. The only way in which a patient can avoid all surgical risk is by not proceeding with surgery.

Despite all our efforts, when a complications occurs, patients sometimes feel they did not fully comprehend the risks outlined. For this reason we have put together this comprehensive consent form.

In this document we have attempted to clearly outline the potential risks associated with the photorefractive keratectomy procedure. This is an elective procedure. Any patient who does not wish to accept these risks can simply elect to not have surgery.

Patient Initials_____

BACKGROUND:
Excimer Laser Eye Surgery or Photorefractive Keratectomy (PRK) is an investigational procedure utilizing an Excimer laser. The Excimer laser reshapes the front surface of the eye known as the cornea, to possibly reduce or eliminate the need for glasses or contact lenses in cases of myopia (nearsightedness), hyperopia (farsightedness), and astigmatism (ovalness).

Currently, photorefractive keratectomy for the correction of myopia, hyperopia, and astigmatism is being evaluated within a clinical study protocol in North America to fully determine the effectiveness and safety prior to widespread and general use in an unrestricted manner.

CLINICAL STUDY GUIDELINES:
PATIENTS INCLUDED IN THE STUDY: Included in the study will be patients over 18 years of age, of either sex and any race, who have myopia (nearsightedness), hyperopia (farsightedness), and/or astigmatism (ovalness).

ALTERNATIVE TREATMENTS: Patients must have rejected alternatives to Excimer Photorefractive Keratectomy, which include not having surgery, glasses, contacts lenses, and other refractive procedures such as radial keratotomy.

PATIENTS EXCLUDED FROM THE STUDY: Excluded from the study are patients with any residual, recurrent or active ocular disease or abnormality except for myopia, hyperopia, and astigmatism in either eye. Also excluded from the study protocol are patients with residual, recurrent, or active systemic disease which may affect corneal wound healing. Such diseases include rheumatoid arthritis, lupus, or other autoimmune disorders.

FOLLOW-UP EXAMINATIONS: Patients are requested to return for follow-up several times during the first 6 months following PRK for testing, then every 6 months for the next 2 years in order to monitor healing of the eye and patient progress following surgery.

Patient Initials_____

All patients are to understand and accept the fact that if an enhancement is needed or a complication occurs, they may be required to return or stay longer. A patient may return more frequently if it is medically necessary. Although the laser procedures performed are covered in the procedure fee, any additional travel and hotel costs incurred are not.

VOLUNTARY PARTICIPATION IN CLINICAL STUDY: By signing this Informed Consent Form, the undersigned understands that he/she will be entered into the study protocol. The undersigned further acknowledges that his/her agreement to participate in the study protocol is a completely voluntary decision.

WITHDRAWAL: Patients are free to withdraw from the study protocol at any time, and their refusal to continue in the study protocol will not in any way jeopardize or prevent their continued medical care now or in the future. If a patient decides to withdraw, it is important to inform the TLC surgeon so that he/she can plan for the patient's continuing care.

CONFIDENTIALITY: Each patient gives permission for the medical data concerning their operation and any subsequent treatment to be submitted to the manufacturer of the Excimer laser and to Health and Welfare Canada. Patient identity will be kept strictly confidential in any reports or journal articles. The patient gives permission for videos and photos which may be used in educational texts, articles, or at conferences.

Patient Initials_____

GOVERNING LAW: The patient (by name) agrees that the relationship between himself/herself and the surgeon shall be governed by and constructed in accordance with the laws of the Province of Ontario.

Patient Initials_____

JURISDICTION: The patient acknowledges that the treatment/service was performed in the Province of Ontario and that the Courts of the Province of Ontario shall have jurisdiction to entertain and complaint, demand, claim, or cause of action, whether based on alleged breach of contract or alleged negligence arising out of treatment. The patient hereby agrees that he/she will commence any such legal proceedings in the Province of Ontario and hereby submits to the jurisdiction of the Courts of the Province of Ontario.

Patient Initials_____

RECOVERY/RISKS
There are five major risks involved with Photorefractive Keratectomy:

1) The risk of **INFECTION** is 1/500, during the healing of the protective layer. This generally takes 3 days, however, it can take a week or even longer. The patient is at risk for infection until the epithelium is completely grown back. The vision remains blurry during the surface healing. Make-up, swimming and possible contamination should be avoided during this time. A serious corneal infection can result in scarring, a permanent reduction in vision and even complete loss of vision. The incidence of severe corneal infections is 1/1000.

Patient Initials_____   TLC Initials_____

2) The risk of **PAIN** is 1/10, during the first 48 to 72 hours after surgery. It is very common to experience a foreign body sensation during this time similar to an eyelash in your eye. Patients may be light sensitive. Eye tearing is common and the eye may be red or swollen. Patients experiencing pain will be provided with medication to take only if required. Fortunately, pain is not always a sign of complication, but daily or more frequent examinations are required if pain is persistent.

Patient Initials_____   TLC Initials_____

3) The risk of developing **SCAR TISSUE** or **SEVERE HAZE** if the prescription is mild 0.5% to 1%, moderate 1% to 3%, severe 3% to 5%, and following radial keratotomy 5%. Severe haze or scar tissue consists of collagen proteins which develop on the surface of the eye. It presents usually as a dirty windshield type of appearance to your vision. Haze is not the initial blurriness you will experience, but may become evident after surgery, developing over weeks or months. Even if scar tissue develops, it can be treated with another laser procedure. Scarring may be persistent or infrequently recurrent, requiring multiple surgeries and possibly producing loss of visual sharpness or overcorrection.

Patient Initials_____   TLC Initials_____

4) **NIGHT GLARE** is very common early on in the healing process and is more common when only one eye has been treated. Typically, 6 months after both eyes have been treated, only 2% of patients still experience significant night glare which interferes with their night driving. Patients with large pupils and severe myopia are at greatest risk for night glare.

Patient Initials_____   TLC Initials_____

5) **BLURRINESS** is *very* common in the healing process. It generally requires 3 to 4 days until the vision is clear enough to drive, however, patients should recognize it may even take longer in certain cases. Patients having both eyes done simultaneously may require 10 to 14 days before they will be able to drive. Full recovery takes 4 to 6 months. Approximately, 1% to 2% of patients independent of the procedure performed will develop corneal irregularities reducing the sharpness, crispness, and clarity to their vision preventing them from reading the bottom two or more lines on an eye chart, that glasses, contacts or another surgery cannot restore. That is, the initial blurriness resolves in 98% to 99% of patients within 6 to 12 months, however, in 1% to 2% of people, the blurriness is permanent. There is no way to predict or predetermine who will be in this 1% to 2%. If you lose sharpness you must understand that your vision will be permanently worse. All forms of eye surgery carry the same risk.

Patients Initials_____   TLC Initials_____

COMPLICATIONS:
One percent of patients develop significant complications. **NO ONE** ever believes they will be in the 1% of people who have complications. PRK, performed for severe myopia is associated with a much higher risk of complications between 2% to 5%.

Patient Initials_____   TLC Initials_____

No one has ever gone blind from the Excimer Laser Surgery BUT you can always be the first. Theoretical risks mean they just have not happened as yet. There are no guarantees. No guarantees of perfect vision. No guarantees of zero glasses or contact. No guarantees that you will not be in the 1% of people that have significant complications.

Patient Initials_____   TLC Initials_____

EXPECTATIONS:
The Goal is to achieve the best visual result the safest way. The goal is NOT to eliminate glasses and contacts completely, but to dramatically reduce the dependence upon them in an attempt to help improve your quality of life. Night driving glasses and readers may always be needed.

     Patient Initials_____   TLC Initials_____

Even 90% clarity of vision is 10% blurry. Enhancement surgeries can be performed when stable UNLESS unwise or unsafe. Typically, if -1.00 D or higher or 20/40 or worse an enhancement may be performed. Enhancement surgeries cannot be performed for at least 4 months, usually after 6 months.

If there is inadequate tissue, it may not be possible to perform an enhancement. An assessment and consultation will be held with the surgeon at which time the benefits and risks of an enhancement surgery will be discussed.

     Patient Initials_____   TLC Initials_____

Currently Photorefractive Keratectomy for the correction of myopia and astigmatism is being evaluated within a clinical study protocol in North America to fully determine the effectiveness and safety prior to widespread and general use. Thousands of these procedures are currently being performed outside North America with considerable success. The potential advantages and disadvantages have been reviewed with me, detailing the above information during my educational consultation.

IMPROVEMENT OF VISUAL POTENTIAL:
Patients who do not see 100% before surgery even with the strongest prescription cannot expect or anticipate 100% after surgery. That is, after surgery the best vision you can possibly attain is 20/____. This surgery does not improve visual potential. Nearsightedness represents multiple visual problems, of which your prescription is only one. The fact that some individuals do not see 20/20 is due to several other factors, primarily the retinal nerve tissue quality that this surgery does not affect. That is why each patient will continue to require routine annual eye examinations to rule out several other conditions associated with nearsightedness.

Approximately 20/40 is legal driving vision, if you cannot achieve corrected vision of 20/40 or better you may not qualify to renew your driver's license.

Monovision: We aim to have the non-dominant eye a little undercorrected to help reading vision. This involves giving up a little distance sharpness. Night driving glasses are more common, and readers may still be required for fine print or prolonged reading BUT overall dependence is still dramatically reduced. In our experience, people over 35 years should consider monovision, over 40 years a slight mono may be helpful, and for patients over 50 years of age full mono may be recommended.

YES _____   NO _____   SLIGHT_____

BILATERAL SURGERY: (Surgery on both eyes simultaneously.)

There are advantages and disadvantages of having bilateral surgery.

Benefits: It is more convenient to have both eyes treated during the same visit.
    Balance is restored quicker.
    Night glare tends to go away quicker.
    Anxiety may be reduced.

Risks: Blurriness may continue in both eyes from 1 to 2 weeks to the point that driving may not be possible. It is advisable to take at least 1 week off work, possibly 2 weeks. It is important to realize that patients who heal abnormally have taken several weeks to heal, whether they have surgery on one eye or both eyes. There is no way of predicting who will take longer to heal. The risk of infection or other healing complications is applicable to both eyes simultaneously, therefore, if an infection occurs in one eye, it may spread to the other eye. By correcting both eyes simultaneously, there is no opportunity to learn from the healing patterns of the first eye before performing the second eye. Therefore, if there is an overcorrection or undercorrection in one eye, chances are there will be in both eyes. If a retreatment is required in one eye, it is quite possible that your fellow eye will also require retreatment.

Patient Initials_____   TLC Initials_____

I wish to have "both my eyes treated during the same procedure."

Steroid Complications:
Topical Steroids:

Postoperative drops are typically used for 4 months in total, tapering monthly. Patients must be monitored monthly while on the topical steroid drops. To achieve the best results, patients must use the medication as prescribed, in general, the minimum dose for the minimum time is recommended.

Your doctor may stop the drops early if you appear to be healing slowly. Your doctor may continue drops once a day after 4 months, if needed, to help stabilize the final result.

Purpose: Early on: Reduces redness, swelling, light sensitivity.
               Later: Promotes normal healing, reduces haze. Slows healing to
                    fine tune results.

Caution: Excessive use can increase eye pressure, produce eyelid drooping,
               promote farsightedness, and rarely promote cataract changes.

Rapid discontinuation can promote regression towards nearsightedness and can increase haze. Patient monitoring while on topical steroid drops will reduce the risk of such occurrences.

Patient Initials_____   TLC Initials_____

PATIENT CONSENT:
PLEASE WRITE IN EACH BOX IN YOUR OWN HANDWRITING AS INDICATED:

1. I understand the basic nature of the procedure and clinical study protocol as well as the possible risks and benefits of photorefractive keratectomy. All of my questions have been answered to my satisfaction. I understand that it is impossible for my surgeon to inform me of every conceivable complication that may occur.

I understand that there are "no guarantees."

[ ]

2. I understand that as a result of surgery using the excimer laser that there is a small risk that my vision may be made worse.

I understand "my vision may be made worse" from the laser surgery.

[ ]

3. I understand that as with any form of surgery the outcome can never be guaranteed. I specifically understand that the benefits of PRK also cannot be guaranteed. PRK may be of no benefit to me and may in fact be harmful.

I understand that "I may not achieve the vision quality I hope for."

[ ]

4. I understand that the correction obtained may not eliminate all of my myopia, farsightedness, or astigmatism and that additional correction with glasses, contact lenses, or further surgery may be needed.

I understand "I may still need to wear glasses."

[ ]

5. Complications that may occur include corneal infection, intraocular infection, corneal scarring, recurrent corneal erosions (breakdown of the protective surface layer), permanent loss of sharpness, night glare or halos, and corneal decompensation (persistent corneal swelling).

Although vision-threatening complications are quite rare, it is possible that if a significant reduction in vision is produced as a result of a complication, I may require a corneal transplant. Blindness resulting from PRK may occur as a result of infection or other sight-threatening condition under very rare conditions.

6. I understand that partially and fully sighted eyes have been treated with the Excimer laser since 1987. The very long-term effects associated with this procedure are not known.

7. Since PRK is an investigational procedure, I understand that no financial compensation or reimbursement is available to me from my surgeon, my ophthalmologist or optometrist, any doctor involved in my care, TLC The Windsor Laser Center Inc., TLC The Laser Center Inc., or the laser manufacturer in the event of any complication related to excimer laser surgery or my dissatisfaction with the results of the PRK procedure.

8. A copy of this consent form is available to me upon request.

Patient Initials _____   TLC Initials _____

VOLUNTARY CONSENT:

In signing this Informed Consent Form I certify that I have read the preceding information and understand the contents. Any questions I have concerning the consent form have been answered by the patient consultant or my surgeon to my satisfaction. I fully understand the possible risks, complications and benefits that can result from the Excimer laser surgery. My decision to participate in this study and proceed with Excimer laser photorefractive keratectomy has been voluntarily and freely given:

PATIENT FULL NAME (print):_____

PATIENT SIGNATURE:_____

WITNESS FULL NAME (print):_____

WITNESS SIGNATURE:_____

CONSULTANT:_____

TLC - THE LASER CENTER INC.

Informed Consent Form for Laser In Situ Keratomileusis

Please read the following consent form very carefully. Please initial each page where indicated. Do not sign this form unless you read and understand each page.

PATIENT'S NAME:_____

SURGEON'S NAME:_____

DATE OF PROCEDURE:_____

TREATMENT: (circle) **Left Eye Right Eye Both Eyes**

Patient Initials_____

SURGEON WILL REVIEW:

SUCCESS RATE FOR 20/ OR BETTER _____%

RETREATMENT RATE _____%

MONOVISION (circle) **Yes No Slight**

SURGEON
COMMENTS:_____

_____

INTRODUCTION:
It is our hope to fully inform you concerning the side effects, limitations, and complications of laser surgery. We continually struggle to balance the benefits of laser surgery with the known and unknown risks. The first important message to understand is that it is impossible to perform any form of surgery without the patient accepting a certain degree of risk and responsibility.

This consent form in combination with the extensive educational materials provided and the entire consultation procedure is designed to enhance your understanding of the potential for difficulties which may be encountered during both the procedure and the healing process.

Many of our patients are surprised and some are upset by the extent to which we attempt to inform them of the potential for complications. It is not our intention to frighten or dissuade someone from pursuing laser surgery, as most of our patients will never encounter any serious complications and the vast majority are pleased with the improvement they achieve. It is our intention, however, to accurately outline the associated risks to all candidates so that they may either elect not to accept the risks associated or be better prepared to deal with any unexpected complication or side effects. The only way in which a patient can avoid all surgical risks is by not proceeding with surgery.

Despite all our efforts, when a complication occurs, patients sometimes feel they did not fully comprehend the risks outlined. For this reason we have put together this comprehensive consent form.

In this document we have attempted to clearly outline the potential risks associated with the laser in situ keratomileusis procedure. This is an elective procedure. Any patient who does not wish to accept these risks can simply elect not to have the surgery. This is the only way to guarantee no complications will occur.

Patient Initials _____

BACKGROUND:
The Excimer laser reshapes the cornea to possibly reduce or eliminate the need for glasses or contact lenses in cases of myopia (nearsightedness), hyperopia (farsightedness), and astigmatism (ovalness). The curvature of the eye must be reshaped. There are two ways it can be accomplished. On the surface with **PRK** (photorefractive keratectomy) or beneath the surface with **LASIK**. The surface cells of the eye are more reactive; they may produce more pain, infection, and scarring. By going underneath a flap of tissue with the LASIK procedure, the risks associated with healing are all reduced. The intraoperative risks, however, are greater with LASIK than PRK alone. The disadvantages of this procedure are those associated with the microkeratome. In severe cases of myopia and astigmatism where more healing complications are encountered, LASIK may be the treatment of choice.

Photorefractive keratectomy (PRK) and Laser in situ keratomileusis (LASIK) are investigational procedures utilizing an Excimer laser. The techniques of Lamellar Keratoplasty have been performed for over two decades, but the use of Automated Lamellar Keratoplasty (ALK) has only recently been combined with Excimer Laser PRK. In the **LASIK** technique, an instrument known as a microkeratome is used to cut a 160-micron flap from the surface of the cornea. The self-propelled instrument is extremely fine and precise with delicate gears which run within tracks of the suction ring. The corneal flap is approximately three hairs thick, with the entire cornea typically 11 hairs thick. A suction ring is attached to the eye, securing it for the microkeratome cut. When the suction is applies, the vision will appear completely gray–patients cannot see or feel the incision. The laser application is performed within the corneal bed instead of on the corneal surface with PRK. Most people state that they do not feel any pain, but rather experience a slight pressure around the eye. The laser application is associated with a clicking sound and pungent odor. The cap is typically hinged and replaced following the laser surgery. The cap is believed to be held into position through an almost immediate suction-type action within the cornea and by the protective epithelial layer, which rapidly envelopes the surface within days. After 6 months a firm seal forms along the flap edge.

CLINICAL STUDY GUIDELINES
PATIENTS INCLUDED IN THE STUDY:
Included in the study will be patients over 18 years of age, preferably over 21, of either sex and any race, who have myopia (nearsightedness), hyperopia (farsightedness), and/or astigmatism (ovalness).

ALTERNATIVE TREATMENTS:
Patients must have rejected alternatives to LASIK, which include: having no surgery, glasses, contact lenses, photorefractive keratectomy alone, and other refractive procedures, such as radial keratotomy.

PATIENTS EXCLUDED FROM THE STUDY:
Excluded from the study are patients with any residual, recurrent, or active ocular disease or abnormality except for myopia, hyperopia, and astigmatism in either eye. Also excluded from the study protocol are patients with residual, recurrent, or active eye disease. Systemic disease which may affect corneal wound healing, such diseases include keloid formers, rheumatoid arthritis, lupus, or other autoimmune disorders, which are routinely excluded with PRK, may possibly be included with LASIK. The healing problems that these patients are subject to are theoretically avoided with the LASIK technique, however there is no data proving this to be the case. Therefore, these patients must assume greater potential risks.

FOLLOW-UP EXAMINATIONS:
Patients are requested to return for follow-up several times during the first 6 months following LASIK for testing, then every 6 months for the first 2 years in order to monitor healing of the eye and patient progress following surgery. All patients are to understand and accept the fact that if an enhancement is needed or a complication occurs, they may be required to return or stay longer. A patient may return more frequently if medically necessary. Although the laser procedures performed at the TLC facility are covered in the procedure fee, the additional travel and hotel costs are not.

Patient Initials _____

VOLUNTARY PARTICIPATION IN CLINICAL STUDY:
By signing this Informed Consent Form, the undersigned understands that he/she will be entered into the study protocol. The undersigned further acknowledges that his/her agreement to participate in the study protocol is completely a voluntary decision.

WITHDRAWAL:
Patients are free to withdraw from the study protocol at any time, and their refusal to continue in the study protocol will not in any way jeopardize or prevent their continued medical care now or in the future. If a patient withdraws, it is important to inform the TLC surgeon so that he/she can plan for the patient's continued care.

CONFIDENTIALITY:
Each patient gives permission for the medical data concerning their operation and any subsequent treatment to be submitted to the manufacturer of the Excimer laser and to Health and Welfare Canada. Patient identity will be kept strictly confidential in any reports or journal articles. The patient gives permission for videos and photos which may be used in educational tests, articles, or at conferences.

Patient Initials _____

GOVERNING LAW:
The patient (by name) agrees that the relationship between himself/herself and the surgeon shall be governed by and constructed in accordance with the laws of the Province of Ontario.

Patient Initials _____

JURISDICTION:
The patient acknowledges that the treatment/service was performed in the Province of Ontario and that the Courts of the Province of Ontario shall have jurisdiction to entertain any complaint, demand, claim, or cause of action, whether based on alleged breach of contract or alleged negligence arising out of the treatment. The patient hereby agrees that he/she will commence any such legal proceedings in the Province of Ontario and hereby submits to the jurisdiction of the Courts of the Province of Ontario.

Patient Initials _____

RECOVERY/RISKS:
1) The risk of serious **INFECTION** is reduced five-fold from approximately 1/1000 with PRK to 1/5000 with LASIK.

Patient Initials _____   TLC Initials _____

2) The risk of **PAIN** is reduced five-fold from approximately 1/10 with PRK to 1/50 with LASIK. It is common to feel an eyelash sensation. Patients may be light sensitive, with eye tearing. The eye may be red or swollen.

Patient Initials _____   TLC Initials _____

3) The risk of **SCAR TISSUE** or **CORNEAL HAZE** is reduced approximately five- to ten-fold with LASIK compared to PRK. The risk of scar tissue formation with PRK ranges from 1% to 5%, increasing in incidence with the degree of attempted correction. Scar tissue is composed of collagen proteins which develop on the surface of the eye with PRK and beneath the corneal flap with LASIK. It presents usually as a dirty windshield type of appearance to your vision. Haze is not the initial blurriness that is commonly experienced, as scar tissue develops over time.

Patient Initials _____   TLC Initials _____

The two side effects that are similar for both the LASIK and PRK procedures are **NIGHT GLARE** and **BLURRINESS**. They are very common early in the healing process, and are observed by most patients. Both typically, but not always, improve over several months once both eyes have been treated.

4) **NIGHT GLARE** is common in nearsighted individuals even before any refractive procedure is performed, but increases almost immediately in the healing process and is more common when only one eye has been treated. Typically, 6 months after *both* eyes have been treated, only 2% of patients still experience significant night glare which seriously interferes with their night driving. Severe night glare can reduce vision in all reduced lighting conditions producing blurriness, ghosting, or halos. Patients with large pupils and severe myopia are at greatest risk for night glare.

Patient Initials _____   TLC Initials _____

5) Almost all patients describe **BLURRINESS** immediately following surgery. Blurriness to one degree or another is common. With the LASIK procedure there is considerable improvement in vision within the first 24 to 48 hours. Approximately 80% of the visual recovery occurs within the first several days, with the last 20% of vision improving over 3 to 6 months. Patients experience a large Quantitative jump in vision within days, with the Qualitative fine tuning or sharpness of vision taking much longer, in the order of several weeks. Many patients do experience a profound and dramatic visual improvement and become able to read half or more of the eye chart the next day, but most state it is still not clear and crisp, but rather has been described as "Vaseline vision." Approximately, 1% to 2% of patients independent of the procedure performed will develop corneal irregularities reducing the sharpness, crispness, and clarity to their vision preventing them from reading the bottom two or more lines on an eye chart that glasses, contacts, or another surgery cannot restore. That is, the initial blurriness resolves in 98% to 99% patients over 6 to 12 months, however, it may be permanent in 1% to 2% of treated patients. There is no way of predicting or predetermining who will be in this 1% to 2%. A patient that loses sharpness, will have vision that is permanently worse. All forms of eye surgeries alter mother nature and possess the same or higher risk.

Patient Initials _____   TLC Initials _____

6) CORNEAL FLAP COMPLICATIONS: The entire incision time is approximately 2 seconds, but during this brief interval a lot of things need to go right. Primarily, there must be adequate internal suction pressure within the eye. Suction pressure and microkeratome assembly and function determine the thickness of the corneal flap of tissue. There is a 1% risk that the eye will experience a corneal flap complication. The primary result of inadequate suction pressure is a corneal flap that is too thin which may result in (1) postponing the procedure for 3 months, (2) performing the procedure but experiencing a prolonged recovery, and/or (3) temporary or permanent blurred vision. Other potential flap complications include a corneal flap incision which is too long, resulting in a free flap; this may increase the potential for a prolonged visual recovery, blurred vision, and epithelial ingrowth (discussed below). Corneal flap incisions which are too short necessitate postponing surgery for 3 months. The most dangerous risk is if the incision goes too deep, which may result in perforation of the eye and immediate blindness. There is a plate in the microkeratome that prevents the incision from perforating the eye. The plate and microkeratome assembly is checked before each and every procedure and the unit tested for proper functioning. The overwhelming majority of LASIK complications are related to the creation of the corneal flap.

Patient Initials _____   TLC Initials _____

7) EPITHELIAL INGROWTH: During the first 24 hours the epithelial protective layer grows over the corneal flap. There is a 2% risk that epithelial cells may grow underneath the flap. This is more common in people with weak protective layers which bond poorly to the eye surface. Any intraoperative breakdown of the protective layer may increase the incidence epithelial ingrowth. Treatment involves lifting the flap and clearing the cells. Untreated epithelial ingrowth may distort vision and may actually damage the flap if severe and progressive. Small ingrowths do not usually present any visual problems and need only be monitored.

Patient Initials _____   TLC Initials _____

COMPLICATIONS:
One percent of patients develop significant complications. **NO ONE** ever believes they will be in the 1% of people who have complications. LASIK, performed for severe myopia and astigmatism is associated with a higher risk of complications, approximately 2%.

Patient Initials _____   TLC Initials _____

No one has ever gone blind from Excimer laser surgery **BUT** you can always be the first. Theoretical risks mean they just have not happened yet.

Patient Initials _____ TLC Initials _____

There are no guarantees. No guarantees of perfect vision. No guarantees of zero glasses or contacts. No guarantees that you will not be in the 1 % of people that have significant complications.

Patient Initials _____ TLC Initials _____

LASIK carries a higher risk of perforation and blindness than **PRK**, but a lower risk of pain, infection, scarring with faster recovery, and less need for eye drops. Higher intraoperative complications and lower postoperative complications.

Patient Initials _____ TLC Initials _____

EXPECTATIONS:

The Goal of the procedure is to achieve the best visual result the safest way. The goal is NOT to eliminate glasses and contacts completely, but to dramatically reduce the dependence upon them in an attempt to help improve your quality of life. Night driving glasses and readers may always be needed.

Patient Initials _____ TLC Initials _____

The degree of correction required determines both the rate of recovery and the initial accuracy of the procedure. Severe prescriptions require at least two procedures. Patient differences in healing will also greatly affect visual recovery and final visual outcome and is impossible to predict.

Patient Initials _____ TLC Initials _____

Even 90% clarity of vision is 10% blurry. Enhancement surgeries can be performed when stable UNLESS unwise or unsafe. Typically, if -1.00 D or greater or 20/40 or worse an enhancement may be performed. Enhancement surgeries are generally performed no sooner than 3 months after the first surgery. Generally, at this point their is no need to make another cut with the microkeratome, the original flap can usually be lifted with specialized techniques. After 6 months of healing, a new LASIK incision is usually required, incurring greater risk.

In order to perform an enhancement surgery, there must be adequate tissue remaining. If there is inadequate tissue, it may not be possible to perform an enhancement. An assessment and consultation will be held with the surgeon at which time the benefits and risks of an enhancement surgery will be discussed.

Patient Initials _____ TLC Initials _____

INVESTIGATIONAL STATUS:

Currently, photorefractive keratectomy (PRK) and Laser in situ keratomileusis (LASIK) for the correction of myopia, hyperopia, and astigmatism is being evaluated within a clinical study protocol in North America to fully determine the effectiveness and safety prior to widespread and general use in an unrestricted manner. Thousands of these procedures are currently being performed outside North America with considerable success. The potential advantages and disadvantages have been reviewed with me, detailing the above information during my educational consultation.

Patient Initials _____ TLC Initials _____

IMPROVEMENT OF VISUAL POTENTIAL:

Patients who do not see 20/20 or 100% before surgery even with the strongest prescription cannot expect or anticipate 100% after surgery. That is, after surgery the best vision a patient can attain is the vision they experienced preoperatively with his/her correction. Rigid gas permeable lenses may actually provide certain patients with better vision than glasses, soft lenses, and refractive surgery. This surgery does not improve visual potential. Nearsightedness represents multiple visual problems, of which your prescription is only one. That is why each patient will continue to require routine annual eye examinations to rule out several other associated conditions, primarily the retinal nerve tissue quality, which this procedure does not directly affect. It is the reduced retinal nerve tissue quality which prevents some individuals from reading 20/20 with full correction

Approximately 20/40 is legal driving vision; if you cannot achieve corrected vision of 20/40 or better you may not qualify to renew your driver's license. Patients with borderline visual function must understand that a loss of sharpness may prevent them from driving legally.

Patient Initials _____   TLC Initials _____

MONOVISION:

Everyone between the ages of 40 and 50 years experiences presbyopia, which is discussed in the accompanying brochure, resulting in the need for reading glasses or bifocals. In monovision the aim is to have the non-dominant eye a little undercorrected to help reading vision. This involves giving up a little distance sharpness. Night driving glasses are more common, and readers may still be required for fine print or prolonged reading BUT overall dependence is still dramatically reduced. Monovision helps with simple near tasks such as opening mail, reading price tags, or looking at one's wrist watch. Patients who desire the best distance or night vision unaided, such as golfers, should avoid monovision. In our experience, people over 35 years should consider monovision, over 40 years a slight mono may be helpful, and for patients over 50 years of age full monovision may be recommended.

YES _____   NO _____   SLIGHT _____

BILATERAL SURGERY: (Surgery on both eyes simultaneously.)

There are advantages and disadvantages of having bilateral surgery.

Benefits: It is convenient to have both eyes treated during the same visit.
Balance is restored quicker.
Night glare tends to go away quicker.
Anxiety may be reduced

Risks: Blurriness may continue in both eyes for anywhere from 1 to 2 weeks to the point that driving may not be possible. It is advisable to take at least 1 week off work, possibly two weeks. It is important to realize that patients who heal abnormally have taken several weeks to heal, whether they have surgery on one eye or both eyes. There is no way of predicting who will take longer to heal. The risk of infection or other healing complications is applicable to both eyes simultaneously, therefore if an infection or complication occurs in one eye, there is a greater chance that it will spread to the other eye. By correcting both eyes simultaneously, there is no opportunity to learn from the healing patterns of the first eye before performing the second eye. Therefore if there is an overcorrection or undercorrection in one eye, chances are there will be in both eyes. If a retreatment is required in one eye, it is quite possible that your fellow eye will also require retreatment.

Patient Initials _____   TLC Initials _____

I wish to have "both my eyes treated during the same procedure."

```
┌─────────────────────────────────────────────────────────────────────┐
│                                                                     │
│                                                                     │
│                                                                     │
└─────────────────────────────────────────────────────────────────────┘
```

PATIENT CONSENT:
PLEASE WRITE IN EACH BOX IN YOUR OWN HANDWRITING AS INDICATED:

1. I understand that basic nature of the procedure and clinical study protocol as well as the possible risks and benefits of LASIK. All of my questions have been answered to my satisfaction. I understand that it is impossible for my surgeon to inform me of every conceivable complication that may occur.

2. I understand that as with any form of surgery the outcome can never be guaranteed. I specifically understand that the benefits of the LASIK also cannot be guaranteed. LASIK may be of no benefit to me and may in fact be harmful.
"I understand that there are no guarantees."

```
┌─────────────────────────────────────────────────────────────────────┐
│                                                                     │
│                                                                     │
│                                                                     │
└─────────────────────────────────────────────────────────────────────┘
```

3. I understand that as a result of surgery using the Excimer laser that there is a small risk that my vision may be made worse.
I understand "my vision may be made worse" from laser surgery.

```
┌─────────────────────────────────────────────────────────────────────┐
│                                                                     │
│                                                                     │
│                                                                     │
└─────────────────────────────────────────────────────────────────────┘
```

4. Complications that may occur include retinal tears, retinal detachments, central retinal artery occlusion (eye stroke), corneal infection, intraocular infection, corneal scarring, recurrent corneal erosions (breakdown of the protective surface layer), decrease in best corrected vision, permanent night vision problems, corneal decompensation (persistent corneal swelling or ectasia), and corneal perforation. Although vision-threatening complications are quire rare, it is possible that if a significant reduction in vision is produced as a result of these complications, I may require a corneal transplant. Blindness resulting from LASIK may occur as a result of perforation and/or infection under very rare circumstances.
I understand that "I may not achieve the level or quality of vision I hope for."

```
┌─────────────────────────────────────────────────────────────────────┐
│                                                                     │
│                                                                     │
│                                                                     │
└─────────────────────────────────────────────────────────────────────┘
```

5. I understand that the correction obtained may not eliminate all of my myopia and astigmatism and that additional correction with glasses, contact lenses, or further surgery may be needed.

I understand "I may still need to wear glasses."

6. I understand that partially and fully sighted eyes have been treated with the Excimer laser since 1987 and that Lamellar Keratoplasty has been performed since the 1970s with the combined LASIK procedure being performed since 1991. The very long-term effects associated with this procedure are not known.

7. Since PRK and LASIK are investigational procedures, I understand that no financial compensation or reimbursement is available to me from my surgeon, my ophthalmologist or optometrist, any doctor involved in my care, TLC The Windsor Laser Center Inc., TLC The Laser Center Inc., or the laser manufacturer in the event of any complication related to Excimer laser LASIK surgery or my dissatisfaction with the results of the LASIK surgery.

8. A copy of this consent form is available to me upon request.

Patient Initials _____   TLC Initials _____

VOLUNTARY CONSENT:
In signing this Informed Consent Form I certify that I have read the preceding information and understand the contents. Any questions I have concerning the consent form have been answered by my surgeon or a TLC patient consultant. I fully understand the possible risks, complications, and benefits that can result from LASIK. My decision to participate in this study and proceed with LASIK has been voluntary and freely given.

PATIENT FULL NAME (print):_____

PATIENT SIGNATURE:_____

WITNESS NAME (print):_____

WITNESS SIGNATURE:_____

PATIENT CONSULTANT:_____

Note

The following companies are acknowledged for their contribution of material:
Alcon Laboratories
Chiron Vision Corporation
CIBA Vision Ophthalmics
Computed Anatomy/Tomey Technology
EyeSys Technology
Humphrey Instruments
Summit Technology Incorporated
VisX Incorporated

The following proprietary drugs mentioned in this work are registered products of these companies:
Acular/Allergan Inc./ketorolac tromethamine .5%
AcuVue/Johnson & Johnson
Alcaine/Alcon Laboratories/proparacaine HCl
Ativan/Wyeth-Ayerst/lorazepam
Celluvisc/Allergan Inc.
Ciloxan/Alcon Laboratories/ciprofloxacin
Demerol/meperidine
Fluor-op/CIBA Vision Ophthalmics
FML/Allergan Inc.
FML Forte/Allergan Inc.
Gravol/dihydraminate
Healon/Pharmacia
Maxidex/Alcon Laboratories/dexamethasone
Merocel/Solan Ophthalmic
NewVue/CIBA Vision Ophthalmics
Norfloxacin/Merck/chibroxin; Merck/noroxin
Ocuflox/Allergan Inc./ofloxacin
Percocet/DuPont/oxycodone HCl
Phenergan/Rhone-Poulenc Rorer/Wyeth-Ayerst/promethazine HCl
Polysporin/Warner Wellcome/polymyxin B sulfate and gramicidin
Polytrim/Allergan Inc./trimethoprim sulfate and polymyxin B sulfate
Predforte/Allergan Inc./prednisolone acetate
TobraDex/Alcon Laboratories/tobramycin
Toradol/Syntex
Valium/Roche/diazepam
Versed/Roche
Voltaren/CIBA Vision Ophthalmics/diclofenac sodium .1%
Xylocaine/Astra/lidocaine

Surgery for the PlanoScan trials was performed by Maria Clara Arbalaez, José Guell, Francis Roy, Michel Kritzinger, Michael Knorz, and Stephen Slade.

Dr. Neal Sher is a paid consultant to CIBA Vision Ophthalmics which provided financial support for the study cited in this book.

Bibliography

Alió JL, Ismail MM. Management of astigmatic keratotomy overcorrections by corneal suturing. *J Cataract Refract Surg.* 1994;20:13-17.

Alió JL, Ismail MM. Management of post-PRK hyperopia by holmium laser. 1995 ISRS Pre-Academy Conference and Exhibition; October 26, 1995; Atlanta, Ga.

Alió JL, Ismail MM. Management of radial keratotomy overcorrections by corneal sutures. *J Cataract Refract Surg.* 1993;19:195-199.

Alió JL, Ismail MM, Artola A. Cirugía de la hipermetropía postqueratotom a radial mediante suturas corneales. *Archivos Sociedad Española de Oftalmologia.* 1994;66:211-218.

Alpins NA. A new method of analyzing vectors for changes in astigmatism. *J Cataract Surg.* 1993;19:524-533.

Amano S, Shimizu K. Excimer laser photorefractive keratectomy for myopia: two year follow-up. *J Refract Surg.* 1995;11(Suppl):S253-S260.

Amano S, Shimizu K, Tsubota K. Corneal epithelial changes after excimer laser photorefractive keratectomy. *Am J Ophthalmol.* 1993;115:441-443.

Amano S, Shimizu K, Tsubota K. Specular microscopic evaluation of the corneal epithelium after excimer laser photorefractive keratectomy. *Am J Ophthalmol.* 1994;117:381-384.

Amano S, Tanaka S, Shimizu K. Topographical evaluation of centration of excimer laser myopia photorefractive keratectomy. *J Cataract Refract Surg.* 1994;20:616-619.

Andrade HA, McDonald M, Liu JC, et al. Evaluation of an opacity lensometer for determining corneal clarity following excimer laser photoablation. *Refract Corneal Surg.* 1990;6:346-351.

Anschutz T. Pupil size, ablation diameter, halo incidence of dependence after PRK. 1995 ISRS Pre-AAO Conference & Exhibition; October 26, 1995; Atlanta, Ga.

Arenas-Archila E, Sanchez-Thorin JC, Naranjo-Uribe JP, Hernandez-Lorano. Myopic keratomileusis in situ: a preliminary report. *J Cataract Refract Surg.* 1987;17:424;435.

Ariyasu RG, Sand B, Menefee R, et al. Holmium laser thermal keratoplasty of 10 poorly sighted eyes. *J Refract Surg.* 1995;11:358-365.

Aron-Rosa DS, Boerner CF, Bath P, et al. Corneal wound healing after excimer laser keratotomy in a human eye. *Am J Ophthalmol.* 1987;103:454-464.

Arshinoff S, D'Addario D, Sadler C, Bilotta R, Johnson TM. Use of topical nonsteroidal anti-inflammatory drugs in excimer laser photorefractive keratectomy. *J Cataract Refract Surg.* 1994;20(Suppl):216.

Assil KK. Halos, starburst and comets: significance of optical aberrations associated with keratorefractive procedures I & II. 1995 ISRS Pre-AAO Conference & Exhibition; October 27, 1995; Atlanta, Ga.

Azzolini M, Vinciguerra P, Epstein D, et al. Laser thermokeratoplasty for the correction of hyperopia, a comparison of two different application patterns. *Invest Ophthalmol Vis Sci.* 1995;36(4):S716.

Baek SH, Kim WJ, Chang JH, Lee JH. The effect of topical corticosteroids on refractive outcome and corneal haze after excimer laser photorefractive keratectomy: comparison of the effects on low-to-moderate and high myopia groups. *Invest Ophthalmol Vis Sci.* 1995;36(4):S713.

Bas AM, Nano HD: In-situ myopic keratomileusis results in 30 eyes at 15 months. Refract Corneal Surg 7:223-231, 1991.

Bende T, Seiler T, Wollensak J. Side effects in excimer corneal surgery. *Graefes Arch Clin Exp Ophthalmol.* 1988;226:277-288.

Beuerman R, McDonald M, Shofner R, et al. Quantitative histological studies of primate corneas after excimer laser photorefractive keratectomy. *Arch Ophthalmol.* 1994;112:1103-1110.

Binder PS. A multicenter trial of photorefractive keratectomy for residual myopia after previous ocular surgery. *Ophthalmology.* 1995;102:1042-1053. Discussion.

Bor Z, Hopp B, Racz B, et al. Plume emissions, shock wave, and surface wave formation during excimer laser ablation of the cornea. *Refract Corneal Surg.* 1993;9:S111-S114.

Brancato R, Carones F, Trabucchi G, Scialdone A, Tavula A. The erodible mask in photorefractive keratectomy from myopia and astigmatism. *Refract Corneal Surg.* 1993;9:S125-S129.

Brancato R, Carones F, Venturi E, Bertuzzi A. Corticosteroids vs diclofenac in the treatment of delayed regression after myopic photorefractive keratectomy. *Refract Corneal Surg.* 1993;9:376-379.

Brancato R, Scialdone A, Carones F, Bertuzzi A. Excimer laser ablation of a corneal protuberance. *J Cataract Refract Surg.* 1992;18:112.

Brancato R, Tavola A, Carones F, Scialdone A, Gallus G, Garancini P, Fontanella G. Excimer laser photorefractive keratectomy for myopia: results in 1165 eyes. *Refract Corneal Surg.* 1993;9:95-104.

Brint SF, Ostrick DM, Fisher C, et al. Six-month results of the multicenter phase I study of excimer laser myopic keratomileusis. *J Cataract Refract Surg.* 1994;20:610-615.

Buratto L, Ferrari M. Excimer laser instrastromal keratomileusis: case reports. *J Cataract Refract Surg.* 1992;18:37-41.

Buratto L, Ferrari M. Photorefractive keratectomy for myopia from 6.00 D to 10.00 D. *Refract Corneal Surg.* 1993;9:S34-S36.

Buratto L, Ferrari M, Genisi C. Keratomileusis for myopia with the excimer laser (Buratto technique): short-term results. *J Refract Corneal Surg.* 1993;9:S130-S133.

Buratto L, Ferrari M, Genisi C. Myopic keratomileusis with the excimer laser: one year follow-up. *Refract Corneal Surg.* 1993;9:12-19.

Buratto L, Ferrari M, Rama P. Excimer laser intrastromal keratomileusis. *Am J Ophthalmol.* 1992;113:291-295.

Campos M, Cuenas K, Garbus J, et al. Corneal wound healing after excimer ablation: effects of nitrogen gas blower. *Ophthalmology.* 1992;99:893-897.

Campos M, Cuevas K, Lee M, et al. Ocular integrity after photorefractive keratectomy and radial keratotomy. *Invest Ophthalmol Vis Sci.* 1992;33(Suppl):999.

Campos M, Cuevas K, Shieh E, et al. Corneal wound healing after excimer laser ablation in rabbits: expanding versus contracting apertures. *Refract Corneal Surg.* 192;8:378-381.

Campos M, Garbus J, McDonnell PJ. Corneal sensitivity after photorefractive keratectomy. *Am J Ophthalmol.* 1992;114:51-54.

Campos M, Hertzog L, Garbus J, Lee M, McDonnell PJ. Photorefractive keratectomy for severe postkeratoplasty astigmatism. *Am J Ophthalmol.* 1992;114:429-436.

Campos M, Hertzog L, Garbus J, McDonnell PJ. Corneal sensitivity after photorefractive keratectomy. *Am J Ophthalmol.* 1992;114:51-54.

Campos M, Wang X, Hertzog L, Lee M, Clapham T, Trokel SL, McDonnell PJ. Ablation rates and surface ultrastructure of 193 nm excimer laser keratectomies. *Invest Ophthalmol Vis Sci.* 1993;34:2493-2500.

Cantera E, Cantera I, Olivieri L. Corneal topographic analysis of photorefractive keratectomy in 175 myopic eyes. *Refract Corneal Surg.* 1993;9:S19-S21.

Carey BE. Synthetic keratophakia: corneal surgery. In: Brightbill FS. St. Louis, Mo: CV Mosby; 1986.

Carones F, Brancato R, Venturi E, Morico A. The corneal endothelium after myopia excimer laser photorefractive keratectomy. *Arch Ophthalmol.* 1994;112:920-924.

Carones F, Brancato R, Venturi E, Scialdone A, Bertuzzi A, Tavola A. Efficacy of corticosteroids in reversing regression after photorefractive keratectomy for myopia. *Refract Corneal Surg.* 1993;10:S52-S60.

Carson C, Taylor H, Melbourne Excimer Laser and Research Group. Excimer laser treatment for high and extreme myopia. *Arch Ophthalmol.* 1994;113:431-437.

Caubet E. Cause of subepithelial corneal haze over 18 months after photorefractive keratectomy for myopia. *J Refract Corneal Surg.* 1993;9:S65-S69.

Cavanaugh TB, Durrie DS, Riedel SM, Hunkeler JD, Lesher MP. Centration of excimer laser photorefractive keratectomy relative to the pupil. *J Cataract Refract Surg.* 1993;19(Suppl):144-148.

Cavanaugh TB, Durrie DS, Riedel SM, Hunkeler JD, Lesher MP. Topographical analysis of the centration of excimer laser photorefractive keratectomy. *J Cataract Refract Surg.* 1993;19(Suppl):136-143.

Chan W-K, Heng WJ, Tseng P, et al. Photorefractive keratectomy for myopia of 6 to 12 diopters. *J Refract Surg.* 1995;11(Suppl):S286-S292.

Cherry PMH. Holmium:YAG laser to treat astigmatism associated with myopia or hyperopia. *J Refract Surg.* 1995;11(Suppl):S349-S357.

Cherry PMH, Tutton MK, Adhikary H, Banerjee D, Garston B, Hayward JM, Ramsell T, Tolia J, Chipman ML, Bell A, Neave C, Fichte C. The treatment of pain following photorefractive keratectomy. *J Refract Corneal Surg.* 1994;10:222-225.

Cho YS, Kim CG, Kim WB, Kim CW. Multistep photorefractive keratectomy for high myopia. *J Refract Corneal Surg.* 1993;9:S37-S40.

Corbett MC, O'Brart DPS, Marshall J. Do topical corticosteroids have a role following excimer laser photorefractive keratectomy? *J Refract Surg.* 1995;11(5):380-387.

Dausch D, Klein R, Schroder E. Excimer laser photorefractive keratectomy for hyperopia. *Refract Corneal Surg.* 1993;9:20-28.

David T, Serdarevic O, Salvoldelli M, Pouliquen Y. Effects of topical corticosteroids and nonsteroidal anti-inflammatory agents on corneal wound healing after myopic photorefractive keratectomy in rabbits. *J Refract Corneal Surg.* 1994;10:299.

Dehm EJ, Puliafito CA, Adler CM, Steinert RF. Corneal endothelial injury in rabbits following excimer laser ablation at 193 and 248 nm. *Arch Ophthalmol.* 1986;104:1364-1368.

Del Pero RA, Gigstad JE, Roberts AD, et al. A refractive and histopathologic study of excimer laser keratectomy in primates. *Am J Ophthalmol.* 1990;109:419-429.

DeVore DP, Scott JB, Nordquist RE, Hoffman RS, Nguyen H, Ditzen K, Anschutz T, Schroder E. Photorefractive keratectomy to treat low, medium, and high myopia: a multicenter study. *J Cataract Refract Surg.* 1994;20(Suppl):234-238.

Doane JF, Cavanaugh TB, Durrie DS, Hassanein KM. Relation of visual symptoms to topographic ablation zone decentration after excimer laser photorefractive keratectomy. *Ophthalmology.* 1995;102:42-47.

Dougherty PJ, Wellish KL, Maloney RK. Excimer laser ablation rate and corneal hydration. *Am J Ophthalmol.* 1994;118169-176.

Durrie DS, Lesher MP, Hunkeler JD. Treatment of overcorrection after myopic photorefractive keratectomy. *J Refract Corneal Surg.* 1994;10:295.

Durrie DS, Schumer J, Cavanaugh TB. Holmium:YAG laser thermokeratoplasty for hyperopia. *J Refract Corneal Surg.* 1994;10(Suppl):S227-S280.

Durrie DS, Schumer J, Cavanaugh TB. Photorefractive keratectomy for residual myopia after previous refractive keratotomy. *J Refract Corneal Surg.* 1994;10:235-238.

Durrie DS, Schumer J, Cavanaugh TB, Gubman DT. Correction of high myopia with the excimer laser: VisX 20/15, VisX 20/20, and the Summit experience. The Summit experience. In: Salz JJ, ed. *Corneal Laser Surgery.* St. Louis, Mo: Mosby; 1995.

Dutt S, Steinert RF, Raizman MB, Puliafito CA. One-year results of excimer laser photorefractive keratectomy for low to moderate myopia. *Arch Ophthalmol.* 1994;112:1427-1436.

Eiferman RA. Rapidly polymerized collagen gel as a smoothing agent in excimer laser photoablation. *J Refract Surg.* 1995;1:50.

Eiferman RA, Hofmann RS, Sher NA. Topical diclofenac reduces pain following photorefractive keratectomy. *Arch Ophthalmol.* 1993;111:1022. Letter.

Epstein D, Fagerholm P, Hamberg-Nystrom H, Tengroth B. Twenty-four month follow-up of excimer laser photorefractive keratectomy for myopia. Refractive and visual acuity results. *Ophthalmology.* 1994;101:1558-1564.

Epstein D, Hamberg-Nystrom H, Fagerholm P, Tengroth B. Stability of refraction 18 months after photorefractive keratectomy with excimer laser. *Klin Monatsbl Auen Heilkd.* 1993;202:245-248.

Epstein RJ, Robin JB. Corneal graft rejection episode after excimer laser phototherapeutic keratectomy. *Arch Ophthalmol.* 1994;112:157. Letter.

Epstein D, Tengroth B, Fagerholm P, Hamberg-Nystrom H. Excimer retreatment of regression after photorefractive keratectomy. *Am J Ophthalmol.* 1994;117:456-461.

Fagerholm P, Hamberg-Nystrom H, Tengroth B, Epstein D. Effect of postoperative steroids on the refractive outcome of photorefractive keratectomy for myopia with the Summit excimer laser. *J Cataract Refract Surg.* 1994;20(Suppl):212.

Fantes FE, Hanna KD, Waring GO III, et al. Wound healing after excimer laser keratomileusis in monkeys. *Arch Ophthalmol.* 1990;108:665-675.

Fitzsimmons TD, Fagerholm P, Tengroth B. Steroid treatment of myopic regression: acute refractive and topographic changes in excimer photorefractive keratectomy patients. *Cornea.* 1993;12:358-361.

Forster W. Time-delayed, two-step excimer laser photorefractive keratectomy to correct high myopia. *Refract Corneal Surg.* 1993;9:465-467.

Frangie JP, Park SB, Kim J, Aquavella JV. Excimer laser keratectomy after radial keratotomy. *Am J Ophthalmol.*1993;115:634-639.

Friedlander MH, Werblin TP, Kaufman HE. Clinical results of keratophakia and keratomileusis. *Ophthalmol.* 1981;88:716-720.

Fucigna RJ, Gelber E, Belmont S. Laser thermal keratoplasty for the correction of hyperopia: a retrospective study of 35 patients. 1995 ISRS Pre-Academy Conference and Exhibition; October 26, 1995; Atlanta, Ga.

Fyodorov SN. A new technique for the treatment of hyperopia. In: Schachar RA, Levy NS, Schachar L, eds. *Keratorefractive Surgery.* Denison, Texas: LAL Publishing; 1989.

Gartry DS, Kerr Muir MG. Photorefractive keratectomy with an argon fluoride excimer laser: a clinical study. *Refract Corneal Surg.* 1991;7:420-435.

Gartry D, Kerr Muir M, Lohmann C, Marshall J. The effect of topical corticosteroids on refractive outcome and corneal haze after photorefractive keratectomy: a prospective, randomized, double-blind trial. *Arch Ophthalmol.* 1992;110:944-952.

Gartry D, Kerr Muir MG, Marshall J. Excimer laser photorefractive keratectomy. *Ophthalmology.* 1992;99:1209-1219.

Gimbel HV, DeBroff BM, Beldavs RA, van Westenbrugge JA, Ferensowicz M. A comparison of laser and manual removal of corneal epithelium for photorefractive keratectomy. *J Refract Surg.* 1995;11:36.

Gimbel HV, van Westenbrugge JA, Johnson H, et al. Visual, refractive, and patient satisfaction results following bilateral photorefractive keratectomy for myopia. *Refract Corneal Surg.* 1993;9(Suppl):S5-S10.

Gomes M. Keratomileusis in situ using manual dissection of corneal flap for high myopia. *J Refract Corneal Surg.* 1994;10:255-257.

Goodman GL, Trokel SL, Stark WJ, et al. Corneal healing following laser refractive keratectomy. *Arch Ophthalmol.* 1989;107:1799-1803.

Green H, Bold J, Parrish JA, et al. Cytotoxicity and mutagenicity of low intensity, 248 and 193 nm excimer laser radiation in mammalian cells. *Cancer Res.* 1987;47:410-413.

Green HA, Margolis R, Bold J, et al. Unscheduled DNA synthesis in human skin after in vitro ultraviolet excimer laser ablation. *J Invest Dermatol.* 1987;89:201-204.

Hahn TW, Kim JH, Lee YC. Photorefractive keratectomy to correct residual myopia after radial keratotomy. *Refract Corneal Surg.* 1993;9:S25-S28.

Hanna KD, Pouliquen Y, Waring GO III, et al. Corneal stromal wound healing in rabbits after 193-nm excimer laser surface ablation. *Arch Ophthalmol.* 1989;107:895-901.

Hardten DR, Lindstrom RL. Treatment of low moderate and high myopia with the 193-nm excimer laser. *Klin Monatsbl Auen Heilkd.* 1994;205:259-265.

Hardten DR, Sher NA, Lindstrom RL. Correction of high myopia with the excimer laser. VisX 2015. In: Salz JJ, McDonnell PJ, McDonald MB, eds. *Corneal Laser Surgery.* St. Louis, Mo: Mosby-Year Book; 1995:77.

Heitzman J, Binder PS, Kassar BS, Nordan LT. The correction of high myopia using the excimer laser. *Arch Ophthalmol.* 1993;111:1627-1634.

Hennekes R. Holmium:YAG laser thermokeratoplasty for correction of astigmatism. *J Refract Surg.* 1995;11(Suppl):S358-S360.

Herschel MK, McDonald MB, Ahmed SD, Klyce SD, Varnell HW, Thompson HW. Voltaren for treatment of discomfort after excimer ablation. *Invest Ophthalmol Vis Sci.* 1993;34:893.

Hersh PS, Patel R. Correction of myopic and astigmatism using an ablatable mask. *J Refract Corneal Surg.* 1994;10:250-254.

Hogan C, McDonald MB, Byrd T, et al. Effect of excimer laser photorefractive keratectomy on contrast sensitivity. *Invest Ophthalmol Vis Sci.* 1991;32(Suppl):721.

Ishikawa T, Park SB, Cox C, del Cerro M, Aquavella JC. Corneal sensation following excimer laser photorefractive keratectomy in humans. *J Refract Corneal Surg.* 1994;10:417-422.

Ismail MM. Non-contact LTK by holmium laser for hyperopia: 15 month follow-up. 1995 ISRS Mid-Summer Symposium and Exhibition; July 28-30, 1995; Minneapolis, Minn.

Ismail MM, Alió JL. Correction of hyperopia by holmium laser. ESCRS Congress; October 2-5, 1994; Lisbon, Portugal.

Ismail MM, Alió JL, Artola A. Tratamiento de las hipercorreciones postqueratotomía astigmatica. *Archivos Sociedad Española de Oftalmologia.* 1994;67:167-172.

Jester JV, Rodrigues MM, Villasenor RA, et al. Keratophakia and keratomileusis: Histopathologic, ultrastructural and experimental studies. Ophthalmology. 1984;91:793-805.

Kassar B, Heitzman J. Correction of high myopia with the excimer laser: VisX 2020. In: Salz JJ, McDonnell PJ, McDonald MB, eds. *Corneal Laser Surgery.* St. Louis, Mo: Mosby Year Book; 1995:77.

Kim JH, Hahn TW, Lee YC, et al. Photorefractive keratectomy in 202 myopic eyes: one year results. *Refract Corneal Surg.* 1993;9(Suppl 2):S11-S16.

Kim JH, Hahn TW, Lee YC, Sah WJ. Clinical experience of two-step photorefractive keratectomy in 19 eyes with high myopia. *J Refract Corneal Surg.* 19939:S44-S47.

Kim JH, Hahn TW, Lee YC, Sah WJ. Excimer photorefractive keratectomy for myopia: two year follow-up. *J Cataract Refract Surg.* 1994;20(Suppl):229-233.

Kim JH, Sah WJ, Hahn TW, et al. Some problems after photorefractive keratectomy. *Refract Corneal Surg.* 1994;10(Suppl):S226-S230.

Koch DD. Holmium laser thermal keratoplasty with slit-lamp delivery system. American Academy of Ophthalmology Meeting; October 30-November 3, 1995; Atlanta, Ga.

Koch DD, Abarca A, Menefee RF, et al. Holmium:YAG laser thermal keratoplasty (LTK) for corrections of spherical refractive errors. Current Research: Refractive and Cataract Surgery Symposium; November 1993; Minneapolis, Minn.

Koch DD, Berry MJ, Vassiliadis A, Abarca AA, Villarreal R, Haft EA, Laser correction of hyperopia: Sunrise holmium laser results. In: Salz JJ, McDonnell PJ, McDonald MB, eds. *Corneal Laser Surgery.* St. Louis, Mo: Mosby Year Book; 1995:237.

Koch DD, Villarreal R, Abarca A, et al. Two-year follow-up of holmium:YAG thermal keratoplasty for the treatment of hyperopia. *Invest Ophthalmol Vis Sci.* 1995;36(4):S2.

Koch JW, Lang GK, Naumann GOH. Endothelial reaction to perforating and non-perforating excimer laser excisions in rabbits. *Refract Corneal Surg.* 1991;7:214-222.

Kochevar I. Cytotoxicity and mutagenicity of excimer laser radiation. *Lasers Surg Med.* 1989;9:440-444.

Kremer FB, Dufek M. Excimer laser in situ keratomileusis. *J Refract Surg.* 1995;11:S244-S247.

Kremer FB, Suscavage P. Radial keratotomy—improved predictability. *Annals of Ophthalmology.* 1992;24:299-302.

Krueger RR, Campos M, Wang XW, Lee M, McDonnell PJ. Corneal surface morphology following excimer laser ablation with humidified gases. *Arch Ophthalmol.* 1993;111:1131-1137.

Krueger RR, Talamo JH, McDonald M, Varnell RY, Wagoner MD, McDonnell PJ. Clinical analysis of excimer laser photorefractive keratectomy using a multiple zone technique for severe myopia. *Am J Ophthalmol.* 1995;119:263-274.

Kwitko ML, Gow JA, Bellavance F. Excimer photorefractive keratectomy after undercorrected radial keratotomy. *J Refract Surg.* 1995;11(Suppl):S280-S283.

L'Esperance FA Jr. History and development of the excimer laser. In: Thompson FB, McDonnell PJ, eds. *Excimer Laser Surgery: The Cornea.* New York, NY: Igaku-Shain; 1993;1-18.

LaFond G, Balazsi G, Kadambi D, et al. Photorefractive keratectomy for low and medium myopia and astigmatism with the Chiron Technolas Keracor 116 excimer laser system: the Canadian experience. ISRS

Mid-Summer Symposium and Exhibition; July 28, 1995; Minneapolis, Minn.

Lans LJ. Experimentelle Untersuchungen uber die Entstehung von Astigmatismus durch nicht-perforierende Corneawunden. *Graefes Arch Clin Ophthalmol.* 1898;45:117-152.

Lavery FL. Photorefractive keratectomy in 472 eyes. *Refract Corneal Surg.* 1993;9:S98-S100.

Lawless MA, Cohen PR, Rogers CM. Retreatment of undercorrected photorefractive keratectomy for myopia. *J Refract Corneal Surg.* 1994;10:174-177.

Lee YC, Park CK, Sah WJ, et al. Photorefractive keratectomy for undercorrected myopia after radial keratectomy: two year follow-up. *J Refract Surg.* 1995;11(Suppl):S274-S279.

Leibowitz HM. Clinical evaluation of ciprofloxacin 0.3% ophthalmic solution for treatment of bacterial keratitis. *Am J Ophthalmol.* 1991;112(4):34S-47S.

Lin DTC. Corneal topographic analysis after excimer photorefractive keratectomy. *Ophthalmology.* 1994;101:1432-1439.

Lin DT, Suton HF, Beman M. Corneal topography following excimer photorefractive keratectomy for myopia. *J Cataract Refract Surg.* 1993;19:149-154.

Lindstrom RL, Sher NA, Barak M, DeMarchi J, Tucci A, Daya S, Hardten DR, Frantz JM, Eiferman RA, Parker P, et al. Excimer laser photorefractive keratectomy in high myopia: a multicenter study. *Trans Am Ophthalmol Soc.* 1992;90:277-296.

Lindstrom RL, Sher NA, Chen V, Bowers RA, Frantz JM, Brown DCK, Eiferman R, Lane SS, Parker P, Ostrov C, et al. Use of the 193 nm excimer laser for myopic photorefractive keratectomy in sighted eyes. A multicenter study. *Trans Am Ophthalmol Soc.* 1991;89:155.

Loewenstein A, Lipshitz I, Lazar M. Scraping of epithelium for treatment of undercorrection and haze after photorefractive keratectomy. *Refract Corneal Surg.* 1994;10:274-276.

Lohmann C, Fitzke F, O'Brart D, Kerr Muir M, Marshall J. Halos—a problem for all myopes? A comparison between spectacles, contact lenses, a photorefractive keratectomy. *J Refract Corneal Surg.* 1993;9:S72-S75.

Lohmann CP, Fitzke F, O'Brart D, Kerr Muir MK, Timberlake G, Marshall J. Corneal light scattering and visual performance in myopic individuals with spectacles, contact lenses, or excimer laser photorefractive keratectomy. *Am J Ophthalmol.* 1993;115:444-453.

Lohmann CP, Gartry D, Kerr Muir M, et al. Corneal haze after excimer laser refractive surgery: objective measurements and functional results. *Eur J Ophthalmol.* 1991;1:173-180.

Lohmann CP, Gartry D, Kerr Muir M, et al. Haze in photorefractive keratectomy: its origins and consequences. *Lasers and Light in Ophthalmology.* 1991;4:15-34.

Lohmann CP, Marshall J. Plasmin- and plasminogen-activator inhibitors after excimer laser photorefractive keratectomy: new concepts in the prevention of myopic regression and haze. *Refract Corneal Surg.* 1993;9(Suppl):300-301.

Lohmann CP, Timberlake GT, Fitzke FW, et al. Corneal light scattering after excimer photorefractive keratectomy: the objective measurements of haze. *Refract Corneal Surg.* 1992;8:114-121.

Ludwig K, Schafer P, Gross H, Lasser TH. Influence of decentration and saccadic eye movements during photorefractive keratectomy (PRK) on the retinal image contrast. *Invest Ophth Vis Sci.* 1994;35(4)2019.

Machat JJ. Double-blind corticosteroid trial in identical twins following photorefractive keratectomy. *Refract Corneal Surg.* 1993;9:S105-S107.

Machat JJ. Multizone PRK versus multizone LASIK for high myopia: principles and results. ISRS Mid-Summer Symposium and Exhibition; July 29, 1995; Minneapolis, Minn.

Machat JJ, Tayfour F. Photorefractive keratectomy for myopia: preliminary results in 147 eyes. *Refract Corneal Surg.* 1993;9:S16-S18.

Maguen E, Machat JJ. Complications of photorefractive keratectomy, primarily with the VisX excimer laser. In: Salz JJ, McDonnell PJ, McDonald MB, eds. *Corneal Laser Surgery.* St. Louis, Mo: Mosby Year Book; 1995:143.

Maguen E, Salz J, Nesburn A, et al. Results of excimer laser photorefractive keratectomy for the correction of myopia. *Ophthalmology.* 1994;101:1548-1557.

Maguire LJ, Klyce SD, et al. Visual distortion after myopic keratomileusis: Computer analysis of keratoscopy photography. *Ophthalmic Surgery.* 1987;18:352-356.

Maguire LJ, Zabel RW, Parker P, Lindstrom RL. Topography and raytracing analysis of patients with excellent visual acuity 3 months after excimer laser photorefractive keratectomy for myopia. *Refract Corneal Surg.* 1991;7:122-128.

Maloney RK. Corneal topography and optical zone location in photorefractive keratectomy. *Refract Corneal Surg.* 1990;6:363-371.

Maloney RK, Chan W-K, Steinert R, et al. A multicenter trial of photorefractive keratectomy for residual myopia after previous ocular surgery. *Ophthalmology.* 1995;102:1042-1053.

Marshall J, Trokel S, Rothery S, Krueger RR. A comparative study of corneal incision induced by diamond and steel knives and two ultraviolet radiations from an excimer laser. *Br J Ophthalmol.* 1986;7:482-501.

Marshall J, Trokel SL, Rothery S, Krueger RR. Long-term healing of the central cornea after photorefractive keratectomy using an excimer laser. *Ophthalmology.* 1988;95:1411-1421.

Marshall J, Trokel S, Rothery S, Krueger RR. Photoablation reprofiling of the cornea using an excimer laser: photorefractive keratectomy. *Lasers and Light in Ophthalmology.* 1986;1:21-48.

Marshall J, Trokel S, Rothery S, Schubert H. An ultrastructural study of corneal incisions induced by an excimer laser at 193 nm. *Ophthalmology.* 1985;92:758.

Mathys B, Van Horenbeeck R. Contact holmium laser thermokeratoplasty (LTK) for hyperopia surgery: follow-up of our first clinical cases. 1995 ISRS Pre-Academy Conference and Exhibition; October 26, 1995; Atlanta, Ga.

McDonald MB, Frantz JM, Klyce SD, et al. Central photorefractive keratectomy for myopia. The blind eye study. *Arch Ophthalmol.* 1990;108:799-808.

McDonald MB, Frantz JM, Klyce SD, et al. One-year refractive results of photorefractive keratectomy for myopia in the nonhuman primate cornea. *Arch Ophthalmol.* 1990;108:40-47.

McDonald M, Kaufman HE. Excimer laser ablation in nine human eyes. *Arch Ophthalmol.* 1989;107:641.

McDonald M, Kaufman HE, Frantz JM, et al. Excimer laser ablation in a human eye. *Arch Ophthalmol.* 1989;107:641.

McDonald M, Liu J, Byrd RJ, et al. Central photorefractive keratectomy for myopia: partially sighted and normally sighted eyes. *Ophthalmology.* 1991;98:1327-1337.

McDonald MB, Talamo JH. Myopic photorefractive keratectomy: the experience in the United States with the VisX excimer laser. In: Salz JJ, ed. *Corneal Laser Surgery.* St. Louis, Mo: Mosby; 1995.

McDonnell PJ, Garbus JJ, Salz JJ. Excimer laser myopic photoradial keratectomy after undercorrected radial keratotomy. *Refract Corneal Surg.* 1991;7:146-150.

McGhee CNJ, Weed KH, Bryce IG, Anastas CN. Results of three zone, single pass PRK and PARK in eyes with greater than -8.00 D of myopia. ISRS Mid-Summer Symposium and Exhibition; July 28, 1995; Minneapolis, Minn.

Menezo JL, Martinez-Costa R, Navea A, et al. Excimer laser photorefractive keratectomy for high myopia. *J Cataract Refract Surg.* 1995;21:393-397.

Meza J, Perez-Santonja JJ, Moreno E, et al. Photorefractive keratectomy after radial keratotomy. *J Cataract Refract Surg.* 1994;20:485-489.

Moreira H, Campos M, Sawusch MR, et al. Holmium laser thermokeratoplasty. *Ophthalmology.* 1993;100:752-761.

Moreira H, McDonnell PJ, Fasano AP, Silverman DL, Coates TD, Sevanian. Treatment of experimental pseudomonas keratitis with cyclo-oxygenase and lipoxygenase inhibitors. *Ophthalmology.* 1991;96:1693-1697.

Muller-Stolzenbert N, Muller G, Buchwald H. UV exposure of the lens during 193 nm excimer laser corneal surgery. *Arch Ophthalmol.* 1990;108:915-916.

Munnerlyn CR, Koons SJ, Marshall J. Photorefractive keratectomy: a technique for laser refractive surgery. *J Refract Surg.* 1988;14:46-52.

Nassaralla BA, Szerenyi K, Wang XW, et al. Effect of diclofenac on corneal haze after photorefractive keratectomy in rabbits. *Ophthalmology.* 1995;102(3):469-474.

Nordan LT, Binder PS, Kassar BS, Heitzmann J. Photorefractive keratectomy to treat myopia and astigmatism after radial keratotomy and penetrating keratoplasty. *J Cataract Refract Surg.* 1995;21:268-273.

Nordan LT, Fallor MK. Myopia keratomileusis: 74 corrected non-amblyopic cases with one year follow-up. *J Refract Corneal Surg.* 1986;2:124-128.

Nuss RC, Puliafito CA, Dehm E. Unscheduled DNA synthesis following excimer laser ablation of the cornea in vivo. *Invest Ophthalmol Vis Sci.* 1987;28:287-294.

O'Brart D, Corbett M, Lohmann C, Kerr Muir M, Marshall J. The effects of ablation diameter on the outcome of excimer laser photorefractive keratectomy: a prospective, randomized, double-blind study. *Arch Ophthalmol.* 1994;113:438-443.

O'Brart DPS, Gartry DS, Lohmann CP, Kerr Muir MG, Marshall J. Photorefractive keratectomy for myopia: comparison of 4.00 mm and 5.00 mm ablation zones. *J Refract Corneal Surg.* 1994;10:281.

O'Brart DP, Lohmann CP, Fitzke FW, et al. Disturbances of night vision after excimer laser photorefractive keratectomy. *Eye.* 1994;8(Pt 1):46-51.

O'Brart D, Lohmann C, Fitzke FW, et al. Night vision disturbances after excimer laser photorefractive keratectomy: haze and halos. *Eur J Ophthalmol.* 1994;4:43-51.

O'Brart DPS, Lohmann CP, Fitzke FW, Klonos G, Corbett MC, Kerr-Muir MG, Marshall J. Discrimination between the origins and functional implications of haze and halo at night after photorefractive keratectomy. *J Refract Corneal Surg.* 1994;10:300.

O'Brart DPS, Lohmann CP, Klonos G, et al. The effects of topical corticosteroids and plasmin inhibitors on refractive outcome, haze, and visual performance after photorefractive keratectomy. A prospective, randomized, observer masked study. *Ophthalmology.* 1994;101(9):1565-1574.

O'Brien TP, Maguire MG, Fink NE, et al. Efficacy of ofloxacin vs cefazolin and tobramycin in the therapy for bacterial keratitis. *Arch Ophthalmol.* 1995;113:1257-1265.

Ohman L, Fagerholm P, Tengroth B. Treatment of recurrent corneal erosions with the excimer laser. *Acta Ophthalmol* (Copenh). 1994;72:461-463.

Pallikaris I, Papatzanaki M, Georgiadis A, Frenschock O. A comparitive study of neural regeneration following corneal wounds induced by an argon fluoride excimer laser and mechanical methods. *Lasers Light Ophthalmol.* 1990;3(2):89-95.

Pallikaris IG, Papatzanaki ME, Siganos DE, et al. A corneal flap technique for laser in situ keratomileusis: human studies. *Arch Ophthalmol.* 1991;109:1699-1702.

Pallikaris IG, Papatzanaki ME, Siganos DS, Tsilimbaris MK. Tecnica de colajo corneal para la queratomileusis in situ mediante laser. Estudios en Humanos. *Arch Opthalmol* (Ed Esp). 1992;3(3):127-130.

Pallikaris IG, Papatzanaki ME, Stathi EZ, et al. Laser in situ keratomileusis. *Lasers Surg Med.* 1990;10:463-468.

Pallikaris IG, Papatzanaki M, Stathi E, Frenschock O, Georgiadis A. Laser in situ keratomileusis. *Lasers Surg Med.* 1990;10:463-468.

Pallikaris IG, Siganos DS. Corneal flap technique for excimer laser in situ keratomileusis to correct moderate and high myopia: two year follow-up. Best papers of Sessions. ASCRS symposium on Cataract, IOL, and Refractive Surgery. 1994;9-17. *J Cataract Refract Surg.* In press.

Palikaris IG, Siganos DS. Excimer laser in situ keratomileusis and photorefractive keratectomy for correction of high myopia. *J Refract Corneal Surg.* 1994;10:498-510.

Pepose JS, Laycock KA, Miller JK, et al. Reactivation of latent herpes virus by excimer laser photorefractectomy. *Am J Ophthalmol.* 1992;116:101-102.

Peyman GA. Modification of rabbit corneal curvature with the use of carbon dioxide laser burns. *Ophthalmic Surg.* 1980;11:325-329.

Piebenga LW, Matta CS, Deitz MR, et al. Excimer photorefractive keratectomy for myopia. *Ophthalmology.* 1993;100:1335-1345.

Pop M, Aras M. Multizone/multipass photorefractive keratectomy: six month results. *J Cataract Refract Surg.* 1995;21:633-643.

Pop M, Aras M. Regression after hyperopic correction with the holmium laser: one year follow-up. 1995 ISRS Mid-Summer Symposium and

Exhibition; July 28-30, 1995; Minneapolis, Minn.

Puliafito CA, Stern D, Krueger RR, et al. High-speed photography of excimer laser ablation of the cornea. *Arch Ophthalmol.* 1987;105:1255-1259.

Puliafito CA, Stern D, Krueger RR, et al. High speed photography of excimer laser ablation of the cornea. *Arch Ophthalmol.* 1991;109:1141-1146.

Puliafito CA, Wong K, Steinert RF. Quantitative and ultrastructural studies of excimer laser ablation of the cornea at 193 and 248 nanometers. *Lasers Surg Med.* 1987;7:155-159.

Pureskin N. Weakening ocular refraction by means of partial stromectomy of the cornea under experimental conditions. *Vestn Oftalmol.* 1967;8:1-7.

Rajendran B, Janakiraman P. Multizone photorefractive keratectomy for myopia of 8 to 23 diopters. *J Refract Surg.* 1995;11(Suppl):S298-S301.

Rashid ER, Waring GO III. Complications of radial and transverse keratotomy. *Surv Ophthalmol.* 1989;34:73-106.

Roberts CW, Koeller CJ. Optical zone diameters for photorefractive corneal laser surgery. *Invest Ophthalmol Vis Sci.* 1993;34:2275-2281.

Rogers CM, Lawless MA, Cohen PR. Photorefractive keratectomy for myopia of more than -10 diopters. *J Refract Corneal Surg.* 1994;10(Suppl):S171-S173.

Rowsey JJ, Doss. Electrosurgical keratoplasty: update and retraction. *Invest Ophthalmol Vis Sci.* 1987;28:224.

Ruiz L, Slade SG, Updegraff SA, Brint S. Excimer laser keratomileusis, II: excimer myopic keratomileusis: Bogota experience. In: Salz JJ, McDonnell PJ, McDonald MB, eds. *Corneal Laser Surgery.* St. Louis, Mo: Mosby Year Book; 1995:187.

Salah T, Waring GO III, El-Maghraby A. Excimer laser keratomileusis, I: excimer laser keratomileusis, I: excimer laser keratomileusis in the corneal bed under a hinged flap: results in Saudi Arabia at the El-Maghraby Eye Hospital. In: Salz JJ, McDonnell PJ, McDonald MB, eds. *Corneal Laser Surgery.* St. Louis, Mo: Mosby Year Book; 1995:187.

Salz JJ. Radial keratotomy vs photorefractive keratectomy. In: Thompson FB, McDonnell PJ, eds. *Excimer Laser Surgery: The Cornea.* New York, NY: Igaku-Shoin; 1993:63-76.

Salz JJ, Maguen E, Nesburn AB, et al. A two-year experience with excimer laser photorefractive keratectomy for myopia. *Ophthalmology.* 1993;100:873-882.

Schipper I, Senn P, Thomann U, Suppiger M. Intraocular pressure after excimer laser photorefractive keratectomy for myopia. *J Refract Surg.* 1995;11(5):366-370.

Schwartz-Goldstein BH, Hesh PS, The Summit Photorefractive Keratectomy Topography Study Group. Corneal topography of phase III excimer laser photorefractive keratectomy. Optical zone centration analysis. *Ophthalmology.* 1995;10(2):951-962.

Seiler T, Derse M, Pham T. Repeated excimer laser treatment after photorefractive keratectomy. *Arch Ophthalmol.* 1992;110:1230-1233.

Seiler T, Genth U, Holschbach A, Derse M. Aspheric photorefractive keratectomy with excimer laser. *Refract Corneal Surg.* 1993;9:166-172.

Seiler T, Holschbach A. Central corneal iron deposit after photorefractive keratectomy. *Ger J Ophthalmol.* 1993;2:143-145.

Seiler T, Holschbach A, Derse M, et al. Complications of myopic photorefractive keratectomy with the excimer laser. *Ophthalmology.* 1994;101:153-160.

Seiler T, Jean B. Photorefractive keratectomy as a second attempt to correct myopia after RK. *Refract Corneal Surg.* 1992;8:211-214.

Seiler T, Kahle G, Kriegerowski M. Excimer laser (193 nm) myopic keratomileusis in sighted and blind human eyes. *Refract Corneal Surg.* 1990;6:165-169.

Seiler T, Matallana M, Bende T. Laser thermokeratoplasty by means of a pulsed holmium:YAG laser for hyperopic correction. *Refract Corneal Surg.* 1990;63:355-359.

Seiler T, Schmidt-Petersen H, Wollensak J. Complications after myopic photorefractive keratectomy, primarily with the Summit excimer laser. In: Salz JJ, ed. *Corneal Laser Surgery.* St. Louis, Mo: Mosby; 1995.

Seiler T, Wollensak J. Myopic photorefractive keratectomy (PRK) with the excimer laser (193 nm): one year follow up. *Ophthalmology.* 1991;98:1156-1163.

Seiler T, Wollensak J. Results of a prospective evaluation of photorefractive keratectomy one year after surgery. *Ger J Ophthalmol.* 1993;2:135-142.

Shaninian L, Lin DTC. Clinical analysis of excimer laser photorefractive keratectomy using a multiple zone technique for severe myopia. *Am J Ophthalmol.* 1995;120(4):546-547. Letter.

Shaw EL, Gasset AR. Thermokeratoplasty (TKP) temperature profile. *Invest Ophthalmol.* 1974;13:181-186.

Sher NA, et al. The use of the 193 nm excimer laser for myopic photorefractive keratectomy in sighted eyes: a multicenter study. *Arch Ophthalmol.* 1991;109:1525-1530.

Sher NA, Barak M, Daya S, et al. Excimer laser photorefractive keratectomy in high myopia. *Arch Ophthalmol.* 1992;110:935-943.

Sher NA, Frantz JM, Talley A, et al. Topical diclofenac in the treatment of ocular pain after excimer photorefractive keratectomy. 1993;9:425-436.

Sher NA, Hardten DR, Fundingsland B, et al. 193 nm excimer photorefractive keratectomy in high myopia. *Ophthalmology.* 1994;101:1575-1582.

Sher NA, Krueger R, Teal P, Jans R. Are steroids necessary after excimer photorefractive keratectomy? ISRK Pre-American Academy of Ophthalmology; October 28-29, 1994.

Sher NA, Krueger R, Teal P, Jans RG, Edmison D. Role of topical corticosteroids and nonsteroidal antiinflammatory drugs in the etiology of stromal infiltrates after excimer photorefractive keratectomy. *J Refract Corneal Surg.* 1994;10:588. Letter.

Shimizu K, Amano S, Tanaka S. Photorefractive keratectomy for myopia: one-year follow-up in 97 eyes. *Refract Corneal Surg.* 1994;10(Suppl):S178-S187.

Siganos DS, Pallikaris IG. Laser in situ keratomileusis in partially sighted eyes. *Invest Ophthalmol Vis Sci.* 1993;34(4):800.

Slade SG, et al. Keratomileusis in-situ: a prospective evaluation. Poster presentation of the American Academy of Ophthalmology meeting; 1993.

Slade SG, Brint SF. Excimer laser myopic keratomileusis. In Rozakis G, ed. *Refractive Lamellar Keratoplasty.* Thorofare, NJ: SLACK Inc; 1994.

Slade SG, Brint SJ, et al. Phase I myopic keratomileusis with the Summit Excimer Laser. In preparation.

Slade SG, Ruiz L, Updegraff SA. A prospective single-center clinical trial to evaluate ALK and ALK combined with PRK using the excimer laser versus PRK alone for the surgical correction of moderate to high myopia. Bogota, Colombia. In preparation.

Sliney D. Safety of ophthalmic excimer lasers with an emphasis on compressed gases. *Refract Corneal Surg.* 1991;7:308-314.

Sliney D, Krueger R, Trokel S, et al. Photokeratitis from 193 nm argon-fluoride laser radiation. *Photochem Photobiol.* 1991;53:739-744.

Spadea L, Sabetti L, Balestrazzi E. Effect of centering excimer laser after PRK on refractive results: a corneal topography study. *Refract Corneal Surg.* 1993;9:S22-S24.

Srinivasan R, Braren B, Dreyfus RW, et al. Mechanism of the ultraviolet laser ablation of polymethyl methacrylate at 193 and 248 nm: laser-induced fluorescent analysis, chemical analysis, and doping studies. *J Opt Soc Am [B].* 1986;3:785-791.

Statmost version 2.5 for Windows. Salt Lake City, Utah: Datamost Corp: 1994-1995.

Stein R, Stein HA, Cheskes A, et al. Photorefractive keratectomy and postoperative pain. *Am J Ophthalmol.* 1994;117:403-404.

Swinger CA, Barker BA: Prospective evaluation of myopic keratomileusis. Ophthalmol 91:785-792, 1984.

Talley AR, Hardten DR, Sher NA, et al. Results one year after using the 193-nm excimer laser for photorefractive keratectomy in mild to moderate myopia. *Am J Ophthalmol.* 1994;118(3):304-311.

Taylor DM, L'Esperance FA, Warner JW, et al. Experimental corneal studies with the excimer laser. *J Refract Surg.* 1989;15:384-389.

Taylor D, Stern A, Romanchuk K. Keratophakia: Clinical evaluation. *Ophthalmology.* 1981;88:1141-1150.

Taylor HR, Kelly P, Alpins N. Excimer laser correction of myopic astigmatism. *J Cataract Refract Surg.* 1994;20(Suppl):243.

Teal P, Breslin C, Arshinoff S, Edmison D. Corneal subepithelial infiltrates following excimer laser photorefractive keratectomy. *J Cataract Refract Surg.* 1995;21:516-518.

Tengroth B, Epstein D, Fagerholm P, et al. Excimer laser photorefractive keratectomy for myopia. Clinical results in sighted eyes. *Ophthalmology.* 1993;100(5):739-745.

Tengroth B, Epstein D, Fagerholm P, Soderberg P, Hamberg-Nystrom H, Epstein D. Effect of corticosteroids in postoperative care following photorefractive keratectomies. *Refract Corneal Surg.* 1993;9:S61-S64.

Tervo T, Mustonen R, Tarkkanen A. Management of dry eye may reduce haze after excimer laser photorefractive keratectomy. *Refract Corneal Surg.* 1993; 9(Suppl):306. Letter.

Thompson KP, Steinert RF, Daniel J, Stulting D. Photorefractive keratectomy with the Summit excimer laser: The phase III US results. In: Salz JJ, ed. *Corneal Laser Surgery.* St. Louis, Mo: Mosby; 1995.

Thompson VM, Seiler T, Durrie DS, Cavanaugh T. Holmium:YAG laser thermokeratoplasty for hyperopia and astigmatism: an overview. *Refract Corneal Surg.* 1993;9:S134-S137.

Tong C, Karn JTK, Lam RHS, et al. Excimer laser photorefractive keratectomy for myopia: six-month follow-up. *J Cataract Refract Surg.* 1995;21:150-155.

Trokel SL. Evolution of excimer laser corneal surgery. *J Cataract Refract Surg.* 1989;15:373-383.

Trokel S, Srinivasan R, Braren R. Excimer laser surgery of the cornea. *Am J Ophthalmol.* 1983;97:710-715.

Tsubota K, Toda I, Itoh S. Reduction of subepithelial haze after photorefractive keratectomy by cooling the cornea. *Am J Ophthalmol.* 1993;115:820-821.

Tuft SJ, Gartry DS, Rawe IM, Meek KM. Photorefractive keratectomy: implications of corneal wound healing. *Br J Ophthalmol.* 1993;77:243-247.

Tuft S, Marshall J, Rothery S. Stromal remodeling following photorefractive keratectomy. *Lasers and Light in Ophthalmology.* 1987;1:177-183.

Tuft SJ, Zabel RW, Marshall J. Corneal repair following keratectomy. *Invest Ophthalmol Vis Sci.* 1989;30:1769-1777.

Uozato H, Guyton DL. Cantering corneal surgical procedures. *Am J Ophthalmol.* 1987;103:264-275.

Updegraff SA, Kritzinger MS. *A Prospective Evaluation of Flow Tectonic Lamellar Keratoplasty: A New Technique fo LASIK and ALK.* International Society of Refractive Surgery (ISRS); October 1995; Atlanta, Ga.

Updegraff SA, Kritzinger MS, Slade SG. *Therapeutic Lamellar Surgery: ALK Homoplastic Grafting and LASIK.* International Society of Refractive Surgery (ISRS); July 1995; Minneapolis, Minn.

Updegraff SA, Ruiz LA, Slade SG. Corneal topography in lamellar refractive surgery. In: Sanders DR, Koch DD, eds. *Corneal Topography.* Thorofare, NJ: SLACK Inc; 1994.

van Westenbrugge JA, Gimbel HV. A comparison of the Summit and VisX excimer lasers: clinical experience at the Gimbel Eye Center. In: Salz JJ, McDonnell PJ, McDonald MB, eds. *Corneal Laser Surgery.* St. Louis, Mo: Mosby Year Book; 1995:201.

Verma S, Corbett MC, Marshall J. A prospective, randomized, double-masked trial to evaluate the role of topical anesthetics in controlling pain after photorefractive keratectomy. *Opthalmology.* 1995;102:1918-1924.

Vrabec MP, Durrie DS, Chase DS. Recurrence of herpes simplex after excimer laser keratectomy. *Am J Ophthalmol.* 1992;116:101-102.

Waring GO III, Lynn MJ, Gelender H, et al. Results of the Prospective Evaluation of Radial Keratotomy (PERK) study one year after surgery. *Ophthalmology.* 1985;92:177-198.

Weinstock SJ, Weinstock VM. Photorefractive keratectomy for myopia: 6-month results in 193 eyes. *Refract Corneal Surg.* 1993;9:S142.

Yang H, Toda I, Bissen-Miyajima H, et al. Allergic conjunctivitis is a risk factor for regression and haze after PRK. 1995 ISRS Pre-AAO Conference & Exhibition; October 26, 1994; Atlanta, Ga.

Yanoff M. Holmium laser hyperopia thermokeratoplasty update. *Eur J Implant Ref Surg.* 1995;7:89-91.

Zabel R, Tuft S, Marshall J. Excimer laser photorefractive keratectomy: endothelial morphology following area ablation of the cornea. *Invest Ophthalmol Vis Sci.* 1988;29(Suppl):390.

Index